Alcohol Use Disorder: Diagnosis and Management

Alcohol Use Disorder: Diagnosis and Management

Edited by Nadia Ruiz

AMERICAN
MEDICAL PUBLISHERS
www.americanmedicalpublishers.com

American Medical Publishers,
41 Flatbush Avenue,
1st Floor, New York,
NY 11217, USA

Visit us on the World Wide Web at:
www.americanmedicalpublishers.com

ISBN: 978-1-63927-088-0

Cataloging-in-Publication Data

Alcohol use disorder : diagnosis and management / edited by Nadia Ruiz.
p. cm.
Includes bibliographical references and index.
ISBN 978-1-63927-088-0
1. Alcoholism. 2. Alcoholism--Diagnosis. 3. Alcoholism--Treatment. 4. Alcoholism--Complications.
5. Alcoholic liver diseases. I. Ruiz, Nadia.
RC565 .A43 2021
616.861--dc23

Table of Contents

Preface

Alcohol use disorder refers to a condition where a person drinks excessive alcohol resulting in mental and physical health problems. It can be categorized into two types, alcohol abuse and alcohol dependence. It occurs due to the constant intake of a large amount of alcohol. The person faces difficulty in cutting down alcohol intake and desires alcohol strongly. Genetic and environmental factors increase the risk of the development of alcoholism. The diagnosis, prevention and treatment of alcohol use disorder are under the domain of addiction medicine. The diagnosis of alcohol use disorder is done with the help of screening, social barriers, urine and blood test, etc. Alcoholism can be managed by detoxification, medication, psychological therapy, etc. The book presents researches and studies performed by experts across the globe. It aims to shed light on some of the unexplored aspects of alcohol use disorder and recent researches in this field. Those in search of information to further their knowledge will be greatly assisted by this book.

This book unites the global concepts and researches in an organized manner for a comprehensive understanding of the subject. It is a ripe text for all researchers, students, scientists or anyone else who is interested in acquiring a better knowledge of this dynamic field.

I extend my sincere thanks to the contributors for such eloquent research chapters. Finally, I thank my family for being a source of support and help.

Editor

1

Non-Employment Histories of Middle-Aged Men and Women Who Died from Alcohol-Related Causes

Tapio Paljärvi[1]*, Pekka Martikainen[2], Taina Leinonen[2], Tiina Pensola[3], Pia Mäkelä[1]

1 Alcohol and Drugs Unit, National Institute for Health and Welfare, Helsinki, Finland, **2** Population Research Unit, University of Helsinki, Helsinki, Finland, **3** Health and Work Ability, Finnish Institute of Occupational Health, Helsinki, Finland

Abstract

Background: Long-term patterning of non-employment among problem drinkers is poorly understood. We determined the level and timing of non-employment, and the relative contribution of various types of non-employment among middle-aged persons who died of alcohol-related causes.

Methods: We conducted a longitudinal retrospective register-based study of Finnish men and women aged 45–64 years who died of alcohol-related causes (n = 15 552) or other causes (n = 39 166) in the period 2000–07, or who survived (n = 204 422) until the end of 2007. We traced back the number of days in employment and non-employment for up to 17 years before death or before the end of the study period for the survivors.

Results: The majority (≥56%) of persons who died of alcohol-related causes were in employment up to ten years before death. Over the 17-year period before death, those who died of alcohol-related causes were in employment on average two years less (mean 6.3 years, 95%CI 6.2–6.4) than those dying of other causes (8.2, 8.1–8.3), and five years less than survivors (11.6, 11.5–11.7), when sex and age were adjusted for. The relative role of various types of non-employment differed markedly across the two mortality groups. Among those who died of alcohol-related causes, unemployment accounted for 54% of the total burden of non-employment, in comparison with 29% among those who died of other causes. In contrast, disability pension accounted for 41% of the total burden of non-employment among those who died of alcohol-related causes, but 65% among those who died of other causes.

Conclusions: The results indicate the feasibility of preventing movement out of employment among middle-aged men and women with severe alcohol-related harm, provided that they are identified early on during their working careers and offered effective interventions.

Editor: Thomas Behrens, Universität Bochum, Germany

Funding: This work was supported by a grant from the Academy of Finland (grant no. 259289) and the Commission of the European Communities Seventh Framework Programme (grant no. 278511). This study is part of the DEMETRIQ project. The study does not necessarily reflect the Commission's views and in no way anticipates the Commission's future policy in this area. The funders had no role in study design, data collection and analysis, decision to publish, or preparation of the manuscript.

Competing Interests: The authors have declared that no competing interests exist.

* E-mail: tapio.paljarvi@thl.fi

Introduction

Labour force non-participation has become highly relevant to public policy because governments try to address budget deficits by cutting costs of welfare systems, and because projected changes in population structures in many Western countries have prompted concerns over long-term sustainability of public finances.[1,2] One potential solution to these financial demands is to increase the employment rate by tackling causes of labour force non-participation.

Due to the well-established acute and chronic adverse effects of excessive alcohol use,[3,4] problem drinking impacts both the overall probability of becoming employed and the mechanisms of temporary and permanent movement out of labour force.[5–14] Overall, the effect of problem drinking on the probability of being in employment is likely to be time-dependent, particularly among those with a less severe condition: when unemployment rate is low, especially mild forms of problem drinking may have little adverse effect on employment, but when the unemployment rate increases, problem drinkers may be more severely affected.[11] It has been claimed that the labour force non-participation of problem drinkers is not only a burden to the benefits system,[15] but also that at an individual level, being in employment facilitates successful recovery from alcohol misuse, and therefore interventions should support problem drinkers to gain employment.[16]

However, it is unclear to what extent problem drinkers are employable in terms of their long-term functional capability for work.[17] In addition to potentially incapacitating health problems, severe forms of problem drinking frequently co-occur with various aspects of social dysfunction likely affecting the ability to gain and maintain employment.[18–20] For developing effective interventions promoting sustained employment among problem drinkers, we need information on how labour market disadvantage is accumulated over the life course of these persons. By establishing the long-term employment histories of problem drinkers we can assess to what extent there is potential to prevent movement out of employment among them that could be capitalized on by effective interventions. For example, if problem drinkers are outside the labor force for the most part of their life, their employability will be low and interventions less effective due to persistent marginalization. Furthermore, information on the timing of different types of non-employment could be used to identify windows of opportunity during which interventions aimed to prevent alcohol-related premature exit from the labour force should be implemented.

The long-term patterning of non-employment among problem drinkers is poorly understood mainly because of lack of suitable data. Therefore, the purpose of this register-based study is to retrospectively examine the non-employment histories of middle-aged men and women who died from alcohol-related causes. Comparisons with survivors (general population) and those who died from other than alcohol-related causes enable us to make conclusions on the special characteristics of the employment trajectories of problem drinkers who are at risk of experiencing severe alcohol-related health outcomes. Survivors represent the normative general population employment trajectory and those who died from other than alcohol-related causes represent the general employment trajectory related to poor health in the years before death. Using this novel design we established the average level and timing of non-employment before alcohol-related death, and the relative contributions of unemployment, medically certified sick leave, and disability pension to the total burden of non-employment. To our knowledge our study is the first to establish the long-term patterning and the relative contribution of various types of non-employment in the life course of problem drinkers at risk of experiencing severe alcohol-related health outcomes.

Materials and Methods

Ethics statement

The sampling and data linkage was approved by the ethics committee of Statistics Finland.

Data

The register-based study data consists of an 11% random sample of the population living in Finland during the period of 1987 to 2007. Because our focus was in the employment histories of persons who died from alcohol-related causes (a proxy for a history of problem drinking), we collected an additional sample of persons who died in 2000–07 in order to increase precision. This oversample of deaths enabled us to capture 80% of all deaths that occurred in Finland during the study period, which was the maximum representation of deaths retrievable from the records of Statistics Finland due to data protection rules. In addition, information from the nation-wide registers of Statistics Finland (employment, unemployment, sociodemographic factors, and causes of death), Social Insurance Institution of Finland (medically certified sick leaves and disability pensions), and Finnish Centre for Pensions (disability pensions) were linked to the data. Statistics Finland carried out the sampling and data linkage using the unique personal identity code issued to all Finnish residents, which was available in all registers used in this study.

Men and women aged 45–64 years at the time of death were eligible for the present analyses because in this age group alcohol-related mortality is at its highest and the employment histories are at their longest. Survivors were of the same age group as the deceased and were alive at the end of 2007. Employment histories were traced back for up to 17 years before death or the end of study period. The study data consisted of 204422 persons who survived until the end of 2007 and 54718 persons who died in 2000–07 (figure 1). Of the deceased, 15552 died from alcohol-related causes and 39166 died without alcohol involvement (other deaths). Persons who emigrated during the study period were excluded (<4%) from the data.

Causes of death were identified using the International Classification of Diseases, tenth revision (ICD–10) codes. In identifying alcohol-related causes we used the following codes F10, mental and behavioural disorders due to use of alcohol; G312, degeneration of nervous system due to alcohol; G4051, epileptic seizures related to alcohol; G621, alcoholic polyneuropathy; G721, alcoholic myopathy; I426, alcoholic cardiomyopathy; E244, alcohol-induced pseudo-Cushing syndrome; K292, alcoholic gastritis; K70, alcoholic liver disease; K852, alcohol-induced acute pancreatitis; T51, toxic effects of alcohol; X45, accidental poisoning by and exposure to alcohol, X65, intentional self-poisoning by and exposure to alcohol; Y15, poisoning by and exposure to alcohol, undetermined intent). In order to improve the coverage of identifying problem drinkers, we used information on recorded underlying and contributory causes of death. Using also contributory causes of death has been shown to improve the coverage of the role of alcohol in mortality.[21] The most important groups that will be identified by using contributory causes are persons who died from external causes and cardiovascular diseases with alcohol intoxication as a contributory cause, and persons who died from various diseases with alcohol dependence as a contributing factor. In other words, persons defined as problem drinkers were either harmful or dependent drinkers at the time of death.

For each calendar year, time in employment and unemployment was recorded as months and converted to days. Time on medically certified sick leave was recorded as number of days. For sick leaves we had information on those periods eligible for sickness allowance from the Social Insurance Institution of Finland, i.e. medically certified sick leave periods lasting over 10 working days (long spells). For disability pensions, end-of-year information was used to determine disability pension status. Those who were on disability pension at the end of each year were assigned to have 365 days of disability pension during that year. Total non-employment was calculated as the sum of days of unemployment, medically certified sick leave, and disability pension.

Information on socioeconomic status was recorded in five-year intervals, and to ensure comparability, we used the most recent information that was available for all year-of-death groups, which was socioeconomic status in 1995; categorized as 1) upper and lower white collar workers, 2) manual workers, and 3) others. Similarly, for marital status we used the most recent information available for all subjects, which was marital status in 1999; dichotomized as 1) married and 2) non-married (single, divorced, or widowed).

Statistical analyses

For those who died of alcohol-related causes and other causes of death in year y_i ($_i$ = 2000–07), time before death was calculated in years. In order to avoid confounding by period effects, the comparison group of survivors was formed separately for each year y_i by randomly assigning each survivor to one of the eight years.

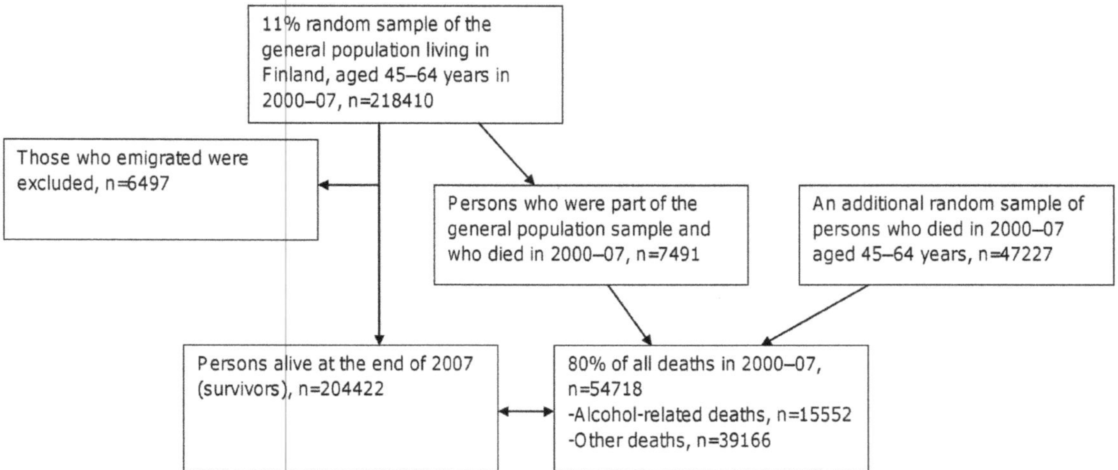

Figure 1. Flow chart of the study population.

By using generalized estimating equations (GEE) we estimated the group-level mean trajectory over all individual trajectories. This method adjusts the standard errors for the within-subject clustering of data over repeated measurements. We used an autoregressive correlation structure on the assumption that within-subject measurements closer in time are more highly correlated than measurements further apart. The results are presented as estimated marginal means with their 95% confidence intervals adjusted for sex and age, and plotted against time before death for the deceased or time before end of follow-up for survivors. Analysis weight variable was used in all the analyses to correct for the different sampling probability between survivors (11%) and the deceased (80%). SAS/STAT software's GENMOD procedure was used to perform the GEE analyses.

Results

Of those who died from alcohol-related causes a larger proportion were men 12694/15 552 (82%), compared to those who died of other causes 25262/39 160 (65%). Furthermore, of those who died of alcohol-related causes a larger proportion were manual workers and non-married, compared to those who died from other causes and survivors, both in men and women (table 1). Of those who died of alcohol-related causes, 26% were in employment at one year before death, 41% at the fifth year before death, 56% at the tenth year, and 79% were in employment at the 17th year before death (figure 2). Thus, at the tenth year before death, the majority (56%) of those who died of alcohol-related causes were still in employment. In comparison, at the tenth year the proportion of persons in employment was only slightly higher among those who died of other causes (63%), but markedly higher among survivors (82%).

The average sex and age adjusted annual number of days of employment was lower among persons dying of alcohol-related causes than among survivors, or among those dying of other causes (table 2). In terms of years of employment accumulated over the 17-year period, those who died of alcohol-related causes were in employment on average two years less (mean 6.3 years, 95%CI 6.2–6.4) than those dying of other causes (8.2, 95%CI 8.1–8.3), and over five years less than survivors (11.6, 95%CI 11.5–11.7). The higher level of non-employment among those who died of alcohol-related causes was mainly explained by unemployment. Among those who died of alcohol-related causes, unemployment accounted for 54% (95.5/177.5) of the total burden of non-employment, in comparison with 29% (42.9/146.0) among those who died of other causes (table 2). In contrast, the average number of days on disability pension was lower among those who died of alcohol-related causes compared to those who died of other causes. Disability pension accounted for 41% (72.4/177.5) of the total burden of non-employment among those who died of alcohol-related causes, but 65% (94.5/146.0) among those who died of other causes (table 2). No marked differences were observed in the average number of days on medically certified sick leaves (long spells) between those who died of alcohol-related causes and who died of other causes, and its contribution to total non-employment was small in both mortality groups.

The employment trajectories declined already at 16 years before death in both mortality groups, but for persons dying of alcohol-related causes the trajectory decreased more steeply (figure 3A). The average rate of decline of days of employment was eight days per year among those who died from alcohol-related causes, in comparison with four days among those who died from other causes. As expected based on the employment trajectory, the total non-employment trajectory increased with the decreasing time to death in both mortality groups, and the trajectory increased more steeply among those who died of alcohol-related causes (figure 3B). The average annual number of days of unemployment was higher among those who died of alcohol-related causes already at 17 years before death compared to survivors, and to those who died of other causes (figure 3C). Taking into account the secular population trend caused by the early 1990's recession and comparing the two mortality groups, it can be seen that the level of unemployment among those who died of alcohol-related causes was disproportionally affected by the economic recession. The average rate of increase in unemployment from the beginning of the follow-up (17th year before death/end of follow-up) to the peak unemployment (7th year before death/end of follow-up) was eight days per year among those who died from alcohol-related causes, in comparison with four days per year among those who died from other causes. At the year when unemployment peaked (7th year before death/end of follow-up), unemployment among those who died from alcohol-related causes was around two-fold higher compared to those who died from other causes and around three-fold higher compared to the survivors (general population). Relative to the unemployment level of those dying from other

Table 1. Characteristics of the study population.

	Men (n = 137980)			Women (n = 120116)		
	Alcohol-related death	Other death	Survivor	Alcohol-related death	Other death	Survivor
No. of subjects[a]	12 694	25 262	100 024	2 858	13 898	103 360
Mean age in years at death/ end of study period (SD)	55 (2.8)	57 (2.7)	54 (7.7)	55 (2.8)	57 (2.7)	54 (7.8)
Manual workers[b]	8013 (63%)	13 662 (54%)	44 309 (45%)	1191 (42%)	4697 (34%)	26 596 (26%)
Non-married[c]	8818 (69%)	12 772 (51%)	35 264 (35%)	1732 (61%)	6555 (47%)	36 850 (36%)

[a]Unweighted, [b]year 1995 status, [c]year 1999 status.

causes, the excess unemployment among those dying from alcohol-related causes was two-fold at the 17th year before death and three-fold at the preceding year before death. The average annual number of days of medically certified sick leave did not differ to any considerable extent during the study period between the two mortality groups, with the exception of the last few years before death (figure 3D). Among those who died of other than alcohol-related causes, the average number of days on medically certified sick leave increased more steeply during the final four to three years before death compared to those who died of alcohol-related causes. The average annual number of days of disability pension was higher among those who died of other causes already at 17 years before death compared to those who died of alcohol-related causes (figure 3E). The increase in number of days of disability pension with the decreasing time to death was comparable between the two mortality groups, but the number of days on disability pension was lower among those who died of alcohol-related causes throughout the study period.

Sensitivity analyses

The age adjusted average annual number of days of non-employment was highest among manual workers and lowest among white collar workers (table 3). This applied to all three types of non-employment, to survivors, and the two mortality groups, both among men and women.

We explored heterogeneity in the level of non-employment across diagnostic groups of alcohol-related causes and causes without alcohol involvement (other deaths). For this, alcohol-related causes of death (n = 15552) were divided according to the ICD–10 codes into diseases of the liver or pancreas (n = 6221; 40%), mental and behavioral disorders (n = 3577; 23%), injury due to external causes with alcohol intoxication as a contributing factor (n = 2644; 17%), alcohol poisoning (n = 2022; 13%), and other

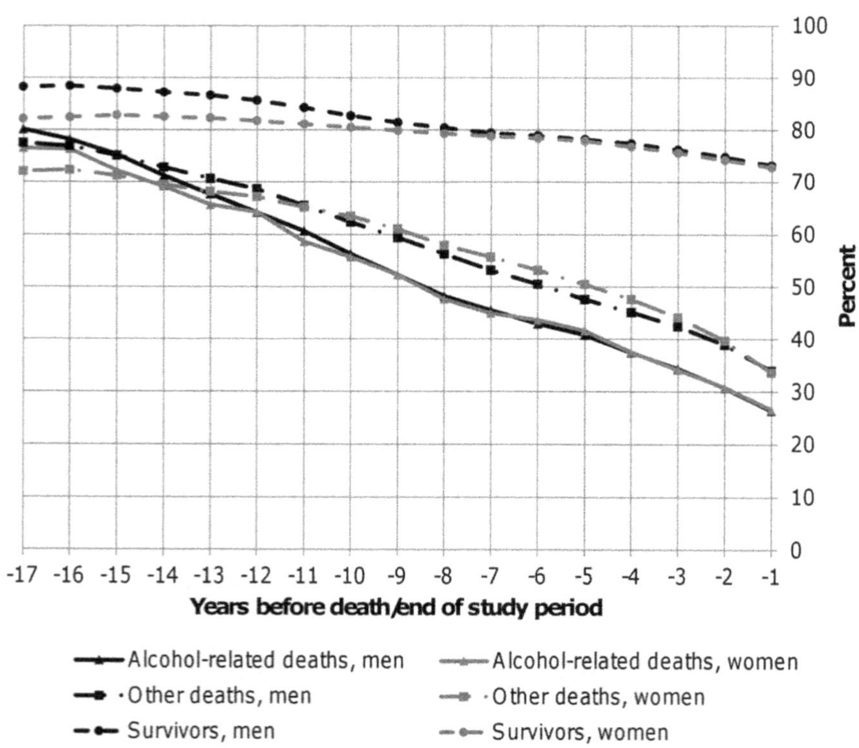

Figure 2. Proportion of men and women in employment at a given year before death/end of study period.

Table 2. Sex and age adjusted average annual number of days of employment, total non-employment, unemployment, medically certified sick leave, and disability pension over the 17-year study period, among those who died of alcohol-related causes and those who died of other causes, and among survivors.

	Average annual number of days[a]		
	Alcohol-related death	**Other death**	**Survivor**
	Mean (95%CI)	**Mean (95%CI)**	**Mean (95%CI)**
Employment	134.9 (132.9–137.0)	175.4 (174.0–176.9)	248.5 (247. 6–249.4)
Total non-employment	177.5 (175.7–179.4)	146.0 (144.7–147.3)	71.1 (70.3–71.9)
Unemployment	95.9 (94.3–97.4)	42.9 (42.1–43.7)	32.2 (31.8–32.7)
Sick leave	9.3 (9.1–9.5)	8.2 (8.1–8.4)	3.8 (3.7–3.8)
Disability pension	72.4 (70.8–74.1)	94.5 (93.1–95.8)	35.2 (34.5–36.0)

[a]Days for employment and total non-employment do not add up to 365 days because total non-employment does not include all possible types of non-employment, and because number of days for unemployment and disability pension were extrapolated using monthly or end-of-year information.

alcohol-related causes (n = 1088; 7%). Causes without alcohol involvement (n = 39166) we divided according to the ICD-10 codes into neoplasms (n = 16450; 42%), diseases of the circulatory system (n = 12925; 33%), external causes of death (n = 3916; 10%), and other diseases (n = 5875; 15%). In identifying neoplasms, diseases of the circulatory system, and external causes of death we used the following ICD-10 codes C00-D48, I00-I99, and V01-Y34, respectively.

Figure 4 shows the mean annual number of days of non-employment over the 17-year study period by type of non-employment for the various diagnostic sub-groups. The level of unemployment did not markedly vary within the combined cause of death groups used in the main analyses (i.e. within alcohol-related and other deaths). Therefore, the overall observation of excess unemployment among those who died of alcohol-related causes was not markedly affected by heterogeneity in cause of death sub-groups.

However, a somewhat less clear picture emerged when the overall level of disability pension was compared across the various diagnostic sub-groups than what was seen in terms of unemployment. Among those who died without alcohol involvement, the sub-group 'other diseases' had a markedly higher level of disability pension than any other sub-group. This cause of death sub-group consisted of diagnoses such as (chronic) diseases of the respiratory system (23%), diseases of the nervous system (20%), and diabetes mellitus (9%). The highest level of disability pension was among those whose underlying cause of death was diabetes (mean annual number of days 166.3, 95%CI 156.6–175.9). When the group of 'other diseases' was removed from the combined group of deaths without alcohol involvement (other deaths) the mean annual number of days of disability pension fell from 94.5 (95%CI 93.1–95.8) to 80.5 (95%CI 79.2–81.7; but was still higher than that among those who died of alcohol-related causes 72.4 (95%CI 70.8–74.1). Much (63%) of the overall excess in disability pension among those who died without alcohol involvement compared to those who died from alcohol-related causes was, therefore, explained by certain chronic conditions which can involve long-term incapacitating symptomatology, such as symptoms related to degeneration of the nervous system and chronic obstructive pulmonary disease.

Furthermore, we tested how the potential effect of the economic recession in Finland in the first half of the 1990's affected the shape of the observed unemployment trajectory. For this, we selected only those who died in 2007 and traced back their unemployment for ten years. In this analysis, which included days of unemployment only after the economic recession, the average annual number of days of unemployment showed steadily decreasing trends in both mortality groups as a function of proximity to death (models not shown). This analysis thus confirmed that the observed shape of the unemployment trajectory in figure 3C is affected by the economic recession.

Discussion

We assessed the long-term patterning of various types of non-employment, and their relative contribution to the total burden of non-employment, in the life course of persons who experienced the most severe possible outcome of problem drinking, i.e. those who died of alcohol-related causes. We showed that the majority of these persons who died at the age of 45–64 years were in employment up to ten years before death. This means that these persons were not marginalized early on during their life course, but were actively participating in the labour market. However, they also experienced disproportionate unemployment. Compared to the level of unemployment among the general population and those who died from other than alcohol-related causes, those who died from alcohol-related causes experienced excess unemployment already at the beginning of the study period, i.e. at the 17th year before death/end of follow-up. The relative contribution of the various types of non-employment differed markedly between the two mortality groups. Among those who died from alcohol-related causes, unemployment accounted for 54% of the total burden of non-employment, in comparison with 29% among those who died of other causes. Relative to the unemployment level of those dying from other causes, the excess unemployment among those dying from alcohol-related causes was two-fold at the 17th year before death and three-fold at the preceding year before death.

Methodological considerations

The strength of this study was that it was based on longitudinal information retrieved directly from various administrative registers of the institutions granting the benefits in question (for unemployment, sick leave, and disability pension). This means that we were able to reliably identify all persons who received these benefits. The 17-year retrospective study period enabled us to gain understanding of the long-term employment trajectories with the opportunity to identify potential time-dependent effects. Informa-

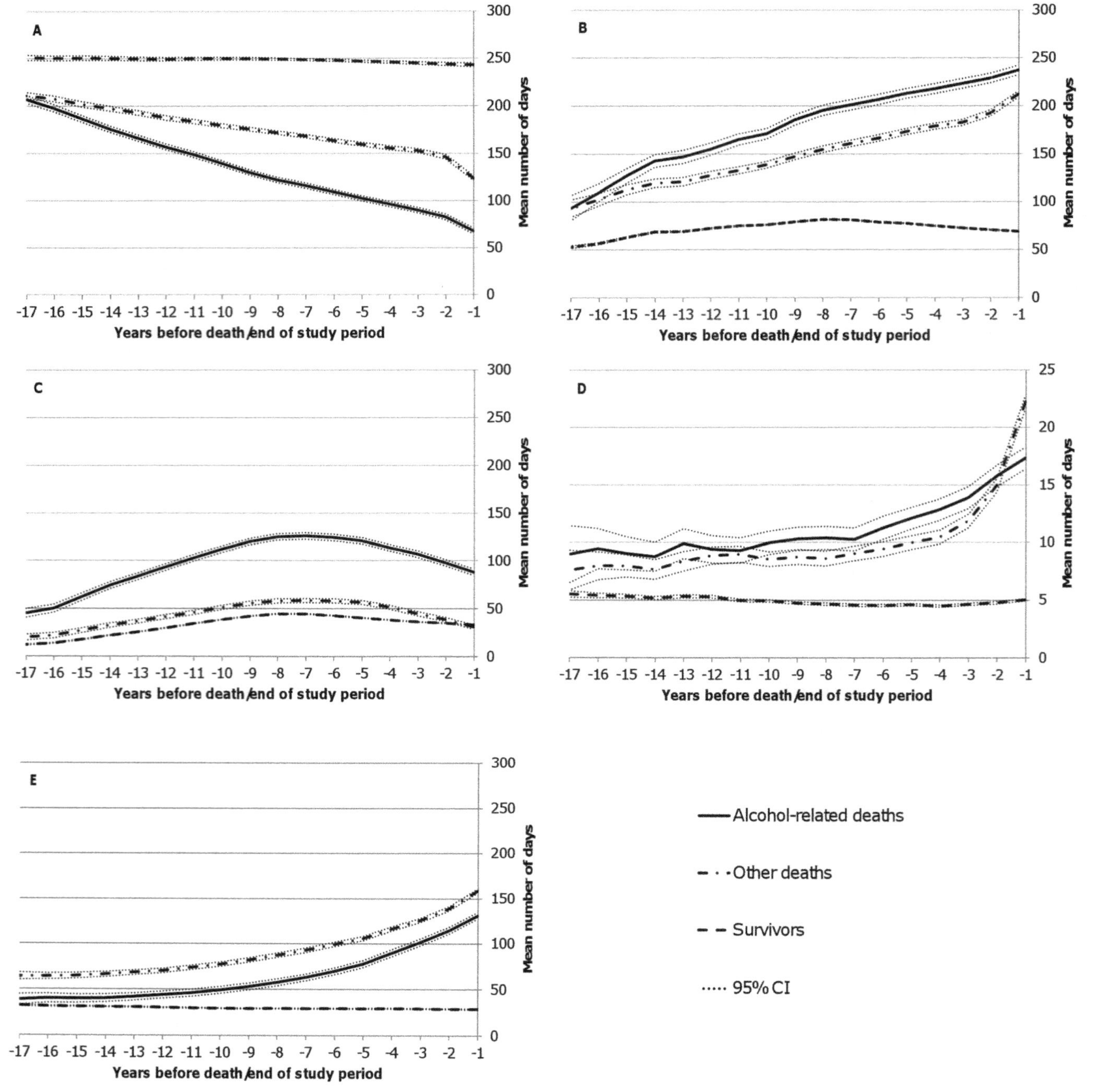

Figure 3. Average annual number of days of employment and non-employment. Sex and age adjusted average annual number of days of A) employment, B) total non-employment, C) unemployment, D) medically certified sick leave, and E) disability pension in the preceding 17 years before death/end of study period for those who died of alcohol-related causes, other causes, and for those who survived the 17-year period.

tion on the three different types of non-employment enabled us, to our knowledge for the first time, to compare the importance of the various types of non-employment in the life course of problem drinkers who eventually died from alcohol-related causes. Comparisons with survivors (general population) and those who died from other than alcohol-related causes enabled us to identify employment histories characteristic to persons dying from alcohol-related causes. The assumption behind the comparison with those who died without alcohol involvement was that their employment trajectory represented the trajectory of those with declining health status in general. The differences between these two mortality groups can therefore highlight the special characteristics related to the typical employment trajectories of problem drinkers who eventually died from alcohol-related causes while taking into account for the effects of declining overall health status with proximity to death.

The sensitivity analyses for diagnostic sub-groups showed that in terms of unemployment, the findings were consistent. In other words, the heterogeneity in causes of death and their etiological correlates did not markedly affect the conclusions. However, in

Table 3. Age adjusted average annual number of days of unemployment, medically certified sick leave, and disability pension over the 17-year study period by socioeconomic status, separately for men and women.

	Men (n = 137 980)			**Women (n = 120 116)**		
	Alcohol-related death	**Other death**	**Survivor**	**Alcohol-related death**	**Other death**	**Survivor**
	Mean (95%CI)	**Mean (95%CI)**	**Mean (95%CI)**	**Mean (95%CI)**	**Mean (95%CI)**	**Mean (95%CI)**
Unemployment						
White collar worker	68.0 (64.9–71.1)	33.2 (31.7–34.6)	21.4 (20.8–22.0)	70.1 (65.9–74.3)	28.3 (27.1–29.6)	24.0 (23.6–24.5)
Manual worker	112.2 (110.1–114.3)	60.7 (59.4–62.1)	48.4 (47.6–49.2)	103.4 (98.3–108.6)	43.9 (42.0–45.8)	45.3 (44.4–46.2)
Other	65.7 (62.0–69.3)	26.1 (24.6–27.6)	24.3 (23.5–25.1)	76.7 (68.0–85.4)	23.5 (21.6–25.4)	30.8 (29.9–31.8)
Sick leave						
White collar worker	8.9 (8.5–9.3)	7.5 (7.2–7.7)	2.5 (2.4–2.6)	10.7 (10.0–11.3)	11.3 (11.0–11.6)	3.9 (3.8–4.0)
Manual worker	10.0 (9.7–10.2)	8.8 (8.6–9.0)	5.1 (5.0–5.3)	10.8 (10.1–11.4)	10.2 (9.9–10.5)	6.0 (5.9–6.2)
Other	9.3 (8.8–9.8)	7.6 (7.3–7.9)	3.7 (3.6–3.9)	11.0 (9.7–12.4)	8.6 (8.1–9.1)	4.4 (4.2–4.6)
Disability pension						
White collar worker	71.9 (68.6–75.2)	74.8 (72.4–77.2)	27.4 (26.7–28.2)	77.0 (72.0–81.9)	87.6 (85.2–89.9)	29.2 (28.6–29.9)
Manual worker	90.9 (88.8–93.0)	110.9 (109.0–112.8)	48.5 (47.6–49.5)	96.8 (91.1–102.5)	128.1 (124.7–131.4)	50.0 (48.8–51.3)
Other	80.7 (76.4–84.9)	109.8 (106.5–113.0)	42.1 (40.8–43.4)	84.0 (73.8–94.1)	137.1 (132.1–142.0)	44.0 (42.4–45.5)

terms of disability pension the conclusions are less clear. Particularly within the group of deaths without alcohol involvement there was considerable variation in the level of disability pension by diagnostic sub-group.

Because this was a register-based study we did not have information on alcohol consumption that could have been used in determining problem drinking status. Instead, we used information on alcohol-related causes of death to identify problem drinkers. By this approach, we identified persons who had a long history of problem drinking, indicated e.g. by diagnoses of alcohol-induced liver cirrhosis and alcohol dependence. The majority of the alcohol-related diagnoses in our data were related to such diagnoses, which means that the majority were problem drinkers for a substantial time before death. We also identified persons who were problem drinkers at least at the time of death, e.g. if they died from external causes with alcohol intoxication as a contributing factor. Not all of these persons were necessarily problem drinkers for a substantial period before death, because even a single heavy drinking occasion can potentially lead to death from external causes. However, it is likely that many of those who died from external causes while intoxicated were problem drinkers earlier in their life course. This assumption is supported by a Finnish study,

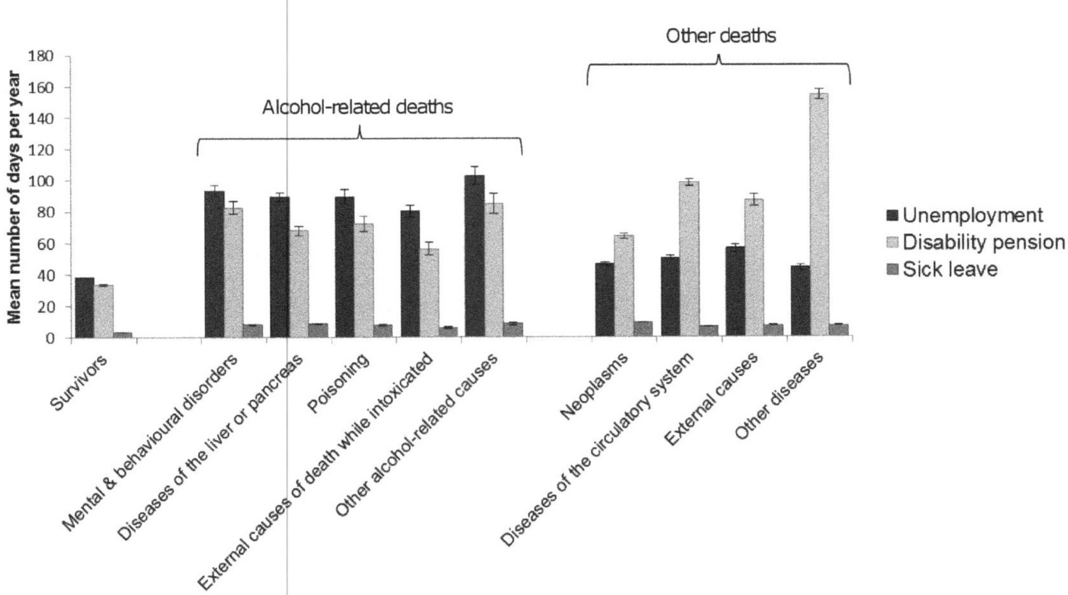

Figure 4. Average annual number of days of non-employment by cause of death. Sex and age adjusted average annual number of days of unemployment, disability pension, and sick leave over the 17-year study period separately by major cause-of-death groups. Error bars represent 95% confidence intervals.

which showed that binge drinking predicted deaths from external causes over a 16-year period.[22] We did not have information on other health behaviours either, such as smoking. Despite the fact that many problem drinkers are known to be also heavy smokers, it does not seem plausible that problem drinkers would e.g. lose their employment mainly due to the effects of smoking and not due to problem drinking. However, the adverse synergistic effect of smoking and heavy drinking on ill health may well explain some of the observed differences in non-employment trajectories.

Not all problem drinkers die from alcohol-related causes. This means that there were problem drinkers among survivors and among those who died from causes without alcohol involvement. In relation to those who died from other than alcohol-related causes, this has probably diluted the observed differences particularly in terms of unemployment, because the level of unemployment is much higher among problem drinkers. A similar dilution effect probably applies also to comparisons with survivors, but because the group of non-problem drinkers is considerably larger than that of problem drinkers, the dilution effect on the observed trajectories is likely very limited. Furthermore, persons who die from alcohol-related causes at the age of 45–64 years are likely to suffer from a less severe progression of alcohol problems compared to those who die from alcohol-related causes at a younger age. Therefore, the employment histories of younger problem drinkers who experience severe alcohol-related harm may be even more strongly characterized by non-employment than those observed here.

In summary, because we used alcohol-related deaths as a proxy for history of problem drinking, these results probably apply only to those middle-aged problem drinkers who are at risk of experiencing similar alcohol-related health outcomes during their life course as those included in this study. Because this was a register-based study with limited information on potential confounders, the reasons for the observed differences in employment trajectories remain unclear. However, a substantial body of evidence particularly on the association between problem drinking and unemployment,[11] supports the conclusion that problem drinking and its correlates are important factors explaining the observed employment disadvantage of those who eventually died from alcohol-related causes. Future studies using prospective design should aim to replicate these findings. Given the current lack of such studies, this retrospective register-based study can provide important insights into the feasibility of preventing alcohol-related non-employment among middle-aged problem drinkers at risk of experiencing severe alcohol-related health outcomes.

Interpretation and implications

When the non-employment trajectories were explored separately by types of non-employment (i.e. unemployment, medically certified sick leaves, and disability pensions), we found that those dying of alcohol-related conditions were markedly more likely to be unemployed at any time point during the 17-year study period before death, and among them the effect of the early 1990's economic recession on unemployment seemed to be much stronger. This finding suggests that the higher probability of unemployment among those with a severe form of problem drinking may be determined by factors that have a long-term effect during the life-course,[23,24] and that the effect of problem drinking on the probability of being in employment is intensified during economic downturns.[11] The comparison with survivors suggests that persons dying prematurely at ages 45–64 years, for any cause, are disadvantaged in terms of unemployment; but the magnitude of the disadvantage is markedly larger and disproportionate among those dying of alcohol-related causes compared to those dying of other causes. The lower level of employment among problem drinkers who eventually died from alcohol-related causes is in line with previous research among problem drinkers without non-fatal outcomes.[5,8,9]

A steep increase in the annual average number of days on medically certified sick leave (periods lasting over 10 working days) during the few final years before death was seen among those dying of other than alcohol-related causes, whereas among those who died of alcohol-related causes a more modestly linearly increasing trend was observed. However, medically certified sick leaves had only a marginal role as a form of non-employment before death in both mortality groups. This can partly be explained by the fact that sickness allowance is paid approximately for one year after which, in the case of continued work disability, these persons apply for disability pension, which means that they move to other types of non-employment.

The average annual number of days on disability pension was constantly lower throughout the study period among those who died of alcohol-related causes than among those who died of other causes. The medical criteria for granting disability pension in Finland may have affected the likelihood of receiving disability benefits among these problem drinkers, because alcohol misuse per se is not accepted as the basis of disability pension. However, the lower level of disability pensions among those who died of alcohol-related causes was probably partly compensated by other non-employment pathways, such as unemployment.

Majority of risky drinkers are in employment,[25] and as we showed, also the majority of problem drinkers who eventually died of alcohol-related causes were in employment up to ten years before death. This means that workplace interventions could have an important role in reducing alcohol-related premature exit from employment. The feasibility of workplace alcohol screening and brief intervention is supported by its expected positive impact e.g. on employee productivity,[26] and by the fact that alcohol screening seems to be widely accepted by the public.[27] However, while the effectiveness of alcohol screening and brief intervention has been consistently shown in health care settings, effectiveness studies in workplace settings are almost non-existent.[28,29]

One key challenge in preventing alcohol-related exit from labour force is that the perceived need for treatment among persons with alcohol use disorders (AUD) is low, and thus most individuals with an AUD are not in treatment or actively seek treatment.[30,31] Those with more severe AUD symptoms may be more likely to perceive a need for treatment than others,[32] but among these persons markedly progressed ill health may affect their ability to gain and maintain employment.[33] Persons with AUDs are also frequently disadvantaged in terms of recovery capital meaning that these persons often lack various personal and social resources needed in overcoming substance abuse disorders.[17,34] Furthermore, accumulation of factors potentially producing synergistic adverse effects among persons with AUDs, such as living alone and being unemployed,[35] also contribute to the increased risk of experiencing alcohol-related harm. Also in our data the majority of problem drinkers who eventually died from alcohol-related causes were manual workers and non-married. However, based on their long-term employment histories, our results suggest that even the majority of these persons are employable, provided that they are identified and treated early enough.

Conclusions

Our results add to the understanding of the relation between a severe form of problem drinking and non-employment by showing that the majority of persons who died from alcohol-related causes were in employment up to ten years before death. Therefore, based on their long-term employment history, these persons should not be seen as 'hopeless cases',[20] but instead they represent a group of persons who can be part of the productive workforce, provided that they are identified for prevention early enough during their working career. However, their disproportionate movement to unemployment is problematic from the point of view of prevention because utilization of health care services is known to be low among unemployed despite their various unmet health needs.[36,37] The results, therefore, also suggest that integrating alcohol screening, brief intervention, and referral to treatment as part of employment services could prove to be effective in preventing alcohol-related permanent exit from the labour force.

Author Contributions

Conceived and designed the experiments: P. Mäkelä P. Martikainen. Analyzed the data: T. Paljärvi. Contributed reagents/materials/analysis tools: TL. Wrote the paper: T. Paljärvi P. Martikainen TL T. Pensola P. Mäkelä.

References

1. United Nations (2013) World population prospects: the 2012 revision, key findings and advance tables. Department of economic and social affairs, population division. New York.
2. Rechel B, Grundy E, Robine JM, Cylus J, Machenbach JP, et al. (2013) Ageing in the European Union. Lancet 381: 1312–22.
3. Room R, Babor T, Rehm J (2005) Alcohol and public health. Lancet 365: 519–30.
4. Whiteford HA, Degenhardt L, Rehm J, Baxter AJ, Ferrari AJ, et al. (2013) Global burden of disease attributable to mental and substance use disorders: findings from the Global Burden of Disease Study 2010. Lancet 382: 1575–86.
5. Mullahy J, Sindelar J (1996) Employment, unemployment, and problem drinking. J Health Econ 15: 409–34.
6. Upmark M, Möller J, Romelsjö A (1999) Longitudinal, population-based study of self-reported alcohol habits, high levels of sickness absence, and disability pensions. J Epidemiol Community Health 53: 223–9.
7. Månsson NO, Råstam L, Eriksson KF, Israelsson B (1999) Alcohol consumption and disability pension among middle-aged men. Ann Epidemiol 9: 341–8.
8. MacDonald Z, Shields MA (2004) Does problem drinking affect employment? Evidence from England. Health Econ 13: 139–55.
9. Johansson E, Alho H, Kiiskinen U, Poikolainen K (2007) The association of alcohol dependency with employment probability: evidence from the population survey 'Health 2000 in Finland'. Health Econ 16: 739–754.
10. Roche AM, Pidd K, Berry JG, Harrison JE (2008) Workers' drinking patterns: the impact on absenteeism in the Australian work-place. Addiction 103: 738–48.
11. Henkel D (2011) Unemployment and substance use: a review of the literature (1990–2010). Curr Drug Abuse Rev 4: 4–27.
12. Skogen JC, Knudsen AK, Mykletun A, Nesvåg S, Øverland S (2011) Alcohol consumption, problem drinking, abstention and disability pension award. The Nord-Trøndelag Health Study (HUNT). Addiction 107: 98–108.
13. Ahola K, Virtanen M, Honkanen T, Isometsä E, Aromaa A, et al. (2011) Common mental disorders and subsequent work disability: a population-based Health 2000 study. J Affect Disord 134: 365–72.
14. Sidorchuk A, Hemmingsson T, Romelsjö A, Allebeck P (2012) Alcohol use in adolescence and risk of disability pension: a 39 year follow-up of a population-based conscription survey. Plos One 7:e42083.
15. Hay G, Bauld L (2010) Population estimates of alcohol misusers who access DWP benefits. Working Paper No. 94. Department for Work and Pensions, HM Government.
16. Home Office (2010) Drug strategy 2010: Reducing demand, restricting supply, building recovery: supporting people to live a drug free life. HM Government.
17. Cloud W, Granfield R (2008) Conceptualizing recovery capital: expansion of a theoretical construct. Subst Use Misuse 43: 1971–86.
18. Maurage P, Joassin F, Philippot P, Heeren A, Vermeulen N, et al. (2012) Disrupted regulation of social exclusion in alcohol-dependence: an fMRI study. Neuropsychopharmacology 37: 2067–75.
19. Thoma P, Friedmann C, Suchan B (2013) Empathy and social problem solving in alcohol dependence, mood disorders and selected personality disorders. Neurosci Biobehav Rev 37: 448–70.
20. McCormack RP, Williams AR, Goldfrank LR, Caplan AL, Ross S, et al. (2013) Commitment to assessment and treatment: comprehensive care for patients gravely disabled by alcohol use disorders. Lancet 382: 995–7.
21. Durkin A, Connolly S, O'Reilly D (2010) Quantifying alcohol-related mortality: should alcohol-related contributory causes of death be included? Alcohol Alcohol 45: 374–8.
22. Paljärvi T, Mäkelä P, Poikolainen K (2005) Pattern of drinking and fatal injury: a population-based follow-up study of Finnish men. Addiction 100:1851–9.
23. Kokko K, Pulkkinen L (2000) Aggression in childhood and long-term unemployment in adulthood: a cycle of maladaptation and some protective factors. Dev Psychol 36: 463–72.
24. Osler M, Nordentoft M, Andersen AM (2006) Childhood social environment and risk of drug and alcohol abuse in a cohort of Danish men born in 1953. Am J Epidemiol 163: 654–61.
25. Halme JT, Seppä K, Alho H, Pirkola S, Poikolainen K, et al. (2008) Hazardous drinking: prevalence and associations in the Finnish general population. Alcohol Clin Exp Res 32: 1615–22.
26. Selvik R, Stephenson D, Plaza C, Sugden B (2004) EAP impact on work, relationship and health outcomes. J Employee Assist 2nd Quarter: 18–22.
27. Mäkelä P, Havio M, Seppä K (2011) Alcohol-related discussions in health care – a population view. Addiction 106: 1239–48.
28. Roman PM, Blum TC (1996) Alcohol: a review of the impact of worksite interventions on health and behavioral outcomes. Am J Health Promot 11: 136–49.
29. Hermansson U, Helander A, Brandt L, Huss A, Rönnberg S (2010) Screening and brief intervention for risky alcohol consumption in the workplace: results of a 1-year randomized controlled study. Alcohol Alcohol 45: 252–7.
30. Grant BF (1997) Barriers to alcoholism treatment: reasons for not seeking treatment in a general population sample. J Stud Alcohol 58: 365–71.
31. Edlund MJ (2009) Perceived need for treatment for alcohol use disorders: results from two national surveys. Psychiatr Serv 60: 1618–28.
32. Hedden SL, Gfroerer JC (2011) Correlates of perceiving a need for treatment among adults with substance use disorder: results from a national survey. Addictive Behav 36: 1213–22.
33. John U, Rumpf HJ, Bischof G, Hapke U, Hanke M, et al. (2013) Excess mortality of alcohol-dependent individuals after 14 years and mortality predictors based on treatment participation and severity of alcohol dependence. Alcohol Clin Exp Res 37: 156–63.
34. Bauld L, Templeton L, Silver K, McKell J, Novak C, et al. (2013) Pathways back to work for problem alcohol users. Policy Studies 34: 360–76.
35. Herttua K, Martikainen P, Vahtera J, Kivimäki M (2011) Living alone and alcohol-related mortality: a population-based cohort study from Finland. Plos Medicine 8:e1001094.
36. Harris E, Harris MF (2009) Reducing the impact of unemployment on health: revisiting the agenda for primary health care. Med J Aust 191: 119–22.
37. Åhs A, Burell G, Westerling R (2012) Care or not care-that is the question: predictors of healthcare utilisation in relation to employment status. Int J Behav Med 19: 29–38.

2

Cue Reactivity Is Associated with Duration and Severity of Alcohol Dependence: An fMRI Study

Zsuzsika Sjoerds[1,2]*, Wim van den Brink[2], Aartjan T. F. Beekman[1], Brenda W. J. H. Penninx[1,3,4], Dick J. Veltman[1]

1 Department of Psychiatry, Neuroscience Campus Amsterdam, VU University Medical Center, Amsterdam, The Netherlands, **2** Department of Psychiatry, Academic Medical Center, University of Amsterdam, Amsterdam, The Netherlands, **3** Department of Psychiatry, Leiden University Medical Center, Leiden, The Netherlands, **4** Department of Psychiatry, University Medical Center of Groningen, Groningen, The Netherlands

Abstract

Introduction: With the progression of substance dependence, drug cue-related brain activation is thought to shift from motivational towards habit pathways. However, a direct association between cue-induced brain activation and dependence duration has not yet been shown. We therefore examined the relationship between alcohol cue-reactivity in the brain, cue-induced subjective craving and alcohol dependence duration and severity. Since alcohol dependence is highly comorbid with depression/anxiety, which may modulate brain responses to alcohol cues, we also examined the relation between comorbid depression/anxiety and cue-reactivity.

Methods: We compared 30 alcohol dependent patients with 15 healthy controls and 15 depression/anxiety patients during a visual alcohol cue-reactivity task using functional magnetic resonance imaging blood oxygenated level-dependent responses and subjective craving as outcomes. Within the alcohol dependent group we correlated cue-reactivity with alcohol dependence severity and duration, with cue-induced craving and with depression/anxiety levels.

Results: Alcohol dependent patients showed greater cue-reactivity in motivational brain pathways and stronger subjective craving than depression/anxiety patients and healthy controls. Depression/anxiety was not associated with cue-reactivity, but depression severity in alcohol dependent patients was positively associated with craving. Within alcohol dependence, longer duration of alcohol dependence was associated with stronger cue-related activation of the posterior putamen, a structure involved in habits, whereas higher alcohol dependence severity was associated with lower cue-reactivity in the anterior putamen, an area implicated in goal-directed behavior preceding habit formation.

Conclusion: Cue-reactivity in alcohol dependence is not modulated by comorbid depression or anxiety. More importantly, the current data confirm the hypothesis of a ventral to dorsal striatal shift of learning processes with longer dependence duration, which could underlie increasingly habitual substance use with progressing substance dependence.

Editor: Leonardo Fontenelle, Institute of Psychiatry at the Federal University of Rio de Janeiro, Brazil

Funding: Funding for this study was provided by grant 31160004 from the Netherlands Organization for Health Research and Development (Zon-Mw), commissioned by the Netherlands Organization for Scientific Research (NWO). The funders had no role in study design, data collection and analysis, decision to publish, or preparation of the manuscript.

Competing Interests: The authors have declared that no competing interests exist.

* E-mail: sjoerds.zs@gmail.com

Introduction

Substance use disorders like alcohol dependence (AD) are considered chronic, relapsing brain disorders [1,2], characterized by compulsive drug use despite negative consequences [3,4]. The development of drug dependence is thought to follow a gradual transition during which initial hedonic effects of drugs decrease [4], and the gradual formation of drug habits contributes to the compulsive character of dependence [5], leading to relapse even after longer periods of abstinence. According to the incentive salience theory [6], repeated drug exposure renders cues to become associated with drug use through Pavlovian conditioning, resulting in an increased salience of drugs and drug-related stimuli, which initiates drug-related responses such as craving [7]. Consequently, the presence of drug-related cues alone can act as a conditioned reinforcer and precipitate instrumental drug-seeking and drug-using behavior, also described as Pavlovian-instrumental transfer [8]. Through this mechanism, cue-elicited craving is implicated in theories of relapse [9], and greater insight into its neurobiological substrate could improve treatments.

Imaging studies in human alcohol abusers have shown alcohol cue-induced activation of brain areas involved in motivational pathways, including orbitofrontal cortex (OFC), medial prefrontal cortex (MPFC) and adjacent anterior cingulate cortex (ACC) and ventral striatum (VS) (for a review see [10]). These areas have shown reactivity to natural rewards such as food and sex in healthy samples [11], and to high-calorie food in obese individuals [12], suggesting a more generalizable involvement of these areas in motivational drives. However, the formation of drug habits following prolonged drug use is thought to be associated with further neural adaptations over time. In rodent studies, prolonged drug use results in a shift in brain involvement from the ventral to the dorsomedial and dorsolateral striatum through a dopamine-dependent cascading loop between sub-regions of the striatum [13,14]. Similarly, in humans, a study in very experienced crack cocaine users (mean duration 11 years) showed strong activation in the dorsal striatum in response to cocaine cues [15]. PET studies in cocaine abusers show that this dorsal striatal activation is associated with significantly increased dopamine levels in the dorsal striatum, which is in turn positively associated with cocaine craving [16–18]. However, these studies did not provide information on a possible time-dependent gradual shift away from reward-related towards more habit driven drug use and its neural correlates. This knowledge is until now almost exclusively based on pre-clinical animal studies [5], and there is currently only one study in humans that has tried to address this issue [19]. In accordance with the hypothesis of a shift of learning processes from ventral to dorsal parts of the striatum with progressing alcohol dependence, this study showed that light social drinkers had higher cue-induced fMRI activations in the ventral striatum (VS) compared with heavy – mostly alcohol dependent – drinkers, whereas heavy drinkers showed significantly higher activations compared with light drinkers in the dorsal striatum (DS). Moreover, VS activation in this study was negatively correlated with a self-report measure of compulsive drinking, whereas DS activation showed a positive correlation with this measure, indicating a shift from VS to DS cue-induced activation when alcohol use becomes compulsive. However, a direct association with the duration of alcohol dependence was not made in this study. Of note, a recent coordinate-based meta-analysis, using activation likelihood estimation [20], analyzed 28 alcohol cue-reactivity imaging studies and found that reactivity to alcohol cues (visual, odor, taste) in the VS was typically reported in heavy alcohol users and less so in individuals with an established diagnosis of alcohol dependence. This further corroborates the hypothesis that the VS is predominantly involved during early stages of (problematic) alcohol use, whereas with a longer drinking history, cue-reactivity shifts towards the DS.

However, the association between the duration of alcohol dependence and cue-reactivity has, to the best of our knowledge, not been examined yet, and the influence of Pavlovian cues on the neurobiological processes towards habitual drug use in humans still needs to be elucidated, especially in relation to addiction characteristics such as duration and severity of dependence. Therefore, the current study aimed to investigate the association between alcohol cue-reactivity during fMRI scanning, craving and alcohol dependence characteristics such as duration and severity. Within a large sample of AD patients we focused on striatal activation and we hypothesized to observe larger involvement of posterior and dorsolateral striatal areas at the expense of VS involvement with a longer history of AD, indicating a cue-induced shift from reward pathways to habit pathways with longer AD duration.

An often overlooked characteristic of alcohol dependence is the high comorbidity with depression/anxiety disorders [21]. Most neurobiological studies in AD, however, either exclude AD patients with comorbid depressive and/or anxiety disorders, thus collecting data on a very specific sample of limited clinical relevance, or fail to consider the presence of comorbid depression and/or anxiety as a potential confounder. This is important, because depression/anxiety disorders are often characterized by anhedonia with reduced brain reward responses towards external, potentially rewarding cues compared with healthy subjects [22,23]. In order to account for this complexity, we included a clinically relevant group of AD patients without excluding AD patients with comorbid depression/anxiety disorders and studied the effect of depression/anxiety within the AD group on cue-reactivity. In addition, we added two comparison groups: a group of healthy controls (HC) and a group of patients with depression/anxiety (D/A). We hypothesized stronger regional brain activation and craving in reaction to alcohol-related cues in AD patients compared with both D/A patients and HCs, an effect that would be mainly associated with alcohol dependence characteristics such as duration and severity and not, or only weakly, with depression/anxiety severity. In addition, we expected reduced regional brain activation in reaction to alcohol-related cues in D/A patients compared with HCs.

Materials and Methods

Participants

Forty-two patients were included with a current (<6 months) DSM-IV diagnosis of AD and no comorbid lifetime Axis-I diagnosis other than major depressive disorder (MDD) and/or anxiety disorders. Twenty-two patients with a current (<6 months) DSM-IV diagnosis of major depression and/or anxiety disorder (generalized anxiety disorder, panic disorder, social anxiety disorder), but no other lifetime diagnosis of Axis-I disorders were included as a psychiatric comparison group (D/A). A group of 21 individuals without any lifetime psychiatric disorder was included as a healthy control group (HC). Both comparison groups were matched on age, gender and education with the AD group.

In order to study a heterogeneous sample of AD subjects with regard to the duration and severity of the disorder, the AD group was recruited from two sources. One half of the AD group was recruited from local addiction treatment clinics; the other half of the AD group was recruited from the Netherlands Study of Depression and Anxiety (NESDA) [24], a large multi-site naturalistic cohort study including patients from primary care and outpatient mental health services. The D/A and HC groups were also recruited from NESDA.

After data collection was completed, we excluded the following participants: subjects with: a) missing data (3 AD, 2 D/A, 1 HC); b) imaging data of poor quality (4 AD, 3 D/A, 2 HC); c) excessive movement during scanning (1 AD); d) not-earlier reported coma (1 HC); or e) testing positive for cocaine or benzodiazepines (5AD, 2D/A, 0 HC). In addition, two HC subjects with substantial alcohol problems (AUDIT score >10) were excluded. The final dataset included 30 AD, 15 D/A, and 15 HC participants for data analyses.

Ethics Statement

The research protocol was approved by the medical ethical review board of the participating universities, and conducted according to the principles expressed in the Declaration of Helsinki. All participants provided written informed consent. All potential participants who declined to participate or otherwise did not participate were eligible for treatment (if applicable) and were not disadvantaged in any other way by not participating in the study.

Procedure and clinical assessments

Participants were screened for current and lifetime psychiatric diagnosis using the Composite International Diagnostic Interview (CIDI, version 2.1) [25]. All participants were free of major

Table 1. Sample Characteristics.

	Alcohol Dependent patients N = 30	Depression/Anxiety patients N = 15	Healthy Controls N = 15			
	Mean (SD)	**Mean (SD)**	**Mean (SD)**	*test*	*test-statistic*	*p-value*
Demographics						
Age	46.5 (8.5)	48.4 (10.6)	46.8 (10)	*H*	*0.94*	*0.626*
Males, N (%)	16 (53.3)	6 (40)	11 (73.3)	X^2	*3.43*	*0.18*
Right handed, N (%)	27 (90)	14 (93.3)	12 (80)	X^2	*1.46*	*0.483*
Years of education	13.1 (3.5)	13.3 (3.9)	14.1 (3.6)	*H*	*1.02*	*0.6*
Clinical characteristics						
Depression severity (IDS score)	20.5 (10.2)	18.8 (12.4)	3.1 (3.9)	*F*	*17.18*	*<0.001*
Anxiety severity (BAI score)	11.8 (10.2)	11.1 (9.2)	1.5 (2.6)	*H*	*21.6*	*<0.001*
AD severity (AUDIT score)	18.1 (8)	1.5 (1.4)	3.7 (2.1)	*H*	*40.32*	*<0.001*
Drinks per drinking day	3.1 (1.4)	0.9 (0.7)	1.3 (0.7)	*H*	*29.56*	*<0.001*
Drinking days per week	4.4 (2.9)	0.6 (0.8)	2.7 (2.5)	*H*	*19.11*	*<0.001*
Drinks per week	15.4 (12.5)	0.8 (1.0)	4.4 (4.6)	*H*	*24.15*	*<0.001*
Duration of AD (years)	15 (11.8)	-	-		-	-
Abstinence (days; minimum 24 hrs.)	12.2 (20.4)	31.3 (78.4)	6.8 (16.4)	*H*	*2.74*	*0.254*
Smokers, N (%)	17 (56.7)	5 (33.3)	0 (0)	X^2	*13.92*	*0.001*
Behavioral characteristics						
Craving Before	31 (13.6)	17.9 (5.8)	19.3 (6.2)	*F*	*10.16*	*<0.001*
Craving After	34.5 (16.7)	18.6 (6.7)	21.6 (9.6)			
Mean Valence score	4.7 (1.4)	2.6 (1.5)	3.9 (1.5)	*H*	*15.29*	*<0.001*

Abbreviations: AD, alcohol dependants; AUDIT, Alcohol Use Disorder Identification Test; BAI, Beck Anxiety Inventory; HC, healthy controls; IDS, Inventory of Depressive Symptomatology; M, mean; N, number; SD, standard deviation; *F*, One-way ANOVA; *H*, Non-parametric Kruskall Wallis test; X^2, Chi-square test.

internal or neurologic disorders and MRI contraindications, did not use psychotropic medication other than a stable prescription of selective serotonin reuptake inhibitors or infrequent benzodiazepine use, and were free of current substance abuse or dependence, other than alcohol for the AD group, and smoking for all three groups. All participants were asked to abstain from alcohol 24 hours and from caffeine a few hours prior to the study and had a confirmed breath alcohol level of 0.00% (Alcoscan Daisy-AL7000). Mean abstinence duration in the AD group was 12 days (see Table 1). No participants scored higher than 8 points on the withdrawal symptom-checklist CIWA-Ar, [26] and were therefore considered withdrawal-free.

For sample-description purposes, self-report questionnaires were filled out to assess demographic and clinical information. Handedness was measured by the Hand Preference Questionnaire [27]. The presence and severity of alcohol use disorders and nicotine dependence was assessed by the Alcohol Use Disorder Identification test (AUDIT; [28], and the Fagerstrom Test for Nicotine Dependence [29]. AD duration in years was calculated by subtracting the age of onset as assessed by the CIDI from the age during scanning. Anxiety severity was assessed by the Beck Anxiety Inventory (BAI) [30] and depression severity by the Inventory of Depressive Symptomatology (IDS) [31].

The Desire for Alcohol Questionnaire (DAQ) [32], a 14-item self-report questionnaire measuring craving for the use of alcohol, was assessed immediately before and after scanning to measure baseline craving and cue-induced subjective craving, respectively. A craving difference score was calculated by subtracting the craving score before scanning from the craving score after scanning. A positive difference score indicated an increase in craving after alcohol cue presentation during scanning.

Cue Reactivity Paradigm

To measure cue-induced brain activity, an event-related visual cue-reactivity fMRI task was used, during which 50 alcohol-related pictures and 50 graphically matched affectively neutral pictures were presented to all participants. A large part of the alcohol stimuli were taken from alcohol databases also used by Wrase *et al* (2002) and Grüsser *et al* (2000) and supplemented with alcohol-related pictures from the web, after validation on positive valence by volunteers with alcohol use disorders. Neutral pictures were taken from the International Affective Picture System (IAPS) (Lang *et al*, 2008), after matching for graphic characteristics with the chosen alcohol cues. Participants were asked to watch and attend to the stimuli. To ensure maintained attention, participants were instructed to press a button when a face was shown on the picture. Of every 50 pictures in each set, 10 contained pictures with faces, which were modeled as a regressor of no interest, leaving 40 alcohol and 40 neutral pictures for analysis. Each picture was presented for 5 seconds, with an interstimulus interval jittered between 500 and 1000 ms. To promote cue-induced craving, the pictures were presented in random order in blocks of various lengths (4-6 pictures), neutral and alcohol blocks alternating. Imaging analyses were performed in an event-related fashion. Every block was preceded by a fixation cross (jittered 4 to 6 seconds), which was used as an implicit baseline. All participants were asked to rate the alcohol

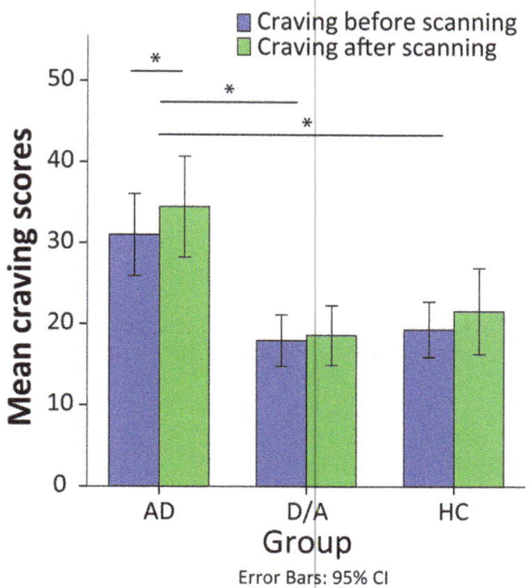

Figure 1. Mean craving scores before and after scanning in the three groups. The AD group showed higher craving scores compared to the D/A ($P=.001$) and HC ($P=.003$) groups. The difference between before and after was only significant for the AD group ($P=.004$). Abbreviations: AD, alcohol dependents; CI, confidence interval; HC, healthy controls; D/A, psychopathology controls.

pictures on positive valence for drinking on a scale from 0 (no valence) to 9 (very salient) immediately after scanning.

Imaging Data Acquisition & Preprocessing

Magnetic resonance imaging was performed at the Academic Medical Centre (AMC) in Amsterdam using a 3T Philips Intera full-body MR system (Philips Medical Systems, Best, the Netherlands) with a phased array SENSE RF 8-channel head coil. Functional blood oxygen level-dependent (BOLD) signals were sequentially acquired with a T2*-weighted, gradient-echo planar imaging (EPI) sequence and an estimated time-course series of approximately 290 volumes (self-paced) per session (TR/TE = 2300 ms/20 ms; matrix size = 96×95, voxel size = 2.29×2.29×2.50 mm; slices = 45). To minimize susceptibility and distortion artifacts in OFC each volume was scanned with an orientation of 30° from the Anterior-Posterior Commissure (AC-PC) line [33]. Three-dimensional T1-weighted images were obtained using a gradient echo sequence for anatomical reference with the EPI data (TR/TE = 9 ms/3.6 ms; matrix size = 256×231; voxel size = 1×1×1 mm; slices = 170).

Imaging data were preprocessed and analyzed using SPM8 (Wellcome Trust Centre for Neuroimaging, London, UK). Images were manually reoriented to the AC-PC line, slicetimed, realigned, warped to Montreal Neurological Institute (MNI) space, and smoothed using a Gaussian kernel of 8 mm at full-width-at-half-maximum.

Statistical analyses

Sample characteristics and behavioral data were analyzed using IBM SPSS Statistics 20 (IBM, New York, NY, USA). Demographic and clinical characteristics were compared between groups using one-way ANOVA procedures, and non-parametric Kruskal-Wallis or Chi-square tests depending on the nature and the distribution of the variables. Craving before and after fMRI scanning was analyzed using repeated measures group (AD, D/A, HC) by session (before and after scanning) ANOVA, and change scores were tested within-groups against a value of 0 (no change) by means of a Student's *t*-test. Follow-up tests were conducted to evaluate pairwise differences among the three groups, controlling for Type-I error across tests by using the Bonferroni approach. Correlation analyses between behavioral parameters, and alcohol use and other clinical characteristics were performed using Spearman's Rho. Significance was set to $P<.05$.

Statistical analysis of individual imaging data was performed using a first-level fixed effects analysis, in the context of the General Linear Model [34], with the onsets of every picture or baseline cross convolved with a canonical hemodynamic response function to model each outcome type. To remove low-frequency signal drift, a high-pass filter (128 Hz) was applied. Two main trial types were distinguished, i.e. alcohol and neutral stimuli, whereas pictures requiring a button press were modeled as a regressor of no interest. For each subject a contrast image Alcohol>Neutral was constructed to examine regional brain activation related to alcohol cue-reactivity. These contrast images were entered into a second level random-effects analysis using a one-way ANOVA design to investigate between-group effects. In addition, we checked for group effects on the Neutral>Baseline contrast, because we previously found that substance dependent patients may show a stronger brain response to neutral compared to baseline pictures [35]. Within the AD group, whole-brain linear regression analyses were performed to study associations between alcohol-cue induced brain activation and duration and severity of AD, and subjective craving. Additionally, we checked for effects of smoking and depression/anxiety severity on cue-induced brain activity by including the amount of smoked cigarettes per day, and IDS and BAI scores in separate regression analyses within the AD group.

To examine the hypothesized striatal shift during cue-reactivity, we performed *a priori* defined region of interest (ROI) analyses in the striatum. Bilateral masks for the putamen, caudate nucleus and globus pallidus were derived from the automatic anatomical labeling (AAL) atlas [36] incorporated in the WFU-PickAtlas Tool v2.5.2 [37]. The WFU-Pickatlas does not provide an anatomical mask for the most ventral part of the striatum, comprising the nucleus accumbens. Therefore we selected a bilateral VS mask [38] defined in the BrainMap database [39], and created a binary mask from the probabilistic mask at $P>.70$ using the ImCalc-tool in SPM8. Following methods in the recent study by Vollstadt-Klein and colleagues [19], this VS mask was subtracted from the AAL-defined striatal areas to distinguish between ventral and dorsal striatal areas. For a visualization of the ROIs, please see Figure S1. Recently, studies focusing on the transfer towards habit-related behavior in healthy human participants indicate that within the putamen an additional distinction can be made between the anterior and posterior putamen [40,41], which may correspond to the dorsomedial versus dorsolateral striatal involvement seen in rodents. Because this distinction is primarily implicated in instrumental rather than Pavlovian conditioning, we did not add this distinction to the statistical ROI analyses, but to explore any (dorsal) putamen findings, we used the anterior vs. posterior demarcation at MNI-coordinate y = 2 proposed earlier [40]. We report significant brain activations within the striatal areas at $P<.05$ that survived family-wise error (FWE) correction for multiple comparisons on the voxel-level within the ROIs using a small volume correction ($P_{SVC\text{-}FWE}<.05$) [42]. Additionally, for explorative reasons we report whole-brain imaging results in the supplementary material at $P<.005$ uncorrected, and to further

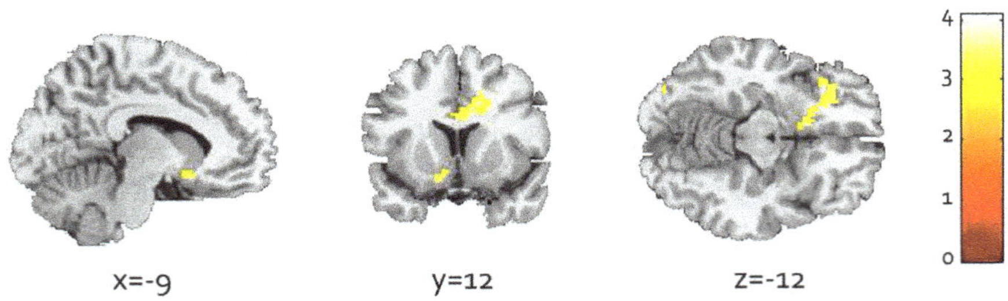

Figure 2. Cue-reactivity in AD patients compared with both comparison groups (D/A patients and HC). Two clusters are visible: Activation of a large cluster reaching from the OFC to the VS, and in the ACC. Colored bar: *Z*-scores from 0 to 4, $P<0.005$, clustersize threshold >= 15 voxels.

protect against type-I error, a voxel extent threshold of 15 voxels [43].

Results

Sample characteristics

As expected, groups differed on alcohol use characteristics ($H_{2,60} = 40.32$; $P<.001$), because the AD group scored significantly higher than the HC and D/A groups (both $P<.001$) whereas the HC and D/A groups did not differ from each other ($P = .919$). The AD and the D/A group reported more depressive and anxiety symptoms than the HC group ($F_{2,57} = 17.175$; $P<.001$, pairwise both $P<.001$; and $H_{2,60} = 21.598$; $P<.001$, pairwise both $P<.001$, respectively). The AD and the D/A group did not differ significantly on depression or anxiety severity (pairwise, $P = 1.000$ and $P = .918$, respectively). The groups differed in the percentage of smokers ($\chi^2_{2,60} = 13.923$; $P<.001$) and number of cigarettes smoked ($H_{2,60} = 14,472$; $P<.001$): none of the HC participants smoked, whereas 17 of the 31 (57%) AD patients and 5 of the 18 (33%) D/A participants did. The number of smoked cigarettes per day, however, did not show associations with other demographic and clinical sample characteristics.

Groups differed in valence ratings ($H_{2,59} = 15.292$; $P<.001$), indicating that AD patients found the alcohol pictures more positively influencing their desire to drink than the D/A group (pairwise, $P<.001$), whereas the AD and the D/A group did not differ from HC (pairwise, $P = .294$ and $P = .153$, respectively).

The mean duration of alcohol dependence in AD patients was 15.0 years with a large variation (SD = 11.8 years), suggesting substantial heterogeneity. Duration of AD was positively associated with alcohol use severity ($r = .441$; $P = .015$).

For detailed information on sample characteristics, see Table 1.

Self-reported craving

Repeated measures ANOVA showed a main effect of group ($F_{2,57} = 10.158$; $P<.001$): the AD group scored significantly higher than the D/A and HC groups both at baseline and after cue-exposure (AD vs. D/A: $P<.001$; AD vs. HC: $P<.001$). A main effect of session showed increased craving after scanning ($F_{1,57} = 6.260$; $P = .015$). No group*session interaction was seen. Within-group one-sample t-tests indicated that the AD group showed significantly increased craving after fMRI scanning (M = 3.3; $P = .004$), whereas this difference in craving before and after the scanning session was not significant for the D/A group ($P = .682$) or the HC group ($P = .167$) (Fig. 1).

Subjective craving scores correlated positively with alcohol severity according to the AUDIT (before scanning: r = .465; $P<.001$; after scanning: r = .494; $P<.001$). Subjective craving scores also correlated positively with depression severity in the total sample (before scanning: r = .439; $P<.001$; after scanning: r = .334; $P<.001$), in the AD group (before scanning: r = .523; $P = .003$; after scanning: r = .403; $P = .027$), and in the HC group (after scanning only: r = .588; $P = .021$).

There were no associations between the number of smoked cigarettes per day and alcohol craving scores, neither in the AD nor in the D/A group.

Imaging data

Group comparisons. The fMRI cue-reactivity paradigm activated a wide network of brain areas implicated in the motivational and reward system, as well as attention and object recognition networks, replicating studies on alcohol cue-reactivity [44,45]. Main effects of Alcohol>Neutral pictures over the whole sample and per group are shown in Table S1.

ANOVA group comparisons on Alcohol>Neutral pictures showed higher cue-induced brain activation in the AD group compared to the D/A and HC groups (See Table S2). Increased VS activation in the comparison between AD and D/A patients approached significance ($P_{FWE}<.1$). Given the similar activation patterns in the two comparison groups (15 D/A, 15 HC), we performed a two-sample t-test comparing 30 AD patients with 30 comparison subjects (15 D/A +15 HC subjects) to further investigate cue-reactivity in AD while increasing statistical power. In AD patients (N = 30) compared with the pooled comparison groups (N = 30), activation of the VS survived ROI FWE-correction ($P_{FWE}<.05$) (see Figure 2). Additionally, during whole-brain exploration of group comparisons at a more liberal threshold (P<0.005 whole-brain uncorrected, cluster extent = 15 voxels), the AD group showed larger activations in previously reported cue-reactivity areas like the ACC, medial PFC, IFG, OFC, VMPFC, caudate body, thalamus and globus pallidus (see Table S2).

The AD group did not show lower activation compared with the two control groups.

Checking for confounding group effects on neutral pictures versus baseline trials only yielded expected results in bilateral occipital cortices ($Z = 3.64$), right hippocampal formation ($Z = 3.58$), right inferior parietal lobule ($Z = 3.63$), and bilateral dorsolateral ($Z = 3.56$) and dorsomedial ($Z = 3.38$) prefrontal cortices, and no effects in ventral prefrontal and striatal areas.

Regression analyses within the AD group. Within the AD group, whole-brain correlation analysis showed no positive correlation between alcohol use disorder severity (AUDIT) and alcohol cue-reactivity in the a priori regions of interest, but a negative association between alcohol use disorder severity and activation of the right anterior putamen after small volume FWE-

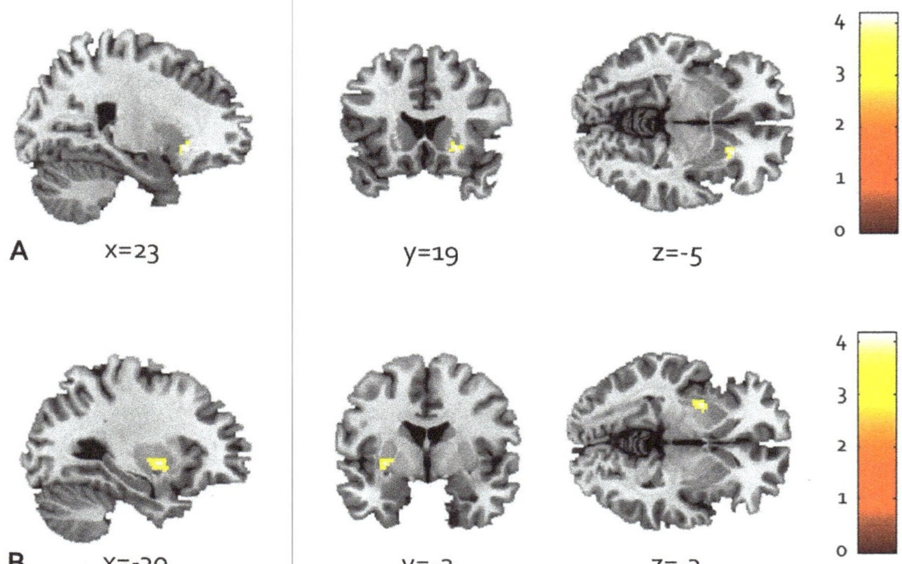

Figure 3. Regression analyses within AD group. a. A negative association between alcohol use disorder severity (AUDIT score) and cue-reactivity in the anterior putamen ($Z = 3.79$; $P_{FWE} < .05$). b. A positive association between alcohol cue-reactivity and duration of alcohol dependence shows activation in the posterior putamen ($Z = 3.64$; $P_{FWE} < .05$). Displayed at $P < 0.005$ uncorrected; cluster size threshold $> = 15$ voxels, masked with bilateral putamen.

correction was found ($P_{SVC\text{-}FWE} < .05$) ($Z = 3.79$) (see Table S3 and Figure 3b).

AD duration showed a positive association with alcohol cue-reactivity in several areas across the brain when exploring the whole-brain (see Table S3), with a significant association in left posterior putamen ($Z = 3.64$; $P_{SVC\text{-}FWE} < .05$). Since AD duration was correlated with age ($\rho = .444$; $P < .014$) we *post-hoc* performed multiple regression analyses in SPM, revealing that posterior putamen activation was correlated with AD duration, but not with age.

Self-reported cue-induced craving scores showed a weak association with alcohol cue-reactivity during whole-brain exploration; however no craving related activation was seen in the striatum.

Depression and anxiety severity within the AD group showed no or only a weak positive association with alcohol cue-reactivity, and a negative association in areas of no a-priori interest during whole-brain explorations. No areas survived small-volume FWE-correction.

Post-hoc analysis showed that the amount of cigarettes was not associated with cue-reactivity in areas seen in the previous analyses or within the *a-priori* ROIs.

For details on the activations of the regression analyses in the a-priori set regions of interest, and additional explorative whole-brain activations at a more liberal threshold see Table S3.

Discussion

In the current study, AD patients showed higher baseline and cue-induced craving than HCs and D/A patients. The increase in craving after alcohol cue-exposure compared with baseline craving before cue-exposure was present in the AD group but not in the two comparison groups, indicating that subjective craving increased disproportionately in AD patients after visual alcohol-cue exposure. In addition, our imaging results showed that exposure to visual alcohol cues during MRI-scanning increased brain activation in AD patients compared with D/A patients and HCs in brain areas that are part of the motivational network, such as the OFC, VS and MPFC.

These findings confirm those of numerous previous studies on cue-reactivity comparing heavy substance users with healthy controls [10,46]. It is hypothesized, however, that motivational pathways such as the VS are mainly involved in the earlier-stage of problematic drug use [20], and that with prolonged drug use a transition towards habit pathways, comprising dorsolateral parts of the striatum, is expected [47]. For example, pharmacological studies have shown that blocking the rewarding effects of drugs by administrating dopamine D2 blockers or the mu-opiate antagonist naltrexone is only successful in non-dependent heavy alcohol users, or 'early-stage' alcohol dependents [4], when rewarding effects of drug intake and the motivational pathways such as the VS still guide alcohol use. Therefore, VS activation would mainly be expected in these 'early stage' AD patients. Our large sample of alcohol dependents comprised a heterogeneous group regarding severity and duration of AD, with about half of the AD patients currently not in treatment, and with less severe and shorter AD. Therefore, the observed effect of cue-exposure on VS activation could be driven by the relatively large group of less chronic AD patients. However, a regression analysis on the possible influence of severity and duration of AD on cue-induced VS activation did not confirm this hypothesis. These analyses did show that with longer lasting AD, the involvement of the posterior putamen during alcohol cue-exposure is more pronounced. Posterior putamen has previously been shown to be involved in habitual behavior [40,41,48], and the current result indicates that, following Pavlovian cues, more chronic AD patients activate habit pathways, which confirms the habit formation theory [5]. Finally, we found lower activation in the anterior putamen, implicated in goal-directed behavior, with higher AD severity, which in turn was positively correlated with AD duration. This finding suggests that the shift from motivational or goal-directed pathways towards pathways involved in habit formation thought to be time dependent (progression over time) is partly mediated by severity of AD. However, future studies using prospective designs should elucidate on the shift away from motivational and goal-directed pathways in favor of increasing involvement of habit pathways as a function of dependence duration as well as severity.

A direct association between craving scores and cue-reactivity in motivational or habitual brain pathways in AD patients was not clearly present. This could be due to a mismatch between self-reported subjective craving and the objective method to assess cue-conditioned brain responses to alcohol-related stimuli. Subjective craving is difficult to measure in human subjects [49] due to denial by detoxified alcohol-dependent patients, despite high relapse rates [9]. Our observation of a lack of association between cue-reactivity and craving, however, is in line with the hypothesis that drug cues can motivate drug intake even in the absence of conscious craving, because habitual drug use has become involved in the maintenance of drug dependence, rather than craving [9]. This could also explain the lack of association between self-reported craving and duration of alcohol dependence in this study.

An additional aim of this study was to examine the effect of depression/anxiety on alcohol cue-reactivity, by directly comparing cue-induced brain activation and subjective craving in AD patients (with and without comorbid depression/anxiety disorders) and D/A patients (without AD), because the latter group is known to show decreased reactivity to rewarding stimuli, a phenomenon also known as reward deficiency or anhedonia [22,23]. In the current study, the D/A group was characterized by lower drinking levels, lower subjective alcohol craving scores, lower valence scores, and lower brain reactivity to alcohol cues compared with the AD group. However, brain reactivity to alcohol cues in D/A patients did not differ from healthy controls. This does not directly confirm a possible blunting effect of depression/anxiety in reactions to alcohol cues. Among heavy drinkers comorbid depression/anxiety symptoms have previously been found to be positively associated with brain activation in response to alcoholic taste cues [50], explaining the association between stress or negative emotional state and relapse after treatment [51]. However, we did not observe a positive association between depression/anxiety symptoms and brain activation in response to visual alcohol cues within our AD group, suggesting that in alcohol dependent populations the presence of depression/anxiety symptoms has no direct effect on neuronal responses to visual alcohol cues. Together, these findings show that the alcohol cue-induced brain activation in our AD group is not influenced by the presence of comorbid D/A disorders, indicating the presence of a strong effect of AD on alcohol cue-induced brain activation even in an ecologically valid and clinically relevant group of AD patients with a high comorbidity with D/A disorders. It should be noted, however, that depressive symptoms were positively correlated with subjective craving rates overall and within the AD group. This is consistent with the idea that depression-related stress induces craving and consequently subsequent relapse [51]. However, we did not show a corresponding association as seen with self-reported craving between depression/anxiety scores and physiological measurements of brain activation, suggesting lower sensitivity of physiological measurements or a more idiosyncratic influence of depression/anxiety severity on craving.

A possible limitation in the current study is, however, that we did not study general positive versus alcohol-specific salient cues, since we were mainly interested in alcohol cue-reactivity in AD patients. Therefore we were not able to test the specificity of a blunted brain response to alcohol cues in D/A patients. We therefore suggest that future cue-reactivity studies should include both alcohol-related cues and non-alcohol related positive and negative cues.

In conclusion, the current study shows that neural responses to drug cues are subject to a change from activation of brain areas involved motivational and goal-directed processes towards activation of brain areas implicated in chronic drug taking habits with increasing severity and longer duration of AD. This observation presumably underlies the instrumental shift from goal-directed towards habitual drug-taking behavior [5], leading to frequent and highly relapsing substance use despite serious negative consequences.

Supporting Information

Figure S1 Regions of interest. Bilateral masks for the putamen, caudate nucleus and globus pallidus were derived from the automatic anatomical labeling (AAL) atlas (Tzourio-Mazoyer et al. 2002) incorporated in the WFU-PickAtlas Tool v2.5.2 (Maldjian et al. 2003). The WFU-Pickatlas does not provide an anatomical mask for the most ventral part of the striatum, comprising the nucleus accumbens. Therefore we selected a bilateral ventral striatal mask (Nielsen and Hansen 2002) defined in the BrainMap database (Fox and Lancaster 1994), and created a binary mask from the probabilistic mask at $P>.70$ using the ImCalc-tool in SPM8. Following methods in the recent study by Vollstadt-Klein and colleagues (Vollstadt-Klein et al. 2010), this VS mask was subtracted from the AAL-defined striatal areas to distinguish between ventral and dorsal striatal areas. References: **Fox** PT, Lancaster JL (1994). Neuroscience on the net. *Science* 266(5187): 994–996. **Maldjian** JA, Laurienti PJ, Kraft RA, Burdette JH (2003). An automated method for neuroanatomic and cytoarchitectonic atlas-based interrogation of fMRI data sets. *Neuroimage* 19(3): 1233–1239. **Nielsen**, F. A. and Hansen, L. K. (2002). Automatic anatomical labeling of Talairach coordinates and generation of volumes of interest via the BrainMap database (Presented at the 8th International Conference on Functional Mapping of the Human Brain, June 2–6, 2002, Sendai, Japan. Available on CD-Rom.). *Neuroimage* 16 (2). **Tzourio-Mazoyer** N, Landeau B, Papathanassiou D, Crivello F, Etard O, Delcroix N, Mazoyer B, Joliot M (2002). Automated anatomical labeling of activations in SPM using a macroscopic anatomical parcellation of the MNI MRI single-subject brain. *Neuroimage* 15(1): 273–289. **Vollstadt-Klein** S, Wichert S, Rabinstein J, Buhler M, Klein O, Ende G, Hermann D, Mann K (2010). Initial, habitual and compulsive alcohol use is characterized by a shift of cue processing from ventral to dorsal striatum. *Addiction* 105(10): 1741–1749.

Table S1 Main effects of Alcohol>Neutral pictures.

Table S2 Group comparisons. Activated areas during alcohol-cue reactivity.

Table S3 Regression analyses during alcohol-cue reactivity within the group of Alcohol Dependent patients.

Acknowledgments

We thank the local treatment clinics Jellinek, De Maliebaan and the Home Clinic for recruitment of alcohol dependent patients, and the Netherlands Study of Depression and Anxiety (NESDA) for the recruitment of alcohol dependent patients, MDD and anxiety patients and healthy controls. We thank Jana Wrase and Sabine Vollstadt-Klein for providing alcohol-cues that we used in the cue-reactivity paradigm.

Author Contributions

Conceived and designed the experiments: ZS DV WvdB BP. Performed the experiments: ZS. Analyzed the data: ZS DV. Contributed reagents/materials/analysis tools: ZS DV WvdB BP. Wrote the paper: ZS. Interpreted the data: ZS DV WvdB AB BP. Critically revised the manuscript: ZS DV WvdB AB BP.

References

1. Leshner AI (1997) Addiction is a brain disease, and it matters. Science 278: 45–47.
2. McLellan AT, Lewis DC, O'Brien CP, Kleber HD (2000) Drug dependence, a chronic medical illness: implications for treatment, insurance, and outcomes evaluation. JAMA 284: 1689–1695.
3. American Psychiatric Association (2001) Diagnostic and Statistical Manual of Mental Disorders, fourth edition. Washington, DC: American Psychiatric Publishing.
4. Heilig M, Thorsell A, Sommer WH, Hansson AC, Ramchandani VA, et al. (2010) Translating the neuroscience of alcoholism into clinical treatments: from blocking the buzz to curing the blues. Neurosci Biobehav Rev 35: 334–344.
5. Everitt BJ, Robbins TW (2005) Neural systems of reinforcement for drug addiction: from actions to habits to compulsion. Nat Neurosci 8: 1481–1489. nn1579 [pii];10.1038/nn1579 [doi].
6. Robinson TE, Berridge KC (1993) The neural basis of drug craving: an incentive-sensitization theory of addiction. Brain Res Brain Res Rev 18: 247–291.
7. Monti PM, Binkoff JA, Abrams DB, Zwick WR, Nirenberg TD, et al. (1987) Reactivity of alcoholics and nonalcoholics to drinking cues. J Abnorm Psychol 96: 122–126.
8. Dickinson A, Smith J, Mirenowicz J (2000) Dissociation of Pavlovian and instrumental incentive learning under dopamine antagonists. Behav Neurosci 114: 468–483.
9. Tiffany ST, Carter BL (1998) Is craving the source of compulsive drug use? Journal of Psychopharmacology 12: 23–30.
10. Heinz A, Beck A, Grusser SM, Grace AA, Wrase J (2009) Identifying the neural circuitry of alcohol craving and relapse vulnerability. Addict Biol 14: 108–118.
11. Demos KE, Heatherton TF, Kelley WM (2012) Individual differences in nucleus accumbens activity to food and sexual images predict weight gain and sexual behavior. J Neurosci 32: 5549–5552.
12. Murdaugh DL, Cox JE, Cook EW, Weller RE (2012) fMRI reactivity to high-calorie food pictures predicts short- and long-term outcome in a weight-loss program. Neuroimage 59: 2709–2721.
13. Ito R, Dalley JW, Robbins TW, Everitt BJ (2002) Dopamine release in the dorsal striatum during cocaine-seeking behavior under the control of a drug-associated cue. J Neurosci 22: 6247–6253. 20026606 [doi];22/14/6247 [pii].
14. Vanderschuren LJMJ, Di Ciano P, Everitt BJ (2005) Involvement of the dorsal striatum in cue-controlled cocaine seeking. J Neurosci 25: 8665–8670.
15. Garavan H, Pankiewicz J, Bloom A, Cho JK, Sperry L, et al. (2000) Cue-induced cocaine craving: neuroanatomical specificity for drug users and drug stimuli. Am J Psychiatry 157: 1789–1798.
16. Volkow ND, Wang GJ, Telang F, Fowler JS, Logan J, et al. (2006) Cocaine cues and dopamine in dorsal striatum: mechanism of craving in cocaine addiction. J Neurosci 26: 6583–6588. 26/24/6583 [pii];10.1523/JNEUROSCI.1544-06.2006 [doi].
17. Volkow ND, Wang GJ, Telang F, Fowler JS, Logan J, et al. (2008) Dopamine increases in striatum do not elicit craving in cocaine abusers unless they are coupled with cocaine cues. Neuroimage 39: 1266–1273. S1053-8119(07)00881-6 [pii];10.1016/j.neuroimage.2007.09.059 [doi].
18. Wong DF, Kuwabara H, Schretlen DJ, Bonson KR, Zhou Y, et al. (2006) Increased occupancy of dopamine receptors in human striatum during cue-elicited cocaine craving. Neuropsychopharmacology 31: 2716–2727. 1301194 [pii];10.1038/sj.npp.1301194 [doi].
19. Vollstadt-Klein S, Wichert S, Rabinstein J, Buhler M, Klein O, et al. (2010) Initial, habitual and compulsive alcohol use is characterized by a shift of cue processing from ventral to dorsal striatum. Addiction 105: 1741–1749.
20. Schacht J, Anton R, Myrick H (2012) Functional neuroimaging studies of alcohol cue reactivity: a quantitative meta-analysis and systematic review. Addict Biol.
21. Boschloo L, Vogelzangs N, Smit JH, van den Brink W, Veltman DJ, et al. (2011) Comorbidity and risk indicators for alcohol use disorders among persons with anxiety and/or depressive disorders Findings from the Netherlands Study of Depression and Anxiety (NESDA). J Affect Disord 131: 233–242. S0165-0327(10)00749-4 [pii];10.1016/j.jad.2010.12.014 [doi].
22. Pizzagalli DA, Iosifescu D, Hallett LA, Ratner KG, Fava M (2008) Reduced hedonic capacity in major depressive disorder: evidence from a probabilistic reward task. J Psychiatr Res 43: 76–87.
23. Eshel N, Roiser JP (2010) Reward and punishment processing in depression. Biol Psychiatry 68: 118–124.
24. Penninx BWJH, Beekman ATF, Smit JH, Zitman FG, Nolen WA, et al. (2008) The Netherlands Study of Depression and Anxiety (NESDA): rationale, objectives and methods. Int J Methods Psychiatr Res 17: 121–140.
25. Robins LN, Wing J, Wittchen HU, Helzer JE, Babor TF, et al. (1988) The Composite International Diagnostic Interview. An epidemiologic Instrument suitable for use in conjunction with different diagnostic systems and in different cultures. Arch Gen Psychiatry 45: 1069–1077.
26. Sullivan JT, Sykora K, Schneiderman J, Naranjo CA, Sellers EM (1989) Assessment of alcohol withdrawal: the revised clinical institute withdrawal assessment for alcohol scale (CIWA-Ar). Br J Addict 84: 1353–1357.
27. Van Strien JW (1992) Classificatie van links- en rechtshandige proefpersonen [Classification of left- and right-handed research participants]. Ned Tijdschr Psychol 47: 88–92.
28. Babor TF, Kranzler HR, Lauerman RJ (1989) Early detection of harmful alcohol consumption: comparison of clinical, laboratory, and self-report screening procedures. Addict Behav 14: 139–157.
29. Heatherton TF, Kozlowski LT, Frecker RC, Fagerstrom KO (1991) The Fagerstrom Test for Nicotine Dependence: a revision of the Fagerstrom Tolerance Questionnaire. Br J Addict 86: 1119–1127.
30. Beck AT, Epstein N, Brown G, Steer RA (1988) An inventory for measuring clinical anxiety: psychometric properties. J Consult Clin Psychol 56: 893–897.
31. Rush AJ, Gullion CM, Basco MR, Jarrett RB, Trivedi MH (1996) The Inventory of Depressive Symptomatology (IDS): psychometric properties. Psychol Med 26: 477–486.
32. Love A, James D, Willner P (1998) A comparison of two alcohol craving questionnaires. Addiction 93: 1091–1102.
33. Deichmann R, Gottfried JA, Hutton C, Turner R (2003) Optimized EPI for fMRI studies of the orbitofrontal cortex. Neuroimage 19: 430–441.
34. Friston KJ, Holmes AP, Poline JB, Grasby PJ, Williams SC, et al. (1995) Analysis of fMRI time-series revisited. Neuroimage 2: 45–53.
35. Zijlstra F, Veltman DJ, Booij J, van den Brink W, Franken IHA (2009) Neurobiological substrates of cue-elicited craving and anhedonia in recently abstinent opioid-dependent males. Drug Alcohol Depend 99: 183–192.
36. Tzourio-Mazoyer N, Landeau B, Papathanassiou D, Crivello F, Etard O, et al. (2002) Automated anatomical labeling of activations in SPM using a macroscopic anatomical parcellation of the MNI MRI single-subject brain. Neuroimage 15: 273–289. 10.1006/nimg.2001.0978 [doi]; S1053811901909784 [pii].
37. Maldjian JA, Laurienti PJ, Kraft RA, Burdette JH (2003) An automated method for neuroanatomic and cytoarchitectonic atlas-based interrogation of fMRI data sets. Neuroimage 19: 1233–1239. S1053811903001691 [pii].
38. Nielsen FA, Hansen LK (2002) Automatic anatomical labeling of Talairach coordinates and generation of volumes of interest via the BrainMap database (Presented at the 8th International Conference on Functional Mapping of the Human Brain, June 2–6, 2002, Sendai, Japan. Available on CD-Rom.). Neuroimage 16.
39. Fox PT, Lancaster JL (1994) Neuroscience on the net. Science 266: 994–996.
40. de Wit S, Watson P, Harsay HA, Cohen MX, van de Vijver I, et al. (2012) Corticostriatal Connectivity Underlies Individual Differences in the Balance between Habitual and Goal-directed Action Control. J Neurosci 32: 12066–12075.
41. Tricomi E, Balleine BW, O'Doherty JP (2009) A specific role for posterior dorsolateral striatum in human habit learning. Eur J Neurosci 29: 2225–2232. EJN6796 [pii];10.1111/j.1460-9568.2009.06796.x [doi].
42. Worsley KJ, Marrett S, Neelin P, Vandal AC, Friston KJ, et al. (1996) A unified statistical approach for determining significant signals in images of cerebral activation. Hum Brain Mapp 4: 58–73.
43. Lieberman MD, Cunningham WA (2009) Type I and Type II error concerns in fMRI research: re-balancing the scale. Soc Cogn Affect Neurosci 4: 423–428. nsp052 [pii];10.1093/scan/nsp052 [doi].
44. Grusser SM, Wrase J, Klein S, Hermann D, Smolka MN, et al. (2004) Cue-induced activation of the striatum and medial prefrontal cortex is associated with subsequent relapse in abstinent alcoholics. Psychopharmacology (Berl) 175: 296–302. 10.1007/s00213-004-1828-4 [doi].
45. Heinz A, Siessmeier T, Wrase J, Hermann D, Klein S, et al. (2004) Correlation between dopamine D(2) receptors in the ventral striatum and central processing of alcohol cues and craving. Am J Psychiatry 161: 1783–1789. 161/10/1783 [pii];10.1176/appi.ajp.161.10.1783 [doi].
46. Braus DF, Wrase J, Grusser S, Hermann D, Ruf M, et al. (2001) Alcohol-associated stimuli activate the ventral striatum in abstinent alcoholics. J Neural Transm 108: 887–894.
47. Fontenelle LF, Oostermeijer S, Harrison BJ, Pantelis C, Yucel M (2011) Obsessive-compulsive disorder, impulse control disorders and drug addiction: common features and potential treatments. Drugs 71: 827–840.

48. Sjoerds Z, de Wit S, van den Brink W, Robbins TW, Beekman AT, et al. (2013) Behavioral and neuroimaging evidence for overreliance on habit learning in alcohol dependent patients. Translational Psychiatry In Press.
49. Sayette MA, Shiffman S, Tiffany ST, Niaura RS, Martin CS, et al. (2000) The measurement of drug craving. Addiction 95 Suppl 2: S189–S210.
50. Feldstein Ewing SW, Filbey FM, Chandler LD, Hutchison KE (2010) Exploring the relationship between depressive and anxiety symptoms and neuronal response to alcohol cues. Alcohol Clin Exp Res 34: 396–403. ACER1104 [pii];10.1111/j.1530-0277.2009.01104.x [doi].
51. Breese GR, Sinha R, Heilig M (2011) Chronic alcohol neuroadaptation and stress contribute to susceptibility for alcohol craving and relapse. Pharmacol Ther 129: 149–171. S0163-7258(10)00191-9 [pii];10.1016/j.pharmthera.2010.09.007 [doi].

3

Disulfiram Efficacy in the Treatment of Alcohol Dependence

Marilyn D. Skinner[1]*, Pierre Lahmek[2], Héloïse Pham[3], Henri-Jean Aubin[4]

1 Centre de Traitement des Addictions, Hôpital Emile Roux, Assistance Publique-Hôpitaux de Paris, Institut National de la Santé et de la Recherche Médicale U669, Limeil-Brévannes, France, **2** Centre de Traitement des Addictions, Hôpital Emile Roux, Assistance Publique-Hôpitaux de Paris, Limeil-Brévannes, France, **3** Centre Médical Marmottan Paris, France, **4** Centre d'Enseignement, de Recherche et de Traitement des Addictions, Hôpital Paul Brousse, Assistance Publique-Hôpitaux de Paris, Université Paris-Sud, Institut National de la Santé et de la Recherche Médicale U669, Villejuif, France

Abstract

Background: Despite its success with compliant or supervised patients, disulfiram has been a controversial medication in the treatment of alcoholism. Often, study designs did not recognize a pivotal factor in disulfiram research, the importance of an open-label design. Our objectives are: (1) to analyze the efficacy and safety of disulfiram in RCTs in supporting abstinence and (2) to compare blind versus open-label studies, hypothesizing that blinded studies would show no difference between disulfiram and control groups because the threat would be evenly spread across all groups.

Methods and Findings: We searched PubMed, EMBASE and the Cochrane Central Register for RCTs on disulfiram use with alcoholics in comparison to any alcoholic control group. The primary outcome was defined by the authors of each trial. Additional analyses included: blind vs. open-label, with or without supervision, cocaine study or not, and type of control. Overall, the 22 included studies showed a higher success rate of disulfiram compared to controls Hedges'g = .58 (95%CI = .35–.82). When comparing blind and open-label RCTs, only open-label trials showed a significant superiority over controls g = .70 (95%CI = .46–.93). RCTs with blind designs showed no efficacy of disulfiram compared to controls. Disulfiram was also more effective than the control condition when compared to naltrexone g = .77, 95%CI = .52–1.02, to acamprosate g = .76, 95%CI = .04–1.48, and to the no disulfiram groups g = .43, 95%CI = .17–.69. Limits include: (1) a population of 89% male subjects and (2) a high but unavoidable heterogeneity of the studies with a substantial I-square in most subgroups of studies.

Conclusions: Blinded studies were incapable of distinguishing a difference between treatment groups and thus are incompatible with disulfiram research. Based on results with open-label studies, disulfiram is a safe and efficacious treatment compared to other abstinence supportive pharmacological treatments or to no disulfiram in supervised studies for problems of alcohol abuse or dependence.

Editor: Jerson Laks, Federal University of Rio de Janeiro, Brazil

Funding: The authors have no support or funding to report.

Competing Interests: All authors have completed the Unified Competing Interest form at www.icmje.org/coi_disclosure.pdf (available on request from the corresponding author) and declare: H-JA has received sponsorship to attend scientific meetings, speaker honorariums, and consultancy fees from Pfizer, Lundbeck, D & A Pharma, Ethypharm, and Merck-Lipha; no other relationships or activities that could appear to have influenced the submitted work.

* E-mail: marilyn.skinner@erx.aphp.fr

Introduction

Disulfiram has been used in the treatment of alcohol dependence with consistently successful results in individuals with high compliance or when medication intake has been directly supervised [1,2,3]. Its mechanism of action for maintaining alcohol abstinence is thought to be primarily psychological [4,5,6,7] and based on a highly disagreeable pharmacological effect if alcohol is consumed. Disulfiram blocks the enzyme aldehyde dehydrogenase (ALDH). If alcohol is present, acetaldehyde accumulates [8,9] usually resulting in an unpleasant reaction, the disulfiram-ethanol reaction (DER), consisting primarily of tachycardia, flushing, nausea, and vomiting [8]. To prevent the first drink, however, the psychological or cognitive threat is thought to be dominant and active and thus dissuade use [5,6,7]. The threat of a DER, indeed the expectancy of negative consequences if alcohol were to be absorbed and ensuing thoughts about avoiding pain and sickness account for the drug's effectiveness.

On the other hand, different pharmacodynamic rather than psychological mechanisms of action have been proposed to explain the success of disulfiram in cocaine addiction [9,10,11], and in one case report of pathological gambling [12]. Several studies have proposed that cocaine use is reduced in subjects taking disulfiram because disulfiram inhibits dopamine beta-hydroxylase (DBH) and the consequent reduction of synaptic norepinephrine release alters the "high" [13,14,15,16].

Despite its apparent success with compliant or supervised alcohol dependent patients, efficacy studies of disulfiram have been all but concordant, leading to confusion and debates that are largely based on poorly designed studies. The principal methodological design flaws are failure to monitor compliance, absence of control groups, unmatched control groups, no clear objective measure of abstinence, and the problem of blinding in disulfiram studies [2,17,18]. The use of double-blind studies has long been considered the standard method of determining drug efficacy. The principal advantages of the blinding procedure are to minimize the effects of disulfiram biases such as perceptions and expectations arising from both patients and researchers about the drug's effects. Disulfiram, however, unlike other medications, is problematic in blind trials for two main reasons. First, the expectation of a DER in the disulfiram treated patients is thought to be directly related to the efficacy of the drug and thus the disulfiram group must be open to their treatment in order to maintain these expectancies. Likewise, the control group(s) must be open to their treatment in order to be free of the DER expectancy. Secondly, participants in a blinded trial can easily unmask the blind by taking a small dose of alcohol, leading to compliance problems. To summarize, the fundamental problem in blinded trials is that the psychological threat of a DER is present and active in both arms of a given trial, impeding a clear distinction between the active and placebo groups. Indeed, if we postulate that the psychological threat of an aversive reaction is the pivotal mechanism of action of the drug as opposed to its actual pharmacodynamic properties when combined with alcohol, then there would be no chance of finding any difference between disulfiram and a control group in a double-blind design [18].

To date, one meta-analysis specifically on disulfiram has been conducted on disulfiram efficacy for the treatment of alcohol use disorder [19]. Of eleven total studies, ten were selected and divided into five forest plots. Not included were trials with co-dependent alcohol and cocaine subjects and trials that combined disulfiram treatment with another treatment (such as a placebo or methadone). They concluded that supervised disulfiram had some effect on short-term abstinence, number of drinking days, and days until relapse compared to placebo, no disulfiram, or other treatments.

While providing results with useful implications, the Jorgensen et al analysis contained a number of shortcomings regarding content and design issues. Although Jorgensen et al proposed a meta-analysis on disulfiram efficacy, one non-efficacy study was included [20] and five eligible trials were absent [21,22,23,24,25]. Furthermore, the critical and determinant factor in disulfiram efficacy – that only open-label trials can show efficacy – was not explored by Jorgensen et al, and they mixed open and blind studies in their meta-analysis.

Our aim is to quantitatively demonstrate that disulfiram treatment is more effective in open-label rather than in blinded experiments, because in the later the psychological effect of the fear of a DER would be expected to have the same effect in both arms of the study. In addition, we expect that this analysis will show disulfiram to be more effective in supervised studies compared to unsupervised studies. Compliance has been a serious impediment in disulfiram research in numerous studies [26,27].

Methods

Search strategy and study selection

We searched all controlled trials on disulfiram use with alcohol dependent patients using the PubMed database (last search date June 2012), EMBASE (last search date July 2012), the Cochrane Central Register (last search November 2012), and a manual search. The details of the search strategies can be found in Search Strategies S1.

Three investigators (MS, PL, HJA) independently read the abstracts in order to select the publications of interest. Included in this study were original, randomized controlled trials (RCTs) comparing the efficacy of orally administered disulfiram to any control group. All studies included subjects with a diagnosis of alcohol abuse or dependence, whatever the classification system. In some studies, the primary inclusion criterion was cocaine dependence. In this case, we performed the analysis in the comorbid alcohol-cocaine subset. These studies consisted of blind and open-label designs, both supervised and unsupervised.

Data extraction

The data extraction was performed by two independent investigators (MS, HJA). Discrepancies were confronted and a consensus was agreed upon. When possible, authors were contacted by e-mail or personally to retrieve missing data, with a special emphasis on the primary endpoint.

We extracted the primary outcome as defined by the authors in their articles (Table 1). Additional variables were extracted for subgroup analysis: blind or open-label, with or without supervision, cocaine study or not, and type of control. We also included meta-regressions to explain heterogeneity (treatment duration, disulfiram dosage, and publication year, with a risk of bias score) [28].

Study quality analysis

The methodological quality of the studies was analyzed according to the Cochrane Collaboration's tool for assessing risk of bias. The 6-item tool assesses the quality of the randomization procedure (adequate sequence generation and allocation concealment), the blinding of treatments, the probability of other bias, the probability of selective reporting, and issues of incomplete data.

Data analysis

Efficacy outcomes were analyzed by calculating the Hedge's g effect-size for each trial with the uncertainty of each result being expressed by their 95% confidence intervals (CI). An effect-size of 0.2 to 0.3 is thought to be a "small" effect, around 0.5 a "medium" effect, and 0.8 to infinity, a "large" effect [28].

Effects were summarized using a random-effects model. The random-effects model was chosen because of the high heterogeneity between trial estimates in each meta-analysis. The underlying assumption of a random-effects model is that the true effect could vary between studies based on characteristics of the study population or intervention. In this case, for example, the primary outcomes may differ as a function of alcohol use disorder severity, intervention duration, comparator type, and associated psychosocial intervention intensity. A random-effect model is more conservative in that it produces wider confidence intervals for the effect estimates than a fixed-effects model.

Initially all studies were included in the analysis in order to have a global assessment of disulfiram efficacy, regardless of blind or open-label design. The second step was to test the hypothesis that disulfiram shows no difference compared to the control condition if its administration is blinded. Validating this hypothesis would signify that only open-label designs could indicate a treatment effect. In this case, the following analyses should be conducted only in the open-label condition: supervised versus non supervised administration, cocaine versus non cocaine studies, and disulfiram versus the various control conditions.

Publication bias was assessed using funnel plots. Heterogeneity was assessed by calculating the I^2 value. I^2 (range = 0–100%) quantifies the degree of variability, with cut-offs suggested as 0% to 40% (probably unimportant heterogeneity), 30% to 60%

Table 1. Study Description.

Study	Participants (Gender), Age (mean)	Principal inclusion criteria	Treatment duration	Intervention Arms (n)	Blind or Open	Super-vision	Particularity	Primary Outcome
Bardeleben et al 1999	60 (44♂), 44.8	Alcohol dependence (DSM-IV criteria)	12 weeks	1) DIS 200 mg/d (20) 2) ACA 1800 mg/d (20) 3) NTX 45 mg/d (20)	Open	Yes		% of abstinent days to treatment days
Carroll et al 1993	18 (13♂), 32	Alcohol dependence or abuse and cocaine dependence (DSM-III-R criteria)	12 weeks	1) DIS 250 mg/d (9) 2) NTX 50 mg/d (9)	Open	Yes		Mean days of alcohol use
Carroll et al 1998	122 (33♀), 30.8	Alcohol dependence or abuse and cocaine dependence (DSM-III-R criteria)	12 weeks	1) DIS 262 mg/d (mean) (78) 2) No DIS (44)	Open	Yes	Combination of arms	3 or more weeks consecutive abstinence
Carroll et al 2004	121 (63 analyzed who were co-dependent, gender & age not available in this subgroup)	Alcohol and cocaine dependence(DSM-IV criteria)	12 weeks	1) DIS 250 mg/d (38)2) Placebo (25)	Blind	No	Combination of arms	3 or more weeks consecutive abstinence
Chick et al 1992	126 (20♀), 43.0	Alcohol dependence (SADQ*)	26 weeks	1) DIS 200 mg/d (64)2) No DIS [Vit C 100 mg/d] (62)	Open	Yes		Days abstinent during last 6 months
De Sousa & De Sousa 2004	100 ♂, 44.4	Alcohol dependence (DSM-IV criteria)	52 weeks	1) DIS 250 mg/d (50) 2) NTX 50 mg/d (50)	Open	Yes		No relapse
De Sousa & De Sousa 2005	100 ♂, 42.2	Alcohol dependence (DSM-IV criteria)	34 weeks	1) DIS 250 mg/d (50) 2) ACA 1998 mg/d (50)	Open	Yes		No relapse
De Sousa et al 2008	100 ♂, 43.3	Alcohol dependence (DSM-IV criteria)	39 weeks	1) DIS 250 mg/d (50)2) TPM 150 mg/d (50)	Open	Yes		No relapse
De Sousa & De Sousa 2008	58 ♂, 17.3	Alcohol dependence (DSM-IV criteria)	26 weeks	1) DIS 250 mg/d (29) 2) NTX 50 mg/d (29)	Open	Yes		Total abstinence
De Sousa & Jagtap 2009	32 ♂, 66.1	Alcohol dependence (DSM-IV criteria)	26 weeks	1) DIS 250 mg/d (16) 2) NTX 100 mg/d (16)	Open	Yes		No relapse
Fuller & Roth 1979	128 ♂, 42.6	Alcohol dependence (No criteria cited)	52 weeks	1) DIS 250 mg/d (43)2) DIS 1 mg/d (43)3) No DIS [riboflavin 50 mg/d] (42)	Blind for comparisons 1 & 2, Open for comparisons 1 & 3	No	3 arms	Continuous abstinence
Fuller et al 1986	605 ♂, 41.7	Alcohol dependence (National Council on Alcoholism criteria)	52 weeks	1) DIS 250 mg/d (202)2) DIS 1 mg/d (204)3) No DIS [riboflavin 50 mg/d] (199)	Blind for comparisons 1 & 2,Open for comparisons 1 & 3	No	3 arms	Continuous abstinence
Gerrein et al 1973	121 (49 analyzed for this meta-analysis, gender & age not available in this subgroup)	Alcohol dependence (No criteria cited)	8 weeks	1) DIS 250 mg/d (26)2) No DIS (23)	Open	Yes (n = 13) No (n = 13)	6 arms	Total abstinence
Grassi et al 2007	12 ♂, 32.87	Alcohol and cocaine dependence (SDS **) criteria	12 weeks	1) DIS 400 mg/d (4)2) No DIS (4)3) NTX 50 mg/d (4)	Open	No	3 arms	4 weeks abstinence

Table 1. Cont.

Study	Participants (Gender), Age (mean)	Principal inclusion criteria	Treatment duration	Intervention Arms (n)	Blind or Open	Super-vision	Particularity	Primary Outcome
Laaksonen et al 2008	243 (71♀), 43.1	Alcohol dependence (ICD-10 criteria)	12 weeks	1) DIS 150 mg/d (mean) (81)2) NTX 50 mg/d (81)3) ACA 1333-1998 mg/d (81)	Open	Yes	3 arms	Time to first heavy drinking day
Ling et al 1983	82 (gender not given), 39.0	Alcohol dependence or abuse (criteria not given)	36 weeks	1) DIS 250 mg/d (41)2) placebo (41)	Blind	Yes for subjects at the clinic. No for those with take home privileges	Methadone patients	No relapse and continued clinic attendance
Nava et al 2006	86 (18♀), 40.0	Alcohol dependence (DSM-IV criteria)	52 weeks	1) DIS 200 mg/d (31)2) NTX 50 mg/d (27)3) GHB 50 mg/kg of body weight/d (28)	Open	Yes	3 arms	No relapse
Niederhofer & Staffen 2003	49 (26 analyzed, 9♀), 17.0	Alcohol dependence, chronic or episodic (DSM-IV criteria)	12 weeks	1) DIS 200 mg/d (13)2) placebo (13)	Blind	No	Adolescents	Total abstinence
Petrakis et al 2000	67 (17 analyzed who were co-dependant, gender & age not available)	Alcohol dependence or abuse and cocaine dependence (DSM-IV criteria or psychiatric evaluation)	12 weeks	1) DIS 250 mg/d (8)2) placebo (9)	Blind	No	Methadone (disulfiram in methadone)	Total abstinence
Petrakis et al 2005	254 (189 analyzed, 5 ♀), 47.0	Alcohol dependence (DSM-IV criteria)	12 weeks	1) DIS 250 mg/d (66) + Placebo2) No DIS (64)3) NTX 50 mg/d (59)	Open	No	Combination of arms	Total abstinence
Pettinati et al 2008	208 (159 analyzed, 46 ♀), 41.0	Alcohol and cocaine dependence (DSM-IV criteria)	11 weeks	1) DIS 250 mg/d (53)2) Placebo (54)3) NTX 100 mg/d (52)	Blind	No	Combination of arms	At least 3 consecutive weeks of abstinence from both alcohol and cocaine
Ulrichsen et al 2010	39 (12♀), 52.0	Alcohol dependence (ICD-10 criteria)	26 weeks	1) DIS 176 mg/d (mean) (19)2) No DIS (20)	Open	Yes		Total abstinence

ACA Acamprosate, DIS disulfiram, NTX Naltrexone, TPM Topimirate, GHB *g*-hydroxybutyrate* SADQ Severity of Alcohol Dependence Questionnaire [66]** SDS- Severity of Dependence Scale questionnaire for cocaine and alcohol dependence.

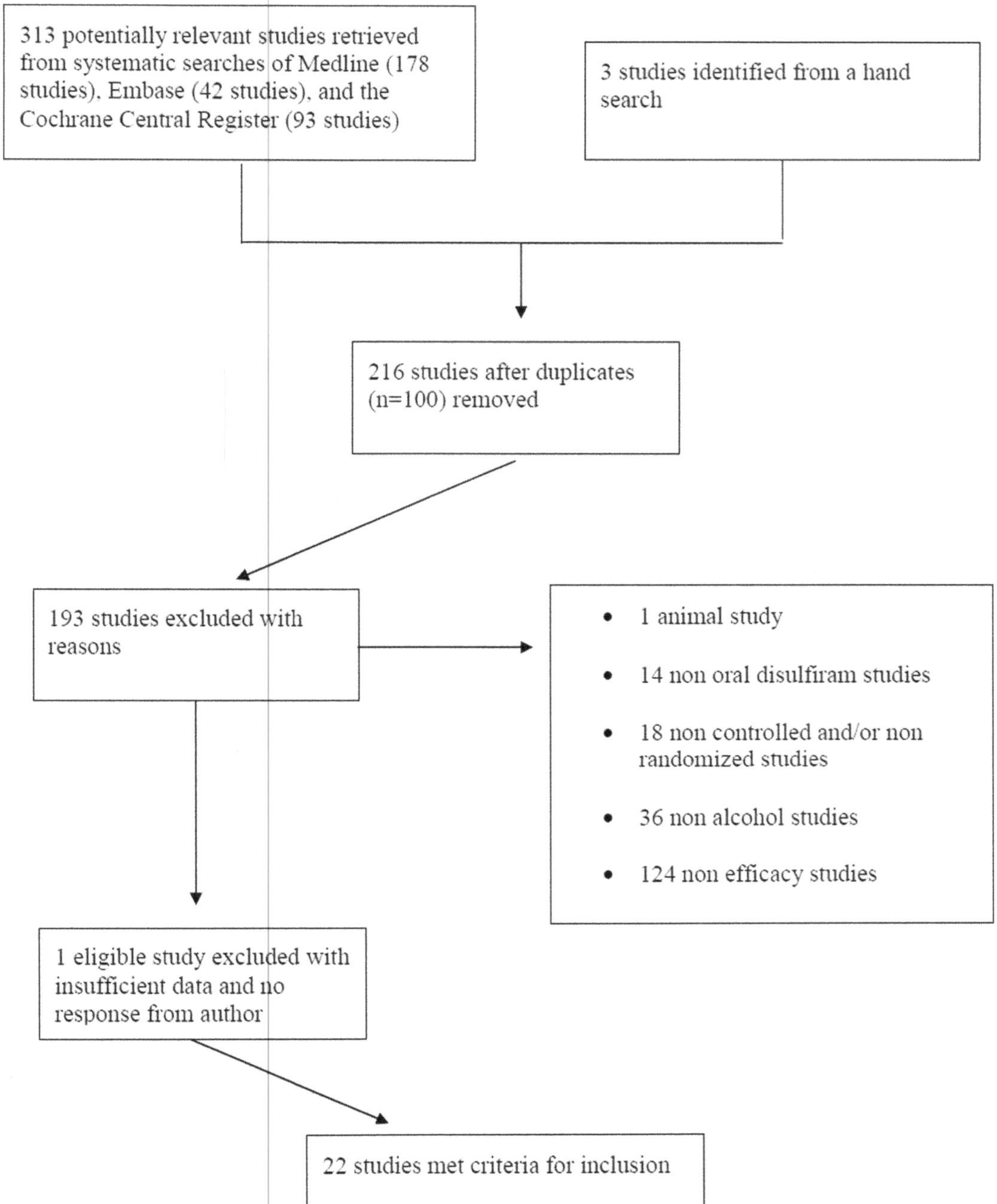

Figure 1. Flowchart of selection of studies for inclusion in the meta-analysis.

(moderate heterogeneity), 50% to 90% (substantial heterogeneity), and 75% to 100% (considerable heterogeneity). The importance of the observed value of I^2 depends on the magnitude and direction of effects and the strength of evidence for heterogeneity (e.g., p-value from the chi-squared test, or a confidence interval for I^2) [29]. Leave-one-out sensitivity analyses were conducted. Sources of bias and heterogeneity were evaluated using meta-regression (for publication year, study quality, treatment duration, and disulfiram dosage). A significance level of $p<.05$ (2-tailed) was used for all analyses.

The forest plot on safety was calculated using the number of events per person years.

All analyses were conducted using the Comprehensive Meta-Analysis statistical program, version 2.2.50 (Englewood, NJ).

Results

Included studies

Systematic searches resulted in 178 references from PubMed, 42 from Embase, and 93 from the Cochrane Central Register. Of these 313 references, 100 were duplicates. A manual search resulted in 3 additional articles bringing the total to 216. After cross-referencing between investigators, 35 were then selected for a detailed review and analysis. From these, 23 were chosen for inclusion in the meta-analysis. In five of these studies, additional

Table 2. Methodological Quality of Included Studies.

	Adequate sequence generation	Allocation concealment	Blinding of participants, personnel and outcome assessors	Free of other bias	Free of selective reporting	Incomplete outcome data addressed	Quality assessment(maximum score: 6/6)
Bardeleben et al 1999	?	-	NA	-	?	?	0
Carroll et al 1993	?	-	NA	-	?	?	0
Carroll et al 1998	?	?	?	-	?	-	0
Carroll et al 2004	+	?	+	+	?	+	4
Chick et al 1992	+	+	-	?	?	+	3
De Sousa & De Sousa 2004	+	?	NA	-	?	+	2
De Sousa & De Sousa 2005	+	?	NA	-	?	+	2
De Sousa et al 2008	+	?	NA	-	?	+	2
De Sousa & De Sousa 2008	+	-	NA	-	?	+	2
De Sousa & Jagtap 2009	+	-	NA	-	?	+	2
Fuller & Roth 1979	+	?	+	-	?	?	2
Fuller et al 1986	+	+	-	?	?	?	2
Gerrein et al 1973	?	?	NA	?	?	?	0
Grassi et al 2007	?	?	NA	-	-	-	0
Laaksonen et al 2008	+	?	NA	+	+	+	4
Ling et al 1983	?	?	+	?	-	-	1
Nava et al 2006	+	?	NA	?	?	+	2
Niederhofer & Staffen 2003	?	+	+	?	?	?	2
Petrakis et al 2005	?	?	NA	-	?	-	0
Petrakis et al 2000	?	?	+	-	+	+	3
Pettinati et al 2008	?	?	+	?	?	+	2
Ulrichsen et al 2010	+	-	NA	-	?	+	2

data were needed on the primary outcome of a subset of the participants. We obtained additional data from the authors in four of these studies. Because we did not obtain a response from the fifth author [30], we were unable to include their trial. The final selection procedure thus allowed us to analyze 22 studies (Figure 1).

Description of the selected studies

The studies selected for this meta-analysis (Table 1) were published between 1973 and 2010. Most were from the United States (10), followed by India (5), Italy (2), and one each from the United Kingdom, Finland, Austria, Denmark, and Switzerland. The cumulative total of subjects analyzed in the 22 studies was 2414, ranging from 12 [13] to 605 [27]. Over half included 100 or more subjects. The subjects were alcohol dependent in 18 of the studies and diagnosed as alcohol abuse or dependent in the other four studies [14,22,31,32]. For the studies indicating gender, 2058 were men and 266 were women (11.4%). The breakdown by gender was not available in a sub sample of two studies in which we analyzed only the arms of the study that were related to our research question [14,25]. In one study, gender was not indicated [32]. Two studies evaluated adolescents (mean age 17) [33,34], one evaluated an older population (>60 years old) [24]. The remaining studies analyzed subjects with a mean age range of 31–52 years.

Six of the studies evaluated a population of cocaine dependent subjects, of which all or a part were also alcohol dependent or abused alcohol [10,13,14,21,26,31]. Where necessary, we extracted for analysis only the co-dependent subjects in these cocaine studies [10,14].

In most studies, subjects were recruited from a center in which they were undergoing treatment for alcohol dependence [22,23,24,33,35,36,37,38,39] or seeking treatment and recruited through the media [10,26,31,34,40,41]. The largest study's subjects (n = 605) were patients participating in VA (Veterans Administration) medical centers [27]. One study included patients admitted to a psychiatric center emergency ward [42], while three others recruited outpatients in alcohol or substance abuse clinics [13,21,25]. Finally in two studies, the subjects were either currently enrolled in a methadone clinic or had been discharged from one because of problems related to drinking [14,32].

Only two of the 22 studies did not require counseling [32,34]. In 20 studies patients generally received weekly group cognitive behavior therapy or less formal alcohol counseling.

Twelve studies required medication intake supervision by a family member, friend, or a member of the clinic staff while eight did not require this supervision. In the remaining two studies, half of the subjects were supervised in one case [25] and in the other, the study medication was to be taken with methadone and was supervised only in those without take home privileges [32]. In ten of the supervised studies, the control arm was also supervised when it consisted of another medication or a placebo. In the three remaining studies, the control arm was "no disulfiram" and thus no supervision was possible [25,31,42].

The most frequent measure of baseline alcohol consumption was the number of drinks consumed per drinking day. In the studies using this criterion, the range was 5–19 drinks with most studies reporting 8–13 drinks per day. The baseline alcohol consumption was not available in four studies [22,34,39,42]. We were unable to obtain the baseline alcohol consumption for the sub sample of codependent patients in the Carroll et al study (2004) [43]. In three of the studies, other consumption measures were provided when the number of drinks per day was not stated: Fuller et al (1986) reported days drank in the prior month (20–21), Gerrein et al (1973) reported the number of years of loss of control drinking (12.83), and Ling et al (1982) reported that 80% of their sample drank daily.

The designs of the studies ranged from two to six arms. Eleven studies contained two arms comparing disulfiram to either placebo [14,32,34], to no disulfiram [23,42], to naltrexone [21,24,33,35], to acamprosate [36], or to topiramate [37]. Six studies had three arms. Four of these compared disulfiram to naltrexone and to one other condition: to no disulfiram [13], to acamprosate [22,40], or to GHB [41]. The control arms in these studies were combined in order to calculate the overall efficacy and the following comparisons: blind versus open-label, supervision versus no supervision, and cocaine versus non cocaine. The control arms were analyzed separately, however, when comparing disulfiram efficacy across the various control conditions. The fifth and sixth studies compared disulfiram to placebo and no disulfiram [27,39]. In these two studies, the control arms were combined in order to calculate the overall efficacy effect-size. In comparisons of efficacy in blind versus open-label, the control arms were analyzed separately. In addition, for comparisons of cocaine versus non cocaine trials, supervised versus non supervised conditions, and across the various control conditions, only the no disulfiram arm was analyzed to determine disulfiram efficacy and this part of both trials was open-label. When appropriate, arms were combined according to Higgins and Green [29].

In the Carroll et al (2004) four arm study in which two types of psychotherapy were combined with disulfiram or placebo in a blind design, we extracted only the patients who were alcohol dependent from the disulfiram and placebo groups regardless of their psychotherapy group allocation to form one comparison. In the Carroll et al (1998) five arm open study, also comparing different types of psychotherapy with disulfiram or with no disulfiram, we again extracted only the patients who were alcohol dependent from the combined disulfiram and no disulfiram groups.

The Gerrein et al (1973) six arm study compared unsupervised and supervised disulfiram intake (groups one and two) to two no disulfiram groups (groups three and four depending upon the frequency of clinic visits). Groups one and three were assigned weekly clinic visits and groups two and four biweekly clinic visits. The last two arms were not randomized and thus not included in our analyses. We compared the supervised (biweekly clinic visit) disulfiram group to the no disulfiram (also biweekly clinic visit) group and the unsupervised (weekly clinic visit) disulfiram group to the other no disulfiram (weekly clinic visit) group.

In the four arm study by Petrakis et al (2005) in which open-label disulfiram + blinded placebo were compared to placebo, naltrexone, or open-label disulfiram + blinded naltrexone, we analyzed two comparisons: disulfiram + placebo compared to naltrexone or compared to placebo. Because the placebos in this study were for naltrexone, we labeled this comparison disulfiram vs "no disulfiram" in our analysis. We did not analyze the comparisons in which disulfiram and naltrexone were administered together.

In the Pettinati et al (2008) double-blind, four arm study, similar comparisons were made. We analyzed disulfiram when administered alone, not with naltrexone. The placebo was double matched for both naltrexone and disulfiram. We analyzed disulfiram compared to naltrexone and the double placebo.

Fifteen of the studies were open-label, five were double-blind, and two contained a blind and an open-label design with the blind arm comparing disulfiram to placebo and the open arm comparing disulfiram to no disulfiram [27,39].

Medication compliance was monitored by self-report (14 studies), friend or family member report (seven studies), a

Table 3. Success Rates on Primary Outcomes.

Study Mean (SD) or %	Disulfiram success Rate	Disulfiram N	Control success rate	Control N
Bardeleben et al 1999	93.3 (16.6)	20	89.6 (18.04)	40
Carroll et al 1993	2.4 (2.3)	9	10.4 (7.7)	9
Carroll et al 1998	53.00%	78	16.00%	44
Carroll et al 2004	87.50%	38	82.60%	25
Chick et al 1992	100 (70)	47	69 (67)	46
De Sousa & De Sousa 2004	82.00%	50	42.00%	50
De Sousa & De Sousa 2005	88.00%	50	46.00%	50
De Sousa et al 2008	90.00%	50	56.00%	50
De Sousa & De Sousa 2008	79.31%	29	51.72%	29
De Sousa & Jagtap 2009	81.25%	16	43.75%	16
Fuller & Roth 1979	21.00%	43	18.58%	85
Fuller et al 1986	18.80%	202	19.34%	403
Gerrein et al 1973	23.07%	26	8.70%	23
Grassi et al 2007	100.00%	4	12.50%	8
Laaksonen et al 2008	46.6 (27.5)	33	17,87 (21,03)	91
Ling et al 1983	9.80%	41	24.40%	41
Nava et al 2006	90.00%	31	80.11%	55
Niederhofer & Staffen 2003	53.80%	13	15.40%	13
Petrakis et al 2000	100.00%	8	57.00%	9
Petrakis et al 2005	77.30%	66	65.02	123
Pettinati et al 2008	17.00%	53	16.13%	106
Ulrichsen et al 2010	26.00%	19	20.00%	20

riboflavin compliance procedure to monitor self-report (three studies), pill count (three studies), linking disulfiram to methadone intake (two studies), using Microelective Events Monitoring (MEM) caps (one study), and supervision (thirteen studies). One study provided weekly clinical management compliance enhancement therapy [38].

The methodological quality of the studies was analyzed according to the Cochrane Collaboration's tool for assessing risk of bias [44]. The 6-item tool assesses the quality of the randomization procedure (adequate sequence generation and allocation concealment), the blinding of treatments, the probability of other bias, the probability of selective reporting, and the issue of incomplete data. When the studies were described as open-label studies, the blinding item was considered as non applicable. With this tool, a high score indicates a low risk of bias.

Among the 22 studies included, two met four of these six criteria, two met three criteria, eleven studies met two criteria, one met one criterion, and six studies met none of them (Table 2).

Primary endpoint

The primary endpoint of this meta-analysis was the effect-size at the end of treatment for the key variable as defined by the authors in their articles. The treatment duration varied from 8 to 52 weeks. The effect-size variable could be: total abstinence, proportion of abstinent days to treatment days, mean days of alcohol use, no relapse, time to first heavy drinking day, or three or more weeks of consecutive abstinence as shown in Table 1. In most cocaine studies, the time point for the effect-size variable was earlier than the total study duration, as previous trials have shown that as little as three consecutive weeks of abstinence from both cocaine and alcohol is predictive of long-term cocaine abstinence [26]. Primary outcome success rates are shown in Table 3.

Disulfiram efficacy

When combining the 22 RCTs, our meta-analysis showed a significant success rate of disulfiram compared to controls: g = .58 (95%CI = .35–.82) (Figure 2). I^2 was 72%. A visual inspection of the funnel plot revealed asymmetry, indicating a possible publication bias. The trim-and-fill analysis indicated that there were 4 potentially missing studies on the left side of the funnel plot. Nevertheless, the summary effect-size remained significant after correcting for the putatively missing studies [adjusted effect-size g = .47 (95%CI = .24–.71)]. The summary effect-size reached significance in all cases in the leave-one-out analysis, with summary effect-sizes varying from g = .53 to g = .63 (all $p < .001$). Meta-regression indicated a significant effect of publication year ($\beta = .03$, $p < .001$) and treatment duration ($\beta = -.01$, $p < .001$), but not of disulfiram dosage or risk of bias score.

The subgroup analysis comparing blind and open-label RCTs indicated that only the open-label trials showed a significant superiority of disulfiram over controls: g = .70 (95%CI = .46–.93), whereas the RCTs with blind designs showed no efficacy of disulfiram as compared to controls: g = .01 (95%CI = .−.29–.32) (Figure 3). I^2 = 65% for open-label studies and I^2 = 43% for blind studies. Having validated our hypothesis that a blind design is unsuitable for assessing disulfiram efficacy, we excluded the blind trials from the subsequent analyses. A visual inspection of the funnel plot for open-label studies revealed asymmetry, indicating possible publication bias. The trim-and-fill analysis indicated that there were 2 potentially missing studies on the left side of the

Study name	Hedges's g	Standard error	Variance	Lower limit	Upper limit	Z-Value	p-Value	Relative weight	Relative weight
	Statistics for each study								
Bardeleben et al 1999	0,193	0,242	0,059	-0,281	0,667	0,798	0,425	5,58	
Carroll et al 1993	1,341	0,501	0,251	0,359	2,323	2,677	0,007	3,22	
Carroll et al 1998	0,974	0,257	0,066	0,470	1,478	3,790	0,000	5,43	
Carroll et al 2004	0,211	0,392	0,154	-0,557	0,979	0,538	0,590	4,10	
Chick et al 1992	0,452	0,208	0,043	0,044	0,860	2,173	0,030	5,93	
De Sousa et al 2008	1,125	0,272	0,074	0,592	1,658	4,136	0,000	5,27	
De Sousa & De Sousa 2004	1,178	0,284	0,081	0,621	1,735	4,148	0,000	5,15	
De Sousa & De Sousa 2005	1,070	0,301	0,091	0,480	1,660	3,555	0,000	4,97	
De Sousa & De Sousa 2008	0,693	0,321	0,103	0,064	1,322	2,159	0,031	4,77	
De Sousa & Jagtap 2009	0,923	0,438	0,192	0,065	1,781	2,107	0,035	3,70	
Fuller & Roth 1979	0,084	0,256	0,066	-0,418	0,586	0,328	0,743	5,44	
Fuller et al 1986	-0,019	0,121	0,015	-0,256	0,218	-0,157	0,875	6,70	
Gerrein et al 1973	0,622	0,474	0,225	-0,307	1,551	1,312	0,189	3,42	
Grassi et al 2007	1,965	0,897	0,805	0,207	3,723	2,191	0,028	1,45	
Laaksonen et al 2008	1,254	0,218	0,048	0,827	1,681	5,752	0,000	5,83	
Ling et al 1983	-0,595	0,349	0,122	-1,279	0,089	-1,705	0,088	4,50	
Nava et al 2006	0,439	0,376	0,141	-0,298	1,176	1,168	0,243	4,24	
Niederhofer & Staffen 2003	0,991	0,506	0,256	-0,001	1,983	1,958	0,050	3,18	
Petrakis et al 2000	1,359	0,837	0,701	-0,281	2,999	1,624	0,104	1,62	
Petrakis et al 2005	0,332	0,192	0,037	-0,044	0,708	1,729	0,084	6,08	
Pettinati et al 2008	0,035	0,247	0,061	-0,449	0,519	0,142	0,887	5,53	
Ulrichsen et al 2010	0,184	0,413	0,171	-0,625	0,993	0,446	0,656	3,91	
	0,583	0,121	0,015	0,346	0,821	4,822	0,000		

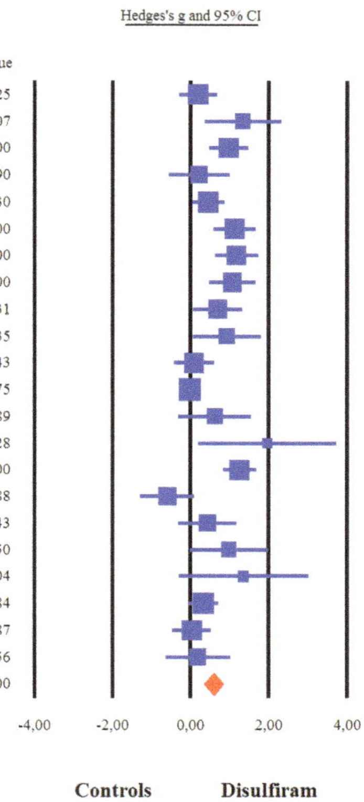

Figure 2. Meta-analysis of Hedges' g effect-size of all RCTs comparing the efficacy of disulfiram and controls.

Group by Subgroup within study	Study name	Study design	Hedges's g	Standard error	Variance	Lower limit	Upper limit	Z-Value	p-Value	Relative weight
			Statistics for each study							
Blind	Carroll et al 2004	Blind	0,211	0,392	0,154	-0,557	0,979	0,538	0,590	11,05
Blind	Fuller & Roth 1979	Blind	-0,124	0,281	0,079	-0,675	0,427	-0,441	0,659	16,83
Blind	Fuller et al 1986	Blind	-0,125	0,135	0,018	-0,390	0,140	-0,926	0,354	29,29
Blind	Ling et al 1983	Blind	-0,595	0,349	0,122	-1,279	0,089	-1,705	0,088	12,94
Blind	Niederhofer & Staffen 2003	Blind	0,991	0,506	0,256	-0,001	1,983	1,958	0,050	7,51
Blind	Petrakis et al 2000	Blind	1,359	0,837	0,701	-0,281	2,999	1,624	0,104	3,14
Blind	Pettinati et al 2008	Blind	0,035	0,247	0,061	-0,449	0,519	0,142	0,887	19,25
Blind			0,013	0,155	0,024	-0,291	0,316	0,082	0,935	
Open	Bardeleben et al 1999	Open	0,193	0,242	0,059	-0,281	0,667	0,798	0,425	7,17
Open	Carroll et al 1993	Open	1,341	0,501	0,251	0,359	2,323	2,677	0,007	3,62
Open	Fuller & Roth 1979	Open	0,365	0,330	0,109	-0,282	1,012	1,106	0,269	5,70
Open	Fuller et al 1986	Open	0,103	0,145	0,021	-0,181	0,387	0,710	0,477	8,86
Open	Carroll et al 1998	Open	0,974	0,257	0,066	0,470	1,478	3,790	0,000	6,90
Open	Chick et al 1992	Open	0,452	0,208	0,043	0,044	0,860	2,173	0,030	7,77
Open	De Sousa & De Sousa 2004	Open	1,178	0,284	0,081	0,621	1,735	4,148	0,000	6,44
Open	De Sousa & De Sousa 2005	Open	1,070	0,301	0,091	0,480	1,660	3,555	0,000	6,16
Open	De Sousa & De Sousa 2008	Open	0,693	0,321	0,103	0,064	1,322	2,159	0,031	5,84
Open	De Sousa & Jagtap 2009	Open	0,923	0,438	0,192	0,065	1,781	2,107	0,035	4,26
Open	De Sousa et al 2008	Open	1,125	0,272	0,074	0,592	1,658	4,136	0,000	6,64
Open	Gerrein et al 1973	Open	0,622	0,474	0,225	-0,307	1,551	1,312	0,189	3,88
Open	Grassi et al 2007	Open	1,965	0,897	0,805	0,207	3,723	2,191	0,028	1,49
Open	Laaksonen et al 2008	Open	1,247	0,217	0,047	0,822	1,672	5,747	0,000	7,61
Open	Nava et al 2006	Open	0,439	0,376	0,141	-0,298	1,176	1,168	0,243	5,04
Open	Petrakis et al 2005	Open	0,332	0,192	0,037	-0,044	0,708	1,729	0,084	8,06
Open	Ulrichsen et al 2010	Open	0,184	0,413	0,171	-0,625	0,993	0,446	0,656	4,56
Open			0,697	0,118	0,014	0,464	0,929	5,878	0,000	

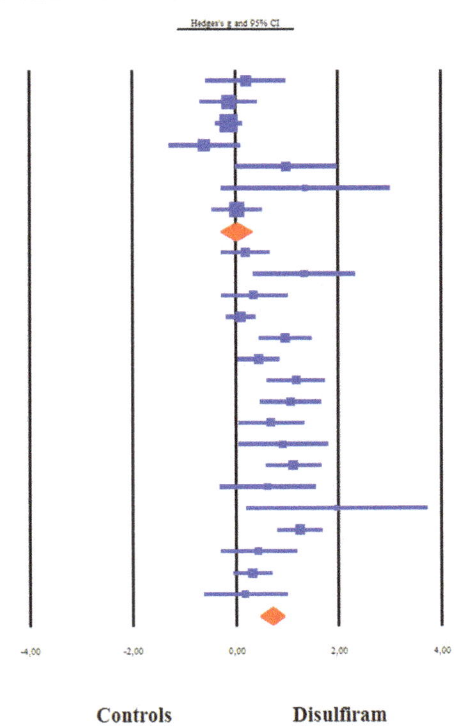

Figure 3. Meta-analysis for blinded versus open-label RCTs. Meta-analysis of Hedges' g effect-size comparing the efficacy of disulfiram and controls in blinded versus open-label RCTs.

Group by / Subgroup within study	Study name	Supervision status	Hedges's g	Standard error	Variance	Lower limit	Upper limit	Z-Value	p-Value	Relative weight
No supervision	Fuller & Roth 1979	No supervision	0,365	0,330	0,109	-0,282	1,012	1,106	0,269	15,05
No supervision	Fuller et al 1986	No supervision	0,103	0,145	0,021	-0,181	0,387	0,710	0,477	46,09
No supervision	Gerrein et al 1973	No supervision	-0,077	0,811	0,658	-1,667	1,513	-0,095	0,924	2,89
No supervision	Grassi et al 2007	No supervision	1,965	0,897	0,805	0,207	3,723	2,191	0,028	2,38
No supervision	Petrakis et al 2005	No supervision	0,332	0,192	0,037	-0,044	0,708	1,729	0,084	33,60
No supervision			0,258	0,140	0,020	-0,016	0,533	1,844	0,065	
Supervision	Gerrein et al 1973	Supervision	1,016	0,637	0,406	-0,232	2,264	1,595	0,111	2,86
Supervision	Bardeleben et al 1999	Supervision	0,193	0,242	0,059	-0,281	0,667	0,798	0,425	10,14
Supervision	Carroll et al 1993	Supervision	1,341	0,501	0,251	0,359	2,323	2,677	0,007	4,21
Supervision	Carroll et al 1998	Supervision	0,974	0,257	0,066	0,470	1,478	3,790	0,000	9,61
Supervision	Chick et al 1992	Supervision	0,452	0,208	0,043	0,044	0,860	2,173	0,030	11,41
Supervision	De Sousa et al 2008	Supervision	1,125	0,272	0,074	0,592	1,658	4,136	0,000	9,11
Supervision	De Sousa & De Sousa 2004	Supervision	1,178	0,284	0,081	0,621	1,735	4,148	0,000	8,73
Supervision	De Sousa & De Sousa 2005	Supervision	1,070	0,301	0,091	0,480	1,660	3,555	0,000	8,21
Supervision	De Sousa & De Sousa 2008	Supervision	0,693	0,321	0,103	0,064	1,322	2,159	0,031	7,65
Supervision	De Sousa & Jagtap 2009	Supervision	0,923	0,438	0,192	0,065	1,781	2,107	0,035	5,13
Supervision	Laaksonen et al 2008	Supervision	1,247	0,217	0,047	0,822	1,672	5,747	0,000	11,06
Supervision	Nava et al 2006	Supervision	0,439	0,376	0,141	-0,298	1,176	1,168	0,243	6,31
Supervision	Ulrichsen et al 2010	Supervision	0,184	0,413	0,171	-0,625	0,993	0,446	0,656	5,57
Supervision			0,820	0,118	0,014	0,589	1,050	6,964	0,000	

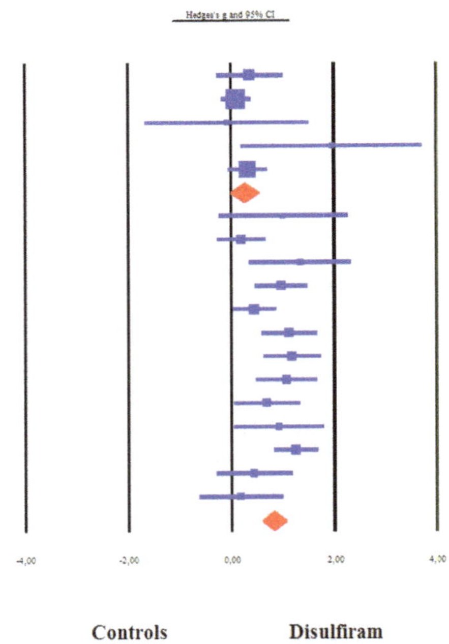

Figure 4. Meta-analysis of RCTs with supervision versus no supervision. Meta-analysis of Hedges' g effect-size comparing the efficacy of disulfiram and controls in RCTs with supervision versus no supervision.

funnel plot. Nevertheless, the summary effect-size remained significant after correcting for the supposedly missing study (adjusted effect-size g = .65 (95%CI = .42–88). The summary effect-size reached significance in all cases in the leave-one-out analysis, with summary effect-sizes varying from g = .64 to g = .75 (all p<.001). Meta-regression indicated no significant effect of publication year, disulfiram dosage, treatment duration, or risk of bias score.

Group by / Subgroup within study	Study name	Cocaine status	Hedges's g	Standard error	Variance	Lower limit	Upper limit	Z-Value	p-Value	Relative weight
Cocaine RCT	Carroll et al 1993	Cocaine RCT	1,341	0,501	0,251	0,359	2,323	2,677	0,007	19,56
Cocaine RCT	Carroll et al 1998	Cocaine RCT	0,974	0,257	0,066	0,470	1,478	3,790	0,000	74,34
Cocaine RCT	Grassi et al 2007	Cocaine RCT	1,965	0,897	0,805	0,207	3,723	2,191	0,028	6,10
Cocaine RCT			1,106	0,222	0,049	0,672	1,541	4,993	0,000	
Non cocaine RCT	Bardeleben et al 1999	Non cocaine RCT	0,193	0,242	0,059	-0,281	0,667	0,798	0,425	8,16
Non cocaine RCT	Chick et al 1992	Non cocaine RCT	0,452	0,208	0,043	0,044	0,860	2,173	0,030	8,88
Non cocaine RCT	De Sousa et al 2008	Non cocaine RCT	1,125	0,272	0,074	0,592	1,658	4,136	0,000	7,55
Non cocaine RCT	De Sousa & De Sousa 2004	Non cocaine RCT	1,178	0,284	0,081	0,621	1,735	4,148	0,000	7,31
Non cocaine RCT	De Sousa & De Sousa 2005	Non cocaine RCT	1,070	0,301	0,091	0,480	1,660	3,555	0,000	6,98
Non cocaine RCT	De Sousa & De Sousa 2008	Non cocaine RCT	0,693	0,321	0,103	0,064	1,322	2,159	0,031	6,61
Non cocaine RCT	De Sousa & Jagtap 2009	Non cocaine RCT	0,923	0,438	0,192	0,065	1,781	2,107	0,035	4,79
Non cocaine RCT	Fuller & Roth 1979	Non cocaine RCT	0,365	0,330	0,109	-0,282	1,012	1,106	0,269	6,45
Non cocaine RCT	Fuller et al 1986	Non cocaine RCT	0,103	0,145	0,021	-0,181	0,387	0,710	0,477	10,18
Non cocaine RCT	Gerrein et al 1973	Non cocaine RCT	0,622	0,474	0,225	-0,307	1,551	1,312	0,189	4,35
Non cocaine RCT	Laaksonen et al 2008	Non cocaine RCT	1,247	0,217	0,047	0,822	1,672	5,747	0,000	8,69
Non cocaine RCT	Nava et al 2006	Non cocaine RCT	0,439	0,376	0,141	-0,298	1,176	1,168	0,243	5,68
Non cocaine RCT	Petrakis et al 2005	Non cocaine RCT	0,332	0,192	0,037	-0,044	0,708	1,729	0,084	9,22
Non cocaine RCT	Ulrichsen et al 2010	Non cocaine RCT	0,184	0,413	0,171	-0,625	0,993	0,446	0,656	5,13
Non cocaine RCT			0,626	0,124	0,015	0,383	0,870	5,036	0,000	

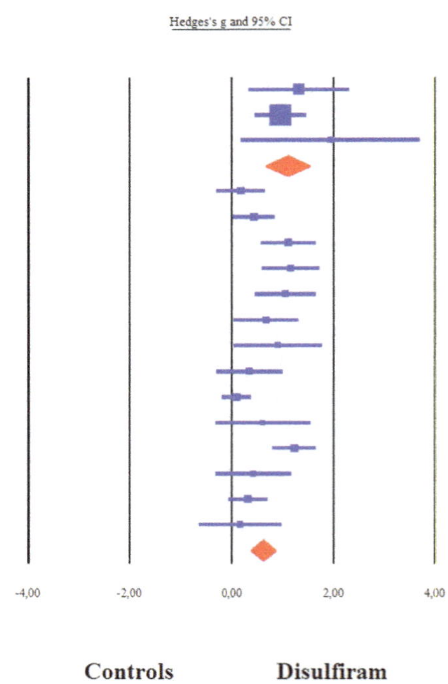

Figure 5. Meta-analysis of RCTs that included cocaine versus non cocaine subjects. Meta-analysis of Hedges' g effect-size comparing the efficacy of disulfiram and controls in RCTs that included alcohol dependent cocaine subjects versus those that did not include cocaine subjects.

Group by / Subgroup within study	Study name	Controls	Hedges's g	Standard error	Variance	Lower limit	Upper limit	Z-Value	p-Value	Relative weight
Acamprosate	Bardeleben et al 1999	Acamprosate	0,018	0,286	0,082	-0,543	0,579	0,063	0,950	32,98
Acamprosate	De Sousa & De Sousa 2005	Acamprosate	1,070	0,301	0,091	0,480	1,660	3,555	0,000	32,28
Acamprosate	Laaksonen et al 2008	Acamprosate	1,172	0,247	0,061	0,688	1,656	4,745	0,000	34,74
Acamprosate			0,759	0,368	0,135	0,038	1,479	2,063	0,039	
GHB	Nava et al 2006	GHB	0,208	0,440	0,194	-0,654	1,070	0,473	0,636	100,00
GHB			0,208	0,440	0,194	-0,654	1,070	0,473	0,636	
Naltrexone	Bardeleben et al 1999	Naltrexone	0,385	0,289	0,084	-0,181	0,951	1,332	0,183	13,73
Naltrexone	Carroll et al 1993	Naltrexone	1,341	0,501	0,251	0,359	2,323	2,677	0,007	5,73
Naltrexone	Laaksonen et al 2008	Naltrexone	0,998	0,238	0,057	0,532	1,464	4,193	0,000	17,69
Naltrexone	Nava et al 2006	Naltrexone	0,626	0,404	0,163	-0,166	1,418	1,550	0,121	8,25
Naltrexone	De Sousa & De Sousa 2004	Naltrexone	1,178	0,284	0,081	0,621	1,735	4,148	0,000	14,06
Naltrexone	De Sousa & De Sousa 2008	Naltrexone	0,693	0,321	0,103	0,064	1,322	2,159	0,031	11,81
Naltrexone	De Sousa & Jagtap 2009	Naltrexone	0,923	0,438	0,192	0,065	1,781	2,107	0,035	7,22
Naltrexone	Grassi et al 2007	Naltrexone	1,516	0,887	0,787	-0,222	3,254	1,709	0,087	2,00
Naltrexone	Petrakis et al 2005	Naltrexone	0,347	0,219	0,048	-0,082	0,776	1,584	0,113	19,51
Naltrexone			0,770	0,128	0,016	0,518	1,022	5,999	0,000	
no disulfiram	Grassi et al 2007	no disulfiram	2,188	1,050	1,103	0,130	4,246	2,084	0,037	1,55
no disulfiram	Petrakis et al 2005	no disulfiram	0,318	0,216	0,047	-0,105	0,741	1,472	0,141	17,42
no disulfiram	Carroll et al 1998	no disulfiram	0,974	0,257	0,066	0,470	1,478	3,790	0,000	14,66
no disulfiram	Chick et al 1992	no disulfiram	0,452	0,208	0,043	0,044	0,860	2,173	0,030	18,01
no disulfiram	Fuller & Roth 1979	no disulfiram	0,365	0,330	0,109	-0,282	1,012	1,106	0,269	10,86
no disulfiram	Fuller et al 1986	no disulfiram	0,103	0,145	0,021	-0,181	0,387	0,710	0,477	23,19
no disulfiram	Gerrein et al 1973	no disulfiram	0,622	0,474	0,225	-0,307	1,551	1,312	0,189	6,39
no disulfiram	Ulrichsen et al 2010	no disulfiram	0,184	0,413	0,171	-0,625	0,993	0,446	0,656	7,91
no disulfiram			0,431	0,134	0,018	0,169	0,694	3,219	0,001	
Topiramate	De Sousa et al 2008	Topiramate	1,125	0,272	0,074	0,592	1,658	4,136	0,000	100,00
Topiramate			1,125	0,272	0,074	0,592	1,658	4,136	0,000	

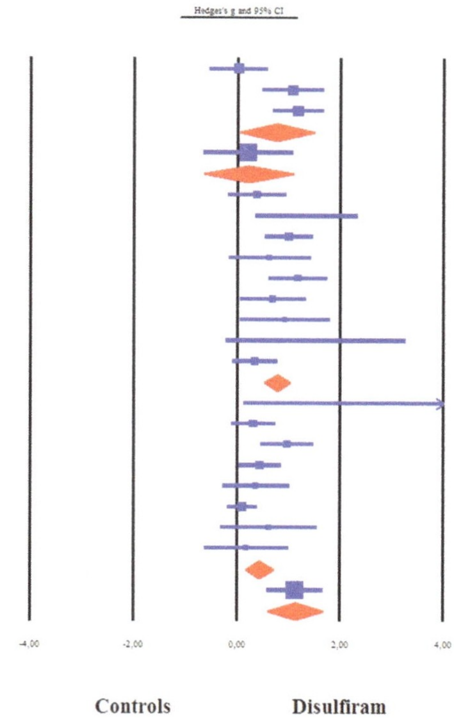

Figure 6. Subgroup analysis of Hedges' g effect-size comparing the efficacy of disulfiram and controls by control types.

The subgroup analysis by supervision categories showed disulfiram to be significantly superior to the control condition when medication compliance was supervised: g = .82, 95%CI = .59–1.05 (Figure 4). I^2 was 46%. When disulfiram treatment was not supervised, however, the treatment showed no significant efficacy as the results fell short of the significance level: g = .26 (95%CI = −.02–.53). In addition these two categories of studies were significantly different from each other. A visual inspection of the funnel plot for supervised studies revealed no asymmetry, indicating no publication bias. The summary effect-size reached significance in all cases in the leave-one-out analysis, with summary effect-sizes varying from g = .74 to g = .89 (all p<.001). Meta-regression indicated no significant effect of treatment duration, publication year, disulfiram dosage, or risk of bias score.

The subgroup analysis by cocaine categories showed a significant disulfiram efficacy as compared to the control condition in both cocaine studies (g = 1.11, 95%CI = .67–1.54) and non cocaine studies primarily enrolling alcoholics (g = .63, 95%CI = .38–.87) (Figure 5). In cocaine studies, I^2 was 0%. In non cocaine studies, I^2 was 66%.

The subgroup analysis by control condition categories showed a significant disulfiram superiority as compared to naltrexone (g = .77, 95%CI = .52–1.02), acamprosate (g = .76, 95%CI = .04–1.48), and to the no disulfiram condition (g = .43, 95%CI = .17–.69) (Figure 6). Our meta-analysis showed that disulfiram was also more effective than topiramate, and no different from GHB, but as only one study could be included for each of two comparisons, our meta-analysis does not add valuable information to this question. Heterogeneity measures were I^2 = 81% for the acamprosate controlled studies; I^2 = 26% for the naltrexone controlled studies; and I^2 = 44% for the no disulfiram controlled studies.

The Safety of Disulfiram

Figure 7 shows the adverse events rate ratio comparisons in disulfiram treated patients and controls. Disulfiram was associated with an increased risk of any adverse events compared with controls: adverse events rate ratio = 1.40 (95%CI 1.01–1.94). Adverse events were reported in 73% of the studies. In the combined disulfiram groups reporting adverse events (n = 962), eight participants reported serious adverse events requiring hospitalization. Of those, two were hospitalized less than one day and then immediately resumed their participation [25]. The other six were from one other study, but according to the authors, three of them returned to complete the study [38]. In the combined control groups, six participants reported serious adverse events requiring hospitalization from three studies [38,39,42]. In one cocaine study, serious adverse events were not specified for those patients with a co-dependency alcohol and cocaine [14].

A total of 13 deaths were reported: one from the combined disulfiram groups [40], six from the control groups [38,40], and six unspecified. Laaksonen et al and Petrakis et al stated that these deaths were not related to their studies. In one large study (n = 605), six deaths were reported, but the authors did not specify if these deaths were from the disulfiram group or the control group [27].

Discussion

Our meta-analysis clearly showed significant efficacy of disulfiram on our primary endpoint that was effect-size. Our first hypothesis that disulfiram should be effective compared to controls only in open-label rather than blinded RCTs was confirmed. In open-label trials, disulfiram was more effective than controls, while there was no difference in the efficacy of disulfiram compared to

Study name	Rate ratio	Lower limit	Upper limit	Z-Value	p-Value	Relative weight
	Statistics for each study					
Carroll et al 1998	1,692	0,069	41,542	0,322	0,747	0,98
Chick et al 1992	3,365	2,020	5,605	4,661	0,000	12,83
De Sousa et al 2004	0,156	0,061	0,401	-3,860	0,000	7,29
De Sousa et al 2005	2,500	0,485	12,886	1,095	0,273	3,26
De Sousa et al 2008	2,000	0,366	10,919	0,800	0,423	3,08
Fuller et al 1986	2,520	1,380	4,600	3,010	0,003	11,42
Gerrein et al 1973	4,423	0,212	92,130	0,960	0,337	1,08
Grassi et al 2007	1,000	0,091	11,028	0,000	1,000	1,68
Laaksonen 2008	1,104	0,739	1,650	0,485	0,628	14,58
Ling et al 1983	6,000	0,722	49,837	1,659	0,097	2,10
Nava et al 2006	1,774	0,444	7,094	0,811	0,417	4,27
Petrakis et al 2005	1,012	0,918	1,115	0,234	0,815	18,41
Pettinati et al 2008	1,107	0,930	1,317	1,142	0,253	17,77
Ulrichsen et al 2010	30,526	1,821	511,722	2,377	0,017	1,25
	1,402	1,012	1,942	2,032	0,042	

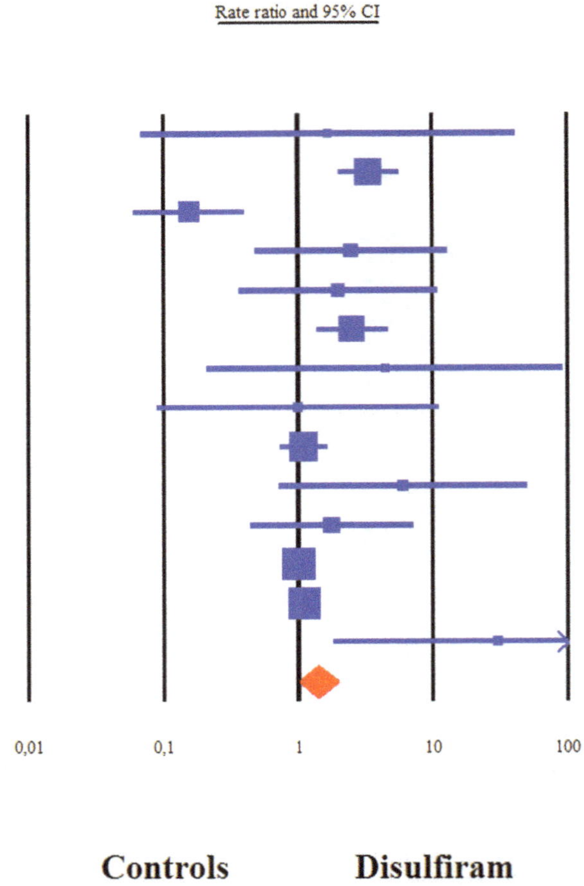

Figure 7. Meta-analysis of adverse events rate ratio comparisons in controls and disulfiram treated patients.

placebo in blinded RCTs. The effect of disulfiram on maintaining abstinence or preventing relapse is mediated by DBH and/or ALDH inhibition as has been proposed in studies mentioned previously on cocaine dependence and pathological gambling. It is noteworthy that our results in double-blind, placebo controlled trials do not advocate for a direct pharmacological effect of disulfiram in preventing alcohol relapse.

In the field of pharmacology, the use of double-blind studies is the gold standard for determining efficacy because blinded trials reduce the influence of outside factors and biases. They help to ensure that all groups are equally matched in terms of possible biases, thus leveling the playing field for all participants. Double-blind studies lower the risk of bias such as social desirability, social support, and perceptions of participants as well as medical and research personnel involved in the study. In the case of disulfiram, the objective of the drug is to prevent consumption of alcohol by psychologically creating an expectancy of being sick if alcohol is consumed. The drug's effectiveness depends directly upon the patient's anticipations. Because the action on potential drinking behavior depends upon a thought process, disulfiram can be considered a pharmacologically assisted psychotherapy. Because of this similarity to psychotherapy, and because psychotherapy studies are necessarily open, only open-label studies could show efficacy in disulfiram RCTs.

Blinded designs for disulfiram research prevent the evaluation of the crucial aspect differentiating the disulfiram and control groups, the psychological threat. Blinding distributes the threat evenly amongst the arms of a study, whereas open-label trials allow the psychological threat to be present in only the disulfiram arm compared to controls. For this reason, we did not include blinded RCTs in our meta-analyses for the subgroups supervision, cocaine, and various controls.

Two of the blinded studies included an open-label and blind design, an admirable originality [27,39]. In the blind portion, while both groups were informed that they were being given disulfiram, the authors dissimulated the dose: one group received 250 mg and the other received 1 mg, a pharmacologically ineffective dose. In the blind portion, as could be expected, no significant difference between disulfiram and the control groups was found. But surprisingly, even in the open-label portion comparing disulfiram to no disulfiram, there were no differences between the groups. Compliance problems rendered the results quasi meaningless. In the larger study (n = 605) [27], only 20% of the 577 who completed the study were compliant. It is noteworthy that a subset of cooperative drinkers reported significantly fewer drinking days when given disulfiram. Supervision might have made a substantial difference in the results of this study and had an important effect on our meta-analysis, as this study alone comprised 26% of the cumulative total of subjects.

Historically, based on this and other blinded trials, disulfiram developed a bad reputation as its detractors perhaps too hastily concluded that disulfiram was not any more effective than controls. But as we have shown, blinded experiments serve no purpose in their attempt to evaluate disulfiram efficacy. Control groups must not be led to believe that they have taken disulfiram so that differences in expectancies appear. Knowledge of disulfiram and its consequences are essential to its function. Disulfiram helps patients learn this new non drinking behavior, this ability to exercise self-control. As described by Brewer and Streel (2003), refraining from alcohol consumption is a learning process and requires intentionally becoming alcohol intolerant through exposure and response prevention [45]. In order to permit the learning phase to proceed despite various temptations, compliance was essential, hence the importance of supervision.

Our second hypothesis was that disulfiram should be more effective in supervised compared to unsupervised studies. We were able to confirm our hypothesis because the difference between the supervised and the unsupervised studies was significant. Our meta-analysis showed that when supervised, disulfiram performed significantly better than controls, while in unsupervised studies, disulfiram was not superior to controls on the main outcome. A closer examination of the unsupervised studies showed that in four out of the five RCTs, disulfiram was not better than the controls. Only in a small pilot study (n = 12) was there a positive disulfiram result against controls [13].

Compliance is a crucial issue in pharmacotherapy in general, but with disulfiram in particular it has been emphasized by many authors [2,17,18,23]. The highest success rates have been with patients who have chosen this type of treatment and are thus highly compliant or are receiving disulfiram under supervision [46]. Some authors have gone so far as to state that unsupervised administration is of limited utility [17,47,48].

This raises the question of bias in supervised studies. Partnership as well as close professional supervision create high functional social support (FSS) [49]. It has been shown that FSS can have a positive effect on the proportion of days abstinent [50] and can predict treatment retention and reduction of alcohol intake [51]. A recent study has shown that FSS is associated with a higher cumulative abstinence [49]. It is probable that the positive influence of strong support had an important impact on compliance and contributed to reducing the use of alcohol. This might explain why supervised treatments had a superior success rate compared to unsupervised treatments. Nevertheless, when bias was eliminated by looking only at supervised studies in which both control and disulfiram arms were supervised, eight out of ten showed a superior performance of disulfiram compared to controls. There seemed to be no bias of social support on the superior performance of disulfiram compared to controls amongst supervised studies in which both arms were supervised.

In two supervised studies [22,42], disulfiram was not different from controls. In the Ulrichsen et al study, the authors attributed this to a small sample size in conjunction with a probable bias of selection. Of the 158 patients who refused to participate, 63 of them refused because they wanted to be treated with disulfiram. This may have resulted in a less than average level of motivation in the sample. In addition, 67% and 41% of the control (no disulfiram) and disulfiram groups, respectively, completed the cognitive behavior therapy sessions, suggesting lower motivation in the disulfiram group. In the Bardeleben et al study, while the number of abstinent days was the same for the three groups, the time to first drink was significantly longer in the disulfiram group compared to the naltrexone and acamprosate groups.

Disulfiram unexpectedly embarked upon a new career in the cocaine dependence treatment field [52]. Most of the trials testing the efficacy of disulfiram in cocaine addicts enrolled subjects with comorbid alcohol and cocaine abuse or dependence, suggesting that the effect of disulfiram on alcohol would have a positive effect on cocaine use. Our decision to include this population is based on the high rates of comorbid alcohol/cocaine use. Numerous studies have shown that the majority of patients who abuse cocaine also abuse alcohol, ranging from 50% to 90% [53,54,55,56,57,58]. This can be explained by the effect of cocaethylene, a pharmacologically active metabolite that is produced when cocaine and alcohol are used together that enhances and prolongs cocaine euphoria [59]. Our meta-analysis showed that treating these subjects with disulfiram for their cocaine problem resulted in a significant improvement of their alcohol condition. Disulfiram also showed its efficacy as compared to a control condition in the studies primarily enrolling alcoholics. The cocaine studies comprised 152 subjects from three studies. We did not include the results of three other cocaine studies because of their blind design [10,14,26].

The subgroup condition by control group categories showed efficacy of disulfiram when compared to (1) the no disulfiram condition (eight studies), (2) naltrexone (nine studies), and (3) acamprosate (three studies). These three studies had a combined total of 403 subjects. Other evidence outside of this meta-analysis in favor of disulfiram compared to acamprosate comes from retrospective data from 2002–2007 with 353 alcoholic patients [60]. In the present study, disulfiram was also superior to topiramate and showed no difference with GHB in these single trial categories, thus providing less useful information as only one study was available. The global picture of this subgroup analysis suggests a favorable image of the efficacy of disulfiram when compared with two of the most evidence based drugs for alcohol dependence.

In sum, the effect-size of disulfiram efficacy compared to various controls can be interpreted as medium ($g = .70$) when combining all open-label studies, or large ($g = .82$) when combining only studies in which compliance was supervised [28].

Safety and Tolerance

Our meta-analysis of the safety and tolerance of disulfiram showed that there was no difference between the disulfiram and control groups in studies reporting deaths and serious adverse events requiring hospitalization. There were, however, significantly more adverse events reported for disulfiram than for controls as shown in Figure 7.

Disulfiram appears to be a safe medication in carefully screened populations. Indeed, as pointed out by Brewer, "compared with the toxicity of alcohol, the toxicity of disulfiram is trivial" [61]. The safety of disulfiram can be attributed primarily to the selection of subjects in RCTs, for the screening process is generally more rigorous than that used for clinical disulfiram use. In a recent systematic review of case reports and clinical trials using disulfiram for alcohol and/or cocaine use or dependence [62], the authors concluded that disulfiram has an acceptable risk profile and is generally safe when used according to the recommendations. They noted that case reports consisted of dermatological, neurological, psychiatric, hepatic, and cardiac adverse events as well as drug-drug interactions and neuroimaging findings. Other authors noted the more common problems of skin rash, halitosis, and fatigue [63].

Iber et al studied liver toxicity in the Fuller et al (1986) study by analyzing the changes in liver status of 605 alcoholics [64]. They found that in those with a liver anomaly, the majority were drinking, concluding that the modest changes that occurred in their liver tests were more related to drinking than to the disulfiram they were taking.

In alcoholics who also abused cocaine, the side effects reported were similar to those reported with the alcoholic only population [65]. In their review of the safety of disulfiram in randomized clinical trials, the authors concluded that use of disulfiram was effective and safe because of adequate medical monitoring. This included attention to comorbid disorders, drug interactions, appropriate dosage, supervision, and clear patient instructions.

Limits

Most subjects in the meta-analysis were men (89%). This should be kept in mind in interpreting these results for women. In three studies, we included subjects who received disulfiram along with another treatment. In one of these trials, the additional treatment was a placebo [38]. In the two others using methadone treated subjects, the disulfiram (given to the experimental group) and the placebo (given to the control group) were placed in the methadone [14] or given with the methadone [32] for compliance purposes. We chose not to analyze any comparisons in which disulfiram was combined with naltrexone or similar abstinence supportive drugs. In addition, we intentionally excluded studies in which all experimental groups received the same dose of disulfiram so as to evaluate other aspects of treatment (i.e., the effects of supervision or behavior therapy) [1].

Limits exist in supervised studies for compliance is often based on self-reports. In the five Indian studies [24,33,35,36,37], family members were asked to supervise, but there was no real method to verify this supervision. The authors noted that India has a good social support system. Negative reinforcement may have helped compliance also as participants were told that they would be excluded for non-compliance.

Studies of disulfiram are heterogeneous. Trial methodologies were highly diverse because since its discovery over 60 years ago no consensus has been reached as to trial methodology. Thus the heterogeneity of the studies was unavoidable, characterized by a substantial I-square. The only subgroups of studies that did not display a high level of heterogeneity were those on cocaine and naltrexone.

As shown by the meta-regressions, the high heterogeneity was partially explained by the wide range of publication years and treatment durations. Notably, heterogeneity was found to be low when disulfiram was compared with each control condition independently, suggesting that the important number of control conditions might explain a substantial amount of heterogeneity.

According to the guidelines of the *Cochrane Handbook for Systematic Reviews of Interventions* [29], a lack of blinding of participants and personnel in randomized trials increases the risk of bias. The areas most affected are performance (i.e., there may be differences in the care that is provided in each arm) and detection bias (i.e., there may be differences between the groups in how outcome is determined). For many reasons discussed previously, while double-blinding is the standard method for medication trials in general, it is unsuitable for disulfiram trials. One might infer that this meta-analysis is biased by using predominantly open-label trials. In disulfiram research, we propose that one revisit the meaning of quality RCTs. A meta-analysis of disulfiram would be of no practical use if it consisted of only double-blind trials. The use of an open-label design in efficacy trials with this atypical medication could be viewed as indispensable rather than as evidence of poor study quality.

Conclusion

The present work focuses on open-label trials to correct the dilutive and misleading effect that blinded trials have had on the question of disulfiram efficacy. In formulating the hypothesis that only open trials can determine disulfiram efficacy, this meta-analysis addresses a cardinal methodological flaw that was not considered in a previous meta-analysis. Disulfiram was shown to be more effective than controls in supervised than non supervised RCTs. Based on a larger sample than a previous meta-analysis [19], adding eleven studies (887 subjects), it broadens the evaluation of disulfiram efficacy to include alcoholics with concomitant cocaine abuse or dependence. In addition, it offers issue to this day.

a meta-analytic evaluation of the safety of disulfiram, a poignant

In summary, how does disulfiram measure up when compared to controls in helping the alcohol dependent stay abstinent or at least relapse free? Overall, this meta-analysis demonstrated evidence in open-label trials of disulfiram efficacy compared to controls in maintaining abstinence or preventing relapse. No efficacy was revealed in blind trials. In terms of safety, there was no difference between the disulfiram and control groups in studies reporting deaths and serious adverse events requiring hospitalization. Adverse events, however, were reported more for disulfiram than for controls. In spite of the limitations mentioned above, our meta-analysis allowed us to draw strong conclusions about the efficacy of disulfiram compared to other abstinence supportive pharmaceutical treatments or to no disulfiram in open-label, supervised studies for problems of alcohol abuse or dependence.

Acknowledgments

We gratefully acknowledge the contributions of Kathleen Carroll and her colleagues for providing us with the data subsets we needed for inclusion of their studies in our meta-analysis.

Author Contributions

Conceived and designed the experiments: MS PL HJA. Analyzed the data: HJA. Wrote the paper: MS HJA HP.

References

1. Azrin NH, Sisson RW, Meyers R, Godley M (1982) Alcoholism treatment by disulfiram and community reinforcement therapy. J Behav Ther Exp Psychiatry 13: 105–112.
2. Brewer C, Meyers R, Johnson J (2000) Does disulfiram help to prevent relapse in alcohol abuse? CNS Drugs 14: 329–341.
3. Wright C, Moore RD (1990) Disulfiram treatment of alcoholism. Am J Med 88: 647–655.
4. Wilson A, Blanchard R, Davidson W, McRae L, Maini K (1984) Disulfiram implantation: a dose response trial. J Clin Psychiatry 45: 242–247.
5. Fuller R, Gordis E (2004) Does disulfiram have a role in alcoholism treatment today? Addiction 99: 21–24.
6. Skinner M, Coudert M, Berlin I, Passeri E, Michel L, et al. (2010) Effect of the threat of a disulfiram-ethanol reaction on cue reactivity in alcoholics Drug Alcohol Depend.

7. Johnson BA (2010) Medication treatment of different types of alcoholism. Am J Psychiatry 167: 630–639.
8. Swift RM (1999) Drug therapy for alcohol dependence. N Engl J Med 340: 1482–1490.
9. Weinshenker D (2010) Cocaine sobers up. Nat Med 16: 969–970.
10. Carroll KM, Fenton LR, Ball SA, Nich C, Frankforter TL, et al. (2004) Efficacy of disulfiram and cognitive behavior therapy in cocaine-dependent outpatients: a randomized placebo-controlled trial. Arch Gen Psychiatry 61: 264–272.
11. Gossop M, Carroll KM (2006) Disulfiram, cocaine, and alcohol: two outcomes for the price of one? Alcohol Alcohol 41: 119–120.
12. Mutschler J, Buhler M, Grosshans M, Diehl A, Mann K, et al. (2010) Disulfiram, an option for the treatment of pathological gambling? Alcohol Alcohol 45: 214–216.
13. Grassi MC, Cioce AM, Giudici FD, Antonilli L, Nencini P (2007) Short-term efficacy of Disulfiram or Naltrexone in reducing positive urinalysis for both cocaine and cocaethylene in cocaine abusers: A pilot study. Pharmacological Research 55: 117–121.
14. Petrakis IL, Carroll KM, Nich C, Gordon LT, McCance-Katz EF, et al. (2000) Disulfiram treatment for cocaine dependence in methadone-maintained opioid addicts. Addiction 95: 219–228.
15. Yao L, Fan P, Arolfo M, Jiang Z, Olive MF, et al. (2010) Inhibition of aldehyde dehydrogenase-2 suppresses cocaine seeking by generating THP, a cocaine use-dependent inhibitor of dopamine synthesis. Nat Med 16: 1024–1028.
16. Gaval-Cruz M, Weinshenker D (2009) mechanisms of disulfiram-induced cocaine abstinence: antabuse and cocaine relapse. Mol Interv 9: 175–187.
17. Hughes JC, Cook CC (1997) The efficacy of disulfiram: a review of outcome studies. Addiction 92: 381–395.
18. Suh JJ, Pettinati HM, Kampman KM, O'Brien CP (2006) The status of disulfiram: a half of a century later. J Clin Psychopharmacol 26: 290–302.
19. Jorgensen CH, Pedersen B, Tonnesen H (2011) The Efficacy of Disulfiram for the Treatment of Alcohol Use Disorder. Alcohol Clin Exp Res.
20. Tønnesen H, Rosenberg J, Nielsen HJ, Rasmussen V, Hauge C, et al. (1999) Effect of preoperative abstinence on poor postoperative outcome in alcohol misusers: randomised controlled trial. BMJ 318: 1311–1316.
21. Carroll C, Ziedonis D, O'Malley S, McCance-Katz E, Gordon L, et al. (1993) Pharmacologic interventions for alcohol and cocaine abusing individuals - a pilot study of disulfiram and naltrexone. American Journal on Addictions 2: 77–79.
22. Bardeleben UK, H.; Biedert, E.; Ihde, T.; Ladewig, D. (1999) Randomized open efficacy study of naltrexone vs. acamprosate vs. disulfiram combined with cognitive-behavioral psychotherapy in preventing alcohol relapse. In: Ladewig D, editor. Basic and Clinical Science of Substance Related Disorders. Basel: Karger. pp. 45–48.
23. Chick J, Gough K, Falkowski W, Kershaw P, Hore B, et al. (1992) Disulfiram treatment of alcoholism. Br J Psychiatry 161: 84–89.
24. De Sousa A, Jagtap J (2009) An open label trial of naltrexone versus disulfiram in elderly patients with alcohol dependence. JPPS 6: 85–89.
25. Gerrein JR, Rosenberg CM, Manohar V (1973) Disulfiram maintenance in outpatient treatment of alcoholism. Arch Gen Psychiatry 28: 798–802.
26. Pettinati HM, Kampman KM, Lynch KG, Xie H, Dackis C, et al. (2008) A double blind, placebo-controlled trial that combines disulfiram and naltrexone for treating co-occurring cocaine and alcohol dependence. Addict Behav 33: 651–667.
27. Fuller RK, Branchey L, Brightwell DR, Derman RM, Emrick CD, et al. (1986) Disulfiram treatment of alcoholism. A Veterans Administration cooperative study. JAMA 256: 1449–1455.
28. Cohen J (1988) Statistical Power Analysis for the Behavioral Sciences: Lawrence Erlbaum Associates.
29. Higgins J, Green Se (2011) Cochrane Handbook for Systematic Reviews of Interventions Version 5.1.0 The Cochrane Collaboration.
30. Oliveto A, Poling J, Mancino MJ, Feldman Z, Cubells JF, et al. (2011) Randomized, double blind, placebo-controlled trial of disulfiram for the treatment of cocaine dependence in methadone-stabilized patients. Drug Alcohol Depend 113: 184–191.
31. Carroll KM, Nich C, Ball SA, McCance E, Rounsavile BJ (1998) Treatment of cocaine and alcohol dependence with psychotherapy and disulfiram. Addiction 93: 713–727.
32. Ling W, Weiss DG, Charuvastra VC, O'Brien CP (1983) Use of disulfiram for alcoholics in methadone maintenance programs. A Veterans Administration Cooperative Study. Arch Gen Psychiatry 40: 851–854.
33. De Sousa A, De Sousa A (2008) An open randomized trial comparing disulfiram and naltrexone in adolescents with alcohol dependence. Journal of Substance Use 13: 382–388.
34. Niederhofer H, Staffen W (2003) Comparison of disulfiram and placebo in treatment of alcohol dependence of adolescents. Drug Alcohol Rev 22: 295–297.
35. De Sousa A, De Sousa A (2004) A one-year pragmatic trial of naltrexone vs disulfiram in the treatment of alcohol dependence. Alcohol Alcohol 39: 528–531.
36. De Sousa A, De Sousa A (2005) An open randomized study comparing disulfiram and acamprosate in the treatment of alcohol dependence. Alcohol Alcohol 40: 545–548.
37. De Sousa AA, De Sousa J, Kapoor H (2008) An open randomized trial comparing disulfiram and topiramate in the treatment of alcohol dependence. J Subst Abuse Treat 34: 460–463.
38. Petrakis IL, Poling J, Levinson C, Nich C, Carroll K, et al. (2005) Naltrexone and disulfiram in patients with alcohol dependence and comorbid psychiatric disorders. Biol Psychiatry 57: 1128–1137.
39. Fuller RK, Roth HP (1979) Disulfiram for the treatment of alcoholism. An evaluation in 128 men. Ann Intern Med 90: 901–904.
40. Laaksonen E, Koski-Jannes A, Salaspuro M, Ahtinen H, Alho H (2008) A randomized, multicentre, open-label, comparative trial of disulfiram, naltrexone and acamprosate in the treatment of alcohol dependence. Alcohol Alcohol 43: 53–61.
41. Nava F, Premi S, Manzato E, Lucchini A (2006) Comparing treatments of alcoholism on craving and biochemical measures of alcohol consumptionst. J Psychoactive Drugs 38: 211–217.
42. Ulrichsen J, Nielsen MK, Ulrichsen M (2010) Disulfiram in severe alcoholism–an open controlled study. Nord J Psychiatry 64: 356–362.
43. Carroll K, Fetnon LR, Bale SA, Nich C, Frankforter TL, et al. (2004) Efficacy of disulfiram and cognitive behavior therapy in cocaine-dependent outpatients. Archives of General Psychiatry 61: 264–272.
44. Higgins JP, Altman DG (2008) Assessing Risk of Bias in Included Studies. In: Higgins JP, Green Se, editors. Cochrane Handbook for Systematic Reviews of Interventions Chichester, UK: John Wiley & Sons.
45. Brewer C, Streel E (2003) Learning the language of abstinence in addiction treatment: some similarities between relapse-prevention with disulfiram, naltrexone, and other pharmacological antagonists and intensive "immersion" methods of foreign language teaching. Subst Abus 24: 157–173.
46. Johnson BA (2008) Update on neuropharmacological treatments for alcoholism: scientific basis and clinical findings. Biochem Pharmacol 75: 34–56.
47. Brewer C (1986) Patterns of compliance and evasion in treatment programmes which include supervised disulfiram. Alcohol Alcohol 21: 385–388.
48. Anton RF (2001) Pharmacologic approaches to the management of alcoholism. J Clin Psychiatry 62 Suppl 20: 11–17.
49. Mutschler J, Eifler S, Dirican G, Grosshans M, Kiefer F, et al. (2013) Functional social support within a medical supervised outpatient treatment program. Am J Drug Alcohol Abuse 39: 44–49.
50. Beattie MC, Longabaugh R (1999) General and alcohol-specific social support following treatment. Addict Behav 24: 593–606.
51. Dobkin PL, De CM, Paraherakis A, Gill K (2002) The role of functional social support in treatment retention and outcomes among outpatient adult substance abusers. Addiction 97: 347–356.
52. Pani PP, Trogu E, Vacca R, Amato L, Vecchi S, et al. (2010) Disulfiram for the treatment of cocaine dependence. Cochrane Database Syst Rev: CD007024.
53. Closser MH, Kosten TR (1992) Alcohol and cocaine abuse. A comparison of epidemiology and clinical characteristics. Recent Dev Alcohol 10: 115–128.
54. Weiss RD, Mirin SM, Griffin ML, Michael JL (1988) Psychopathology in cocaine abusers. Changing trends. J Nerv Ment Dis 176: 719–725.
55. Grant BF, Harford TC (1990) Concurrent and simultaneous use of alcohol with cocaine: results of national survey. Drug Alcohol Depend 25: 97–104.
56. Khalsa H, Paredes A, Anglin MD (1992) The role of alcohol in cocaine dependence. Recent Dev Alcohol 10: 7–35.
57. Regier DA, Farmer ME, Rae DS, Locke BZ, Keith SJ, et al. (1990) Comorbidity of mental disorders with alcohol and other drug abuse. Results from the Epidemiologic Catchment Area (ECA) Study. JAMA 264: 2511–2518.
58. Carroll KM, Rounsaville BJ, Bryant KJ (1993) Alcoholism in treatment-seeking cocaine abusers: clinical and prognostic significance. J Stud Alcohol 54: 199–208.
59. McCance-Katz EF, Price LH, McDougle CJ, Kosten TR, Black JE, et al. (1993) Concurrent cocaine-ethanol ingestion in humans: pharmacology, physiology, behavior, and the role of cocaethylene. Psychopharmacology (Berl) 111: 39–46.
60. Diehl A, Ulmer L, Mutschler J, Herre H, Krumm B, et al. (2010) Why is Disulfiram Superior to Acamprosate in the Routine Clinical Setting? A Retrospective Long-Term Study in 353 Alcohol-Dependent Patients. Alcohol Alcohol.
61. Brewer C (2001) Disulfiram for alcohol abuse: Why is such an effective drug so under-prescribed? Primary Care in the New NHS Autumn: 227–231.
62. Alharbi FFae-G, N. (2013) The relative safety of disulfiram. Addictive Disorders & Their Treatment 12(3) 12: 140–147.
63. Schuckit MA (1996) Recent developments in the pharmacotherapy of alcohol dependence. J Consult Clin Psychol 64: 669–676.
64. Iber FL, Lee K, Lacoursiere R, Fuller R (1987) Liver toxicity encountered in the Veterans Administration trial of disulfiram in alcoholics. Alcohol Clin Exp Res 11: 301–304.
65. Malcolm R, Olive MF, Lechner W (2008) The safety of disulfiram for the treatment of alcohol and cocaine dependence in randomized clinical trials: guidance for clinical practice. Expert Opin Drug Saf 7: 459–472.
66. Stockwell T, Hodgson R, Edwards G, Taylor C, Rankin H (1979) The development of a questionnaire to measure severity of alcohol dependence. Br J Addict Alcohol Other Drugs 74: 79–87.

4

Prenatal and Childhood Growth, and Hospitalization for Alcohol Use Disorders in Adulthood: The Helsinki Birth Cohort Study

Jari Lahti[1]*, Marius Lahti[1], Anu-Katriina Pesonen[1], Kati Heinonen[1], Eero Kajantie[2], Tom Forsén[2], Kristian Wahlbeck[2], Clive Osmond[3], David J. P. Barker[3†], Johan G. Eriksson[2,4], Katri Räikkönen[1]

1 Institute of Behavioural Sciences, University of Helsinki, Helsinki, Finland, **2** National Public Health Institute, Helsinki, Finland, **3** Medical Research Council Lifecourse Epidemiology Unit, University of Southampton, United Kingdom, **4** Department of General Practice and Primary Health Care, University of Helsinki

Abstract

Background: Small birth size - an indicator of a sub-optimal prenatal environment - and variation in growth after birth have been associated with non-communicable diseases in later life. We tested whether birth size or growth in childhood associated with the risk of hospital admission for alcohol use disorders (AUDs) from early to late adulthood.

Methods: The sample comprised 6544 men and 6050 women born between 1934 and 1944 in Helsinki, Finland. Data on anthropometric measures were extracted from medical records and diagnoses of AUD from the Finnish Hospital Discharge Register and Causes of Death Register covering a 40-year period from 1969 to 2008.

Results: Altogether 171 women (2.8%) and 657 men (10.0%) were diagnosed at a hospital with AUD. After adjusting for major confounders, shorter length at birth, shorter height up to two years of age, and lower weight at two years associated with hospitalization for AUD in women. In men, slower growth in height, particularly from 2 to 7 years, and slower weight gain from 7 to 11 years as well as shorter height and lower weight at 7 and 11 years associated with a diagnosis of AUD in men.

Conclusions: Pre- and postnatal growth associates with the risk for AUD later in life differently in women than in men: the fetal period and infancy seem to be the sensitive periods for women, whereas those for men the occur from toddlerhood onwards.

Editor: Natalie Walker, The National Institute for Health Innovation, New Zealand

Funding: Funding for this study was provided by the Academy of Finland, Doctoral Programme of Psychology, Alfred Kordelin foundation, Ella and Georg Ehrnrooths Stiftelse, and Yrjö Jahnsson Foundation. The funders had no role in study design, data collection and analysis, decision to publish, or preparation of the manuscript.

Competing Interests: The authors have declared that no competing interests exist.

* E-mail: jari.lahti@helsinki.fi

† Deceased.

Introduction

In Western European societies, the lifetime prevalence of alcohol dependence is around 5% to 8% with rates four to five times higher for men than for women [1,2]. Alcohol use ranks among the top causes of disease burden [3] and its impact in the developed world is projected to increase [4]. Since alcohol use can be an important causal factor in the development of a multitude of medical conditions [5], identifying early risk factors for alcohol use disorders (AUD) could help in preventive action.

Within the developmental origins of health and disease framework (DOHaD), the associations between small birth size or slower growth in childhood and health outcomes in later life have been attributed to suboptimal environmental conditions during sensitive time periods that alter the structure and function of key organs such as the brain [6]. These environmental conditions include psychosocial stress and malnutrition, which are amenable to intervention [6,7].

Various non-communicable health conditions, such as hypertension and several psychiatric conditions, show high comorbidity with AUDs [5,8–10] and have been linked to small body size at birth [7,11–16] as well as growth patterns in childhood [7,12,15,17,18]. However, whether body size at birth or later in life associates with the risk for AUDs remains uncertain. In addition, the few existing studies show conflicting results and focus on those who were born at the extreme low end of the birth weight distribution [19–23] or on those who were obese in childhood [24]. Birth cohort studies have suggested that those born at the extreme low end of the birth weight distribution are at around 40% higher risk for alcohol abuse or substance-related disorders [19,20] while one study showed an inverse gradient across decreasing birth weight [25]. Studies focusing on those born prematurely and with very low birth weight (<1500 grams;

VLBW) suggest that VLBW is associated with *less frequent* alcohol consumption in young adulthood [21–23]. To our knowledge, no studies have examined the associations between body size or growth in childhood and subsequent AUDs in adulthood, and few studies point to such associations with respect to other psychiatric morbidity [24,26,27].

Our study aimed to investigate whether length of gestation, body size at birth and physical growth measured serially from birth to 11 years of age associate with hospitalization for or death due to AUDs in the Helsinki Birth Cohort Study (HBCS) sample. In addition to testing for linear effects, we examined whether nonlinear associations existed between birth size and hospitalization for AUDs. We also tested whether associations between physical growth and AUDs stem from comorbid mental disorders.

Materials and Methods

Subjects

The original study cohort comprised 13345 subjects who were born in Helsinki, Finland at one of the two public maternity hospitals, who visited child welfare clinics, and who received a Finnish personal ID number. Of these participants, we excluded 191 individuals because they moved abroad or died before data collection for the Finnish Hospital Discharge Register (HDR) began in 1969, 226 who were missing data on AUDs, and 334 who were missing data on childhood socioeconomic position (SEP). The cohort available for the analyses comprised 12 594 subjects (6544 men and 6050 women together comprising 94.3% of the original cohort). The excluded participants had an earlier year of birth ($p<0.02$), were more often women ($p<0.004$) and were lighter ($p = 0.03$) and thinner at birth ($p<0.001$), but showed no differences from the included participants in childhood SEP, length of gestation, placental weight, or length and head circumference at birth (p-values >0.05). Furthermore, 847 participants were excluded from the analysis of neonatal characteristics due to missing data on the length of gestation. The Ethics Committee of the National Public Health Institute and the Ethics Committee of the Helsinki and Uusimaa Hospital District approved the HBCS. The study has was conducted in adherence to the Declaration of Helsinki.

Measures of neonatal characteristics and physical growth

Data on year of birth, weight (g), length (cm), head circumference (cm), placental weight (g), and date of the mother's last menstrual period were collected from the birth records. Data on monthly changes in weight (kg) and height (cm) from birth to 2 years and annual changes from 2 to 11 years were estimated from child welfare clinic and school health records as described previously [28]. From these measures we calculated the ponderal index at birth (kg/m^3) and body mass index (BMI: kg/m^2).

Our primary indicator of SEP in childhood was occupational status of the father. These data were derived from school, child welfare clinic, and birth records (inferred from the last two, respectively, if data from school records were not available) and were classified as low SEP (manual workers: 62.3%), middle SEP (lower middle class: 22.6%), and high SEP (upper middle class: 15.2%). We used highest maternal SEP as secondary indicator of childhood socio-economic environment due to higher number of those belonging to unclassified category (e.g. housewives or students). Of the mothers, 50.9%, 34.2%, 3.8%, 11.1% belonged to low SEP, middle SEP, high SEP, and other/unclassified SEP, respectively [29].

Definition of hospitalization for alcohol use disorder (AUD) and of other mental disorders

Diagnoses were extracted from the HDR, which contained data on all hospitalizations in psychiatric and general hospitals in Finland between 1969 and 2008. The HDR also includes personal and hospital ID numbers, dates of hospital admission and discharge, and primary as well as up to three subsidiary diagnoses at discharge. The HDR is a valid and reliable tool for research [30], and studies have shown that diagnoses based on the HDR are more reliable than those based on medical examination or interview- or questionnaire-based measures, especially when a combined best-estimate diagnosis served as the validation criteria [31]. Accuracy of the HDR data with respect to AUDs proved high [32], and hospitalization for AUDs have served as an outcome in several studies [33,34]. The HDR has also shown high validity with regard to psychotic disorders in general [31] and schizophrenia in particular [35]. We also identified AUDs as causes of death from the National Causes of Death-Register (CDR), which contains records of primary and subsidiary causes of death from all deaths in Finland.

Diagnoses were entered into the HDR and CDR according to the International Classification of Diseases, Eighth Revision (ICD-8) until 1986, according to the ICD-9 using the Diagnostic and Statistical Manual of Mental Disorders, Revised Third Edition (DSM-III-R) criteria until 1995, and according to the ICD-10 since 1996. In the current study, the primary diagnoses of alcohol intoxication (ICD-9: 3050A and ICD-10: F10.0) as well as the primary and subsidiary diagnoses of harmful alcohol use, alcohol dependence, and psychotic disorder due to alcohol abuse (ICD-8/9: 291, 303 and ICD-10 F10.1-F10.9) from either register served to index the AUDs. In our sample, we identified 746 and 34 AUD cases based solely on the HDR and CDR, respectively, and identified 48 based on both registers (6.6% of the total sample).

We examined the different AUDs together as one broad diagnostic outcome rather than as separate entities (such as alcohol dependence and harmful use of alcohol) to make our definition of AUDs more comparable with the definition of AUDs in the DSM-5, that was introduced in 2013. However, in correspondence with ICD-10, our definition of AUDs includes also the primary and subsidiary diagnoses of alcohol psychoses, amnesic syndrome due to alcohol use, and other and unspecified mental and behavioural disorders due to alcohol use, and the primary diagnoses of alcohol intoxification.

The primary and up to three subsidiary diagnoses of mental disorders other than those due to alcohol use were drawn with the following codes: 295–302, 304–305, 306.4–306.5, 306.8, 306.98, and 307 from ICD-8; 292, 295–298, 300–302, 304, 3051–3059, 3071A, 3074, 3075A–3075B, 3078A, 3079X, 3090A, 3092C–3099X, and 312 from ICD-9; and F11–F69 from ICD-10 [36].

Statistical analyses

First, we used logistic regression analyses to test whether neonatal characteristics and body size or growth from birth to age 11 were associated with hospitalization for AUDs in adulthood. We tested for nonlinear associations between birth size and hospitalization for AUDs using a model that included a squared term of the variable centered around the grand mean together with a non-squared linear variable. We focused on measurements conducted at birth, at 6 months of age, and at 1, 2, 7, and 11 years of age to represent growth in the prenatal period (at birth), in infancy (up to 2 years), and in childhood (up to 11 years). Physical size measurements served as continuous variables to test for linear and nonlinear associations. All the neonatal characteristics and the measures on attained size at different ages were converted to z-scores by sex. Postnatal growth variables were standardized residuals from linear regression models of weight, height, and BMI where body size at each point in time was regressed on corresponding measures at all earlier points in time, creating completely uncorrelated residuals reflecting growth conditional on history (i.e. conditional growth) [37]. In Model 1, we adjusted for year of birth and SEP in childhood in all analyses, and in analyses of birth size, we further adjusted for length of gestation. In Model 2, we further adjusted for maternal SEP. To test whether associations between physical growth and AUDs are attributable to comorbid mental disorders, in Model 3 we adjusted for other mental disorders in addition to those variables in Model 1. In addition, we reran all the Model 1 analyses in a sample comprising only those with any mental disorder (i.e. contrasting those with AUDs to those with other mental disorders).

Although we found no statistically significant interactions between body size or growth by sex (p-values for interactions > 0.08), we conducted all the analyses separately for men and women, since previous studies have found major sex differences in the prevalence of AUDs [2] and in factors influencing alcohol use [38] as well as sex-specific associations between body size or growth and mental disorders [11,24,26,27,39–47].

Results

Table 1 presents neonatal and adulthood characteristics according to sex. In men, low childhood SEP associated with 46.1% higher odds (95% Confidence Interval [CI] 11.4–86.6%, p = 0.002) for AUDs than for high childhood SEP. We found no associations between childhood SEP and AUDs in women (p> 0.54).

Neonatal characteristics and hospitalization for AUDs

Table 2 shows that after adjusting for birth year, SEP in childhood and length of gestation, shorter length at birth increased the risk of hospitalization for AUDs linearly (p = 0.03) among women, and birth weight also shows a similar trend (p = 0.054). The ponderal index and head circumference at birth showed no association with the risk of hospitalization for AUDs in women (p-values>0.17; data not shown). Birth size showed nonlinear associations with the risk of hospitalization for AUDs in women (p-values >0.25). In men, we found neither linear (p-values >0.11) nor nonlinear (p-values >0.054) associations between body size at birth and the risk of hospitalization for AUDs. These associations are further illustrated in Figure 1. Moreover, we found no associations between gestational age and AUDs in men (linear: Odd's Ratio [OR] = 1.04, 95% CI = 0.95 to 1.12, p = 0.39; non-linear: OR = 1.03, 95% CI = 0.98 to 1.09, p = 0.30) or in women (linear: OR = 1.03, 95% CI = 0.88 to 1.21, p = 0.70; non-linear: OR = 1.01, 95% CI = 0.91 to 1.13, p = 0.80). Further adjusting for maternal SEP (Model 2) or comorbid mental disorders (Model 3) changed none of the significance levels (Table 2), but restricting the sample to those with mental disorders rendered non-significant all associations between neonatal characteristics and AUDs in women (p-values >0.09) and in men (p-values >0.25).

Body size and conditional growth after birth and hospitalization for AUDs

Table 2 also shows that after adjusting for birth year and SEP in childhood, increased risk of hospitalization for AUDs was associated with shorter height from six months to two years in women (p-values<0.03). Moreover, in women, lower weight at two years increased the risk of hospitalization for AUDs (p = 0.02), and weight at six months showed a similar trend (p = 0.057). In men, shorter height and lower weight at 7 and 11 years associated with increased risk of hospitalization for AUDs (p-values<0.05; Figure 1). Further adjusting for maternal SEP (Model 2) or comorbid mental disorders (Model 3) did not change the significance levels (Table 2), except for one: in men, the association between lower weight at seven years and AUDs became non-significant in both models (p-values >0.07). Restricting the sample to those with mental disorders had no effect on the significance levels of the associations between body size after birth and AUDs in women (p-values<0.04), whereas in men, it rendered all associations non-significant (p-values >0.21).

We then tested whether growth conditional on history associated with hospitalization for AUDs. Among men we found that after adjusting for birth year and SEP in childhood, hospitalization for AUDs was associated with slower growth in height from two to seven years (OR = 1.10, 95% CI = 1.00 to 1.22, p = 0.048) and with slower weight gain from seven to 11 years (OR = 1.12, 95% CI = 1.01 to 1.23, p = 0.03), while weight gain from two to seven years showed a similar trend (OR = 1.10, 95% CI = 1.00 to 1.21, p = 0.06). We found no significant associations between growth conditional on history and AUDs in women. Further adjusting for maternal SEP (Model 2) or comorbid mental disorders (Model 3) yielded only one change in significance levels: in men, slower growth in height from two to seven years became non-significant (Model 2: OR = 1.1, 95% CI = 1.00 to 1.22, p = 0.06; and Model 3: OR = 1.09, 95% CI = 1.00 to 1.21, p = 0.09). Restricting the sample to those with mental disorders rendered all significant associations non-significant (p-values > 0.19).

Discussion

We explored whether length of gestation and body size or physical growth up to 11 years of age associated with hospitalization for AUDs in adulthood in 12594 women and men participating in the Helsinki Birth Cohort Study. Different growth periods were associated with increased risk for AUDs in both women and men. After adjusting for gestational age, birth year, and SEP in childhood, shorter length at birth associated linearly with increased risk of hospitalization for AUDs in women. This association was unattributable to maternal SEP or comorbid other mental disorders, although restricting the sample to those with any mental disorders rendered the association non-significant. AUDs showed no association with growth after birth, although women who were hospitalized for AUDs remained on average shorter up to two years of age, and weighed less at two years of age. These results were unattributable to maternal SEP or comorbid mental disorders. In men, birth characteristics showed no association with the risk for AUDs. However, men who were hospitalized because of AUDs had slower growth in height between two and seven years of age; they also gained less weight from seven to 11 years and, as a consequence, were shorter and weighed less at age 7 and 11 years. Similar findings related to weight and height are likely the result of slower growth in height, as there was no relationship with BMI in childhood. In men, maternal SEP or comorbid mental disorders had little effect on these associations, but restricting the sample to those with any mental disorders rendered the associations non-significant.

These results are in line with those of previous studies on population-based birth cohorts that have shown an inverse gradient between birth weight and substance-related disorders in young adulthood [25], and increased risk for AUDs [19] or substance-related disorders [20,25]_ENREF_15 in those who were born with low birth weight [19] or were small for their

Table 1. Characteristics of the sample.

Characteristic	Males		Females	
	N	Mean (SD)	N	Mean (SD)
At Birth:				
Weight (kg)	6544	3.5 (0.5)	6050	3.3 (0.5) #
Length (cm)	6490	50.6 (1.9)	5995	49.9 (1.8) #
Body Mass Index (kg/m^2)	6484	13.5 (1.2)	5992	13.4 (1.2) #
Ponderal index (kg/m^3)	6490	26.7 (2.2)	5995	26.8 (2.2)
Head circumference (cm)	6474	35.3 (1.5)	5988	34.7 (1.4) #
Gestational age (days)	6420	279.0 (14.3)	5935	279.7 (13.7)#
Placental weight (g)	6520	651.2 (119.9)	6040	639.2 (118.9)#
At age 6 months:				
Height (cm)	6534	67.8 (2.3)	6043	66.1 (2.3) #
Weight (kg)	6539	7.9 (0.9)	6049	7.4 (0.8) #
Body Mass Index (kg/m^2)	6535	17.2 (1.4)	6045	16.8 (1.4) #
At age 1 year:				
Height (cm)	6534	76.5 (2.6)	6043	74.8 (2.6) #
Weight (kg)	6539	10.5 (1.1)	6049	9.8 (1.0) #
Body Mass Index (kg/m^2)	6535	17.9 (1.4)	6045	17.5 (1.4) #
At age 2 years:				
Height (cm)	6536	86.6 (3.2)	6044	85.5 (3.2) #
Weight (kg)	6542	12.4 (1.2)	6049	11.9 (1.2) #
Body Mass Index (kg/m^2)	6538	16.7 (1.2)	6046	16.4 (1.2) #
At age 7 years:				
Height (cm)	4909	120.7 (4.9)	4521	119.9 (4.8) #
Weight (kg)	4917	22.5 (2.7)	4527	22.2 (2.9) #
Body Mass Index (kg/m^2)	4903	15.5 (1.1)	4512	15.5 (1.2)
At age 11 years:				
Height (cm)	4814	141.3 (6.0)	4409	141.4 (6.4)
Weight (kg)	4817	33.6 (4.6)	4407	34.3 (5.7) #
Body Mass Index (kg/m^2)	4809	16.8 (1.5)	4403	17.1 (1.9) #
Father's SEP				*
Low	4022 (61.5%)		3819 (63.1%)	
Middle	1469 (22.4%)		1372 (22.7%)	
High	1053 (16.1%)		859 (14.2%)	
Mother's SEP				
Low	3290 (56.4%)		3120 (58.2%)	
Middle	2299 (39.4%)		2008 (37.4%)	
High	247 (4.2%)		234 (4.4%)	
Other (e.g.housewives)	708 (10.8%)		688 (11.4%)	
In adulthood				
Hospitalization for alcohol use disorders (yes)	657 (10.0%)		171 (2.8%) #	
Hospitalization for other mental disorders (yes)	565 (8.6%)		506 (8.4%)	

*: $p<0.05$; #: $p<0.001$.

gestational age [20,25]. Our results add the previous literature by showing not only that the associations extend beyond birth weight, but also that slower intrauterine skeletal growth seemed to play a role in increasing the risk of hospitalization for AUDs in adulthood. Furthermore, the follow-up periods in previous research extend only into young adulthood, while our findings show that the effects persist across several decades into older adulthood. Our findings disagree with those found in young adults born prematurely: in previous studies, those born at VLBW reported less frequent heavy alcohol use or lower consumption of alcohol than did their peers born at term [21,22]. However, these findings may be limited to those born the smallest and most immature, who were unlikely to survive when the subjects in the present cohort were born. As in this study, previous research has

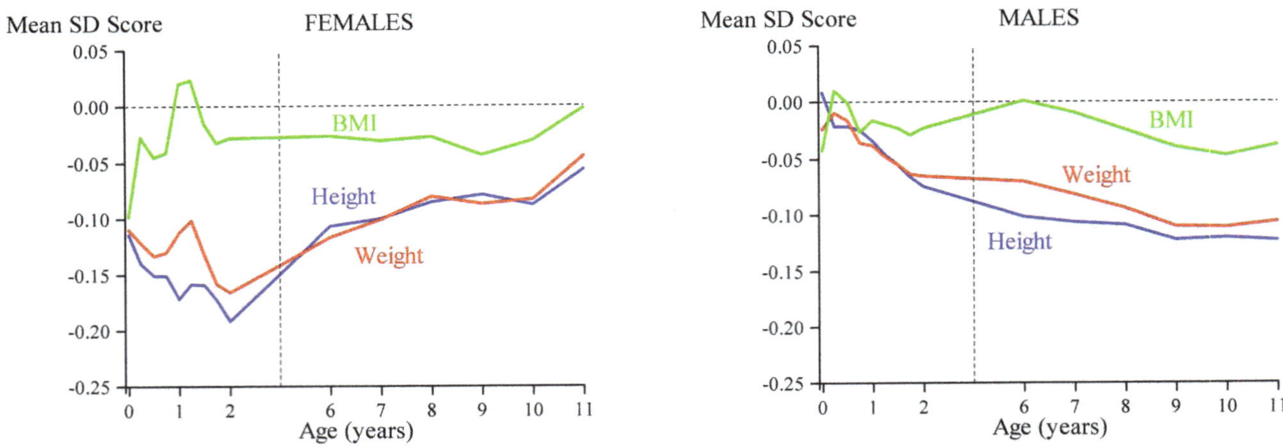

Figure 1. Trajectories of height (blue line), weight (red line), and BMI (green line) in those who were hospitalized for alcohol use disorder in adulthood. The mean values for height, weight and BMI of the monthly measures from birth to 2 years, and the yearly measures from 6 to 11 years, are set at zero with deviations from the mean expressed as standard deviations (*z* scores).

also shown that associations of birth size with mental health vary between men and women: some studies have reported stronger inverse associations between birth weight and emotional or attention problems in women than in men [40–43], while other studies show links between lower birth weight and depression in men, but not in women [44–47].

To the best of our knowledge, this study is the first to explore body size or physical growth in childhood with respect to AUDs in

Table 2. Odd's ratio (OR) of hospitalization for alcohol use disorders according to the decrease in standardized weight, length/height, and BMI from birth to 11 years of age.

Men								**Women**							
	Model 1					**Model 2**	**Model 3**		**Model 1**					**Model 2**	**Model 3**
	N	**OR**	**95% CI**		**p**	**p**	**p**	**p**	**N**	**OR**	**95% CI**		**p**	**p**	**p**
Height/Length															
Birth	6055	1.02	0.93	1.12	0.72	0.77	0.66	Birth	5609	1.22	1.02	1.46	0.03	0.03	0.05
6 months	6534	1.02	0.94	1.11	0.57	0.57	0.61	6 months	6043	1.18	1.02	1.38	0.03	0.03	0.05
1 year	6534	1.04	0.96	1.12	0.40	0.39	0.50	1 year	6043	1.20	1.03	1.40	0.02	0.02	0.02
2 years	6536	1.08	0.99	1.17	0.07	0.07	0.11	2 years	6044	1.22	1.05	1.42	0.01	0.01	0.01
7 years	4909	1.13	1.03	1.24	0.01	0.02	0.03	7 years	4521	1.12	0.95	1.33	0.18	0.21	0.30
11 years	4814	1.14	1.04	1.26	0.01	0.01	0.01	11 years	4409	1.07	0.90	1.27	0.44	0.49	0.64
Weight															
Birth	6094	1.06	0.97	1.17	0.21	0.25	0.18	Birth	5653	1.19	1.00	1.42	0.05	0.06	0.05
6 months	6539	1.03	0.95	1.11	0.55	0.55	0.88	6 months	6049	1.16	1.00	1.35	0.06	0.06	0.07
1 year	6539	1.04	0.96	1.13	0.32	0.33	0.44	1 year	6049	1.13	0.97	1.32	0.11	0.12	0.13
2 years	6542	1.07	0.99	1.16	0.10	0.11	0.14	2 years	6049	1.19	1.02	1.50	0.02	0.03	0.02
7 years	4917	1.10	1.00	1.20	0.05	0.07	0.09	7 years	4527	1.13	0.95	1.34	0.16	0.18	0.23
11 years	4817	1.13	1.03	1.24	0.01	0.01	0.03	11 years	4407	1.07	0.90	1.26	0.46	0.49	0.75
BMI															
Birth	6049	1.07	0.98	1.17	0.13	0.16	0.11	Birth	5606	1.12	0.95	1.33	0.17	0.18	0.15
6 months	6535	1.01	0.93	1.10	0.81	0.83	0.87	6 months	6045	1.05	0.90	1.23	0.51	0.51	0.50
1 year	6535	1.02	0.94	1.10	0.66	0.69	0.56	1 year	6045	0.99	0.85	1.15	0.87	0.86	0.85
2 years	6538	1.03	0.95	1.11	0.51	0.55	0.49	2 years	6046	1.04	0.89	1.21	0.65	0.66	0.55
7 years	4903	1.01	0.92	1.11	0.84	0.88	0.88	7 years	4512	1.05	0.88	1.24	0.61	0.61	0.56
11 years	4809	1.05	0.95	1.15	0.35	0.35	0.50	11 years	4403	1.02	0.86	1.21	0.79	0.79	0.97

CI: Confidence interval.
All models are adjusted for year of birth and socioeconomic position in childhood, and models pertaining to body size at birth are also adjusted for gestational age (Model 1). In addition to those variables in Model 1, Model 2 and Model 3 are adjusted for maternal socioeconomic position or other mental disorders, respectively.

adulthood; consequently, the current findings cannot be directly compared to the previous ones. Cross-sectional studies on associations between body size and psychiatric morbidity show conflicting results, with some linking obesity with psychiatric problems [26,48–51], and others showing no association [52] or an inverse association between BMI and mental disorders [53,54]. Longitudinal studies suggest sex-specificity in associations between childhood body size or physical growth and psychiatric morbidity in later life [24,26,27]. In girls, but not in boys, higher BMI and gain in BMI in childhood linked with anxiety disorders and depression in adulthood [26]. Moreover, chronic obesity in childhood increased the risk for depression in adolescence only in boys, but for oppositional disorder in both sexes [24]. Another study also found no association between childhood overweight and subsequent depression [52]. Furthermore, still other studies have shown that these associations may be not only sex-specific, but also specific to a particular growth period. Physical growth in infancy and in childhood show different patterns with respect to risk of hospitalization for personality disorders in adulthood in both boys and girls [27]. Thus, some of the inconsistencies in the findings may stem from a lack of physical growth data on specific age periods.

Our finding that restricting the sample to those with mental disorders attenuated many of the associations is in line with earlier findings that smaller birth size associates with a wide range of mental disorders [25] and may therefore be considered a marker more for overall vulnerability than for a specific disorder. However, our findings that in women shorter height in early childhood and lower weight at two years associated with increased risk of hospitalization for AUDs after adjusting for other mental disorders and after restricting the sample to those with any mental disorder, suggest that these associations may be more specific and confined to AUDs.

Our results cannot determine the biological and psychosocial mechanisms that underlie the associations between smaller body size and the risk for AUDs. The DOHaD framework postulates that these conditions may relate to environmental psychosocial stress and/or malnutrition that alter the structure and function of the brain [6,7]. Indeed, in animal studies, prenatal stress [55,56] and the prenatal administration of synthetic glucocorticoids [57], probably mediated via hypothalamic pituitary adrenocortical (HPA) axis activity, have associated with a variety of alterations in hormonal axes, in monoamine neurotransmission, and in the morphology of the offspring [56]. In addition, human studies have linked several indicators of extreme small birth size with structural or functional alterations in the brain. Greater birth weight within the normal range was recently linked with generalized increase in brain volume, which in the cortical sheet, seems to be driven by increased surface area [58] as well as with increase in the volume of several striatal areas [59]. Similar results were found in monozygotic twins, suggesting that environmental factors underlie these associations [58], and in singletons [59]. Intrauterine growth retardation has been linked with metabolic disturbances in brain serotonin synthesis [60], low birth weight with increased lateral ventricular volume [61], and preterm birth with a smaller hippocampus [62,63]. Moreover, a recent meta-analysis showed children who were very premature and/or of very low birth weight to have significantly smaller total brain volume than term-born comparison group, less white and grey matter volume, and smaller cerebellum, hippocampus, and corpus callosum [64]. Roza et al. [65] showed that reduced fetal growth in head circumference and biparietal diameter predicted lower ventricular volume in infancy. Interestingly, previous studies have implicated serotonin genes in alcohol dependence [66] and have linked alcohol use with alterations in HPA axis activity [67] and hippocampal volume [68] in adolescents.

Our findings suggest that sensitive periods with respect to the risk for AUDs may differ for men and women. Exposures *in utero* and in infancy may have greater effects for women, whereas for men, the sensitive periods occur later, from toddlerhood onwards. Consistent with these results, exposure to prenatal stress associated with larger alterations in monoamine neurotransmission [69] and HPA axis function [70], and increased anxiety-like behaviors [71] in female animals, whereas males exhibited more learning deficits [71].

The strengths of our study are its longitudinal study design, its relatively large sample of participants derived from the general population, and its use of comprehensive register data. Moreover, we measured growth at several points in time, which permitted us to track critical periods of growth with respect to subsequent AUDs. Our study also has its limitations. First, we have no data on parental mental disorders or risk behaviors such as alcohol use or smoking. Since smoking or alcohol use during pregnancy may increase the risk for small birth size [72] as well as the risk for psychiatric disorders in the offspring [73,74], the associations observed may have resulted from prenatal exposures. Moreover, the lack of data on parental alcohol use after birth for our sample precluded us from investigating and accounting for the role of social learning in the development of AUDs. Second, our data on diagnoses were based on hospital records and not everyone with AUD requires hospitalization. Moreover, the HDR data do not cover the years between 1934 and 1969. Consequently, participants with AUDs may have had severe disorders, so our results may not be generalized to less severe disorders. However, the proportion of participants in our sample diagnosed with AUDs (6.6%) is only slightly lower than the lifetime prevalence of 7.9% reported recently in a population-based sample of Finns over 30 years of age [1]. Third, although our participants correspond to 94.3% of the original cohort, one limitation of the external validity of our findings is that they do not include those who died or emigrated before assignment of personal ID numbers and those who did not attend free-of-charge, voluntary child welfare clinics. Moreover, loss to follow-up is inevitable. Compared with the original cohort, participation was unrelated to childhood SEP, length of gestation, placental weight, or length and head circumference at birth, but the participants of this study were born later, were more often men, and tended to be heavier at birth. These differences could, however, introduce bias only if the associations between growth and AUDs in people included in the sample differed from such associations in those who were not. Furthermore, one should be cautious about generalizing our findings to people living in other types of societies or to those born in later decades.

In summary, the associations between anthropometric traits, indicators of the prenatal and childhood nutritional and psychosocial environment, and AUDs showed differences between women and men: shorter length/height at birth and in infancy in girls and in childhood in boys, associated with increased risk for AUDs in later life.

Acknowledgments

Professor Barker (now deceased) contributed actively to the design of this study, to discussion of the interpretation of the results, and he saw drafts up to the latest Researchers interested in using HBCS data must obtain approval from the Steering Committee of the Helsinki Birth Cohort Study. Researchers using the data are required to follow the terms in a number of clauses designed to ensure protection of privacy and compliance with relevant Finnish laws. For further information, contact Johan Eriksson (johan.eriksson@helsinki.fi).

Author Contributions

Conceived and designed the experiments: KR JGE DJPB CO. Performed the experiments: JL ML AKP KH EK TF KW JGE KR. Analyzed the data: JL ML KW CO KR. Contributed reagents/materials/analysis tools: JL ML KW KR. Wrote the paper: JL ML AKP KH EK TF KW CO DJPB JGE KR.

References

1. Pirkola SP, Poikolainen K, Lönnqvist JK (2006) Currently active and remitted alcohol dependence in a nationwide adult general population–results from the Finnish Health 2000 study. Alcohol Alcohol 41: 315–320.
2. Bijl RV, Ravelli A, van Zessen G (1998) Prevalence of psychiatric disorder in the general population: results of The Netherlands Mental Health Survey and Incidence Study (NEMESIS). SocPsychiatry PsychiatrEpidemiol 33: 587–595.
3. Lopez AD, Mathers CD, Ezzati M, Jamison DT, Murray CJ (2006) Global and regional burden of disease and risk factors, 2001: systematic analysis of population health data. Lancet 367: 1747–1757.
4. Murray CJ, Lopez AD (1997) Alternative projections of mortality and disability by cause 1990-2020: Global Burden of Disease Study. Lancet 349: 1498–1504.
5. Rehm J, Room R, Graham K, Monteiro M, Gmel G, et al. (2003) The relationship of average volume of alcohol consumption and patterns of drinking to burden of disease: an overview. Addiction 98: 1209–1228.
6. Gillman MW (2005) Developmental origins of health and disease. New England Journal of Medicine 353: 1848–1850.
7. Barker DJ (2004) The developmental origins of chronic adult disease. Acta Paediatrica Supplement 93: 26–33.
8. Ohlmeier MD, Peters K, Te Wildt BT, Zedler M, Ziegenbein M, et al. (2008) Comorbidity of alcohol and substance dependence with attention-deficit/ hyperactivity disorder (ADHD). Alcohol Alcohol 43: 300–304.
9. Green AI, Brown ES (2006) Comorbid schizophrenia and substance abuse. J Clin Psychiatry 67: e08.
10. Trull TJ, Jahng S, Tomko RL, Wood PK, Sher KJ (2010) Revised Nesarc Personality Disorder Diagnoses: Gender, Prevalence, and Comorbidity with Substance Dependence Disorders. J Pers Disord 24: 412–426.
11. Costello EJ, Worthman C, Erkanli A, Angold A (2007) Prediction from low birth weight to female adolescent depression: a test of competing hypotheses. Archives of General Psychiatry 64: 338–344.
12. Lahti J, Räikkönen K, Pesonen AK, Heinonen K, Kajantie E, et al. (2009) Prenatal growth, postnatal growth and trait anxiety in late adulthood - the Helsinki Birth Cohort Study. Acta Psychiatr Scand 121: 227–235.
13. Lahti J, Räikkönen K, Sovio U, Miettunen J, Hartikainen AL, et al. (2009) Early-life origins of schizotypal traits in adulthood. Br J Psychiatry 195: 132–137.
14. Lahti J, Raikkonen K, Kajantie E, Heinonen K, Pesonen AK, et al. (2006) Small body size at birth and behavioural symptoms of ADHD in children aged five to six years. J Child Psychol Psychiatry 47: 1167–1174.
15. Wahlbeck K, Forsen T, Osmond C, Barker DJ, Eriksson JG (2001) Association of schizophrenia with low maternal body mass index, small size at birth, and thinness during childhood. Archives of General Psychiatry 58: 48–52.
16. Lahti M, Räikkönen K, Wahlbeck K, Heinonen K, Forsen T, et al. (2010) Prenatal origins of hospitalization for personality disorders: the Helsinki birth cohort study. Psychiatry Res 179: 226–230.
17. Schlotz W, Phillips DI (2009) Fetal origins of mental health: evidence and mechanisms. Brain Behav Immun 23: 905–916.
18. Räikkönen K, Pesonen AK, Roseboom TJ, Eriksson JG (2012) Early determinants of mental health. Best Pract Res Clin Endocrinol Metab 26: 599–611.
19. Osler M, Kriegbaum M, Christensen U, Holstein B, Nybo Andersen AM (2008) Rapid report on methodology: does loss to follow-up in a cohort study bias associations between early life factors and lifestyle-related health outcomes? AnnEpidemiol 18: 422–424.
20. Gustafsson WM, Josefsson K, Selling KE, Sydsjö G (2009) Preterm birth or foetal growth impairment and psychiatric hospitalization in adolescence and early adulthood in a Swedish population-based birth cohort. Acta Psychiatrica Scandinavica 119: 54–61.
21. Cooke RW (2004) Health, lifestyle, and quality of life for young adults born very preterm. ArchDisChild 89: 201–206.
22. Strang-Karlsson S, Räikkönen K, Pesonen AK, Kajantie E, Paavonen EJ, et al. (2008) Very low birth weight and behavioral symptoms of attention deficit hyperactivity disorder in young adulthood: the helsinki study of very-low-birth-weight adults. AmJPsychiatry 165: 1345–1353.
23. Hallin AL, Stjernqvist K (2011) Adolescents born extremely preterm: behavioral outcomes and quality of life. Scand J Psychol 52: 251–256.
24. Mustillo S, Worthman C, Erkanli A, Keeler G, Angold A, et al. (2003) Obesity and psychiatric disorder: developmental trajectories. Pediatrics 111: 851–859.
25. Abel KM, Wicks S, Susser ES, Dalman C, Pedersen MG, et al. (2010) Birth weight, schizophrenia, and adult mental disorder: is risk confined to the smallest babies? Arch Gen Psychiatry 67: 923–930.
26. Anderson SE, Cohen P, Naumova EN, Must A (2006) Association of depression and anxiety disorders with weight change in a prospective community-based study of children followed up into adulthood. ArchPediatrAdolescMed 160: 285–291.
27. Lahti M, Räikkönen K, Wahlbeck K, Heinonen K, Forsen T, et al. (2011) Growth in infancy and childhood and hospitalization for personality disorders in adulthood: the Helsinki Birth Cohort Study. J Pers Disord 25: 620–633.
28. Osmond C, Kajantie E, Forsen TJ, Eriksson JG, Barker DJP (2007) Infant growth and stroke in adult life the Helsinki birth cohort study. Stroke 38: 264–270.
29. Mikkonen M, Salonen MK, Häkkinen A, Pesonen AK, Räikkönen K, et al. (submitted) Mother's marital status and offspring's socio-economic status in adulthood - the Helsinki Birth Cohort Study 1934–11944.
30. Keskimäki I, Aro S (1991) Accuracy of data on diagnoses, procedures and accidents in the Finnish Hospital Discharge Register. Int J Health Serv 2: 15–21.
31. Perälä J, Suvisaari J, Saarni SI, Kuoppasalmi K, Isometsä E, et al. (2007) Lifetime prevalence of psychotic and bipolar I disorders in a general population. ArchGenPsychiatry 64: 19–28.
32. Poikolainen K (1983) Accuracy of hospital discharge data: five alcohol-related diseases. Drug Alcohol Depend 12: 315–322.
33. Veijola J, Laara E, Joukamaa M, Isohanni M, Hakko H, et al. (2008) Temporary parental separation at birth and substance use disorder in adulthood. A long-term follow-up of the Finnish Christmas Seal Home Children. Soc Psychiatry Psychiatr Epidemiol 43: 11–17.
34. Mäkelä P, Paljärvi T (2008) Do consequences of a given pattern of drinking vary by socioeconomic status? A mortality and hospitalisation follow-up for alcohol-related causes of the Finnish Drinking Habits Surveys. J Epidemiol Community Health 62: 728–733.
35. Mäkikyrö T, Isohanni K, Moring J, Hakko H, Lönnqvist J (1998) Accuracy of register-based schizophrenia diagnoses in a genetic study. Eur Psychiatry 13: 57–62.
36. Räikkönen K, Lahti M, Heinonen K, Pesonen AK, Wahlbeck K, et al. (2011) Risk of severe mental disorders in adults separated temporarily from their parents in childhood: the Helsinki birth cohort study. J Psychiatr Res 45: 332–338.
37. Barker DJ, Osmond C, Forsen TJ, Kajantie E, Eriksson JG (2005) Trajectories of growth among children who have coronary events as adults. N Engl J Med 353: 1802–1809.
38. Schulte MT, Ramo D, Brown SA (2009) Gender differences in factors influencing alcohol use and drinking progression among adolescents. Clin Psychol Rev 29: 535–547.
39. Perrin MA, Chen H, Sandberg DE, Malaspina D, Brown AS (2007) Growth trajectory during early life and risk of adult schizophrenia. Br J Psychiatry 191: 512–520.
40. O'Keeffe MJ, O'Callaghan M, Williams GM, Najman JM, Bor W (2003) Learning, cognitive, and attentional problems in adolescents born small for gestational age. Pediatrics 112: 301–307.
41. Hack M, Youngstrom EA, Cartar L, Schluchter M, Taylor HG, et al. (2004) Behavioral outcomes and evidence of psychopathology among very low birth weight infants at age 20 years. Pediatrics 114: 932–940.
42. Alati R, Lawlor DA, Mamun AA, Williams GM, Najman JM, et al. (2007) Is there a fetal origin of depression? Evidence from the Mater University Study of Pregnancy and its outcomes. AmJEpidemiol 165: 575–582.
43. Rice F, Jones I, Thapar A (2007) The impact of gestational stress and prenatal growth on emotional problems in offspring: a review. Acta Psychiatr Scand 115: 171–183.
44. Kelly YJ, Nazroo JY, McMunn A, Boreham R, Marmot M (2001) Birthweight and behavioural problems in children: a modifiable effect? International Journal of Epidemiology 30: 88–94.
45. Thompson C, Syddall H, Rodin I, Osmond C, Barker DJ (2001) Birth weight and the risk of depressive disorder in late life. British Journal of Psychiatry 179: 450–455.
46. Wiles NJ, Peters TJ, Leon DA, Lewis G (2005) Birth weight and psychological distress at age 45-51 years: results from the Aberdeen Children of the 1950s cohort study. British Journal of Psychiatry 187: 21–28.
47. Schlotz W, Jones A, Phillips NM, Godfrey KM, Phillips DI (2007) Size at birth and motor activity during stress in children aged 7 to 9 years. Pediatrics 120: e1237–1244.
48. Lumeng JC, Gannon K, Cabral HJ, Frank DA, Zuckerman B (2003) Association between clinically meaningful behavior problems and overweight in children. Pediatrics 112: 1138–1145.

49. Bjerkeset O, Romundstad P, Evans J, Gunnell D (2008) Association of adult body mass index and height with anxiety, depression, and suicide in the general population: the HUNT study. AmJEpidemiol 167: 193–202.
50. Becker ES, MargrafJ, Turke V, Soeder U, Neumer S (2001) Obesity and mental illness in a representative sample of young women. IntJObesRelat Metab Disord 25 Suppl 1: S5–S9.
51. Simon GE, Von Korff M, Saunders K, Miglioretti DL, Crane PK, et al. (2006) Association between obesity and psychiatric disorders in the US adult population. ArchGenPsychiatry 63: 824–830.
52. Goodman E, Whitaker RC (2002) A prospective study of the role of depression in the development and persistence of adolescent obesity. Pediatrics 110: 497–504.
53. Crisp AH, McGuiness B (1976) Jolly fat: relation between obesity and psychoneurosis in general population. BrMedJ 1: 7–9.
54. Stewart AL, Brook RH (1983) Effects of being overweight. AmJPublic Health 73: 171–178.
55. Huizink AC, Mulder EJ, Buitelaar JK (2004) Prenatal stress and risk for psychopathology: specific effects or induction of general susceptibility? PsycholBull 130: 115–142.
56. Charil A, Laplante DP, Vaillancourt C, King S (2010) Prenatal stress and brain development. Brain Res Rev 65: 56–79.
57. Slotkin TA, Kreider ML, Tate CA, Seidler FJ (2006) Critical prenatal and postnatal periods for persistent effects of dexamethasone on serotonergic and dopaminergic systems. Neuropsychopharmacology 31: 904–911.
58. Raznahan A, Greenstein D, Lee NR, Clasen LS, Giedd JN (2012) Prenatal growth in humans and postnatal brain maturation into late adolescence. Proc Natl Acad Sci U S A 109: 11366–11371.
59. Walhovd KB, Fjell AM, Brown TT, Kuperman JM, Chung Y, et al. (2012) Long-term influence of normal variation in neonatal characteristics on human brain development. Proc Natl Acad Sci U S A 109: 20089–20094.
60. Manjarrez G, Cisneros I, Herrera R, Vazquez F, Robles A, et al. (2005) Prenatal impairment of brain serotonergic transmission in infants. Journal of Pediatrics 147: 592–596.
61. Allin M, Henderson M, Suckling J, Nosarti C, Rushe T, et al. (2004) Effects of very low birthweight on brain structure in adulthood. Developmental Medicine and Child Neurology 46: 46–53.
62. Nosarti C, Al Asady MH, Frangou S, Stewart AL, Rifkin L, et al. (2002) Adolescents who were born very preterm have decreased brain volumes. Brain 125: 1616–1623.
63. Lodygensky GA, Seghier ML, Warfield SK, Tolsa CB, Sizonenko S, et al. (2008) Intrauterine growth restriction affects the preterm infant's hippocampus. PediatrRes 63: 438–443.
64. de Kieviet JF, Zoetebier L, van Elburg RM, Vermeulen RJ, Oosterlaan J (2012) Brain development of very preterm and very low-birthweight children in childhood and adolescence: a meta-analysis. Dev Med Child Neurol 54: 313–323.
65. Roza SJ, Govaert PP, Vrooman HA, Lequin MH, Hofman A, et al. (2008) Foetal growth determines cerebral ventricular volume in infants The Generation R Study. Neuroimage 39: 1491–1498.
66. Enoch MA, Gorodetsky E, Hodgkinson C, Roy A, Goldman D (2011) Functional genetic variants that increase synaptic serotonin and 5-HT3 receptor sensitivity predict alcohol and drug dependence. Mol Psychiatry 16: 1139–1146.
67. Evans BE, Greaves-Lord K, Euser AS, Franken IH, Huizink AC (2012) The relation between hypothalamic-pituitary-adrenal (HPA) axis activity and age of onset of alcohol use. Addiction 107: 312–322.
68. De Bellis MD, Clark DB, Beers SR, Soloff PH, Boring AM, et al. (2000) Hippocampal volume in adolescent-onset alcohol use disorders. Am J Psychiatry 157: 737–744.
69. Bowman RE, MacLusky NJ, Sarmiento Y, Frankfurt M, Gordon M, et al. (2004) Sexually dimorphic effects of prenatal stress on cognition, hormonal responses, and central neurotransmitters. Endocrinology 145: 3778–3787.
70. Mccormick CM, Smythe JW, Sharma S, Meaney MJ (1995) Sex-Specific Effects of Prenatal Stress on Hypothalamic-Pituitary-Adrenal Responses to Stress and Brain Glucocorticoid Receptor Density in Adult-Rats. Developmental Brain Research 84: 55–61.
71. Weinstock M (2011) Sex-dependent changes induced by prenatal stress in cortical and hippocampal morphology and behaviour in rats: an update. Stress 14: 604–613.
72. Sampson PD, Bookstein FL, Barr HM, Streissguth AP (1994) Prenatal alcohol exposure, birthweight, and measures of child size from birth to age 14 years. Am J Public Health 84: 1421–1428.
73. Sood B, Delaney-Black V, Covington C, Nordstrom-Klee B, Ager J, et al. (2001) Prenatal alcohol exposure and childhood behavior at age 6 to 7 years: I. dose-response effect. Pediatrics 108: E34.
74. Disney ER, Iacono W, McGue M, Tully E, Legrand L (2008) Strengthening the case: prenatal alcohol exposure is associated with increased risk for conduct disorder. Pediatrics 122: e1225–1230.

5

Relationships between Reward Sensitivity, Risk-Taking and Family History of Alcoholism during an Interactive Competitive fMRI Task

Haley L. Yarosh[1,2*], Christopher J. Hyatt[1], Shashwath A. Meda[1], Rachel Jiantonio-Kelly[1], Marc N. Potenza[2,3,4], Michal Assaf[1,2], Godfrey D.Pearlson[1,2,3]

1 Olin Neuropsychiatry Research Center, Institute of Living at Hartford Hospital, Hartford, Connecticut, United States of America, **2** Department of Psychiatry, Yale University School of Medicine, New Haven, Connecticut, United States of America, **3** Department of Neurobiology, Yale University School of Medicine, New Haven, Connecticut, United States of America, **4** Child Study Center, Yale University School of Medicine, New Haven, Connecticut, United States of America

Abstract

Background: Individuals with a positive family history for alcoholism (FHP) have shown differences from family-history-negative (FHN) individuals in the neural correlates of reward processing. FHP, compared to FHN individuals, demonstrate relatively diminished ventral striatal activation during anticipation of monetary rewards, and the degree of ventral striatal activation shows an inverse correlation with specific impulsivity measures in alcohol-dependent individuals. Rewards in socially interactive contexts relate importantly to addictive propensities, yet have not been examined with respect to how their neural underpinnings relate to impulsivity-related measures. Here we describe impulsivity measures in FHN and FHP individuals as they relate to a socially interactive functional magnetic resonance imaging (fMRI) task.

Methods: Forty FHP and 29 FHN subjects without histories of Axis-I disorders completed a socially interactive Domino task during functional magnetic resonance imaging and completed self-report and behavioral impulsivity-related assessments.

Results: FHP compared to FHN individuals showed higher scores ($p = .004$) on one impulsivity-related factor relating to both compulsivity (Padua Inventory) and reward/punishment sensitivity (Sensitivity to Punishment/Sensitivity to Reward Questionnaire). Multiple regression analysis within a reward-related network revealed a correlation between risk-taking (involving another impulsivity-related factor, the Balloon Analog Risk Task (BART)) and right ventral striatum activation under reward >punishment contrast ($p<0.05$ FWE corrected) in the social task.

Conclusions: Behavioral risk-taking scores may be more closely associated with neural correlates of reward responsiveness in socially interactive contexts than are FH status or impulsivity-related self-report measures. These findings suggest that risk-taking assessments be examined further in socially interactive settings relevant to addictive behaviors.

Editor: Daniel Houser, George Mason University, United States of America

Funding: The project was funded by the following sources: National Institute on Alcohol Abuse and Alcoholism (NIAAA) Grant number 5 P50 AA01280; Project 4 (GDP); National Institutes of Health (NIH) Grant number RL1 AA017539 (MNP); and NIH Grant number P20 DA027844 (MNP). The funders had no role in study design, data collection and analysis, decision to publish, or preparation of the manuscript.

Competing Interests: Dr. Potenza has received financial support or compensation for the following: Dr. Potenza has consulted for and advised Somaxon, BoehringerIngelheim, Lundbeck and Ironwood Pharmaceuticals; has had financial interests in Somaxon; has received research support from the National Institutes of Health, Veteran's Administration, Mohegan Sun Casino, the National Center for Responsible Gaming and its affiliated Institute for Research on Gambling Disorders, Glaxo-SmithKline, Psyadon and Forest Laboratories pharmaceuticals; has participated in surveys, mailings or telephone consultations related to drug addiction, impulse control disorders or other health topics; has consulted for gambling and legal entities on issues related to addictions or impulse control disorders; has provided clinical care in the Connecticut Department of Mental Health and Addiction Services Problem Gambling Services Program; has performed grant reviews for the National Institutes of Health and other agencies; has guest-edited journal sections; has given academic lectures in grand rounds, CME events and other clinical or scientific venues; and has generated books or book chapters for publishers of mental health texts. There are no patents, products in development or marketed products to declare.

* E-mail: haley.yarosh@yale.edu

Introduction

Impulsivity is a complex, multi-faceted construct characterized by premature motor responses, decreased inhibition, abnormal reward sensitivity and risk-associated behaviors [1,2]. Aspects of impulsivity-related behaviors are associated with neural responses to rewards and punishments [3–6]. Brain regions implicated in these processes include the amygdala [7], anterior cingulate cortex (ACC) [8], nucleus accumbens (NAcc), orbitofrontal cortex (OFC)[9–12], medial prefrontal cortex (mPFC) [13,14], striatum [12,15,16], insula [4,13,17,18], ventral tegmental area (VTA) [19], hippocampus [20], and subthalamic nucleus (STN) [21]. In particular, ventral striatal (VS) responses during processing of rewards and punishments, more specifically reward anticipation, may represent endophenotypes for disorders characterized by impaired impulse control such as alcoholism, pathological gambling, and binge eating disorder [6,13,22,23].

Several hypotheses have been advanced to explain neural activity underlying reward processing as related to impulse control. The "reward deficiency hypothesis" suggests that individuals compensate for trait-like under-activation of neural-based reward response with risk-taking and impulsive behaviors [24]. This is consistent with observations of blunted VS responses during reward anticipation and lower availability of D2-like dopamine receptors in drug abuse/dependence [25–27].

The term "impulsivity" is sometimes used broadly and imprecisely [28–30]. Although multiple studies discuss 'trait impulsivity' or 'impulsive behavior', few have used multiple standard assessments in the same subjects to examine relationships between behavioral risk-taking, self-reported risk-taking, and social influences on these tendencies and behaviors. Furthermore, few studies investigate multiple impulsivity-related characteristics in a single clinical population. Using principal component analysis, we previously identified five impulsivity-related domains that comprise: 1) self-reported behavioral activation, 2) self-reported compulsivity and reward/punishment sensitivity, 3) self-reported impulsivity, 4) behavioral temporal discounting, and 5) behavioral risk-taking [12,16,18,19,29,31,32].

Lineages with heavy drug and alcohol use disorders (AUDs) show higher prevalence of impulsive behaviors, including those related to reward-processing differences [12,30,33–42]. Children of alcohol-dependent parents (family-history-positive (FHP) for alcoholism) are more likely to demonstrate under-controlled behavior, make impulsive errors, exhibit steeper delay discounting curves and perform more poorly on cognitive-control and decision-making measures compared to family-history-negative (FHN) peers [43–47]. They are also likely to initiate drug and alcohol use earlier [48]. While social environments and time of initial encounter with substances may influence substance-use behaviors, family history of alcoholism (FHA) is arguably the single greatest risk factor for developing substance-use disorders [49,50]. Data suggest heritable factors underlie heightened impulsivity-related behaviors in alcohol abuse/dependence. FHP individuals may express increased hedonic and stimulatory responses to the effects of alcohol and related cues [51,52]. Non-drinking children of alcoholic and drug-abusing parents show risk-taking and sensation-seeking attributes independent of alcohol and drug use [53–56].

In the current study, we investigated relationships between FHA, impulsivity-related domains and brain activations assessed using functional magnetic resonance imaging (fMRI) during performance of an interactive competitive Domino task that includes both risk-taking and rewards/punishments. Each round of the Domino task includes an outcome interval with a notification of reward/punishment. Impulsivity-related domains were examined using a factor analysis approach that we have employed previously [6,29,31,42]. We aimed to investigate whether: a) impulsivity-related domains are associated with reward-related neural activity across all subjects, and b) FHA associated with impulsivity-related factor scores or fMRI reward response during the Domino task. We hypothesized that we would observe between-group differences (FHP/FHN) in reward-related activity in targeted regions of interest (ROIs): ventral and dorsal striatum [54,57]. We also hypothesized that high scores on behavioral risk-taking would be associated with reward-related neural activity based on prior research showing that such brain activity correlated highly with behavioral risk-taking [58].

Materials and Methods

Ethics Statement

The experimental protocol and the study were approved by the Human Research Protections Program (HRPP) of the Hartford Hospital Institutional Review Board (IRB) and Yale University Institutional Review Board (HIC/HSC). The studies were carried out at Hartford Hospital Institute of Living. All study participants provided written informed consent after the study had been fully explained to them. Participants were paid for participating in the imaging study. Sixty-nine healthy individuals, 40 FHP and 29 FHN, were recruited by word-of-mouth, flyers, newspaper, online advertisement and drug abuse programs.

Study Participants

Sixty-nine healthy individuals, 40 FHP and 29 FHN were recruited into two groups based on FHA using detailed interviews. These subjects include 7 FHP and 11 FHN individuals who participated in a prior study employing the MID task, and additionally included 33 FHP and 18 FHN subjects [6]. As previously, FHN was defined as having no first-degree relative with alcohol-abuse history; FHP subjects reported an alcohol-dependent father and alcohol abuse or dependence in one or more first-degree or second-degree relatives. Potential FHP subjects that have mothers with a lifetime history of alcohol abuse were excluded to avoid confounds related to fetal alcohol exposure. Subjects meeting neither group criteria (e.g., alcoholism in several second-degree, but no first-degree, relatives) were excluded. Exclusion criteria included current or past history of any Axis-I diagnosis, assessed by the Structured Clinical Interviewed for DSM-IV Axis-I Disorders (SCID), major physical illness, current or past history of central neurological disease or substance abuse or dependence, history of head trauma causing loss of consciousness>10 min, MRI contraindications, poor understanding of spoken/written English, auditory or visual impairments impeding test-taking, positive urine toxicology for commonly abused substances, positive pregnancy screen, and positive alcohol breath screen at the time of fMRI scanning [59]. Subjects were group-matched for age and sex as detailed in Table 1. Additionally, participants were asked to record on which days they drank, and how many drinks were consumed each day over a one-month period prior to their visit. An independent samples T-test reveals a significant difference between groups ($p = .007$, $F = 8.270$) on number of days participants drank during the month, but no difference between drinks per episode ($p = .491$, $F = .481$).

Domino Task

Subjects performed the Domino task described previously [16,60,61]. This two-player competitive game involves participant- and computer-generated responses, though players are told that they have a human opponent to mimic an interpersonal competitive interaction. This creates a social context for the participant. At the start of each game, 12 random Domino-like chips from a pool of 28are shown face up on the screen and assigned to the player. An opponent's Domino chip (constant throughout the game) shows face-up on the top-corner of the board. Four undisclosed chips are assigned to a bank, leaving 11 remaining chips not used for the current game. The player's goal is to dispose of all assigned chips before the game ends (4 min). Each assigned chip can either match the opponent's (match one of the opponent chip's numbers) or not. Playing a matching chip is considered a 'safe' move because it will not result in punishment. Non-matching chips are considered 'risky' moves or 'bluffs', since they can result in a gain of chips if challenged by the opponent. A

Table 1. Subject Demographics.

Demographic	FHN	FHP	Total	Chi-Square	p Value
Gender (M:F Ratio)	**11:18**	**14:26**	**29:40**	**0.063**	**0.80**
Ethnicity (White/Hispanic/African American/Asian/Other)	27/0/1/0/1	36/1/2/0/1	63/1/3/0/2	1.654	0.80
Age, years (Mean± SD)	25.45±6.33	26.15±5.58	25.86±5.87		

M = male, F = female.
Demographics for FHN, FHP, and total sample used in the study.

player must occasionally bluff to win the game, since he/she will not always have a matching chip to play. Each game is played for a $10 reward bonus; losing a game results in no bonus.

Subjects play two rounds of the game, each 15 min in duration, where the player decides which chip to play next and awaits the opponent's response. The opponent can either challenge the player by asking him/her to reveal (turn face-up) the chosen chip or not challenge, allowing him/her to move on to the next round. Players are given visual and aural instructions throughout the round (Figure 1). (a) 'Choose' instructs the subject to mentally select a chip to be played next (4 sec). (b) 'Ready' instructs the subject to move a cursor (using his/her dominant hand) to the chosen chip (4 sec). (c) 'Go' instructs the player to put the chosen chip face down next to the opponent's chip. The player then awaits the opponent's response (3.4 sec, 5.4 sec or 7.4 sec) of either (d) 'Show' or 'No-Show'. The former command exposes the player's selected chip (revealing whether they played safe or bluffed), while the latter leaves it unexposed. The next round of the game starts by presenting the 'Choose' command.

Based on the players' choice and opponent's response, there are four possible outcomes/consequences. (1) **Show matching chip**: player rewarded by disposal of the selected chip and one additional random chip from the game board (*overt gain*). (2) **Show non-matching chip**: the players' choice of non-matching chip is exposed, and they are punished by receiving back the selected chip plus two additional chips (*overt loss*). (3) **No-show of non-matching chip**: a choice of a non-matching chip remains unexposed, and only the selected chip is disposed of (*relative gain*). (4) **No-show of matching chip**: the choice of a matching chip is not exposed and only the selected matching chip is disposed of (*relative loss*).

Rounds continue until subjects win (by getting rid of all of their chips) or lose (240 sec pass or they receive all the chips from the bank and the board back).

Impulsivity-Related Measures

We administered two behavioral tasks and five self-report questionnaires, used previously to generate factor scores in five domains [29]. The assessments included the: (A) Behavioral Inhibition System/Behavioral Activation System (BIS/BAS) scale [62] B) Barratt Impulsivity Scale (BIS-11) [63], (C) Sensitivity to Punishment/Sensitivity to Reward Questionnaire (SPSRQ) [64], (D) Sensation-Seeking Scale (Form V) [65], and (E)Padua Inventory [66]. The computerized tasks included the (F) Balloon Analog Risk Task [67]and (G) Experiential Discounting Task [68]. To calculate new z-scores for the current subjects, we used a component score coefficient matrix described previously [29]. This matrix generated scores for five factors: Factor 1- "self-reported behavioral activation" (A), Factor 2 - "Self-Reported Compulsivity and Reward/Punishment Sensitivity"(C+E), Factor 3 - "Self-Reported Impulsivity" (B+D), Factor 4 - "Behavioral Temporal Discounting" (A+G), Factor 5 - "Behavioral Risk-Taking" (F).

Behavioral Data Analysis for Domino Task

After completing the Domino game, subjects were administered a 44-question Likert-scale (1–5) questionnaire to assess understanding and emotional response to the task. Four questions measured emotional responses to choice outcome including the following statements: Show match/overt gain: "I felt glad when a matching chip was challenged", No-show non-match/relative gain: "I felt glad when a non-matching chip was not challenged", Show non-match/overt loss: "I felt angry when a non-matching chip was challenged" or No-show match/relative loss: "I felt unhappy when a matching chip was not challenged". Between-group t-tests for each question response were run to determine group differences in response to reward and loss outcome.

To characterize player's choices during the game, a Risk-Taking Index was defined as the ratio of the number of times a player chose a non-matching chip to the total number of choices. This index represents an unbiased choice when equal to 0.5 (exactly half of the choices were non-matching choices), a biased choice for matching chips when smaller than 0.5 or for non-matching chips when greater than 0.5.All behavioral statistics were compiled using SPSS™ software (v19, SPSS Inc., Chicago, IL).

Functional MRI Acquisition for Domino Task

Blood oxygenation level dependent (BOLD) data were collected with a T2*-weighted echo-planar-imaging (EPI) sequence (TR/TE = 1,860/27 msec, Flip angle = 70°, Field of view = 22 cm with a 64×64 acquisition matrix) using a Siemens Allegra 3 Tesla scanner. Thirty-six contiguous axial functional slices of 3 mm thickness with 1 mm gap were acquired, yielding 3.4×3.4×4.0 mm voxels. Overall, 492 images were acquired per run, including six 'dummy' images at the beginning to allow global image intensity to reach equilibrium, which were excluded from data analysis.

Functional MRI Data Analysis for Domino Task

Preprocessing: Imaging data were analyzed using SPM8 (Wellcome Department of Imaging Neuroscience, London, UK). Each individual's data set was realigned to the first 'non-dummy'T2* image using the INRIAlign toolbox [69], spatially normalized to the Montreal-Neurological-Institute space [70] using an EPI template, and spatially smoothed with a 9 mm-isotropic-FWHM Gaussian kernel. A high-pass filter with 128 sec cutoff was used to correct for EPI signal low-frequency drift. Participants with >3.5 mm of movement in x,y, or z direction during the task were excluded, eliminating six FHP and two FHN from assessment, leaving 40 FHP and 29 FHN subjects (Table 1).

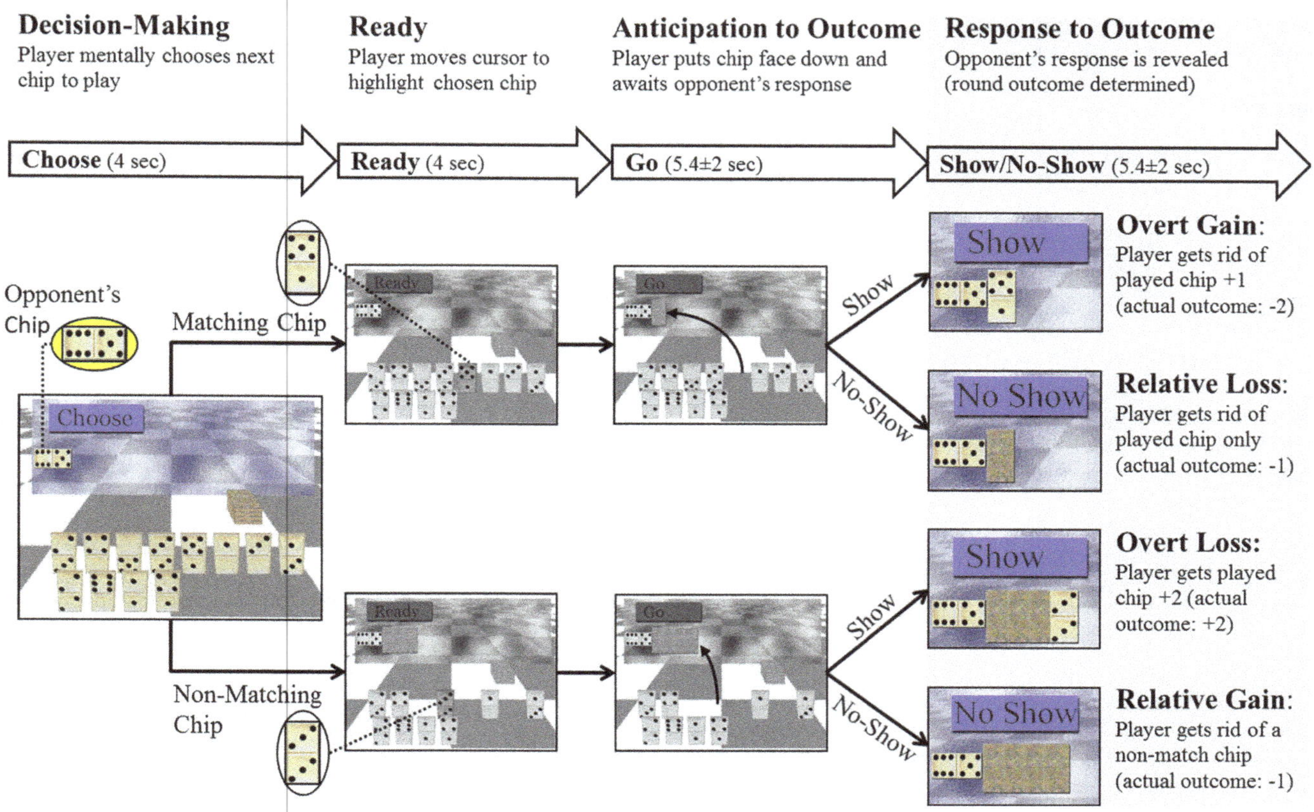

Figure 1. Domino game task. Domino Game Paradigm. The upper panel describes the 4 intervals that comprise each round of the game: Decision Making, Ready, Anticipation to Outcome and Response to Outcome. The latter is the main focus of this study, thus it is highlighted in gray. The duration of each interval and the command (i.e. event) that starts it are described in the bolded arrows below. The lower panel depicts the Domino Game sequence and corresponding consequences. At the beginning of each game the player (participant scanned) gets 12 playing chips and his/her goal is dispose of all 12 within 4 minutes. A constant opponent's chip (in this example 6:5, shown enlarged in the yellow ellipsoid) to which the player matches one chip in each round of the game, is displayed in the upper left corner of the screen throughout the game. Each round starts with the player instructed to decide what chip he/she will play next by the command 'Choose' (Decision-making interval). Then the player is instructed to move the cursor to this chip (Ready interval). The chip can either match the opponent's (i.e. have one of the numbers match those on the opponent's chip, upper row, 5:1 in this example) or not (lower row: 3:3; note that this is a later round in the same game). After placing the selected chip face down next to the opponent's, he/she awaits the opponent's response (Anticipation of Outcome interval). The opponent can either challenge the player's choice ('Show') or not ('No-Show'). Based on the player's choice and the opponent's response there are four possible consequences for each round (Response to Outcome interval): Show Match (overt gain); No-Show Match (relative loss, as the player could have been rewarded if challenged); Show Non-Match (overt loss) and No-Show Non-Match (relative gain, as the player could have been punished if challenged).

Events and regressors: Ten first-level (subject-level) regressors were from the four game intervals described above (Figure 1): (1) choose-match and choose-nonmatch from the 'Decision-making' interval; (2) ready from the 'Ready' interval; (3) pick-match and pick- nonmatch from the 'Anticipation of Outcome' interval; (4) show-match, show-nonmatch, noshow-match and noshow-non-match from the 'Response to Outcome' interval, each regressor corresponding to the four consequences; (5) and a miscellaneous regressor for events of non-interest including Go events and between-game events, during which the subject learned whether they won or lost the last game and then waited for the next game to begin. The miscellaneous regressor also included all events occurring during games of <1 min duration; these were not analyzed.

Data were analyzed using a general-linear-model (GLM) approach using SPM8. Regressors were modeled as boxcar functions convolved with the SPM8 canonical hemodynamic response function (HRF) and included HRF temporal derivatives. All six movement parameters (translation: x, y and z; rotation: pitch, roll and yaw) were included as covariates of no interest in the model.

Contrast images and individual statistical parametric maps were calculated with contrasts from the four 'Response to Outcome' interval regressors in a fixed-effects first-level analysis. These include the Reward contrast, a linear combination of overt and relative win outcomes compared to baseline, the Punishment contrast, a linear combination of overt and relative loss compared with an implicit baseline, and finally the Reward-Punishment difference contrast. Based on previous analyses [16], the last contrast was used to delineate a reward network based on a one-sample t-map of neural activation from all 69 subjects (random effects one-sample t–test) to create a study specific "Reward-mask" ($p_{FWE}<0.05$, corrected at the whole-brain level, $k=10$ voxels). We chose this number to conservatively detect extended clusters of activation rather than isolated voxels.

To assess between-group differences in activation related to response to reward, Reward-Punishment individual contrast maps were entered into a random-effects 2-sample t-test. A random-effects multiple-regression analysis evaluated the association between reward-related brain activations and impulsivity-related factor scores. These group analyses were masked with the Reward-mask and thresholded at $p_{FWE}<0.05$, corrected for voxels within the Reward-mask,$k = 10$ voxels.

Results

Domino Information

Subjects completed two 15 min scanning sessions, where there were 81.1±4.62 and 79.9±4.72 'Response to Outcome' events for each FHP and FHN subject respectively (group differences via t-test F = 3.32, df = 2,68, p = .081) and subjects won 22.0% of their games (group difference via t-test, F = 0.015, df = 1,67, p = .90). There was an average of 52.7% gain events for FHP group and 52.6% gain events for FHN subjects (F = .127, df = 2,68, p = .72).

Domino Debriefing

As in our previous report [16], gain responses were more salient than loss statement responses (p = .029), but there were no significant differences between absolute and relative loss and gain statements, respectively. As such, we grouped relative and absolute game events for task-related neural analysis. There was no mean between-group difference for each of these four responses (Table 2).

Domino Risk-taking Propensity

A Risk-Taking Index was generated by measuring tendency to 'bluff' over time, and a score was generated for each of four 1 min intervals per game. A two-way ANOVA (family-history-by-time-elapsed-into-game) revealed no effect of group (F = .52, df = 1,67, p = .47) and no group-by-time interaction. As we reported previously [16], there was a significant main effect of time for both groups (F = 9.58, df = 3, 201, p<.0001), indicating that players bluffed more often as the game progressed (Figure 2).

Impulsivity-related Constructs

Independent-samples t-test of impulsivity-related factor scores by group revealed significant differences between groups for factor 2 (Self-reported Compulsivity and Reward-Punishment Sensitivity; F = .35, df = 1,67, p = .004), where FHP subjects had higher factor-2 scores. There was no interaction effect with or significant difference by group with factors 1, 3, 4 or 5.

fMRI Analyses

The Reward-mask obtained from contrasting reward and punishment events in the Response-to-Outcome interval included the caudate, putamen and ventral striatum ($p_{FWE}<0.05$, k = 10; Figure 3). The Reward-mask was applied as an explicit mask to two-sample t-tests, but no statistically significant differences were observed between FHP and FHN subjects.

Table 2. Subject Debriefing after Domino Game.

Group	*Overt Gain*	*Relative Gain*	*Overt Loss*	*Relative Loss*
FHN	4.10±1.04	3.72±1.31	2.62±1.20	3.28±1.16
FHP	4.48±0.88	4.15±1.17	2.70±1.32	3.65±1.17
χ^2	5.66	3.75	1.18	3.35
p	0.23	0.44	0.88	0.50

FHN = family history negative, FHP = family history positive.
Domino debriefing scores as Likert scale responses (1–5) to statements regarding salience of gains and losses during game play.

A multiple-regression analysis within the Reward-mask revealed a positive correlation across all subjects between impulsivity-related factor-5 scores and neural activity under the Reward-Punishment contrast in right ventral caudate($r^2 = .26$, T = 4.75, df = 63, $p_{FWE} = .006$ at coordinates x,y,z = 12,4,–8) (Figure 4).

Discussion

Using a previously described interactive, competitive fMRI Domino task [16,60,61], we observed no differences in activation related to FHA in response to reward, focusing on a pre-defined, extended reward/motivation network. However, across all subjects, we observed a significant correlation between right ventral caudate activation to reward (assessed with reward>punishment contrast)and an empirically derived, impulsivity-related factor, "Behavioral Risk-Taking" (involving BART average adjusted number of pumps). In addition, impulsivity-related Factor 2 (Padua-Inventory and SPSRQ scores) comprising self-rated compulsivity and reward-punishment sensitivity, was significantly higher in FHP subjects, but not associated with regional task-related BOLD activation. This component has been associated with alcohol-use measures in a similar population [6]and related to insular/inferior-frontal-gyral activation during response inhibition [18]. Factor 2 also distinguished current cocaine users from both former cocaine users and healthy controls [16,19,71].

Based on previous research [60,61], we expected that the Domino task would demonstrate FHA-related differences in neural reward responses in regions including the mesocorticolimbic circuit [72,73], though the magnitude and direction of the association between impulsivity-related characteristics and these ROIs have been seemingly conflicting in previous studies. For example, during a Monetary Incentive Delay (MID) task performance in a subset of the same subject population, FHP versus FHN participants showed blunted activation in ventral striatum, OFC and insula during reward anticipation, and caudate hyperactivation during potential monetary reward outcome [6]. Ventral striatal hypoactivation during reward anticipation was also seen with an MID task in adolescents ages 18–22 years with AUD diagnoses in one or more parents [54], pathological gamblers [13,74], adults with inattentive attention-deficit/hyperactivity disorder (ADHD) [75] detoxified male alcoholics [22,27], binge-eating adults [23], and adolescent smokers [27]. Monetary rewards in the Domino task are not revealed to subjects until all games end. In contrast, the MID task reveals payment after each trial, which may be more participant-salient and account for group differences. Alternate possibilities include the socially competitive aspects of reward in the Domino but not MID task. The Domino Task is played in a social context, where participants are told that they have a human opponent. Neural activity related to reward and punishment outcomes may have both social and monetary influences; thus, the two tasks assess different aspects of these domains.

Both the VS and a functionally connected brain region, the ventromedial prefrontal cortex, are frequently implicated in reward-processing networks including tasks assessing decision-making under risk [76,77]. We saw no hypoactivity in these regions as predicted by the reward-deficiency hypothesis. We did, however, see greater VS activation related to higher behavioral risk-taking (Factor 5) scores, possibly more consistent with a model of enhanced pro-motivational drive and diminished cognitive control. These findings might explain reward saliency/processing in at-risk individuals, as measured by risk-taking rather than FHA. The positive correlation with risk-taking differs from the inverse correlation seen with self-reported impulsivity and VS activation

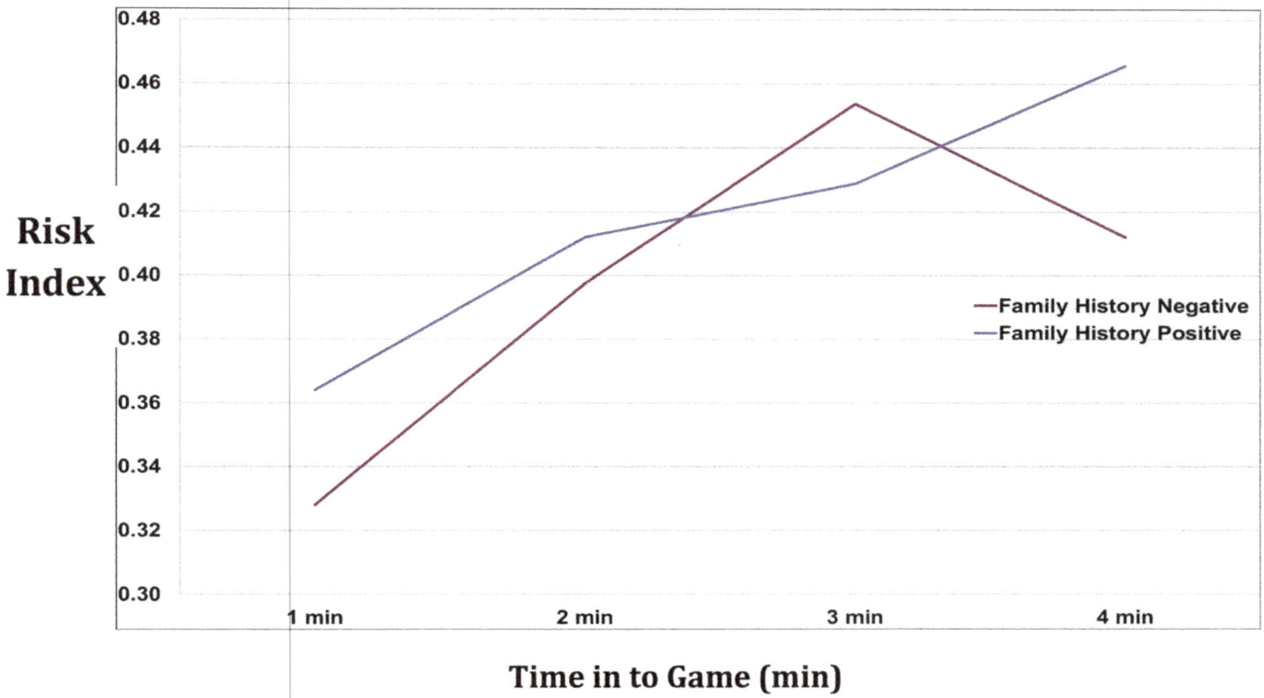

Figure 2. Risk indices by group (Family History Positive and Family History Negative) over time in to game. Risk Index was derived by dividing number of non-match choices by number of total choices when non-match and match choices were available to the player. FHP (a) and FHN (b) data are plotted by minute into game with standard error (averaged for all games for all subjects). No significant differences were found between groups. There was a significant main effect of time across groups ($F = 9.58$, $df = 3, 201$, $p < .0001$).

during reward anticipation during MID performance in individuals with alcohol dependence or pathological gambling [13]. The extent to which this represents differences in subject groups, tasks (including social and/or competitive aspects), risk-taking versus self-reported impulsivity or other factors warrants additional study.

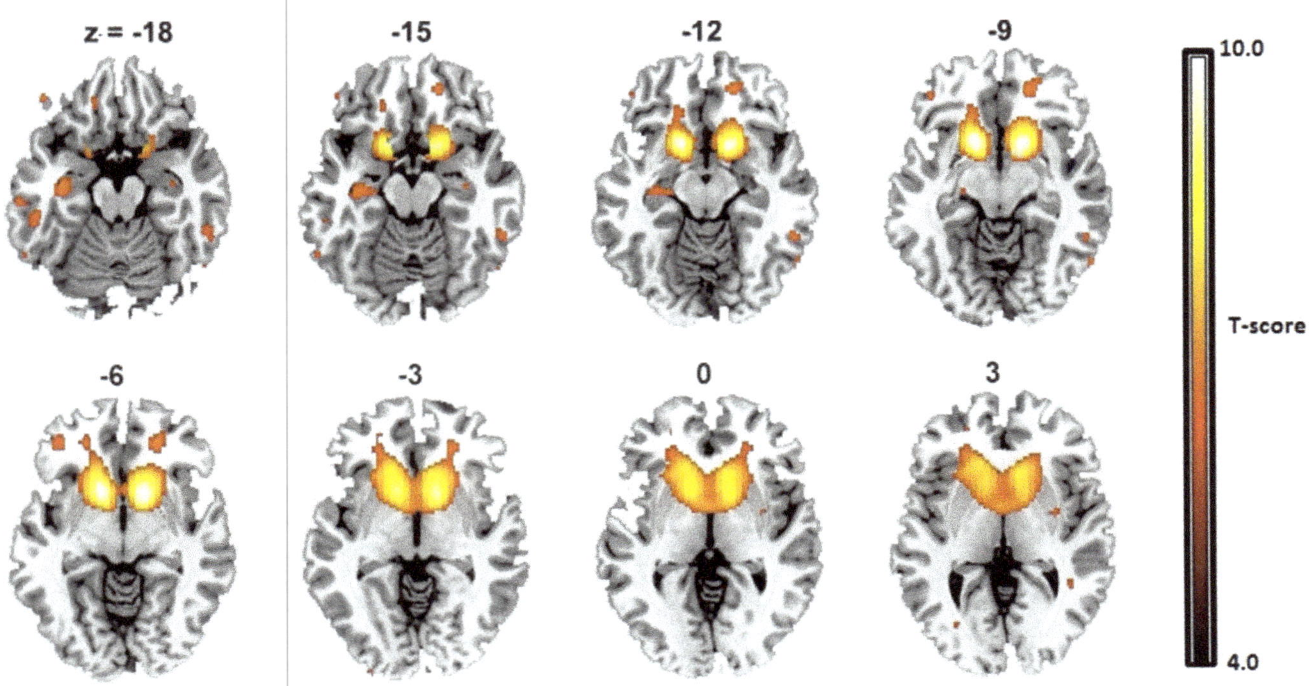

Figure 3. Reward Network. One-sample t-maps of the Reward-Punishment contrast for all subjects ($n = 69$) were used to construct the "reward network". The threshold was set at $p < 0.05$ FWE whole-brain corrected. Axial slices are depicted from $z = -18$ mm to $z = +3$ mm.

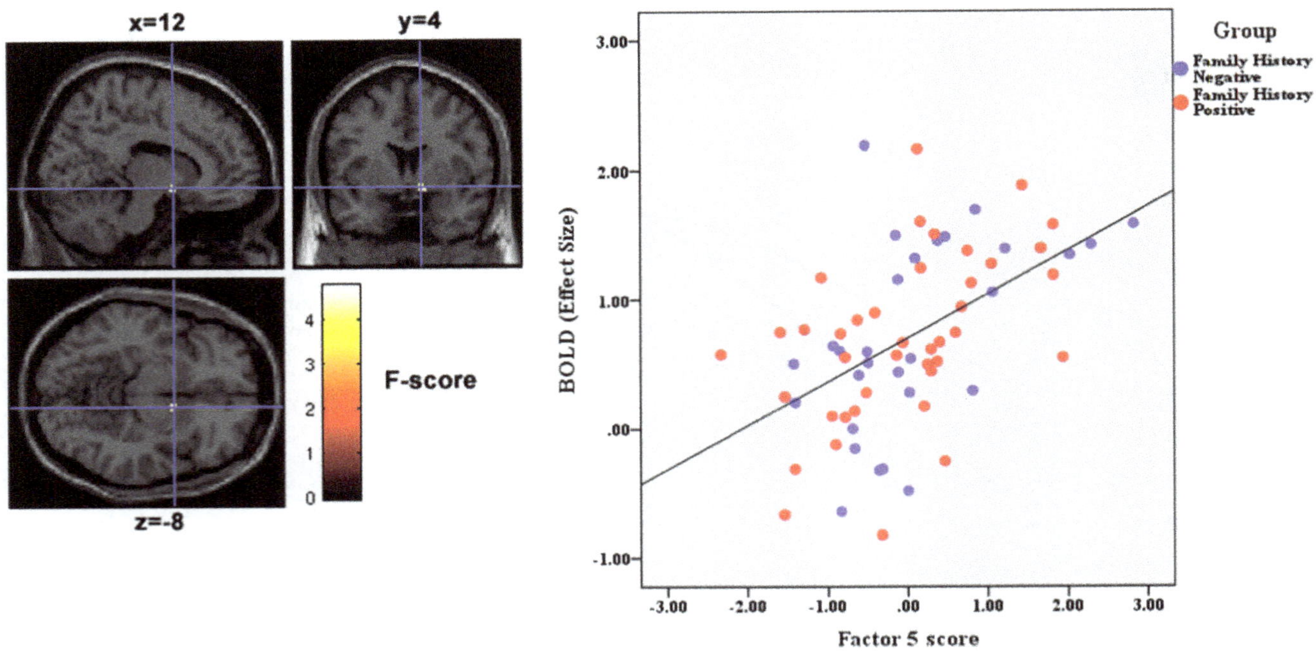

Figure 4. Correlation of Impulsivity-related Factor 5 (Behavorial Risk-Taking) scores with neural activation under the reward-punishment contrast across all subjects. A. Threshold was set at $p<0.05$ FWE for voxels within the reward network mask. Statistical parametric F-maps (sagittal, coronal and axial) of the Reward-Punishment contrast for multiple regression against Factor 5 - "Behavioral Risk-Taking". Crosshairs overlaid on brain slices are at the voxel of peak correlation (MNI coordinates: x,y,z = 12,4,–8). Bottom panel depicts individual factor scores vs. individual peak cluster activation at this voxel. **B**. Linear regression plot at the voxel of peak correlation between reward-punishment BOLD activity in the right ventral caudate and Factor-5 score for each subject.

One interpretation of our data is that individuals with greater BART risk-taking scores display activity in cognitive control and reward regions that is more typical of adolescence, a time when reward-seeking and impulsive behavior is maximal. Impaired adult reward response may be associated with atypical development of reward circuitry[2,38,78–80]. Adolescents engage VS more robustly than both children and adults during reward anticipation [56,57] and receipt [55,81]. However, some publications suggest the opposite is true in adolescents [57]. While this interpretation is speculative, it suggests that some impulsivity-related features might be based in persistently immature mesocorticolimbic circuitry.

FHP versus FHN subjects scored higher on impulsivity-related factor-2. This same factor was inversely correlated with VS BOLD response during the MID anticipation phase in our previous work investigating FHA, highlighting differences in neural responsiveness between reward anticipation and outcome presentation and the different task contexts [6]. In current and former cocaine-dependent subjects, impulsivity-related factor-2 scores correlated with right dorsal caudate BOLD signal under a reward> punishment contrast. Such factor analytically derived impulsivity-related measures are useful in clarifying relationships with brain biology. Additionally, these measures highlight neurobiological differences across at-risk and addicted populations.

A previous study of young adolescents with alcoholism vulnerability also reported no differences in reward-related neural responsiveness, but observed differences in sensation-seeking scores [57]. Impulsive behavior likely subsumes cognitive and motor control, in addition to reward sensitivity, and these neurobiological underpinnings should be parsed when considering the genetic and social influences and/or correlates of AUDs [82], analogous to animal models [83,84]. VS is a germane neural region as it receives input from cortico-limbic regions involved in cognitive control [85]. The current data contribute to a growing literature on aspects of impulsivity-related constructs and FHA, a characteristic representing a possible risk factor for various disorders, including alcoholism, substance abuse, ADHD, binge-eating disorder, pathological gambling, and bipolar disorder.

We recognize study limitations. FHA relies on self-report data from individuals for themselves and family members. We also did not record data on history of subject smoking status, which could influence brain activation patterns. Our FHP subjects have passed early vulnerability ages for substance abuse and therefore may show more similar brain activation patterns to FHN subjects than other FHP individuals with substance-use disorders. As an interpersonal game, the Domino task includes neural activation during reward and punishment events subsuming both social and monetary elements. The ventral caudate has been linked with dysfunctional reward processing in other studies of disorders characterized by poor impulse control; these neural differences may be attributable to variations in motivational drive or cognitive control that should be examined directly in future research.

Conclusions

Impulsivity is a broad trait with subfeatures that are not clearly distinguished by current standardized measurements. In this study, we demonstrate that FHP individuals exhibit risk-taking behavior that is different from FHN individuals by one impulsivity component. Also, behavioral risk-taking scores correlate with neural activity during reward responsiveness in the VS during an interactive competitive fMRI task in all subjects. This is a brain region that shows consistent association with impulsivity measures in previous tasks, and across several disorders. These findings show that impulsivity components may better highlight differences in disease states than a single measure.

Author Contributions

Conceived and designed the experiments: MA GP. Performed the experiments: RJK. Analyzed the data: HY CH SM. Contributed reagents/materials/analysis tools: GP MA. Wrote the paper: HY. Edited manuscript: MP GP MA CH. Advised on analysis: GP MA.

References

1. Robbins T, Curran H, de Wit H (2012) Special issue on impulsivity and compulsivity. Psychopharmacology (Berl) 219: 251–252.
2. Dalley JW, Everitt BJ, Robbins TW (2011) Impulsivity, compulsivity, and top-down cognitive control. Neuron 69: 680–694.
3. Everitt BJ, Parkinson JA, Olmstead MC, Arroyo M, Robledo P, et al. (1999) Associative processes in addiction and reward. The role of amygdala-ventral striatal subsystems. Ann N Y Acad Sci 877: 412–438.
4. Tanaka SC, Doya K, Okada G, Ueda K, Okamoto Y, et al. (2004) Prediction of immediate and future rewards differentially recruits cortico-basal ganglia loops. Nat Neurosci 7: 887–893.
5. Heimer L, Van Hoesen GW (2006) The limbic lobe and its output channels: implications for emotional functions and adaptive behavior. Neurosci Biobehav Rev 30: 126–147.
6. Andrews MM, Meda SA, Thomas AD, Potenza MN, Krystal JH, et al. (2011) Individuals family history positive for alcoholism show functional magnetic resonance imaging differences in reward sensitivity that are related to impulsivity factors. Biol Psychiatry 69: 675–683.
7. Zalla T, Koechlin E, Pietrini P, Basso G, Aquino P, et al. (2000) Differential amygdala responses to winning and losing: a functional magnetic resonance imaging study in humans. Eur J Neurosci 12: 1764–1770.
8. Sallet J, Quilodran R, Rothe M, Vezoli J, Joseph JP, et al. (2007) Expectations, gains, and losses in the anterior cingulate cortex. Cogn Affect Behav Neurosci 7: 327–336.
9. Winstanley CA (2007) The orbitofrontal cortex, impulsivity, and addiction: probing orbitofrontal dysfunction at the neural, neurochemical, and molecular level. Ann N Y Acad Sci 1121: 639–655.
10. Pattij T, Vanderschuren LJ (2008) The neuropharmacology of impulsive behaviour. Trends Pharmacol Sci 29: 192–199.
11. Goldstein RZ, Tomasi D, Alia-Klein N, Cottone LA, Zhang L, et al. (2007) Subjective sensitivity to monetary gradients is associated with frontolimbic activation to reward in cocaine abusers. Drug Alcohol Depend 87: 233–240.
12. Ahmadi A, Pearlson GD, Meda SA, Dager A, Potenza MN, et al. (2013) Influence of Alcohol Use on Neural Response to Go/No-Go Task in College Drinkers. Neuropsychopharmacology.
13. Balodis IM, Kober H, Worhunsky PD, Stevens MC, Pearlson GD, et al. (2012) Diminished frontostriatal activity during processing of monetary rewards and losses in pathological gambling. Biol Psychiatry 71: 749–757.
14. Knutson B, Cooper JC (2005) Functional magnetic resonance imaging of reward prediction. Curr Opin Neurol 18: 411–417.
15. Liu X, Powell DK, Wang H, Gold BT, Corbly CR, et al. (2007) Functional dissociation in frontal and striatal areas for processing of positive and negative reward information. J Neurosci 27: 4587–4597.
16. Hyatt CJ, Assaf M, Muska CE, Rosen RI, Thomas AD, et al. (2012) Reward-related dorsal striatal activity differences between former and current cocaine dependent individuals during an interactive competitive game. PLoS One 7: e34917.
17. Knutson B, Westdorp A, Kaiser E, Hommer D (2000) FMRI visualization of brain activity during a monetary incentive delay task. Neuroimage 12: 20–27.
18. Devito EE, Meda SA, Jiantonio R, Potenza MN, Krystal JH, et al. (2013) Neural Correlates of Impulsivity in Healthy Males and Females with Family Histories of Alcoholism. Neuropsychopharmacology.
19. Patel KT, Stevens MC, Meda SA, Muska C, Thomas AD, et al. (2013) Robust Changes in Reward Circuitry During Reward Loss in Current and Former Cocaine Users During Performance of a Monetary Incentive Delay Task. Biol Psychiatry.
20. Adcock RA, Thangavel A, Whitfield-Gabrieli S, Knutson B, Gabrieli JD (2006) Reward-motivated learning: mesolimbic activation precedes memory formation. Neuron 50: 507–517.
21. Eagle DM, Baunez C, Hutcheson DM, Lehmann O, Shah AP, et al. (2008) Stop-signal reaction-time task performance: role of prefrontal cortex and subthalamic nucleus. Cereb Cortex 18: 178–188.
22. Beck A, Schlagenhauf F, Wustenberg T, Hein J, Kienast T, et al. (2009) Ventral striatal activation during reward anticipation correlates with impulsivity in alcoholics. Biol Psychiatry 66: 734–742.
23. Balodis IM, Kober H, Worhunsky PD, White MA, Stevens MC, et al. (2013) Monetary reward processing in obese individuals with and without binge eating disorder. Biol Psychiatry 73: 877–886.
24. Blum K, Braverman ER, Holder JM, Lubar JF, Monastra VJ, et al. (2000) Reward deficiency syndrome: a biogenetic model for the diagnosis and treatment of impulsive, addictive, and compulsive behaviors. J Psychoactive Drugs 32 Suppl: i-iv, 1–112.
25. Volkow ND, Wang GJ, Fowler JS, Telang F (2008) Overlapping neuronal circuits in addiction and obesity: evidence of systems pathology. Philos Trans R Soc Lond B Biol Sci 363: 3191–3200.
26. Volkow ND, Fowler JS, Wang GJ, Swanson JM (2004) Dopamine in drug abuse and addiction: results from imaging studies and treatment implications. Mol Psychiatry 9: 557–569.
27. Peters J, Bromberg U, Schneider S, Brassen S, Menz M, et al. (2011) Lower ventral striatal activation during reward anticipation in adolescent smokers. Am J Psychiatry 168: 540–549.
28. Congdon E, Canli T (2008) A neurogenetic approach to impulsivity. J Pers 76: 1447–1484.
29. Meda SA, Stevens MC, Potenza MN, Pittman B, Gueorguieva R, et al. (2009) Investigating the behavioral and self-report constructs of impulsivity domains using principal component analysis. Behav Pharmacol 20: 390–399.
30. Acheson A, Richard D.M., Mathias C.W. and D.M Dougherty (2011) Adults with a family history of alcohol related problems are more impulsive on measures of response initiation and response inhibition. Drug Alcohol Depend 117: 198–203.
31. Ginley MK, Whelan JP, Meyers AW, Relyea GE, Pearlson GD (2013) Exploring a Multidimensional Approach to Impulsivity in Predicting College Student Gambling. J Gambl Stud.
32. Patel K, Stevens, M C., Meda, S A., Muska C., Thomas, A D., Potenza, M N., Pearlson, G D. (2013) Robust Changes in Reward Circuitry During Reward Loss in Current and Former Cocaine Users During Performance of a Monetary Incentive Delay Task. Biol Psychiatry.
33. Saunders B, Farag N, Vincent AS, Collins FL, Jr., Sorocco KH, et al. (2008) Impulsive errors on a Go-NoGo reaction time task: disinhibitory traits in relation to a family history of alcoholism. Alcohol Clin Exp Res 32: 888–894.
34. Hill SY, Shen S, Lowers L, Locke-Wellman J, Matthews AG, et al. (2008) Psychopathology in offspring from multiplex alcohol dependence families with and without parental alcohol dependence: a prospective study during childhood and adolescence. Psychiatry Res 160: 155–166.
35. Chen AC, Porjesz B, Rangaswamy M, Kamarajan C, Tang Y, et al. (2007) Reduced frontal lobe activity in subjects with high impulsivity and alcoholism. Alcohol Clin Exp Res 31: 156–165.
36. McGue M (1997) A behavioral-genetic perspective on children of alcoholics. Alcohol Health Res World 21: 210–217.
37. Galvan A (2010) Adolescent development of the reward system. Front Hum Neurosci 4: 6.
38. Doremus-Fitzwater TL, Varlinskaya EI, Spear LP (2010) Motivational systems in adolescence: possible implications for age differences in substance abuse and other risk-taking behaviors. Brain Cogn 72: 114–123.
39. Spear LP, Varlinskaya EI (2010) Sensitivity to ethanol and other hedonic stimuli in an animal model of adolescence: implications for prevention science? Dev Psychobiol 52: 236–243.
40. Sigvardsson S, Bohman M, Cloninger CR (1996) Replication of the Stockholm Adoption Study of alcoholism. Confirmatory cross-fostering analysis. Arch Gen Psychiatry 53: 681–687.
41. Ruocco AC, Laporte L, Russell J, Guttman H, Paris J (2012) Response inhibition deficits in unaffected first-degree relatives of patients with borderline personality disorder. Neuropsychology 26: 473–482.
42. Jamadar S, DeVito EE, Jiantonio RE, Meda SA, Stevens MC, et al. (2012) Memantine, an NMDA receptor antagonist, differentially influences Go/No-Go performance and fMRI activity in individuals with and without a family history of alcoholism. Psychopharmacology (Berl) 222: 129–140.
43. Sher KJ, Walitzer KS, Wood PK, Brent EE (1991) Characteristics of children of alcoholics: putative risk factors, substance use and abuse, and psychopathology. J Abnorm Psychol 100: 427–448.
44. Herting MM, Schwartz D, Mitchell SH, Nagel BJ (2010) Delay discounting behavior and white matter microstructure abnormalities in youth with a family history of alcoholism. Alcohol Clin Exp Res 34: 1590–1602.
45. Lovallo WR, Yechiam E, Sorocco KH, Vincent AS, Collins FL (2006) Working memory and decision-making biases in young adults with a family history of alcoholism: studies from the Oklahoma family health patterns project. Alcohol Clin Exp Res 30: 763–773.
46. Cservenka A, Nagel BJ (2012) Risky decision-making: an FMRI study of youth at high risk for alcoholism. Alcohol Clin Exp Res 36: 604–615.
47. Cservenka A, Herting MM, Nagel BJ (2012) Atypical frontal lobe activity during verbal working memory in youth with a family history of alcoholism. Drug Alcohol Depend 123: 98–104.
48. Dougherty DM, Mathias CW, Tester ML, Marsh DM (2004) Age at first drink relates to behavioral measures of impulsivity: the immediate and delayed memory tasks. Alcohol Clin Exp Res 28: 408–414.
49. Hansell NK, Agrawal A, Whitfield JB, Morley KI, Zhu G, et al. (2008) Long-term stability and heritability of telephone interview measures of alcohol consumption and dependence. Twin Res Hum Genet 11: 287–305.
50. Yan J, Aliev F, Webb BT, Kendler KS, Williamson VS, et al. (2013) Using genetic information from candidate gene and genome-wide association studies in risk prediction for alcohol dependence. Addict Biol.

51. Soderpalm Gordh AH, Soderpalm B (2011) Healthy subjects with a family history of alcoholism show increased stimulative subjective effects of alcohol. Alcohol Clin Exp Res 35: 1426–1434.
52. Dager AD, Anderson BM, Stevens MC, Pulido C, Rosen R, et al. (2013) Influence of alcohol use and family history of alcoholism on neural response to alcohol cues in college drinkers. Alcohol Clin Exp Res 37 Suppl 1: E161–171.
53. Elkins IJ, McGue M, Malone S, Iacono WG (2004) The effect of parental alcohol and drug disorders on adolescent personality. Am J Psychiatry 161: 670–676.
54. Yau WY, Zubieta JK, Weiland BJ, Samudra PG, Zucker RA, et al. (2012) Nucleus accumbens response to incentive stimuli anticipation in children of alcoholics: relationships with precursive behavioral risk and lifetime alcohol use. J Neurosci 32: 2544–2551.
55. Padmanabhan A, Geier CF, Ordaz SJ, Teslovich T, Luna B (2011) Developmental changes in brain function underlying the influence of reward processing on inhibitory control. Dev Cogn Neurosci 1: 517–529.
56. Geier CF, Terwilliger R, Teslovich T, Velanova K, Luna B (2010) Immaturities in reward processing and its influence on inhibitory control in adolescence. Cereb Cortex 20: 1613–1629.
57. Bjork JM, Knutson B, Hommer DW (2008) Incentive-elicited striatal activation in adolescent children of alcoholics. Addiction 103: 1308–1319.
58. Bornovalova MA, Cashman-Rolls A, O'Donnell JM, Ettinger K, Richards JB, et al. (2009) Risk taking differences on a behavioral task as a function of potential reward/loss magnitude and individual differences in impulsivity and sensation seeking. Pharmacol Biochem Behav 93: 258–262.
59. First MB SR, Gibbon M, Williams JBW. (2002) Structured Clinical Interview for DSM-IV-TR axis I disorders, research version, patient edition. (SCID-I/P) Biometrics Research. New York New York State Psychiatric Institute.
60. Assaf M, Kahn I, Pearlson GD, Johnson MR, Yeshurun Y, et al. (2009) Brain Activity Dissociates Mentalization from Motivation During an Interpersonal Competitive Game. Brain Imaging Behav 3: 24–37.
61. Kahn I, Yeshurun Y, Rotshtein P, Fried I, Ben-Bashat D, et al. (2002) The role of the amygdala in signaling prospective outcome of choice. Neuron 33: 983–994.
62. Carver CS, White TL (1994) Behavioral inhibition, behavioral activation, and affective responses to impending reward and punishment: The BIS/BAS Scales. Journal of Personality and Social Psychology 67: 319–333.
63. Patton JH, Stanford MS, Barratt ES (1995) Factor structure of the Barratt impulsiveness scale. J Clin Psychol 51: 768–774.
64. Torrubia R, Avila C, Molto J, Caseras X (2001) The Sensitivity to Punishment and Sensitivity to Reward Questionnaire (SPSRQ) as a measure of Gray's anxiety and impulsivity dimensions. Personality and Individual Differences 31: 837–862.
65. Zuckerman M (1979) Abbreviated Manual with Scoring Keys and Forms for Form V of the Sensation Seeking Scale. Newark, Delaware.
66. Sternberger LG, Burns GL (1990) Obsessions and compulsions: Psychometric properties of the Padua Inventory with an American college population. Behaviour Research & Therapy 28: 341–345.
67. Lejuez CW, Read JP, Kahler CW, Richards JB, Ramsey SE, et al. (2002) Evaluation of a behavioral measure of risk taking: the Balloon Analogue Risk Task (BART). J Exp Psychol Appl 8: 75–84.
68. Reynolds B, Schiffbauer R (2004) Measuring state changes in human delay discounting: an experiential discounting task. Behav Processes 67: 343–356.
69. Leroy PJRaAM (1987) Robust Regression and Outlier Detection. Wiley Series in Probability and Mathematical Statistics.
70. Friston KJ AJ, Frith CD, Poline JB, Heather JD, Frackowiak RSJ (1995) patial registration and normalization of images. Human Brain Mapping 3: 165–189.
71. KT. Patel MS, SA Meda, C Muska, AD Thomas, MN Potenza, GD Pearlson (2013) Robust Changes in Reward Circuitry during Reward Loss in Current and Former Cocaine Users during Performance of a Monetary Incentive Delay Task. BIological Psychiatry in press.
72. Wolen AR, Miles MF (2012) Identifying gene networks underlying the neurobiology of ethanol and alcoholism. Alcohol Res 34: 306–317.
73. Hill SY, Wang S, Kostelnik B, Carter H, Holmes B, et al. (2009) Disruption of orbitofrontal cortex laterality in offspring from multiplex alcohol dependence families. Biol Psychiatry 65: 129–136.
74. Choi JS, Shin YC, Jung WH, Jang JH, Kang DH, et al. (2012) Altered brain activity during reward anticipation in pathological gambling and obsessive-compulsive disorder. PLoS One 7: e45938.
75. Edel MA, Enzi B, Witthaus H, Tegenthoff M, Peters S, et al. (2012) Differential reward processing in subtypes of adult attention deficit hyperactivity disorder. J Psychiatr Res.
76. Bechara A (2003) Risky business: emotion, decision-making, and addiction. J Gambl Stud 19: 23–51.
77. Knutson B, Fong GW, Adams CM, Varner JL, Hommer D (2001) Dissociation of reward anticipation and outcome with event-related fMRI. Neuroreport 12: 3683–3687.
78. Fareri DS, Martin LN, Delgado MR (2008) Reward-related processing in the human brain: developmental considerations. Dev Psychopathol 20: 1191–1211.
79. Whelan R, Conrod PJ, Poline JB, Lourdusamy A, Banaschewski T, et al. (2012) Adolescent impulsivity phenotypes characterized by distinct brain networks. Nat Neurosci 15: 920–925.
80. Duka T (2011) Deficits in reward system activation and impulsivity: a predisposing condition to alcoholism? Biol Psychiatry 69: 612–613.
81. Somerville LH, Hare T, Casey BJ (2011) Frontostriatal maturation predicts cognitive control failure to appetitive cues in adolescents. J Cogn Neurosci 23: 2123–2134.
82. Tessner KD, Hill SY (2010) Neural circuitry associated with risk for alcohol use disorders. Neuropsychol Rev 20: 1–20.
83. Hayton SJ, Olmstead MC, Dumont EC (2011) Shift in the intrinsic excitability of medial prefrontal cortex neurons following training in impulse control and cued-responding tasks. PLoS One 6: e23885.
84. Bryden DW, Burton AC, Kashtelyan V, Barnett BR, Roesch MR (2012) Response inhibition signals and miscoding of direction in dorsomedial striatum. Front Integr Neurosci 6: 69.
85. E. Camara AR-F, Z Ye, T.F Munte (2009) Reward networks in the brain as captured by connectivity measures. Front Hum Neurosci 3: 350–362.

6

Depressive Symptoms in People with and without Alcohol Abuse: Factor Structure and Measurement Invariance of the Beck Depression Inventory (BDI-II) Across Groups

Cecilie Skule[1]*, Pål Ulleberg[2], Hilde Dallavara Lending[1], Torkil Berge[1], Jens Egeland[2,3], Tim Brennen[2], Nils Inge Landrø[2]

1 Community Mental Health Center Vinderen, Diakonhjemmet Hospital, Oslo, Norway, **2** Department of Psychology, University of Oslo, Oslo, Norway, **3** Vestfold Mental Health Care Trust, Tønsberg, Norway

Abstract

This study explored differences in the factor structure of depressive symptoms in patients with and without alcohol abuse, and differences in the severity of depressive symptoms between the two groups. In a sample of 358 patients without alcohol problems and 167 patients with comorbid alcohol problems, confirmatory factor analysis revealed that the same factor structures, Beck et al.'s two-factor Somatic Affective-Cognitive (SA-C) model, and Buckley et al.'s three-factor Cognitive-Affective- Somatic (C-A-S) model, demonstrated the best fit to the data in both groups. The SA-C model was preferred due to its more parsimonious nature. Evidence for strict measurement invariance across the two groups for the SA-C model was found. MIMIC (multiple-indicator-multiple-cause) modeling showed that the level of depressive symptoms was found to be highest on both factors in the group with comorbid alcohol problems. The magnitude of the differences in latent mean scores suggested a moderate difference in the level of depressive symptoms between the two groups. It is argued that patients with comorbid depression and alcohol abuse should be offered parallel and adequate treatment for both conditions.

Editor: Brett Thombs, McGill University, Canada

Funding: The research was funded by the Regional Competence Centre for Double Diagnoses, South Eastern Norway, and the research fund in the Community Mental Health Center, Vinderen, Diakonhjemmet Hospital, Oslo. The funders had no role in study design, data collection and analysis, decision to publish, or preparation of the manuscript.

Competing Interests: The authors have declared that no competing interests exist.

* E-mail: cecilie9@diakonsyk.no

Introduction

The co-occurrence of mood symptoms and the abuse of alcohol and other drugs is common [1,2,3]. Patients with comorbid major depression and substance abuse tend to be more severely depressed than those without the combined condition [4]. Among medical inpatients, more severe depressive symptoms are associated with unhealthy drinking [5].

Self-report instruments, such as the Beck Depression Inventory-II (BDI-II), are often used in clinical practice and research. However, research on the BDI-II and other self-report instruments in patients with comorbid depression and substance use disorders is scarce [6]. Studies have investigated the factor structure of the BDI-II [8,9]. A three-factor model consisting of a cognitive, affective and somatic factor seems to usually give the best fit [10,11,12], but there are exceptions [7,9]. It has been claimed that the factor structure of BDI-II scores differ among various clinical populations [13]. If the BDI-II measure fails to operate in the same manner across groups (i.e. there is a lack of measurement invariance of the construct), the between-group differences in the mean scores of the BDI-II may be misleading. However, no previous study has compared the severity of depressive symptoms and the factor structure of depressive symptoms between a clinical sample of depressed participants with and without comorbid alcohol abuse.

It is often assumed that the clinical implications of depressive symptoms in patients with substance abuse are different than those in depressed patients without substance abuse. This study examines the factor structure of the BDI-II in a large clinical sample of people seeking treatment for depression. Some of the participants have concurrent problems of alcohol abuse, therefore allowing a comparison of the two samples.

In this study we have two research aims: to identify differences in the factor structure of depressive symptoms in patients with and without alcohol abuse, and to identify differences in the severity of depressive symptoms between the two groups.

Subjects and Methods

Participants

Participants were recruited from the attendees of cognitive-behavioral courses of treatment for depression either via individual consultations or in groups. In the preconsultation or during information meetings held by group leaders/therapists conducted before treatment start, the participants were informed about the study and asked if they would like to participate in this research project. They were informed that participation was voluntary and were informed that they could leave the project at any time, and if they decided not to participate in the project, it would not have any consequences for the treatment they were offered. Participation in the project was not paid for. Exclusion criteria for taking part in the treatment program were psychotic or acute suicidal symptoms. The participants were from the same health region in the south and east part of Norway. Most of the participants were recruited from community mental health centers. A small group was recruited from a substance abuse clinic. In total 525 patients provided written informed consent, and all participants were considered to possess competent consent. The project was approved by Regional Committees for Medical and Health Research Ethics in the South East Health Region in Norway. The research was funded by the Regional Competence Centre for Double Diagnoses, South Eastern Norway and the research fund in the Community Mental Health Center, Vinderen, Diakonhjemmet Hospital, Oslo. The funders had no role in study design, data collection and analysis, decision to publish, or preparation of the manuscript.

Instruments

The Beck Depression Inventory - Second Edition (BDI-II) [7] is one of the most commonly used self-report instruments for estimating the severity of depression. The total score indicates whether the individual presents a mild, moderate or major depression. The BDI-II consists of 21 items, each of which is scored on a scale from 0 to 3. The maximum score is 63. The recommended cutoff for minimal depression is 13, whereas a score of 14–19 indicates mild, 20–28 moderate and 29–63 serious depression.

The Alcohol Use Disorders Identification Test (AUDIT) [14] consists of ten items and can be self-administered by the patient. Each item is scored on a 4-point scale. The total ranges from 0–40, and a score larger than 7 indicates an alcohol problem. Based on research the following categories have been identified for the total score: 0–7 low risk, 8–15 moderate risk and 16–19 major risk.

Procedure

A total of 525 patients provided informed consent. In addition to the BDI-II and substance abuse screening using the AUDIT, participants answered questions on their demographics and their history of depression. The patients completed the screening before the cognitive-behavioral course of treatment for depression started.

Statistical Analyses

Confirmatory factor analyses based upon maximum likelihood estimation were applied to test the fit of the various models to the data of both samples (descriptive statistics and intercorrelations among the 21 items is presented separately for each sample in Appendix A and B). All models were estimated using the statistical software Mplus 6.1 [15]. Because the data were expected to have a non-normal distribution, the models were estimated using maximum likelihood estimation and tested with the Satorra-Bentler scaled chi-square [16]. The fit of the models was evaluated using several $\chi 2$ goodness-of fit-statistics; the comparative fit index (CFI), the root mean square error of approximation (RMSEA) and the standardized root mean squared residual (SRMR). As a general rule, a CFI above .95, and a RMSEA/SRMR below .06 indicates a very good fit between the model and the data, whereas a RMSEA below .08, SRMR below .09 and a CFI above .90 is conventionally regarded as a reasonable fit [17,18]. The fit of the various factor structures were estimated separately for each sample.

Measurement invariance across groups of the best-fitting factor structures was tested in several models, using Multigroup Confirmatory Factor Analysis. The procedure involved examining changes in model fit measures after imposing increasingly restrictive conditions of invariance [19]. The first model tested whether the same items are associated with the same factor in both groups. This is commonly referred to as configural invariance. The second model involved examining the invariance of the factor loadings, meaning that the loadings are the equal in both groups. The equality of covariance between residuals was also included in this model. The third model tested for invariance at the intercept level of the items. This level of invariance (together with measurement invariance established in the previous models) is required to compare differences in the latent mean scores between groups. The fourth model involved invariance of the item residuals, signifying that all group differences on the items are due to group differences on the level of the common factors. This model is, however, regarded as representing a very stringent criterion, and is rarely fulfilled in practice [20,21]. Two additional models were also estimated; model 5 tested for invariance in factor variances and model 6 for invariance in the covariance between factors across groups.

Traditionally, evidence supporting measurement invariance has been based on non-significant differences in the chi-square value ($\Delta\chi 2$) relative to the change in the degrees of freedom (Δdf) between nested models. If the $\Delta\chi 2$ is significant for the more restrictive model, it can be assumed that that the two models are not equivalent (i.e. non-invariant) across groups. However, the $\Delta\chi 2$ value is highly sensitive to the sample size, and based on simulation studies, researchers [20,21] have recommended alternative criteria for evaluating measurement invariance across groups. According to Chen [21], the following cutoff values have been suggested to indicate non-invariance in large samples ($N>300$): a change of $\geq -.01$ in CFI, supplemented by a change of $\geq .015$ in RMSEA or a change of $\geq .030$ in SRMR.

Differences in the severity of depressive symptoms between the groups with and without comorbid alcohol problems was examined using MIMIC (multiple-indicator-multiple-cause) modeling. MIMIC modeling is comparable to a multivariate regression model in which latent variables (e.g. latent scores on factors of depression) are "caused" by independent variables. The main independent variable in this case the grouping variable separating between those with and without comorbid alcohol problems. Possible systematic differences between the two groups on other variables potentially related to depression scores (e.g. gender, age) may also be included in such an analysis as independent variables and thereby serve as covariates.

Results

Descriptive Statistics

Table 1 shows descriptive statistics for both samples. There were no significant differences in age and educational level between the two samples. There were significantly more men among the participants with a comorbid alcohol problem, and they were less likely to be married or have a registered partner compared to the sample without comorbid alcohol problems. The level of depression (as measured by the total BDI-II score) was 3.5 points higher in the sample with comorbid alcohol problems.

Table 1. *Patient demographics, AUDIT-score, and BDI-II-score.*

	Without comorbid alcohol problem (n = 358)	*With comorbid alcohol problem (n = 167)*	*t or χ^2-value*
Age (*M, SD*)	42.2 (11.3)	41.8 (13.0)	0.37
% Men	29.5	50.3	
% Women	70.5	49.7	22.09***
Highest educational level attained			
% Lower secondary	7.4	6.1	
% Upper secondary/vocational	11.6	9.8	
% Upper secondary/academic	13.3	20.2	
% Tertiary	67.7	63.8	4.57
Marital status			
% Single	29.1	39.0	
% Married/reg. partner	57.1	37.2	
% Divorced	12.4	23.2	
% Widow/widower	1.4	0.6	20.9***
AUDIT-score (*M, SD*)	3.2 (2.0)	14.5 (5.8)	−32.0***
Total BDI-II-score (*M, SD*)	23.1 (11.1)	26.6 (10.1)	−3.40***

***$p<.001$.

Model Testing

The alternative models presented in Figure 1 were separately estimated for each sample using confirmatory factor analysis. Table 2 shows that all models had good or acceptable RMSEA/SRMR values in both samples. In the sample without comorbid alcohol problems, the CFI for the one-factor model and the Beck et al.'s [7] CA-S model was below the conventional limits for acceptable fit (>.90). In the sample with concurrent alcohol problems, only the model proposed by Ward [9] had a CFI value above the threshold for acceptable fit.

The model formulated by Ward [9] was therefore the only one able to fulfill all the criteria for good or acceptable fit in both samples. However, a closer inspection of the factor loadings in Ward's model revealed the cognitive factor had several non-significant loadings in both samples. The proposed error covariance between Item 7 and Item 8 in the sample with concurrent alcohol problems was also nonsignificant. Furthermore, the residual variance was negative for item 20 and had to be constrained to zero to allow the model to converge. This feature suggested that Ward's [9] model was problematic due to inadequate factor loadings, and was therefore abandoned from further analyses. This justify studying the modification indices of the alternative models more closely. In all alternative models, the modification indices indicated that a rather large reduction in *SB*-chi square value could be obtained by allowing two pairs of correlated residuals: the first between Item 5 (guilty feelings) and Item 8 (self-criticalness): and the second between Item 15 (loss of energy) and item 20 (tiredness or fatigue). Both modifications were regarded as theoretically meaningful, because the items semantically overlapped and both pair of items clustered on the same factor in all models. No further modifications were found necessary.

Table 2 shows that the fit indices for all models improved after the modifications were implemented. In the sample without concurrent alcohol problems, all models demonstrated an acceptable or good fit to the data. In particular, Beck et al.'s [7] SA-C model and Buckley et al.'s [10] C-A-S model were regarded as better-fitting than the CA-S and one-factor model due to the difference in CFI-value (>.01) between these models. Although a Satorra-Bentler scaled chi-square difference test demonstrated that the Buckley et al. [10] model fitted significantly better to the data than the Beck et al. [7] SA-C model (SB χ^2_{diff} (2) = 13.2, $p<.01$), this difference was regarded as trivial due to the small differences in model fit measures between the two models.

In the sample with comorbid alcohol problems, Beck et al.'s [7] SA-C model and Buckley et al.'s [10] C-A-S model also demonstrated the best fit to the data compared to the two other modified models (e.g. ΔCFI≥.01). However, only the RMSEA and SRMR suggested adequate fit to the data for the two models, whereas the GFI and CFI were close to, but did not reach the threshold for acceptable values. Buckley et al.'s [10] model was significantly better fitting than Beck et al.'s [7] SA-C (SB χ^2_{diff} (2) = 10.3, $p<.01$) in this sample also. However, the comparison of the other model fit indices suggested that the difference between the two models was small (e.g. ΔCFI<.01).

Based on the small difference in model fit indices between the two models, Beck et al.'s [7] SA-C model was chosen as the preferred one due to its more parsimonious nature, i.e. represented by two factors instead of three factors as in the C-A-S model [10].

Measurement Invariance across Samples

Beck et al. [7] SA-C model was tested for measurement invariance across the two samples. As shown in Table 3, the change in fit indices fell well below the recommended cutoff values (ΔRMSEA≥.015, ΔCFI≥−.01 and ΔSRMR≥.030) at all six steps for testing invariance. Therefore, the results demonstrated support for measurement invariance across groups for the SA-C model. The same procedure for testing measurement invariance

Model 1: One-factor model

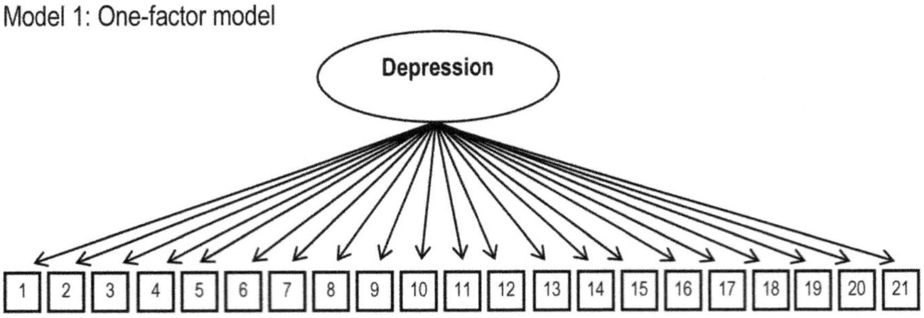

Model 2: Beck et al.'s [7] Cognitive and Somatic-affective factor model

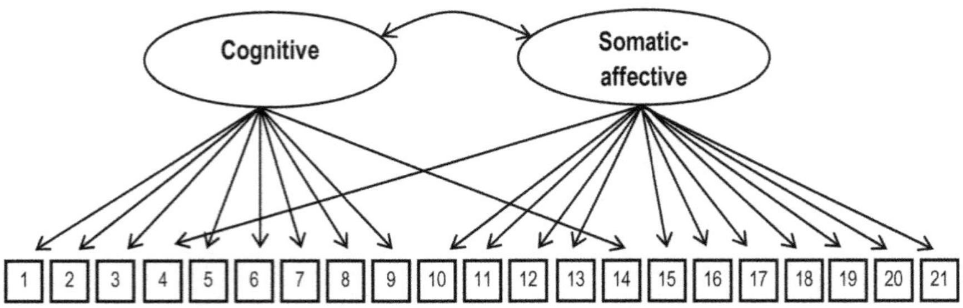

Model 3: Beck et al.'s [7] Cognitive-affective and Somatic factor model

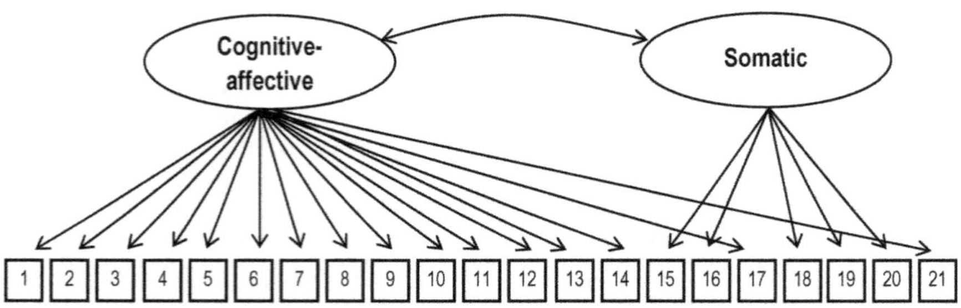

Model 4: Buckely et al.'s [10] Cognitive, Affective and Somatic factor model

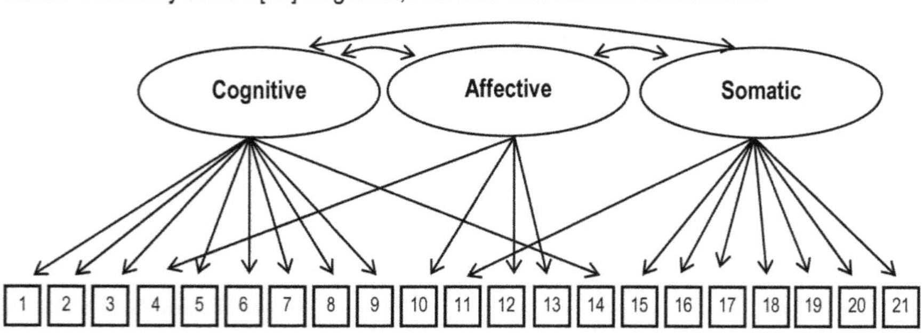

Model 5: Ward's [9] General, Cognitive and Somatic factor model

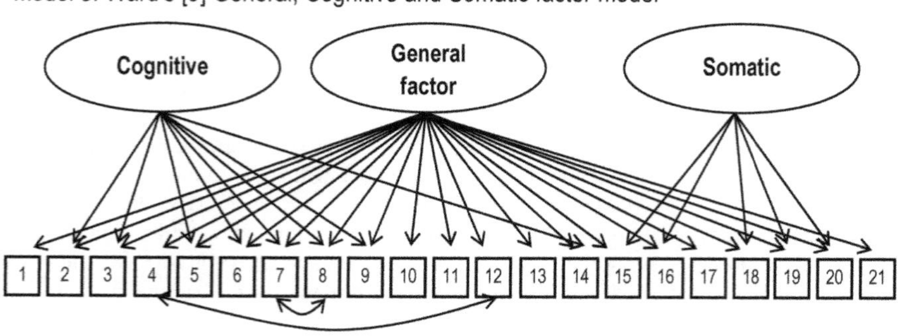

Figure 1. Factor structure of the different models tested.

was also applied for the C-A-S model [10], and this gave the same conclusion as for the SA-C model, i.e. support for measurement invariance across groups.

Table 4 shows the standardized factor loadings, factor correlations and error term correlations for the SA-C Beck model [7]. All parameters presented in Table 4 are significant at the 5% level.

Differences in Level of Depression Between the Samples

To test whether the level of depression on the Somatic-Affective and the Cognitive factor was different in the two samples, MIMIC modeling was applied using group (without vs. with comorbid alcohol problems) as the independent variable, and gender and marital status as covariates (due to significant differences between groups on these two variables). The results of the analysis showed that the latent mean score was significantly higher on both the Somatic-Affective (0.185 (0.053), $p<.001$) and the Cognitive factor (0.175 (0.044), $p<.001$) for patients with comorbid alcohol problems compared to those without alcohol problems. These differences indicate that although the factor structure is very similar in the two samples, the level of depression varies.

In order to examine the magnitude of the difference in latent mean scores, differences between groups in terms of standard deviation on the latent variables was estimated by setting the variance in each factor equal to 1. The results showed that the relative differences between groups were of about the same size on both factors, i.e. 0. 418 and 0.348 standard deviation on the Cognitive factor and Somatic-Affective factor, respectively. According to the criteria suggested by Cohen [22], this represents a moderate effect size.

Table 2. *Confirmatory factor analysis fit indices for five different factor models. Separately for the samples with and without comorbid alcohol problems.*

	SB χ^2	df	RMSEA	SRMR	CFI
Without comorbid alcohol problem (*n* = 358)					
Model 1: One factor model	557.6	189	.074	.056	.867
Modified model[b]	396.4	187	.056	.049	.919
Model 2: Beck et al. [7] SA-C	431.1	188	.060	.048	.936
Modified model[b]	312.0	186	.043	.042	.950
Model 3: Beck et al. [7] CA-S	464.1	188	.064	.054	.893
Modified model[b]	360.7	186	.051	.046	.932
Model 4: Buckley et al. [10] C-A-S	399.4	186	.057	.047	.917
Modified model[b]	299.1	184	.042	.040	.955
Model 5: Ward [9] G-C-S[a]	306.7	174	.046	.041	.949
With comorbid alcohol problem (*n* = 167)					
Model 1: One factor model	363.5	189	.074	.069	.836
Modified model[b]	331.7	187	.068	.067	.864
Model 2: Beck et al. [7] SA-C	335.1	188	.068	.069	.862
Modified model[b]	311.1	186	.063	.067	.882
Model 3: Beck et al [7] CA-S	339.1	188	.069	.070	.858
Modified model[b]	325.5	186	.067	.067	.869
Model 4: Buckley et al [10] C-A-S	316.7	186	.065	.067	.877
Modified model[b]	301.0	184	.062	.066	.890
Model 5: Ward [9] G-C-S[a, c]	261.9	175	.055	.061	.918

SB χ^2 = Satorra-Bentler corrected χ^2; *df* = degrees of freedom; RMSEA = root mean square of approximation; SRMR = Standardized root mean square; CFI = comparative fit index.
[a]Correlated residuals allowed for Items 4–12 and 7–8,
[b]Correlated residuals allowed for Items 5–8 and 15–20.
[c]Residual variance of item 20 constrained to zero.

Discussion

The results showed that the same models (i.e. Beck et al.'s [7] SA-C model and Buckley et al.'s [10] C-A-S model), gave the best fit to the data in both groups. The similarity in the factor structure of the BDI-II was further supported by the finding of measurement invariance across groups for both models. Although there are exceptions [see 13], this finding corroborates other studies examining samples of various drug abuse populations [10,11,12].

The two proposed factor structures are identical with regard to the Cognitive factor. The difference between the two models is that the Somatic-Affective factor in Beck et al.'s model is split into two factors in Buckley et al.'s [10] model: one Somatic factor and one Affective factor. Based on the small difference in model fit indices between the two models, one might argue that Beck et al.'s [7] SA-C model should be the preferred model due to its more parsimonious nature.

Patients with comorbid alcohol problems reported on average a higher degree of depressive symptoms on both the Somatic-Affective and the Cognitive factor. A higher score on depressive symptoms among patients with comorbid alcohol abuse has also described by Ostacher [4]. The magnitude of the difference in depressive symptoms on the two factors between the two groups was found to be of equal size, suggesting that alcohol abuse has an overall effect upon depressive symptoms. Others have claimed that the somatic factor in depression is closely related to abstinence and the intoxication of alcohol or other substances in patients with

Table 3. *Tests for measurement invariance across the sample without alcohol problems and the sample with comorbid alcohol problems for the SA-C model.*

	SB $\chi 2$	*Df*	RMSEA	SRMR	CFI
Beck et al. [7] SA-C:					
Model 1: Configural model	623.2	372	.051	.050	.932
Model 2a: Factor loadings invariant	659.8	391	.051	.062	.927
Model 2b: Residual cov. Invariant	664.1	393	.051	.066	.926
Model 3: Item intercepts invariant	694.4	412	.051	.064	.923
Model 4: Item residual variance invariant	726.4	433	.051	.064	.920
Model 5: Factor variance invariant	729.8	435	.051	.072	.920
Model 6: Factor covariance invariant	731.0	436	.051	.071	.920

SB χ^2 = Satorra-Bentler corrected χ^2; *df* = degrees of freedom; RMSEA = root mean square of approximation;
SRMR = Standardized root mean square; CFI = comparative fit index.

Table 4. *Multigroup confirmatory factor analysis with robust maximum likelihood estimation. Standardized factor loadings, factor correlation and error correlations for the modified SA-C model [7].*

	Standardized loadnings/ correlations
Cognitive	
1 Sadness	.659
2 Pessimism	.607
3 Past Failure	.691
5 Guilty Feelings	.587
6 Punishment Feelings	.462
7 Self-Dislike	.679
8 Self-Criticalness	.663
9 Suicidal Thoughts or Wishes	.530
14 Worthlessness	.732
Somatic-affective	
11 Agitation	.403
15 Loss of Energy	.661
16 Changes in Sleeping Pattern	.394
17 Irritability	.418
18 Changes in Appetite	.511
19 Concentration Difficulty	.707
20 Tiredness or Fatigue	.616
21 Loss of Interest in Sex	.481
4 Loss of Pleasure	.718
10 Crying	.528
12 Loss of Interest	.706
13 Indecisiveness	.686
Correlation C-SA	.859
Correlation e5–e8	.340
Correlation e15–e20	.449

All loadings/correlations are significant at the .001 level.

comorbid substance abuse [11]. On this basis, if is expected that the difference in level of depression between the two groups should primarily be found on the Somatic factor. This claim was not confirmed in our study [see also 12].

The results from the current study support the view that major depression and substance-induced depression differ mainly in the level of depressive symptoms, rather than in the structure of the symptoms [12]. However, it is difficult to determine the direction of causality between depressive symptoms and alcohol abuse. Our study indicates that depression-like symptoms in patients with alcohol problems are not merely transient, alcohol-induced effects. Patients with comorbid depression and alcohol abuse should be offered parallel and adequate treatment for both conditions.

There are some limitations in our study. The participants did not undergo a clinical interview to verify that their symptoms assessed with BDI-II indicated a formal diagnosis of depression. Despite these diagnostic limitations, we improved our understanding regarding the type and strength of symptoms in a sample of patients with depressive symptomatology. This study cannot illuminate the complex ways in which depressive symptoms and alcohol problems continue to interact over time. The strength is the size of the sample, which consists of two groups of depressed subjects with and without comorbid alcohol abuse.

Conclusion

Although there were differences in the symptom load, the basic factor structure is similar in patients with depressive symptoms with and without unhealthy alcohol use. This finding may strengthen the arguments for giving both of these problems clinical attention during treatment.

Supporting Information

Table S1 Beck Depression Inventory-II. Means, standard deviations and inter-item correlations for patients without alcohol problems (n = 358).

Table S2 Beck Depression Inventory-II. Means, standard deviations and inter-item correlations for patients with comorbid alcohol problems (n = 158).

Author Contributions

Conceived and designed the experiments: CS PU HD TB JE TB NIL. Performed the experiments: CS PU HD TB JE TB NIL. Analyzed the data: CS PU HD TB JE TB NIL. Contributed reagents/materials/analysis tools: CS PU HD TB JE TB NIL. Wrote the paper: CS PU HD TB JE TB NIL.

References

1. Davis L, Uezato A, Newell JM, Frazier E (2008) Major depression and comorbid substance disorders. Curr Opin Psychiatry 21: 14–18.
2. Hesse M (2004) Achieving abstinence by treating depression in the presence of substance-use disorders. Addict Behav 29: 1137–1141.
3. Kessler RC, Nelson CB, McGonagle KA, Edlund MJ, Fank RG, et al. (1996) The epidemiology of co-occurring addictive and mental disorders: implications for prevention and service utilization. Am J Orthopsychiatry 66: 17–31.
4. Ostacher MJ (2007) Comorbid alcohol and substance abuse dependence in depression: impact on the outcome of antidepressant treatment. Psychiatr Clin North Am 30: 69–76.
5. Palfai TP, Cheng DB, Samet JH, Kramer KL, Roberts MS, et al. (2007) Depressive symptoms and subsequent alcohol use and problems. A prospective study of medical inpatients with unhealthy alcohol use. J Stud Alcohol Drugs 68: 673–680.
6. Dum M, Pickren J, Sobell IC, Sobell MB (2008) Comparing the BDI-II and the PHQ-9 with outpatient substance abusers. Addict Behav 33: 381–387.
7. Beck AT, Steer RA, Brown GK (1996) Beck Depression Inventory - Second Edition. U.S.A; Haarcourt Assessment Inc.
8. Vanheule S, Desmet M, Groenvynck H, Rosseel Y, Fontaine J (2008) The factor structure of the Beck Depression Inventory-II: a evaluation. Assessment 15: 177–187.
9. Ward CL (2006) Comparison of factor structure models for the Beck Depression Inventory-II. Psychol Assess 18: 81–88.
10. Buckley TC, Jefferson PD, Heggie JA (2001) A psychometric evaluation of BDI-II in treatment seeking substance abusers. J Subst Abuse 20: 197–204.
11. Johnson ME, Neal DB, Brems C, Fisher DG (2006) Depression as measured by the Beck depression inventory-II among injecting drug users. Assessment 66: 17–31.
12. Seignourel PJ, Green C, Schmitz JM (2008) Factor structure and the diagnostic efficiency of the BDI-II in treatment-seeking substance users. Drug Alcohol Depend 93: 271–278.
13. Quilty LC, Zhang AK, Bagby MR (2010) The latent symptoms structure of the Beck Depression Inventory-II in outpatients with major depression. Psychol Assess 22: 603–608.
14. Babor TF, Higgins-Biddle JC, Saunders JB, Monterio MG (2001) The Alcohol Use Disorders Identification Test: Guidelines for use in primary care. 2nd

edition. Geneva; World Health Organization, Department of Mental Health and Substance Dependence.

15. Muthén LK, Muthén BO (2010) Mplus User's Guide. Sixth Edition. Los Angeles, CA: Muthén & Muthén.
16. Satorra A, Bentler PM (2001) A scaled difference chi-square test statistics for moment structure analysis. Psychometrica 66: 507–514.
17. Hu L, Bentler PM (1999) Cutoff criteria for fit indexes in covariance structure analysis: conventional criteria versus new alternatives. Structural Equation Modeling 6: 1–55.
18. Loehlin JC (1998) Latent variable models: an introduction to factor, path, and structural analyses. 3rd Edition. London: Lawrence Erlbaum Associates.
19. Byrne BM (2012) Structural equation modeling with M*plus*, Basic Concepts, Applications, and Programming. New York, NJ; Routledge.
20. Cheung GW, Rensvold RB (2002) Evaluating goodness-of-fit indexes for testing measurement invariance. Structural Equation Modeling, 9, 233–255.
21. Chen FF (2007) Sensitivity of goddness of fit indexes to lack of measurement invariance. Structural Equation Modeling, 14, 464–504.
22. Cohen J (1988) Statistical power analysis for the behavioural sciences. 2 ed, New York: Academic Press.

7

The Gender-Specific Association between Age at First Drink and Later Alcohol Drinking Patterns in Korea

Minsun Kang[1,2], Jae-Hyun Kim[1,2], Woo-Hyun Cho[2,3], Eun-Cheol Park[2,4]*

1 Department of Public Health, Graduate School, Yonsei University, Seoul, Korea, 2 Institute of Health Services Research, Yonsei University, Seoul, Korea, 3 Eulji University, Daejeon, Korea, 4 Department of Preventive Medicine, Yonsei University College of Medicine, Seoul, Korea

Abstract

This study investigated the association between the age at first drink and later alcohol drinking patterns, and analyzed whether differences in the association exist among Korean adults according to gender. The subjects included 10,649 adults (5,405 men and 5,244 women) from the fourth Korean National Health and Nutrition Examination Survey between 2007 and 2009, which extracted the standard survey household by using the proportional systematic sampling method. Baseline individual characteristics, the age at first drink, and individual alcohol drinking patterns were obtained by specially trained interviewers or examiners. The association between the age at first drink and the adult alcohol drinking patterns was summarized with odds ratios and their confidence intervals obtained from multiple logistic regression analysis with sampling weights of KNHANES complex sample survey design. The results of this study show that age, co-habitation, occupation, smoking, and self-rated stress level were significantly related to the drinking patterns for men, whereas education, co-habitation, smoking, and self-rated stress level were significant factors for the drinking patterns of women. The association between the age at first drink and the adult alcohol consumption was significant for both genders and, interestingly, the alcohol drinking patterns were significantly differed by gender even after controlling for the individual characteristics. These results imply a need for gender-specific strategies to prevent hazardous alcohol consumption at a later time for Korean.

Editor: Bernard Le Foll, Centre for Addiction and Mental Health, Canada

Funding: The authors have no support or funding to report.

Competing Interests: The authors have declared that no competing interests exist.

* E-mail: ecpark@yuhs.ac

These authors contributed equally to this work.

Introduction

Alcohol use disorders are leading preventable causes of death and disability worldwide [1,2]. Excessive alcohol consumption causes more than 4,500 deaths annually in Korea, and the alcohol-induced death rate was 9.1 per 100,000 individuals in 2010 [3]. Unhealthy alcohol use is prevalent among a large portion of Korean men, and the prevalence of alcohol dependence and alcohol abuse is much higher in Korea compared to other countries [4,5].

Numerous studies have demonstrated a correlation between the age at first drink and alcohol use disorders later in life [5–8]. Therefore, delaying the onset of drinking behavior would be an important aim in alcohol use disorder prevention programs. However, in reality the adolescent drinking rate gradually increases with age, and female adolescent drinking rates approach those of males [8,9]. These issues are recently of growing international concern.

Starting to drink at an early age may lead to prolonged neurobiological effects specific to the adolescent brain [10], including various cognitive and social problems [11] as well as binge drinking in adulthood. Indeed, there is much evidence converging to support this hypothesis. Significant associations between the age at first drink and later heavy use of alcohol have been found in several studies. Some authors have suggested a positive association between the age at first drink and alcohol consumption [12–14], frequency of drinking at young ages [15], alcohol abuse and dependence in adulthood [16,17], frequency of heavy drinking [18], and consequent binge drinking in adulthood [19]. Additionally, several studies show significant relationships between the age at first drink and the risk for unintentional injury with the use of alcohol [20] and drugs [11,21]. Based on these previous studies, it might seem that the age at first drink would be one of major factors related with later hazardous alcohol consumption, but most studies have not yet assessed for different gender-specific relationships. This study aimed to analyze the gender-specific association between the age at first drink and later alcohol drinking patterns after controlling for possible confounders which may influence alcohol consumption behaviors using the Korea National Health and Nutrition Examination Survey data.

Materials and Methods

Study Data

Data were obtained from the fourth Korean National Health and Nutrition Examination Survey (KNHANES IV) between 2007 and 2009. The KNHANES is a nationwide representative survey using a stratified and multistage probability sampling design for the selection of household units. The survey was conducted by the Korean Ministry of Health and Welfare to establish national health policy based on the evaluation of health risk factors and health indicators. The survey data were obtained by specially trained interviewers or examiners who were not provided with any prior information about the survey participants and all participants signed an informed consent form before the survey was conducted. More details on the research methodology used to gather and analyze the KNHANES are available from the KNHANES website.

Participants over the age of 18 years were identified for this study. A total of 10,649 individuals (5,405 men and 5,244 women) were included as our final study population after excluding persons who never consumed alcohol.

Measures

Baseline individual characteristics regarding gender, age, household income, education level, co-habitation, residential region, occupation, smoking, and self-rated stress level were collected for all cases. Age was categorized into five groups (≤ 29, 30–39, 40–49, 50–59, and ≥60). Household income was classified into four groups: low, middle-low, middle-high, and high. Education level was categorized as follows: elementary school graduate and under, middle school graduate, high school graduate, and college graduate or post-graduate. Co-habitation referred to whether the individual lived with a spouse. With regard to residential region, participants were classified into living in Seoul, living in an urban area, and living in a rural area. Occupation was categorized as follows: white-collar jobs, blue-collar jobs, and unemployed (including student and housewife). Smoking status was categorized into nonsmoker with no past smoking experience, ex-smoker, and current smoker. Self-rated stress level was categorized as follows: very much, much, little, and almost none.

Self-reported questionnaires were used to assess each participant's alcohol related behaviors. For the age at first drink, participants were asked the age at which they first started drinking, not counting tastes or sips, which was classified into eight categories (≤14, separately for each year from 15 through 20 years old, and ≥21). Three indicators of the adult alcohol drinking patterns were used: The Alcohol Use Disorder Identification Test (AUDIT) score, average drinking frequency in past year, and typical drinking quantity per drinking day in past year. AUDIT is a 10-item screening instrument developed by the World Health Organization for the early detection of persons with harmful alcohol consumption behavior [22]. The AUDIT summary score range is 0 to 30. In this study, AUDIT was classified into two categories (≥8 and <8) based on that a score of 8 or higher is usually considered as at-risk drinking level [22]. Average drinking frequency in past year was assessed with five categories(<1/month, 1/month, 2–4/month, 2–3/week, and ≥4/week) and typical drinking quantity per drinking day in past year was assessed with five categories(1 or 2 drinks, 3 or 4 drinks, 5 or 6 drinks, 7–9 drinks, and ≥10 drinks). In these questions, a 'drink' was defined as one serving of alcoholic beverages regardless of the kind including beer, whisky, or Soju which is Korean traditional liquor. One serving of these beverages contains 8–9 g alcohol, even though each drink has different volumes. In this study, we considered participants having ≥8 on the AUDIT, or reporting average drinking ≥2–3 times/week, or consuming more than 5–6 drinks/drinking day as individuals with at-risk drinking level based on previous studies [5,22]. Therefore, average drinking frequency was classified into two groups (≥2–3/week and <2–3/week) and typical drinking quantity per drinking day was classified into two groups (≥5 or 6 drinks and < 5 or 6 drinks).

Statistical analyses

Statistical analyses were performed using SAS version 9.2 (SAS Institute Inc, Cary, NC, USA) to take into account the complex sampling design with sampling weights of KNHANES and provide nationally representative estimates. Descriptive statistics including means, standard deviation, and frequency for estimates of the adult alcohol drinking patterns were calculated for men and women separately since there was no interaction found. Baseline characteristics of the study participants according to the alcohol drinking patterns were compared using the chi-square test. The gender-specific alcohol drinking patterns were compared using a two sample t-test for continuous variables and the chi-square test for categorical variables. The gender-specific effects of the age at first drink on adult alcohol drinking patterns were tested using the chi-square test. Multiple logistic regression analysis was used to find out the relationships between the age at first drink and the adult alcohol drinking patterns after adjusting for potential confounders. Odds ratios and 95% confidence intervals (CIs) were calculated to describe the association between the age at first drink and the drinking patterns for those with age 14 years and under at first drink and each age from 15 through 20 years relative to those with age 21 years or older at first drink, which was the reference group. The sample weights account for sampling variability and adjust the data for differential probability of selection of persons in KNHANES complex sample survey design.

Results

Characteristics of the study participants

The characteristics of 10,649 individuals based on the alcohol drinking pattern are shown in Table 1. There is no significant effect of residential region on the three indicators of the adult alcohol drinking patterns for both genders. Age, co-habitation, occupation, smoking, and self-rated stress level were significantly related to AUDIT, average drinking frequency and typical drinking quantity for men. Household income and education were significantly related to average drinking frequency and typical drinking quantity for men. Education, co-habitation, smoking, and self-rated stress level were significantly related to AUDIT, average drinking frequency and typical drinking quantity for women. There is no significant effect of household income on the women's drinking patterns.

Alcohol drinking patterns and gender

Just over half (59%) of the respondents were men and 41% were women. The mean AUDIT score was significantly higher for the men than the women with a mean AUDIT of 10.9±7.1 for the men and 4.7±5.0 for the women respectively (Table 2). Among men, 43% reported average drinking ≥2–3 times/week in past year and 69% of men consumed more than 5–6 drinks/drinking day. However, only 16% of women reported average drinking ≥ 2–3 times/week in past year and 25% of women consumed more than 5–6 drinks/drinking day (Table 2).

Age at first drink

Table 3 showed inverse associations between the age at first drink and the adult alcohol drinking patterns for both genders. Among those men who first started drinking at age 14 or under, 71% had ≥8 on the AUDIT, 54% reported average drinking ≥2–3 times/week in past year and 73% consumed more than 5–6 drinks/drinking day. Among those men who first started drinking at age 21 or older, only 54% had ≥8 on the AUDIT, 49% reported average drinking ≥2–3 times/week in past year and 47% consumed more than 5–6 drinks/drinking day. In the group of

Table 1. Characteristics of the study population (number, %).

	Men (n = 5405)								
	AUDIT ≥ 8	**AUDIT < 8**	***p*-value**	**ADF ≥2-3/week**	**ADF <2-3/week**	***p*-value**	**TDQ ≥ 5 or 6**	**TDQ < 5 or 6**	***p*-value**
Age									
≤ 29	471 (19.3)	330 (23.8)	<.0001	219 (13.1)	582 (26.9)	<.0001	603 (23.3)	198 (15.9)	<.0001
30–39	780 (26.5)	432 (24.6)		479 (23.2)	733 (27.8)		897 (27.8)	315 (21.3)	
40–49	858 (28.4)	372 (21.1)		627 (29.8)	603 (22.6)		897 (27.6)	333 (21.5)	
50–59	628 (16.7)	301 (15.5)		526 (20.3)	403 (13.2)		596 (15.1)	333 (18.8)	
≥ 60	644 (9.1)	589 (15.0)		672 (13.6)	561 (9.5)		445 (6.2)	788 (22.5)	
Household income									
Low	505 (11.3)	332 (11.3)	0.867	442 (12.6)	395 (10.4)	0.004	428 (10.0)	409 (14.2)	0.001
Middle-low	803 (23.0)	499 (23.8)		655 (25.3)	647 (21.8)		798 (23.0)	504 (24.0)	
Middle-high	989 (31.3)	589 (32.0)		702 (30.6)	876 (32.3)		1,048 (32.0)	530 (30.7)	
High	1,084 (34.3)	604 (32.9)		724 (31.6)	964 (35.5)		1,164 (35.0)	524 (31.1)	
Education									
≤ Elementary school	571 (11.4)	321 (9.6)	0.091	566 (15.7)	326 (6.9)	<.0001	429 (8.5)	463 (15.6)	<.0001
≤ Middle school	412 (10.6)	239 (9.3)		365 (13.1)	286 (7.8)		353 (9.4)	298 (11.7)	
≤ High school	1,320 (43.3)	782 (43.6)		920 (41.0)	1,182 (45.3)		1,445 (45.2)	657 (39.6)	
≥ College	1,078 (34.7)	682 (37.5)		672 (30.1)	1,088 (40.1)		1,211 (37.0)	549 (33.0)	
Co-habitation									
Married	2,615 (73.1)	1,537 (69.7)	0.002	2,071 (78.3)	2,081 (67.0)	<.0001	2,531 (69.6)	1,621 (76.8)	<.0001
Single	574 (22.1)	405 (26.9)		300 (16.5)	679 (29.4)		726 (26.1)	253 (19.0)	
Separated	88 (1.9)	50 (1.7)		74 (2.2)	64 (1.5)		79 (1.6)	59 (2.2)	
Divorced	104 (2.9)	32 (1.7)		78 (3.0)	58 (2.0)		102 (2.7)	34 (2.0)	
Residential region									
Capital city	536 (20.8)	382 (23.5)	0.137	390 (20.4)	528 (22.8)	0.074	590 (21.7)	328 (21.9)	0.802
Urban	1,588 (48.5)	941 (48.2)		1,140 (47.8)	1,389 (48.8)		1,646 (48.7)	883 (47.6)	
Rural	1,257 (30.7)	701 (28.4)		993 (31.8)	965 (28.4)		1,202 (29.6)	756 (30.6)	
Occupation									
White-collar	1,433 (49.0)	748 (43.8)	<.0001	924 (44.6)	1,257 (49.1)	<.0001	1,572 (50.6)	609 (39.5)	<.0001
Blue-collar	1,381 (37.5)	802 (37.1)		1,158 (42.4)	1,025 (33.5)		1,306 (35.5)	877 (41.5)	
None	567 (13.4)	474 (19.0)		441 (13.0)	600 (17.4)		560 (13.9)	481 (19.1)	
Smoking									
Nonsmoker	431 (12.9)	451 (23.0)	<.0001	268 (10.2)	614 (21.5)	<.0001	485 (14.2)	397 (21.8)	<.0001
Ex-smoker	1,118 (30.0)	807 (36.4)		882 (31.2)	1,043 (33.2)		1,081 (29.0)	844 (39.7)	
Current	1,832 (57.2)	766 (40.6)		1,373 (58.6)	1,225 (45.3)		1,872 (56.8)	726 (38.5)	
Self-rated stress									
Very much	183 (5.2)	73 (3.3)	0.002	130 (5.0)	126 (4.1)	0.018	172 (4.7)	84 (4.1)	0.012
Much	791 (24.5)	398 (21.4)		558 (23.7)	631 (23.1)		801 (24.0)	388 (22.0)	
Little	1,900 (57.6)	1,177 (59.8)		1,373 (56.0)	1,704 (60.3)		1,985 (58.8)	1,092 (57.7)	
Almost none	507 (12.7)	376 (15.5)		462 (15.3)	421 (12.5)		480 (12.6)	403 (16.3)	
	Women (n = 5244)								
	AUDIT ≥ 8	AUDIT < 8	*p*-value	ADF ≥2-3/week	ADF <2-3/week	*p*-value	TDQ ≥ 5 or 6	TDQ < 5 or 6	*p*-value
Age									
≤ 29	326 (42.6)	610 (20.2)	<.0001	134 (24.9)	802 (25.2)	0.8571	425 (46.0)	511 (18.3)	<.0001
30–39	273 (23.6)	1,064 (24.8)		210 (25.1)	1,127 (24.4)		320 (24.1)	1,017 (24.6)	
40–49	232 (21.0)	1,022 (26.6)		204 (26.7)	1,050 (25.1)		244 (18.8)	1,010 (27.5)	
50–59	115 (9.2)	724 (16.1)		115 (13.8)	724 (14.8)		119 (8.3)	720 (16.7)	
≥ 60	67 (3.5)	811 (12.3)		124 (9.6)	754 (10.5)		58 (2.7)	820 (12.9)	
Household income									

Table 1. Cont.

	Men (n = 5405)								
	AUDIT ≥ 8	**AUDIT < 8**	***p*-value**	**ADF ≥2-3/week**	**ADF <2-3/week**	***p*-value**	**TDQ ≥ 5 or 6**	**TDQ < 5 or 6**	***p*-value**
Low	155 (12.1)	687 (13.5)	0.0261	144 (14.7)	698 (12.9)	0.0694	168 (12.2)	674 (13.6)	0.3387
Middle-low	287 (29.4)	1,008 (24.2)		198 (26.5)	1,097 (25.2)		305 (27.4)	990 (24.7)	
Middle-high	303 (30.0)	1,214 (29.5)		239 (31.8)	1,278 (29.2)		355 (30.3)	1,162 (29.4)	
High	268 (28.5)	1,322 (32.7)		206 (26.9)	1,384 (32.7)		338 (30.2)	1,252 (32.3)	
Education									
≤ Elementary school	156 (11.0)	1,059 (19.0)	<.0001	192 (18.5)	1,023 (17.0)	<.0001	147 (9.4)	1,068 (19.9)	<.0001
≤ Middle school	121 (11.5)	459 (10.7)		99 (14.1)	481 (10.3)		101 (8.3)	479 (11.7)	
≤ High school	516 (53.3)	1,551 (39.6)		356 (48.0)	1,711 (41.6)		619 (54.4)	1,448 (38.7)	
≥ College	220 (24.2)	1,162 (30.6)		140 (19.5)	1,242 (31.0)		299 (28.0)	1,083 (29.6)	
Co-habitation									
Married	557 (50.1)	3,048 (70.5)	<.0001	513 (63.2)	3,092 (66.6)	0.0041	625 (49.3)	2,980 (71.6)	<.0001
Single	298 (37.5)	525 (16.8)		117 (20.3)	706 (21.5)		382 (39.9)	441 (15.2)	
Separated	85 (6.4)	529 (9.8)		102 (10.4)	512 (8.8)		79 (5.4)	535 (10.2)	
Divorced	73 (6.0)	129 (2.9)		55 (6.1)	147 (3.1)		80 (5.4)	122 (3.0)	
Residential region									
Capital city	196 (22.1)	704 (21.4)	0.8994	145 (22.6)	755 (21.3)	0.4427	223 (21.7)	677 (21.5)	0.8877
Urban	478 (48.8)	2,058 (49.7)		373 (50.8)	2,163 (49.3)		565 (48.8)	1,971 (49.8)	
Rural	339 (29.1)	1,469 (28.9)		269 (26.6)	1,539 (29.4)		378 (29.5)	1,430 (28.8)	
Occupation									
White-collar	476 (51.6)	1,486 (41.5)	<.0001	326 (45.6)	1,636 (43.4)	0.2737	549 (51.4)	1,413 (41.2)	<.0001
Blue-collar	174 (15.5)	886 (18.2)		172 (18.8)	888 (17.3)		174 (13.1)	886 (19.0)	
None	363 (32.9)	1,859 (40.3)		289 (35.7)	1,933 (39.3)		443 (35.5)	1,779 (39.8)	
Smoking									
Nonsmoker	688 (65.6)	3,819 (89.5)	<.0001	561 (67.3)	3,946 (87.4)	<.0001	809 (67.9)	3,698 (89.7)	<.0001
Ex-smoker	106 (11.9)	225 (6.0)		79 (12.3)	252 (6.3)		120 (11.3)	211 (5.9)	
Current	219 (22.5)	187 (4.5)		147 (20.4)	259 (6.2)		237 (20.8)	169 (4.4)	
Self-rated stress									
Very much	86 (9.3)	212 (5.3)	<.0001	59 (8.9)	239 (5.7)	0.0089	88 (8.2)	210 (5.5)	<.0001
Much	348 (34.9)	1,055 (26.0)		234 (30.4)	1,169 (27.5)		385 (33.9)	1,018 (26.0)	
Little	494 (48.1)	2,444 (57.6)		415 (52.5)	2,523 (56.1)		597 (49.8)	2,341 (57.4)	
Almost none	85 (7.7)	520 (11.0)		79 (8.3)	526 (10.7)		96 (8.0)	509 (11.0)	

Abbreviations: AUDIT, Alcohol Use Disorder Identification Test; ADF, average drinking frequency in past year; TDQ, typical drinking quantity (drinks/drinking day).
Note: *p*-values are based on the chi-squared test for categorical variables.

Table 2. The association between alcohol drinking patterns and gender [a].

	Overall		**Men**		**Women**		***p*-value** [b]
n (%)	**10,649**	**(100%)**	**5,405**	**(59%)**	**5,244**	**(41%)**	-
Alcohol drinking patterns in adulthood							
AUDIT score	8.5		10.9	(7.1)	4.7	(5.0)	<.0001
ADF ≥ 2–3/week	3,310		2,523	(43%)	787	(16%)	<.0001
TDQ ≥ 5 or 6 drinks/drinking day	4,604		3,438	(69%)	1,166	(25%)	<.0001

Abbreviations: AUDIT, Alcohol Use Disorder Identification Test; ADF, average drinking frequency in past year; TDQ, typical drinking quantity.
[a]Data are expressed as the mean (SD) or n (%) by weighted number.
[b]*p*-values were calculated using a two sample t-test or chi-square test.

Table 3. Alcohol drinking patterns in adult by the age at first drink and gender [a].

Age at first drink (year)	Men				Women			
	Total	AUDIT ≥ 8 [b]	ADF ≥2-3/week [b]	TDQ ≥ 5 or 6 [b]	Total	AUDIT ≥ 8 [b]	ADF ≥2-3/week [b]	TDQ ≥ 5 or 6 [b]
≤14	350 (8%)	250 (71%)	189 (54%)	255 (73%)	108 (3%)	51 (47%)	24 (22%)	53 (49%)
15	359 (7%)	249 (69%)	189 (53%)	253 (70%)	127 (3%)	48 (38%)	24 (19%)	60 (47%)
16	428 (9%)	307 (72%)	212 (50%)	338 (79%)	144 (3%)	60 (42%)	30 (21%)	69 (48%)
17	641 (13%)	447 (70%)	327 (51%)	468 (73%)	246 (6%)	90 (37%)	57 (23%)	101 (41%)
18	907 (18%)	593 (65%)	419 (46%)	616 (68%)	474 (10%)	127 (27%)	68 (14%)	162 (34%)
19	792 (15%)	467 (59%)	315 (40%)	522 (66%)	732 (15%)	147 (20%)	91 (12%)	183 (25%)
20	1,033 (17%)	586 (57%)	431 (42%)	566 (55%)	1,057 (20%)	165 (16%)	142 (13%)	211 (20%)
21≤	895 (13%)	482 (54%)	441 (49%)	420 (47%)	2,356 (39%)	325 (14%)	351 (15%)	327 (14%)
Total	5,405 (100%)	3,381 (63%)	2,523 (43%)	3,438 (69%)	5,244 (100%)	1,013 (22%)	787 (16%)	1,166 (25%)

Abbreviations: AUDIT, Alcohol Use Disorder Identification Test; ADF, average drinking frequency in past year; TDQ, typical drinking quantity (drinks/drinking day).
[a]Data are expressed as n (%) by weighted number.
[b]*p*-values were significant at the P<0.01 level using chi-square test.
Note: percentages may not add to 100, or to the subgroup total, due to rounding.

women, 47% of those who started drinking at age 14 or under had ≥8 on the AUDIT, 22% reported average drinking ≥2–3 times/week in past year and 49% consumed more than 5–6 drinks/drinking day, whereas 14% of those who started drinking at age 21 or older had ≥8 on the AUDIT, 15% reported average drinking ≥2–3 times/week in past year and 14% consumed more than 5–6 drinks/drinking day (Table 3). The interactions of gender and the age at first drink were not statistically significant at 0.01 level on the AUDIT score (F_{470} = 2.18, P = 0.0347), average drinking frequency (F_{470} = 1.42, P = 0.1939), and typical dinking quantity per drinking day (F_{470} = 2.44, P = 0.0183).

Effect of the age at first drink on alcohol drinking pattern

Odds ratios and 95% CIs from multiple logistic regression analysis revealed that relative to those who waited until age 21 years or older, those who started drinking at an earlier age were more likely to have ≥8 on the AUDIT, report average drinking ≥ 2–3 times/week, and consume more than 5–6 drinks/drinking day (Figure 1). After controlling for age, household income, education, co-habitation, residential region, occupation, smoking, and self-rated stress level, men who first started drinking at age 14 or under had 1.46 (95% CI, 0.99–2.15) times the odds of having ≥8 on the AUDIT, 1.56 (95% CI, 1.08–2.24) times the odds of reporting average drinking ≥2–3 times/week, and 1.50 (95% CI, 1.05–2.16) times the odds of consuming more than 5–6 drinks/drinking day relative to those who waited until they were 21 years or older. For women relative to those who started drinking at age 21 or older, those who first started drinking at age 14 or under had 2.23 (95% CI, 1.27–3.91) times the odds of having ≥8 on the AUDIT, 1.35 (95% CI, 0.71–2.55) times the odds of reporting average drinking ≥2–3 times/week, and 1.82 (95% CI, 0.98–3.37) times the odds of consuming more than 5–6 drinks/drinking day, after controlling for all the mentioned confounders.

Discussion

This study demonstrated that alcohol drinking patterns in regards to AUDIT scores, average drinking frequency, and typical drinking quantity on drinking day in later adulthood were associated with the age at first drink in Korean. Although several studies indicated that the age at first drink is associated with later hazardous alcohol consumption [15,17,23], it is particularly unclear whether those associations differ by gender. An important aim for many prevention programs targeting young people for alcohol-related disorders is to delay the onset of drinking as long as possible [24,25] and many studies have recommended that the prevention of adult heavy drinking should include delaying the onset of drinking [26,27]. Therefore, it is essential to understand differences in the onset age of drinking and alcohol drinking patterns in adulthood between men and women so to inform the construction and evaluation of gender-specific strategies to prevent risky or hazardous alcohol consumption at a later time.

Age, co-habitation, occupation, smoking, and self-rated stress level were significantly related to the drinking patterns for men, whereas education, co-habitation, smoking, and self-rated stress level were significant factors for the drinking patterns of women. Overall, men were more likely to have higher AUDIT score and reported drinking more frequently and more daily consumed alcohol quantity than women. Regardless of gender, our results showed a significant inverse association between the age at first drink and the adult alcohol drinking patterns: persons who first started drinking at earlier age are more likely to have ≥8 on the AUDIT, report average drinking ≥2–3 times/week, and consume more than 5–6 drinks/drinking day, which means individuals with at-risk drinking level [2,5]. Those inverse associations between the age at first drink and the alcohol drinking patterns in regards to AUDIT scores, average drinking frequency, and typical drinking quantity on drinking day in later adulthood were constant except for average drinking frequency of women even after adjusting potential confounders including age, household income, education, co-habitation, residual region, occupation, smoking, and self-rated stress level (Figure 1). Men and women participants who initiated drinking prior to age 17 reported significantly more in at-risk drinking indicators than individuals who began drinking at age 20 or later which is the legal age limit in Korea. Thus the effect of the age at first drink on adult alcohol drinking patterns was similar for both genders.

The results were in accordance with several evidences from previous studies. Both men and women experiencing binge drinking in adulthood most frequently had a drinking onset of age 14 or under, which was an association that rapidly declined after age 21 [19,22]. Significant increasing trends were observed in

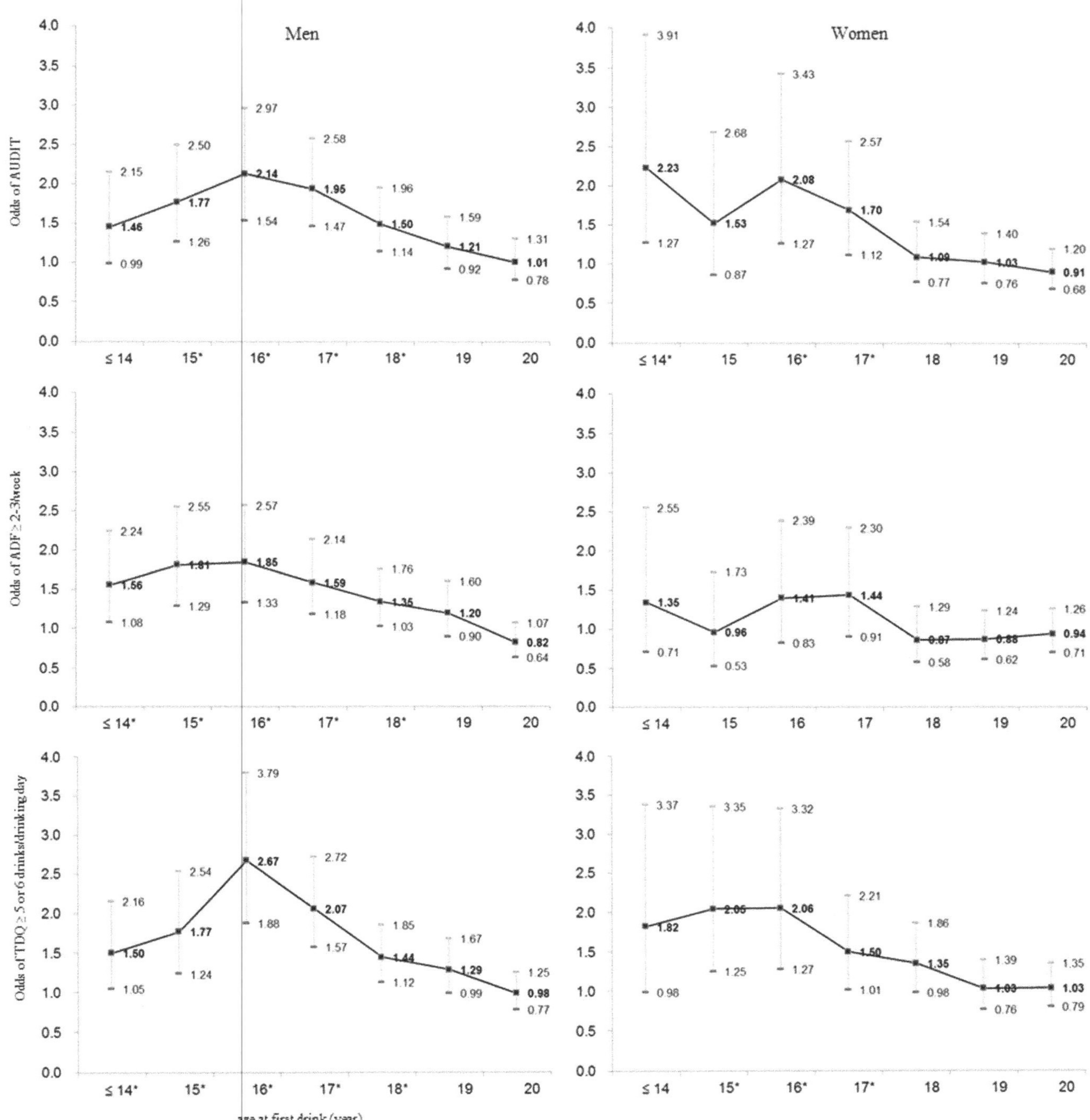

Figure 1. Mean adjusted odds ratios of three indicators of the adult alcohol drinking patterns from multiple logistic regressions. Abbreviations: AUDIT, Alcohol Use Disorder Identification Test; ADF, average drinking frequency in past year; TDQ, typical drinking quantity (drinks/drinking day). * *p*-values were significant at the P<0.05 level using chi-square test. *Note*: odds ratios are relative to those who started drinking at 21 years or older, controlling for age, household income, education, co-habitation, residential region, occupation, smoking, and self-rated stress level by gender. Error bars represent 95% confidence intervals.

the rate of alcohol consumption [5,15,19], frequency of drinking at young ages [1], alcohol abuse and dependence in adulthood [9,20], frequency of heavy drinking [18], and consequent binge drinking in adulthood [16] among participants who initiated drinking at earlier age. Apart from a previous study [16], there was no significant association between the age at first drink and average drinking frequency among women in present study. Only men who initiated drinking at age 18 or under were slightly more likely to report average drinking ≥2–3 times/week and the results were statistically significant. Future study is warranted to better understand the gender-specific association between the onset age of drinking and alcohol drinking patterns.

This study has several limitations that need to be taken into consideration. First, we could not fully exclude the effects of information bias because the measurement of alcohol drinking patterns along with the age at first drink was based on a self-reported questionnaire survey. However, there is an evidence that self-assessment of alcohol consumption is reliable [28]. Second, causal inferences cannot be drawn from this study result using a cross-sectional study design. Third, there may be residual or uncontrolled confounders that influence the associations. For instance, some previous studies suggested that children with particular adverse childhood experiences may be at risk for earlier drinking initiation along with a different pattern of alcohol consumption across their life span [29], suggesting that these unknown confounders might be related to our study results. In addition, a study [30] indicated that higher educational attainment is associated with increased alcohol consumption and the relationship is stronger for women than men. If education attainment was systematically varied between younger and older generation, our analytical model could not capture the residual relationship even though education level and age variables were controlled for the multiple logistic regressions. Finally, the cut-off used to define individuals with at-risk drinking level at ≥8 on the AUDIT and 5–6 drinks/drinking day may be too high and therefore inappropriate in women. We considered the cut-off points based on previous studies [5,22] but those studies were not designed to analyze gender differences. Therefore, those variables might be related to a ceiling effect and the estimates were somehow biased.

In conclusion, the present findings in a representative Korean population demonstrate that the age at first drink is a predictor of adult alcohol drinking patterns in both genders although men report consuming more alcohol and spend more time drinking than women. Our findings suggest that delaying the initiation of drinking might be an appropriate goal for prevention efforts and that the present level for the legal age limit (18 years) for alcohol use is relevant; in some countries it is even higher. Prescott and Kendler [29] have, however, claimed that delaying the age of onset of drinking would not prevent severe alcoholism, because so many other factors are included. By delaying the onset age, at least the hazardous effects of heavy drinking in adolescence could possibly be avoided. As proposed by previous study [12], a change in general attitudes is needed to prevent an increase in problems caused by alcohol in the future. Achieving this result will require a joint effort by everyone, including parents, media, professionals, and politicians, and will necessitate a change in adult drinking culture.

Acknowledgments

The English in this document has been checked by a professional editor, a native speaker of English.

Author Contributions

Conceived and designed the experiments: JHK MK. Analyzed the data: JHK MK. Wrote the paper: JHK MK. Performed statistical analyses: JHK MK. Contributed to discussion: JHK MK. Reviewed the manuscript: ECP WHC. Provided recommendations regarding statistical analysis: JHK MK. Had full access to all the data in the study and is the guarantor of this work: ECP. Takes responsibility for the integrity of the data and the accuracy of the data analysis: ECP.

References

1. Mokdad AH, Marks JS, Stroup DF, Gerberding JL (2004) Actual causes of death in the United States, 2000. JAMA 291: 1238–1245.
2. Ezzati M, Lopez AD, Rodgers A, Vander Hoorn S, Murray CJ (2002) Selected major risk factors and global and regional burden of disease. Lancet 360: 1347–1360.
3. Korea S (2010) Annual Report on the Cause of Death Statistics 2010.
4. Min S, Noh S, Shin J, Ahn JS, Kim TH (2008) Alcohol dependence, mortality, and chronic health conditions in a rural population in Korea. J Korean Med Sci 23: 1–9.
5. Hingson RW, Zha WX (2009) Age of Drinking Onset, Alcohol Use Disorders, Frequent Heavy Drinking, and Unintentionally Injuring Oneself and Others After Drinking. Pediatrics 123: 1477–1484.
6. Dawson DA, Goldstein RB, Chou SP, Ruan WJ, Grant BF (2008) Age at First Drink and the First Incidence of Adult-Onset DSM-IV Alcohol Use Disorders. Alcoholism-Clinical and Experimental Research 32: 2149–2160.
7. Bonomo YA, Bowes G, Coffey C, Carlin JB, Patton GC (2004) Teenage drinking and the onset of alcohol dependence: a cohort study over seven years. Addiction 99: 1520–1528.
8. Donovan JE (2004) Adolescent alcohol initiation: a review of psychosocial risk factors. J Adolesc Health 35: 529 e527–518.
9. Labouvie E, Bates ME, Pandina RJ (1997) Age of first use: Its reliability and predictive utility. Journal of Studies on Alcohol 58: 638–643.
10. Monti PM, Miranda R, Jr., Nixon K, Sher KJ, Swartzwelder HS, et al. (2005) Adolescence: booze, brains, and behavior. Alcohol Clin Exp Res 29: 207–220.
11. DeWit DJ, Adlaf EM, Offord DR, Ogborne AC (2000) Age at first alcohol use: A risk factor for the development of alcohol disorders. American Journal of Psychiatry 157: 745–750.
12. Pitkanen T, Lyyra AL, Pulkkinen L (2005) Age of onset of drinking and the use of alcohol in adulthood: a follow-up study from age 8–42 for females and males. Addiction 100: 652–661.
13. York JL, Welte J, Hirsch J, Hoffman JH, Barnes G (2004) Association of age at first drink with current alcohol drinking variables in a national general population sample. Alcoholism-Clinical and Experimental Research 28: 1379–1387.
14. Pedersen W, Skrondal A (1998) Alcohol consumption debut: predictors and consequences. J Stud Alcohol 59: 32–42.
15. Samson HH, Maxwell CO, Doyle TF (1989) The relation of initial alcohol experiences to current alcohol consumption in a college population. J Stud Alcohol 50: 254–260.
16. Hingson RW, Heeren T, Winter MR (2006) Age at drinking onset and alcohol dependence - Age at onset, duration, and severity. Archives of Pediatrics & Adolescent Medicine 160: 739–746.
17. Grant BF, Stinson FS, Harford TC (2001) Age at onset of alcohol use and DSM-IV alcohol abuse and dependence: A 12-year follow-up. Journal of Substance Abuse 13: 493–504.
18. Werner MJ, Walker LS, Greene JW (1994) Longitudinal Evaluation of a Screening Measure for Problem Drinking among Female College-Freshmen. Archives of Pediatrics & Adolescent Medicine 148: 1331–1337.
19. Jefferis BJ, Power C, Manor O (2005) Adolescent drinking level and adult binge drinking in a national birth cohort. Addiction 100: 543–549.
20. Hingson RW, Heeren T, Jamanka A, Howland J (2000) Age of drinking onset and unintentional injury involvement after drinking. JAMA 284: 1527–1533.
21. Flory K, Lynam D, Milich R, Leukefeld C, Clayton R (2004) Early adolescent through young adult alcohol and marijuana use trajectories: Early predictors, young adult outcomes, and predictive utility. Development and Psychopathology 16: 193–213.
22. Saunders JB AO, Babor TF, De La Fuente JR, Grant M (1993) Development of the alcohol use disorders identification test (AUDIT): WHO Collaborative Project on early detection of persons with harmful alcohol consumption-II. Addiction 88: 791–804.
23. Dubow EF, Boxer P, Huesmann LR (2008) Childhood and adolescent predictors of early and middle adulthood alcohol use and problem drinking: the Columbia County Longitudinal Study. Addiction 103: 36–47.
24. Smyth BP, Kelly A, Cox G (2011) Decline in age of drinking onset in Ireland, gender and per capita alcohol consumption. Alcohol Alcohol 46: 478–484.
25. Ward B, Snow P, Aroni R (2010) Children's alcohol initiation: An analytic overview. Drugs-Education Prevention and Policy 17: 270–277.
26. McGue M, Iacono WG (2005) The association of early adolescent problem behavior with adult psychopathology. Am J Psychiatry 162: 1118–1124.
27. Prescott CA, Kendler KS (1999) Age at first drink and risk for alcoholism: A noncausal association. Alcoholism-Clinical and Experimental Research 23: 101–107.
28. Giovannucci E, Colditz G, Stampfer MJ, Rimm EB, Litin L, et al. (1991) The assessment of alcohol consumption by a simple self-administered questionnaire. Am J Epidemiol 133: 810–817.
29. Rothman EF, Edwards EM, Heeren T, Hingson RW (2008) Adverse childhood experiences predict earlier age of drinking onset: results from a representative US sample of current or former drinkers. Pediatrics 122: e298–304.
30. Huerta MC, Borgonovi F (2010) Education, alcohol use and abuse among young adults in Britain. Social Science & Medicine 71: 143–151.

8

A Heuristic Model of Alcohol Dependence

Zhen Qi[1,2,3], Felix Tretter[4], Eberhard O. Voit[1,2]*

1 Department of Biomedical Engineering, Georgia Institute of Technology and Emory University Medical School, Atlanta, Georgia, United States of America, 2 Integrative BioSystems Institute, Georgia Institute of Technology, Atlanta, Georgia, United States of America, 3 Center for Neurodegenerative Disease, Emory University School of Medicine, Atlanta, Georgia, United States of America, 4 Isar-Amper-Klinikum gemeinnützige GmbH, Klinikum München-Ost, Haar, Landkreis München, Germany

Abstract

Background: Substance dependence poses a critical health problem. Sadly, its neurobiological mechanisms are still unclear, and this lack of real understanding is reflected in insufficient treatment options. It has been hypothesized that alcohol effects are due to an imbalance between neuroexcitatory and neuroinhibitory amino acids. However, glutamate and GABA interact with other neurotransmitters, which form a complicated network whose functioning evades intuition and should be investigated systemically with methods of biomedical systems analysis.

Methods and Results: We present a heuristic model of neurotransmitters that combines a neurochemical interaction matrix at the biochemical level with a mobile describing the balances between pairs of neurotransmitters at the physiological and behavioral level. We investigate the effects of alcohol on the integrated neurotransmitter systems at both levels. The model simulation results are consistent with clinical and experimental observations. The model demonstrates that the drug diazepam for symptoms of alcohol withdrawal effectively reduces the imbalances between neurotransmitters. Moreover, the acetylcholine signal is suggested as a novel target for treatment of symptoms associated with alcohol withdrawal.

Conclusions: Efficient means of integrating clinical symptoms across multiple levels are still scarce and difficult to establish. We present a heuristic model of systemic neurotransmitter functionality that permits the assessment of genetic, biochemical, and pharmacological perturbations. The model can serve as a tool to represent clinical and biological observations and explore various scenarios associated with alcohol dependence and its treatments. It also is very well suited for educational purposes.

Editor: Nestor V. Torres, Universidad de La Laguna, Spain

Funding: This work was supported by a grant from the National Institutes of Health (P01-ES016731, Gary W. Miller, PI) and an endowment from the Georgia Research Alliance (to EOV, PI). The funders had no role in study design, data collection and analysis, decision to publish, or preparation of the manuscript.

Competing Interests: FT is employed by Isar-Amper-Klinikum gemeinnützige GmbH, Klinikum München-Ost, Haar, Landkreis München, Germany.

* E-mail: eberhard.voit@bme.gatech.edu

Introduction

"Substance dependence" describes a physiological and psychological state in which a user has developed a dependence on such drugs as alcohol, tobacco, opiates or amphetamines. Substance dependence is nothing new, as alcohol use and abuse were already observed in ancient Egypt and Greece [1,2]. The *Diagnostic and Statistical Manual of Mental Disorders* [3] defines: "When an individual persists in use of alcohol or other drugs despite problems related to use of the substance, substance dependence may be diagnosed. Compulsive and repetitive use may result in tolerance to the effect of the drug and withdrawal symptoms when use is reduced or stopped." Substance dependence is unfortunately quite prevalent. The lifetime prevalence of alcohol dependence was reported to be 14% in a non-institutionalized adult population (ages: 15–54 years) [3], and alcohol abuse is associated with 85,000 deaths annually in the United States alone [4]. In 2000, there were over 1.2 billion smokers worldwide [5], and it is estimated that there are 24.8 million amphetamine users worldwide [6].

Depending on the type of substance dependence, different neurotransmitters have been suggested as targets. Specifically, alcohol can increase inhibitory neurotransmission (*e.g.*, through gamma-aminobutyric acid (GABA)), while simultaneously reducing excitatory neurotransmission (*e.g.*, through glutamate (Glu)) [7]. Substances like amphetamine increase the dopamine level in the synaptic cleft [8], whereas nicotine mimics psychopharmacological effects of the neurotransmitter acetylcholine and modulates dopamine release [9,10]. In addition to modulation of direct targets, addictive substances can indirectly modulate other neurotransmitters through neuronal projections and metabolic pathways. For example, alcohol can directly reduce glutamate level in the *striatum*, which in turn regulates GABAergic activity in the *nucleus accumbens*. As a consequence, alcohol can have an indirect effect on the GABA level in the *nucleus accumbens*. In this manner, all neurotransmitters interact with each other directly or indirectly, as it is shown in Figure 1. These interactions imply that behavioral effects of addictive substances are not merely associated with direct targets. Instead, both direct and indirect effects should be investigated in an integrated fashion involving all neurotransmitter systems. This conclusion is in line with clinical experience showing that altered function of any individual neurotransmitter alone cannot explain a complex syndrome such as the development of alcoholism, withdrawal craving and relapse.

Alcohol withdrawal syndrome is one of the criteria for alcohol dependence according to DSM-IV [3]. It follows alcohol abuse and exhibits symptoms of autonomic hyperactivity, tremor,

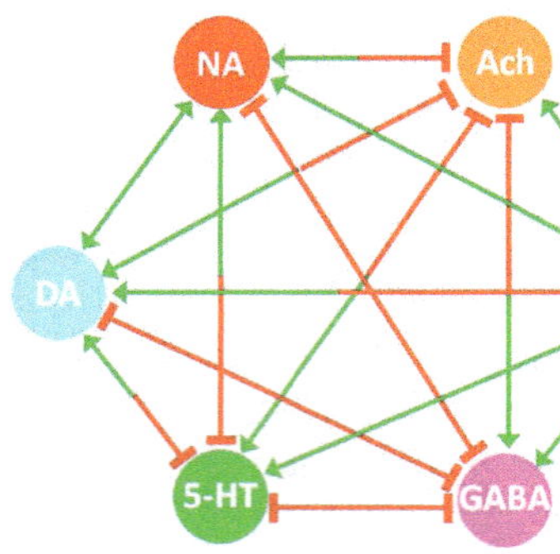

Figure 1. The neurochemical interaction matrix. The interactions among six neurotransmitter systems in the human brain form a fully connected network, which may be represented as a matrix. Arrows represent activation; while bar-headed lines represent inhibition. Abbreviation: dopamine (DA), acetylcholine (ACh), serotonin (5-HT), glutamate (Glu), noradrenaline (NA), and gamma-aminobutyric acid (GABA).

anxiety and restlessness. Some individuals also have seizures, hallucinations and, possibly, delirium. As a common medical problem, alcohol withdrawal syndrome has had a mortality as high as 15% in the past [11], which later improved to 2% due to better recognition and treatment [12].

Studies have shown that alcohol withdrawal is associated with an increase in glutamate in the *striatum* [13], the *nucleus accumbens* [14], the *hippocampus* [15], and the cerebrospinal fluid [16]. Changes in the inhibitory activity of GABA are also observed and connected to hyper-excitability [17]. Since alcohol can affect neurotransmitters in the brain and modify behaviors, a general perturbation of the brain's neurotransmitter systems has been suggested as the effect of alcohol withdrawal [18]. In particular, it was hypothesized that an imbalance between neuroexcitatory and neuroinhibitory amino acids may cause many of the symptoms of alcohol withdrawal, at least partially [19]. This hypothesis pointed to Glu and GABA as the main excitatory and inhibitory neurotransmitters, while other neurotransmitters, such as dopamine (DA), serotonin (5-HT), acetylcholine (ACh), and noradrenaline (NA), were assumed to act as regulators. In line with this observation, DA and 5-HT show a deficit in the *nucleus accumbens* during alcohol withdrawal that can rapidly be reversed by alcohol intake [20]. It is becoming better recognized that the various neurotransmitters are not isolated in their functioning, but instead interact with each other through neuronal projections (such as the DA-GABA-Glu pathway) and metabolic pathways. Therefore, substance abuse should be investigated from a systemic point of view.

Neurotransmitters not only communicate with each other through a "neurochemical interaction matrix" (Fig. 1), but there is also a delicate dynamic balance between these neurotransmitters from a functional point of view. Disruption of this balance can affect brain function, which in consequence may induce mental disorders. The concept of health and disease as being related to balances and imbalances is at least 2,500 years old, as Hippocrates used the metaphor of the "balance of juices" to describe health status. Inspired by this idea, Fritze suggested studying brain health in terms of balances between neurotransmitters [21]. Subsequently, one of us (FT) constructed a "neurochemical mobile" that represents in a consistent manner different clinical observations of symptoms and of actions of psychopharmacological agents. In this model, different pairs of neurotransmitters form a set of hierarchical balances [22]. The mobile, in its simplest form, includes the neurotransmitters DA, 5-HT, NA on one side, and ACh, Glu, and GABA on the other (Fig. 2). These transmitters, from a functional point of view, mainly act in a more or less opposing mode with each other.

Each component of the neurochemical mobile represents the "relative functional weight" of a neurotransmitter, a term which summarily captures its physiological or behavioral importance and will be discussed later. The functional weight profile determines how the neurotransmitter system is balanced during health or off balance if it is perturbed by substance abuse.

In this study, we explore a combined model of the neurochemical mobile and the neurotransmitter interaction matrix. We are primarily interested in the interactions that correspond to clinical syndromes based on experience and on data of global drug action, regardless of the anatomical distribution of neurotransmitters in the human brain. In particular, we use this modeling platform to simulate alcohol abuse, adaptation, and withdrawal, and analyze the consequences of different schemes in comparison with clinical and experimental experience regarding the balance of neurotransmitters. We also use the model simulations to screen for potential treatments of the symptoms of alcohol withdrawal.

The model proposed here is heuristic and may be categorized as mesoscopic, as its complexity and function fall between those of detailed microscopic (molecular) and high-level macroscopic (physiological and behavioral) models [23]. A mesoscopic model can serve as an important conceptual and cognitive tool, as it rigorously formalizes the logic of argumentation within a complex system, which in a detailed mathematical representation would vastly exceed our intuition [24,25]. Here, the mesoscopic model forms a critical functional link between lower and higher levels of brain function and provides a conceptual and technical strategy for merging models that characterize specific functional aspects at multiple levels.

Materials and Methods

The human brain responds differently to the duration and disruption of alcohol intake. Short-term exposure tends to inhibit some brain functions, whereas chronic consumption causes the brain to compensate toward normalcy. When chronic alcohol consumption is disrupted, the direct effects of alcohol disappear, but the compensatory changes are still active, thereby causing symptoms of withdrawal. The model simulations address these mechanisms and processes. They also allow us to explore potential treatments of alcohol withdrawal.

Our modeling framework includes two modules: The first is the neurochemical interaction matrix (Fig. 1) that characterizes interactions between neurotransmitters and their regulations [26]. This model has previously been tested with respect to stability and parameter sensitivities [26]. The second module contains a neurochemical mobile system (Fig. 2) that describes hierarchical functional balances between pairs of neurotransmitters with respect to health and disease [21,27]. The neurochemical interaction matrix is formulated as a dynamic model with six neurotransmitters, namely DA, ACh, 5-HT, Glu, NA, and GABA. These six neurotransmitters correspond to signals that can regulate each other's activity. In our model, the interaction matrix is a fully connected network with bidirectional signals (Fig. 1; *cf.* [26] for details). Neurotransmitter concentrations, which may be used to represent signal strengths regulating each other, are available in the literature [28–39].

The neurochemical mobile system describes hierarchical functional balances between pairs of neurotransmitters and emulates the idea of a hierarchical "balance scale" (Fig. 2). Each

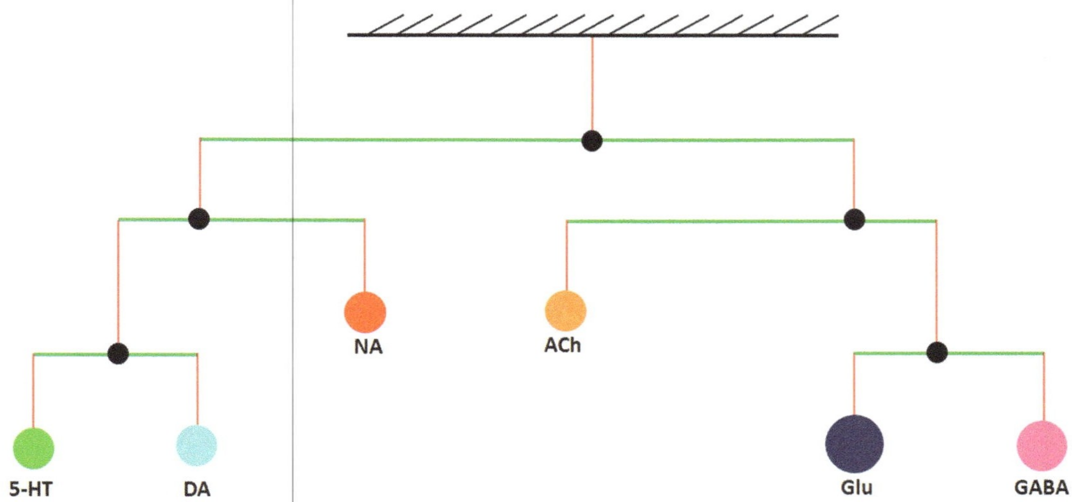

Figure 2. The neurochemical mobile as a system of balanced rods with individual neurotransmitters as weights. The neurochemical mobile represents a hierarchical functional organization of neurotransmitters, along with their relative functional contributions and dynamic imbalances in human brain. The mobile represents synergisms or antagonisms between neurotransmitter systems at the physiological, behavioral, and pathological level, and can be tailored for a specific disease. For illustration, we use a weighting scheme, where the areas of circles are proportional to the relative signal intensities of neurotransmitters 5-HT (100 units), DA (100 units), NA (100 units), ACh (100 units), Glu (200 units), and GABA (150 units). The lengths of the arms of each rod are thus different and reflect corresponding relative signal intensities.

neurotransmitter has a weight representing its relative functional importance, and under normal homeostasis, corresponding to health, all rods are balanced.

The implementation of the neurochemical interaction matrix and the neurochemical mobile system under the categorized weighting scheme is illustrated in Table 1. The implementation presents the ODEs for the neurochemical interaction matrix with specified initial values and the mobile configuration (defined by the lever length profile) for the neurochemical mobile system. As a minimally biased format for the equations, we follow the tenets of Biochemical Systems Theory [40–43]. The information in Table 1 should be sufficient for simulations with the model; nonetheless, Matlab code for the system is available as *Supplement S2*.

To model the acute alcohol usage, we increase GABA synthesis and decrease Glu synthesis in the neurochemical interaction matrix. These direct effects trigger compensatory mechanisms during chronic usage that are implemented as an increase in GABA degradation and a decrease in Glu degradation in the neurochemical interaction matrix. Again, these direct effects trigger secondary responses by the system. During alcohol withdrawal, the alcohol effects are removed, but the compensatory mechanisms of the brain are taken into account.

For the functional weights within the mobile, we assume that the contributions of the different neurotransmitters to alcohol dependence are of comparable impact, even though their actual concentrations in the brain differ quite considerably. The rationale is that neurotransmitters with normally small concentrations are correspondingly more potent. Specifically, we transform the concentrations into low, medium and high magnitudes and assign 100, 150, and 200 as relative signal intensities of neurotransmitters, respectively. These relative signal intensities are used to compute the profile of lever lengths in the mobile during health. In addition, they are used as neurotransmitter "signal intensities" in the neurochemical interaction matrix, which characterizes signal interactions between neurotransmitters.

As an alternative, the functional weights of neurotransmitters could directly be equated with their concentrations. This option and its ramifications are discussed in *Supplement S1*. The length of each lever arm relative to its counterpart is computed under the assumption of perfect balance, which means that the two lever arms of a balance scale in our mobile can have different lengths. To show an imbalance within the mobile properly, and to prevent a rotation angle from reaching $\pm 90°$, we add a resistant force at the end of each lever arm, which is proportional to the vertical displacement of the end of a lever arm from its corresponding balanced position. In this manner, we can properly compute and visualize dynamic imbalances within the mobile. To describe an imbalanced state unambiguously, we define counterclockwise and downward as positive directions for rotation and force, respectively. One should note that the balances within the mobile are governed by both the length profile of the arms (determined by the profile of functional weights) and the intensities of neurotransmitter signals (determined by the neurochemical interaction matrix) in a time-dependent manner. Thus, the mobile is dynamic. The computation of the appropriate rotation angle of a rod in the mobile is shown in Figure S3 in Supplement S1.

Results

The overall state of the mobile is greatly disturbed by alcohol. Indeed, all rods exhibit imbalances, some of which are quite significant (Fig. 3). As a direct consequence of acute exposure to alcohol, the rod connecting Glu and GABA tilts toward GABA. If the acute exposure turns into repeated abuse, the body adapts, but full compensation cannot be achieved, and the rod eventually becomes less slanted than before but still not level. During withdrawal, the mobile tilts back toward the excitatory neurotransmitter Glu (Fig. 4).

In more detail, the top rod, which balances DA, NA, and 5-HT on the left, and Glu, GABA and ACh on the right, tilts toward the right under acute exposure. For repeated abuse, it moves back toward normalcy, thereby reflecting adaptive compensation, which however is not perfect. During withdrawal, the rod tilts back toward DA, NA, and 5-HT. Another significant imbalance is seen in the rod connecting 5-HT and DA, which tilts toward DA during withdrawal. One interesting phenomenon in this context is

Table 1. Implementation of the neurochemical interaction matrix and the neurochemical mobile system[%].

Entity	Implementation
Equations[$]	$DA' = ACh^{0.5} \cdot HT^{0.2} \cdot Glu^{0.5} \cdot NA^{0.5} \cdot GABA^{-0.3} - 7.901101 \cdot DA$
	$ACh' = DA^{-0.3} \cdot HT^{-0.3} \cdot Glu^{0.5} \cdot NA^{-0.3} \cdot GABA^{-0.3} - 0.0004985258 \cdot Ach$
	$HT' = DA^{-0.2} \cdot ACh^{0.5} \cdot Glu^{0.5} \cdot NA^{-0.3} \cdot GABA^{-0.3} - 0.03145485 \cdot HT$
	$Glu' = DA^{-0.3} \cdot ACh^{0.5} \cdot HT^{0.5} \cdot NA^{0.5} \cdot GABA^{-0.3} - 0.2793461 \cdot Glu$
	$NA' = DA^{0.5} \cdot ACh^{0.5} \cdot HT^{0.5} \cdot Glu^{0.5} \cdot GABA^{-0.3} - 31.45485 \cdot NA$
	$GABA' = DA^{-0.3} \cdot ACh^{0.5} \cdot HT^{-0.3} \cdot Glu^{0.5} \cdot NA^{-0.3} - 0.01494252 \cdot GABA$
Initial values[#]	HT = 100; DA = 100; NA = 100;
	Glu = 200; GABA = 150; ACh = 100;
Mobile configuration (Lever length)[&]	Lever_HT = 1; Lever_DA = 1; Lever_NA = 2;
	Lever_HT_DA = 1; Lever_HT_DA_NA = 1;
	Lever_Glu = 1; Lever_GABA = 1.3333; Lever_ACh = 3.5;
	Lever_Glu_GABA = 1; Lever_ACh_Glu_GABA = 0.6667;

%:This implementation of the system uses the categorized weighting scheme, which assumes that the contributions of the different neurotransmitters to alcohol dependence are of comparable impact. Specifically, the concentrations are categorized into classes and transformed into low (100), medium (150), and high (200) values. A Matlab file of the system is presented in *Supplement S2*.
$:Apostrophes on the left-hand sides of the equations indicate derivatives with respect to time.
#:Relative signal intensities of neurotransmitters.
Lever lengths in the mobile for the various neurotransmitters. Please see the Figure 2 for the corresponding positions of levers within the mobile.

that the neurochemical interaction matrices exhibit only subtle differences in dynamic responses for the two alternative definitions of functional weights (Fig. 4B and Figure S1B in Supplement S1), although the two mobiles show distinctly different imbalance profiles (Fig. 3 and Figure S2 in Supplement S1).

The results raise the question of whether a quasi-balance could be regained with proper treatment. Several medications are currently available to treat the symptoms of alcohol withdrawal. Table 2 shows some of these, along with their pharmacological mechanisms. Most of them act on the GABA receptor and enhance GABA signals. Others affect the Glu or NA systems.

As a prominent example, consider diazepam, which activates the $GABA_A$ receptor. It is not difficult to simulate this effect, and the model results directly confirm that diazepam clearly reduces the overall imbalance of the mobile system during alcohol withdrawal (Fig. 5). Even though diazepam only targets the GABA signal directly, all other neurotransmitters are indirectly affected through the neurochemical interaction matrix, as it is shown in Figure 6. For example, the excitatory Glu is reduced and the inhibitory GABA is elevated. These changes help to alleviate perturbations induced by alcohol withdrawal.

In addition to medications acting on the GABA signal, our simulations confirm the beneficial effects of pharmacological actions on the NA signal and suggest a potential target of the ACh system (data not shown). With regard to actions on the NA signal, one medication, Clonidine (Kapvay or Nexiclon), is already in use. The effect on the ACh system is revisited in the discussion section.

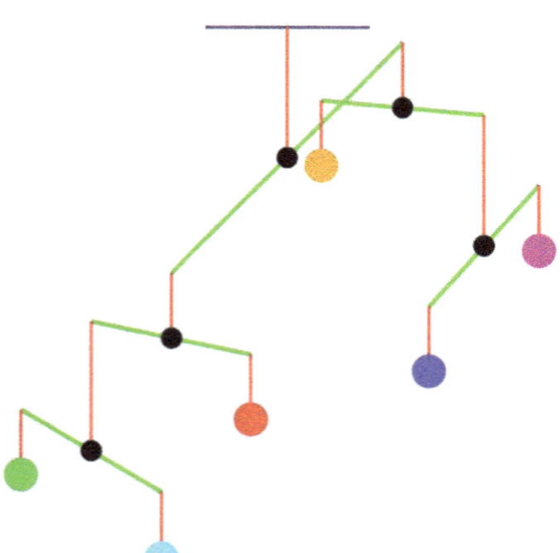

Figure 3. In response to alcohol withdrawal, the mobile system exhibits significant imbalance. Circles from left to right: 5-HT, DA, NA, ACh, Glu, and GABA. For visibility, the lengths of arms in the mobile are adjusted as described, and neurotransmitter concentrations are transformed into comparable relative signal intensities, so that all neurotransmitters have similar functional weights.

Conclusions and Discussion

Over many decades, biologists and clinicians have been accumulating large amounts of data and information on drug abuse and withdrawal, mainly from targeted animal studies, clinical trials, and observations on individual patients. The assemblage of knowledge resulting from these efforts is indeed impressive and very valuable, but also poses the challenge of integrating the diverse and heterogeneous pieces of information into a common functional entity that can be analyzed, interrogated, and used to formulate new hypotheses. Such an integrative investigation of a phenomenon like drug dependency requires a systemic point of view, which in turn mandates the use of computational means of data management and the development of dynamic mathematical models. These computational tools are well suited for the purpose because they are able to accommodate and merge diverse data sets that were obtained from genetic, biochemical, pharmacological, and clinical investigations.

In this study, we presented a systemic model of neurotransmitter interactions to address questions of alcohol abuse and withdrawal. The model is heuristic and intuitive and, while conceptually simple, can simulate the effects of genetic mutations, biochemical interventions, and pharmacological actions. For example, our

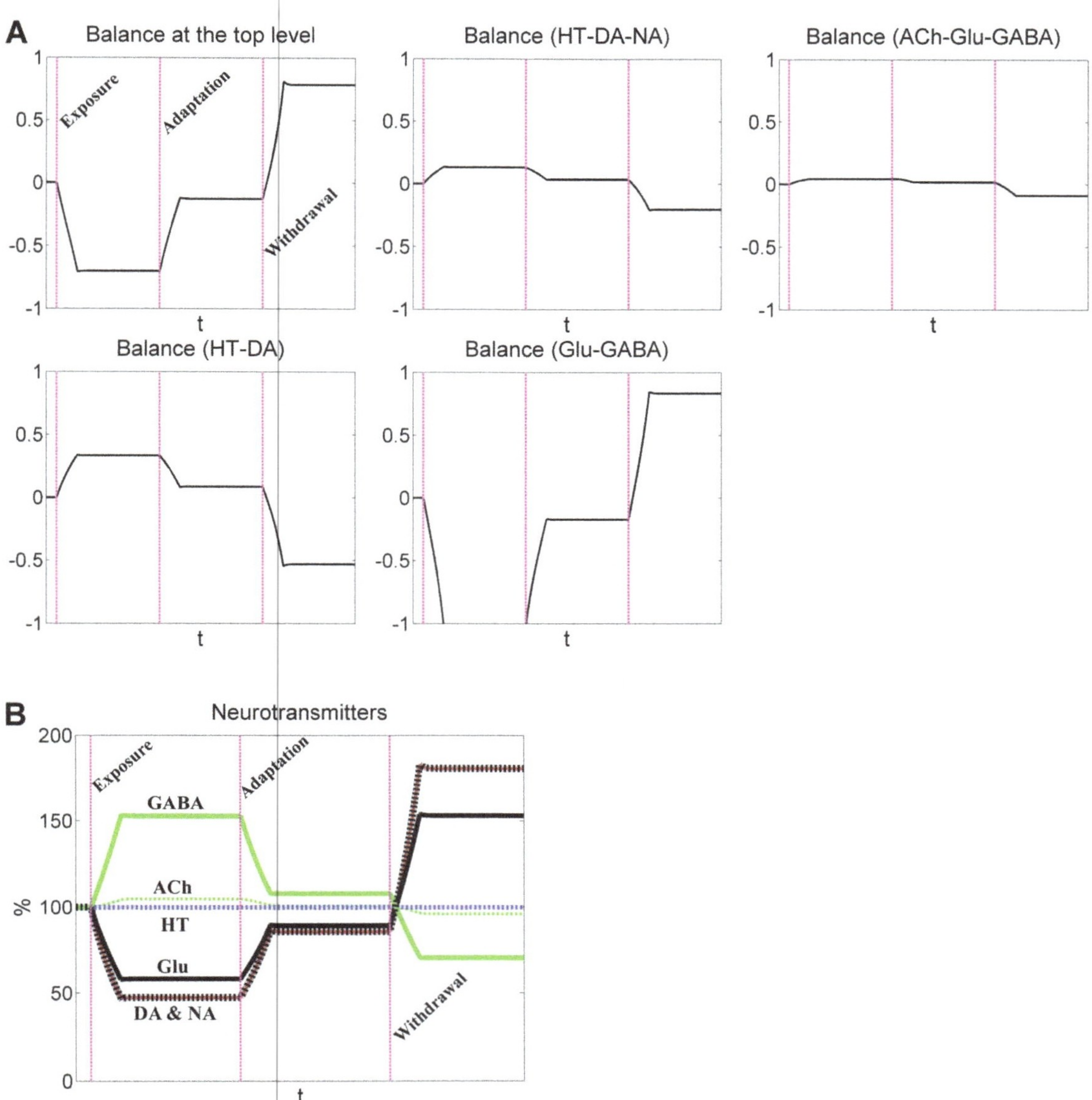

Figure 4. Dynamics of neurotransmitters and rod balances in response to acute alcohol exposure, adaptation, and withdrawal. Neurotransmitters have similar functional contributions in the mobile system. The three vertical dashed lines represent, from left to right, the beginning of acute alcohol exposure, adaptation, and withdrawal, respectively. A: Dynamic imbalances associated with five rods are represented by rotation angles relative to the horizontal position. B: Dynamics of neurotransmitters. Note that the dynamic responses of DA and NA overlap.

simulations demonstrate the actions of the drug diazepam for alcohol withdrawal symptoms quite well. By integrating various pieces of information, the dynamic framework allowed us to search for explanations of the details of alcohol dependency and permitted simulations of currently used as well as hypothesized treatment options.

The heuristic model combines a neurotransmitter interaction matrix with the concept of a neurochemical mobile. It is incomparably simpler than complicated dynamic models of neurotransmitters, such as our detailed nonlinear ordinary differential equation models of the dopamine dynamics in neurons [44–46], but nevertheless capable of connecting molecular events

Table 2. Partial list of medications for symptoms of alcohol withdrawal.

Generic name (brand name)	Pharmacological mechanism
Diazepam (Valium or Diastat)	Binds to the $GABA_A$ receptor and results in enhanced GABA effects
Chlordiazepoxide (Librium or Angirex)	Modifies $GABA_A$ receptor and increases its overall conductance
Clonidine (Kapvay or Nexiclon)	Binds to α_2 receptors and inhibits the release of NA

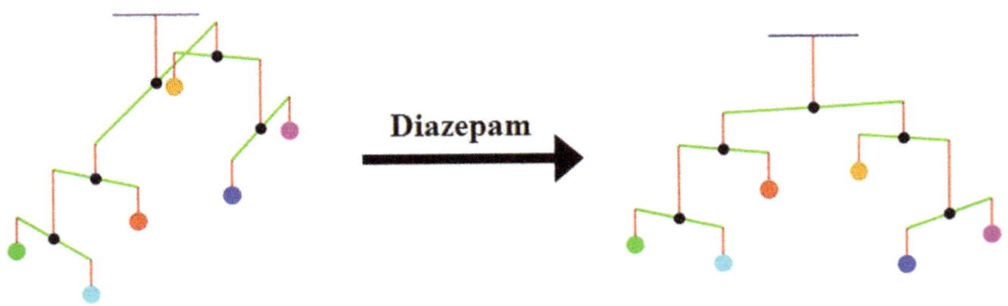

Figure 5. Diazepam reduces imbalances caused by alcohol withdrawal. The mobile confirms that diazepam reduces imbalances during alcohol withdrawal. Circles from left to right: 5-HT, DA, NA, ACh, Glu, and GABA. For better visibility, the lengths of arms in the mobile are adjusted and do not reflect functional contributions of neurotransmitters.

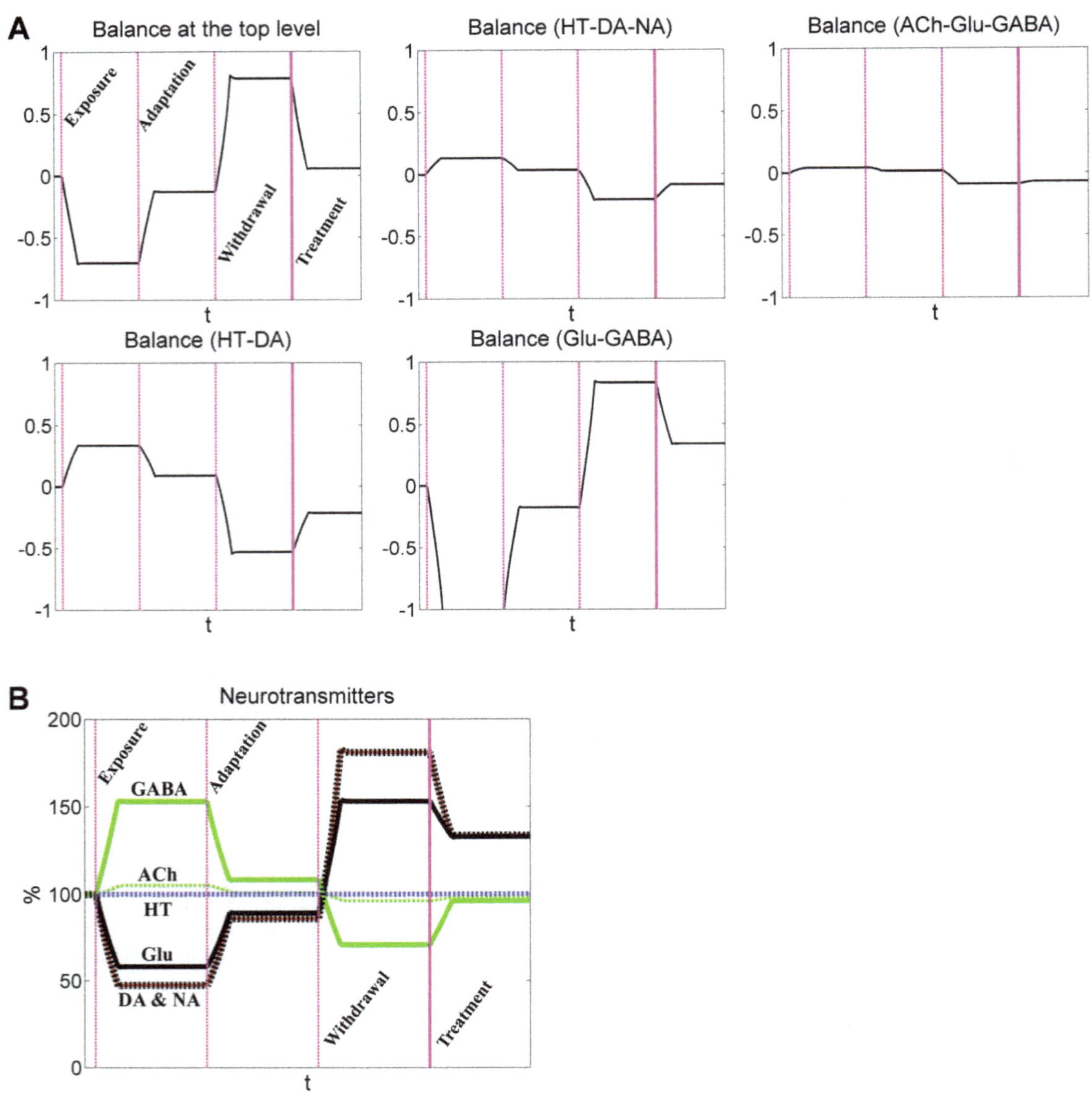

Figure 6. Diazepam partly restores the balance between excitatory and inhibitory neurotransmitters. Neurotransmitters have similar functional contributions in the mobile system. The three dashed vertical lines represent, from left to right, the beginning of acute alcohol exposure, adaptation, and withdrawal, respectively. The solid vertical line represents the application of diazepam. A: Dynamic imbalances associated with five rods are represented by rotation angles relative to the horizontal position. B: Dynamics of neurotransmitters. Note that the dynamic responses of DA and NA overlap.

to the physiological or behavioral deviations from normalcy that are observed during alcohol abuse and withdrawal. The model is mesoscopic and connects otherwise isolated levels of functioning, namely the dynamics of molecular events at the neurotransmitter level and the responses of alcohol usage and withdrawal at the high level of physiology and behavior [23–25]. In doing so, the combined matrix-interaction-mobile model opens new avenues of integrating formerly isolated pieces of information about alcohol dependence that can be attributed to different neurotransmitter systems.

As an example, perturbations may be introduced into a detailed dynamic model of a neurotransmitter at the molecular level, and the perturbed neurotransmitter level can then be fed into the neurotransmitter matrix, which then reveals changes in neurotransmitter balance and consequent mobile imbalance. With this combination, the effects of the perturbation at the physiological or behavioral level are quantified through the mobile model. In a different application, one may use the mobile model and the neurotransmitter interaction matrix to explore different scenarios of neurotransmitter alterations that can induce a particular phenomenon of interest. In this case, the possible causes of the neurotransmitter alterations may be assessed with relevant dynamic models, which in turn may also suggest potential interventions.

The model suggests that, following alcohol exposure, the main inhibitory neurotransmitter GABA is enhanced, while the main excitatory neurotransmitter Glu is suppressed. In response to withdrawal, these changes are opposite to those during the acute exposure phase: Glu is elevated, while GABA is reduced. These simulation results are consistent with experimental observations [13–17,47]. In addition to Glu and GABA, the model identifies DA as being over-active during alcohol withdrawal, a result that is supported by several experiments [48–51], although not by all [20]. Consistent with experimental data, NA is also increased following alcohol withdrawal in our simulations (Fig. 4 and Figure S1 in Supplement S1) [50–52]. Our model does not show significant changes in ACh and 5-HT in response to alcohol abuse and withdrawal. This result is partially supported by a study of the effects of neuropharmacological agents on seizures during withdrawal [53].

The model demonstrates that the drug diazepam for symptoms of alcohol withdrawal effectively reduces the imbalances between neurotransmitters. It also suggests the importance of the NA signal, which is targeted by the prescription drug Clonidine (Kapvay or Nexiclon).

Interestingly, the model suggests the ACh signal as a novel target for treatment of symptoms associated with alcohol withdrawal. It appears that there is currently no drug available that acts on the ACh signal for the treatment of alcohol withdrawal. If the model prediction points into the right direction, this site could be a potential drug target for treating symptoms of alcohol withdrawal and therefore be of pharmaceutical interest. By contrast, our results suggest that DA is not likely an effective drug target, because perturbing DA alleviates the excitatory Glu but exacerbates the inhibitory GABA, or *vice versa* (data not shown). A similar effect is observed if haloperidol is administered as the sole medication to treat a *delirium tremens*. To be effective, a GABA agonist is needed in addition to haloperidol.

Beyond alcohol dependence, the constellation of counteracting transmission systems in the mobile model matches clinical experience with other neurological problems, such as the features of depression, the action of antidepressants, and some side effects of current treatment options. In depression, one encounters low levels of DA, NA and 5-HT transmission, while schizophrenia is associated with high levels of transmission in DA and 5-HT. The mobile permits the investigation of these neurotransmitter profiles, as well as medication strategies for the different states of allostasis.

Neurotransmitter concentrations *in situ* differ greatly; *e.g.*, by three or four orders of magnitude between Glu and DA in the synaptic cleft. This large difference could imply that neurotransmitters with high concentrations, such as Glu and GABA, are the primary players in brain physiology and behavior. Our study, however, suggests that other neurotransmitters seem to be of comparable importance, at least in the case of alcoholism, and that the relative magnitudes to baseline levels, rather than the absolute concentrations, are more appropriate for capturing their physiological and behavioral impact.

The matrix model leaves some questions unresolved. One of them is: What are the primary targets of alcohol, and which neurotransmitters are not directly targeted, although they are greatly affected indirectly through interactions among the neurotransmitters? From experimental observations, both Glu and GABA are frequently and consistently reported to be targeted by alcohol. However, experimental data on DA activity under alcohol withdrawal are contradictory. Since Glu and GABA are mostly reported as alcohol targets, we considered them as the primary targets in our model, but it could as well be the case that NA and DA are first responders. In the future, it might be interesting to investigate systemically whether there could be different scenarios of primary alcohol targets that are consistent with clinical data and provide explanations for so-far contradictory observations.

In this study, we treated each type of neurotransmitters as a single node in the neurotransmitter interaction matrix. However, each type of neurotransmitters has its own subtypes of receptors, which can have opposite actions between two subtypes. In future work, one might account for these subtypes of neurotransmitter receptors and treat them as different nodes in a much larger interaction matrix based on their actions (*e.g.*, grouped into different categories).

Supporting Information

Supplement S1 Supporting text and figures. Figure S1. Dynamics of neurotransmitters and balances in response to acute alcohol exposure, adaptation, and withdrawal. The neurotransmitter concentrations are directly used as functional weights. The three dashed vertical lines represent, from left to right, the beginning of acute alcohol exposure, adaptation, and withdrawal, respectively. A: Dynamic imbalances associated with five rods are represented by rotation angles relative to the horizontal position. B: Dynamics of neurotransmitters. Note that the dynamic responses of DA and NA overlap. **Figure S2.** In response to alcohol withdrawal, the mobile system does not exhibit significant imbalances. Here, the neurotransmitter concentrations are directly used as functional weights. Circles from left to right: 5-HT, DA, NA, ACh, Glu, and GABA. For better visualization, the lengths of the arms in the mobile are adjusted and do not reflect functional contributions of neurotransmitters. **Figure S3.** Computation of a rotation angle of a scale in the mobile system. The scales in the mobile can have different lengths of lever arms. A and B are the signal intensities of two neurotransmitters in this study. θ is the rotation angle, while r_a and r_b are the lengths of lever arms. F_a and F_b are resistant forces, while k is the coefficient of resistant force.

Acknowledgments

Disclaimer: Any opinions, findings, conclusions or recommendations expressed in this material are those of the authors and do not necessarily reflect the views of the sponsoring institutions.

Author Contributions

Conceived and designed the experiments: ZQ FT EOV . Performed the experiments: ZQ EOV . Analyzed the data: ZQ EOV . Wrote the paper: ZQ FT EOV.

References

1. el-Guebaly N, el-Guebaly A (1981) Alcohol abuse in ancient Egypt: the recorded evidence. Int J Addict 16: 1207–1221.
2. Leibowitz JO (1967) Studies in the history of alcoholism. II. Acute alcoholism in ancient Greek and Roman medicine. Br J Addict Alcohol Other Drugs 62: 83–86.
3. American Psychiatric Association (2000) Diagnostic and Statistical Manual of Mental Disorders, Fourth Edition, Text Revision (DSM-IV-TR): Washington, DC: American Psychiatric Association.
4. Carlson RW, Kumar NN, Wong-Mckinstry E, Ayyagari S, Puri N, et al. (2012) Alcohol withdrawal syndrome. Crit Care Clin 28: 549–585.
5. Guindon G, Boisclair D (2003) Past, Current and Future Trends in Tobacco Use. Health, Nutrition and Population (HNP) Discussion Paper (Economics of Tobacco Control Paper No. 6). Nutrition and Population (HNP) Discussion Paper: Washington, World Bank.
6. Greene SL, Kerr F, Braitberg G (2008) Review article: amphetamines and related drugs of abuse. Emerg Med Australas 20: 391–402.
7. Valenzuela CF (1997) Alcohol and neurotransmitter interactions. Alcohol Health Res World 21: 144–148.
8. Kuczenski R, Segal DS (1997) Effects of methylphenidate on extracellular dopamine, serotonin, and norepinephrine: comparison with amphetamine. J Neurochem 68: 2032–2037.
9. Pomerleau OF, Rosecrans J (1989) Neuroregulatory effects of nicotine. Psychoneuroendocrinology 14: 407–423.
10. Barik J, Wonnacott S (2009) Molecular and cellular mechanisms of action of nicotine in the CNS. Handb Exp Pharmacol: 173–207.
11. Victor M, Adams RD (1953) The effect of alcohol on the nervous system. Res Publ Assoc Res Nerv Ment Dis 32: 526–573.
12. Ferguson JA, Suelzer CJ, Eckert GJ, Zhou XH, Dittus RS (1996) Risk factors for delirium tremens development. J Gen Intern Med 11: 410–414.
13. Rossetti ZL, Carboni S (1995) Ethanol withdrawal is associated with increased extracellular glutamate in the rat striatum. Eur J Pharmacol 283: 177–183.
14. Dahchour A, Quertemont E, De Witte P (1996) Taurine increases in the nucleus accumbens microdialysate after acute ethanol administration to naive and chronically alcoholised rats. Brain Res 735: 9–19.
15. Dahchour A, De Witte P, Bolo N, Nedelec JF, Muzet M, et al. (1998) Central effects of acamprosate: part 1. Acamprosate blocks the glutamate increase in the nucleus accumbens microdialysate in ethanol withdrawn rats. Psychiatry Res 82: 107–114.
16. Tsai G, Coyle JT (1998) The role of glutamatergic neurotransmission in the pathophysiology of alcoholism. Annu Rev Med 49: 173–184.
17. Devaud LL, Fritschy JM, Sieghart W, Morrow AL (1997) Bidirectional alterations of GABA(A) receptor subunit peptide levels in rat cortex during chronic ethanol consumption and withdrawal. J Neurochem 69: 126–130.
18. Lovinger DM, White G, Weight FF (1989) Ethanol inhibits NMDA-activated ion current in hippocampal neurons. Science 243: 1721–1724.
19. De Witte P (2004) Imbalance between neuroexcitatory and neuroinhibitory amino acids causes craving for ethanol. Addict Behav 29: 1325–1339.
20. Weiss F, Parsons LH, Schulteis G, Hyytia P, Lorang MT, et al. (1996) Ethanol self-administration restores withdrawal-associated deficiencies in accumbal dopamine and 5-hydroxytryptamine release in dependent rats. J Neurosci 16: 3474–3485.
21. Fritze J (1989) Biologische Psychiatrie. Stuttgart: Fischer.
22. Bender W, Albus M, Moller HJ, Tretter F (2006) Towards systemic theories in biological psychiatry. Pharmacopsychiatry 39 Suppl 1: S4–9.
23. Noble D (2011) The aims of systems biology: between molecules and organisms. Pharmacopsychiatry 44 Suppl 1: S9–S14.
24. Voit EO, Qi Z, Kikuchi S (2012) Mesoscopic models of neurotransmission as intermediates between disease simulators and tools for discovering design principles. Pharmacopsychiatry 45 Suppl 1: S22–30.
25. Voit EO (2014) Mesoscopic modeling as a starting point for computational analyses of cystic fibrosis as a systemic disease. Biochim Biophys Acta 1844: 258–270.
26. Qi Z, Fieni D, Tretter F, Voit EO (2013) The neurochemical mobile with non-linear interaction matrix: an exploratory computational model. Pharmacopsychiatry 46 Suppl 1: S53–63.
27. Tretter F, Albus M (2004) Einfürhung in die Psychiopharmakotherapie. Stuttgart Thieme.
28. Goldstein DS, Eisenhofer G, Kopin IJ (2003) Sources and significance of plasma levels of catechols and their metabolites in humans. J Pharmacol Exp Ther 305: 800–811.
29. Nirogi R, Mudigonda K, Kandikere V, Ponnamaneni R (2010) Quantification of acetylcholine, an essential neurotransmitter, in brain microdialysis samples by liquid chromatography mass spectrometry. Biomed Chromatogr 24: 39–48.
30. Uutela P, Reinila R, Piepponen P, Ketola RA, Kostiainen R (2005) Analysis of acetylcholine and choline in microdialysis samples by liquid chromatography/tandem mass spectrometry. Rapid Commun Mass Spectrom 19: 2950–2956.
31. Church WH, Justice JB Jr, Byrd LD (1987) Extracellular dopamine in rat striatum following uptake inhibition by cocaine, nomifensine and benztropine. Eur J Pharmacol 139: 345–348.
32. Meldrum BS (2000) Glutamate as a neurotransmitter in the brain: review of physiology and pathology. J Nutr 130: 1007S–1015S.
33. Popa D, Cerdan J, Reperant C, Guiard BP, Guilloux JP, et al. (2010) A longitudinal study of 5-HT outflow during chronic fluoxetine treatment using a new technique of chronic microdialysis in a highly emotional mouse strain. Eur J Pharmacol 628: 83–90.
34. Bunin MA, Wightman RM (1998) Quantitative evaluation of 5-hydroxytryptamine (serotonin) neuronal release and uptake: an investigation of extrasynaptic transmission. J Neurosci 18: 4854–4860.
35. Smith TD, Kuczenski R, George-Friedman K, Malley JD, Foote SL (2000) In vivo microdialysis assessment of extracellular serotonin and dopamine levels in awake monkeys during sustained fluoxetine administration. Synapse 38: 460–470.
36. Zhang X, Rauch A, Lee H, Xiao H, Rainer G, et al. (2007) Capillary hydrophilic interaction chromatography/mass spectrometry for simultaneous determination of multiple neurotransmitters in primate cerebral cortex. Rapid Commun Mass Spectrom 21: 3621–3628.
37. Steinberg LL, Sposito MM, Lauro FA, Tufik S, Mello MT, et al. (1998) Serum level of serotonin during rest and during exercise in paraplegic patients. Spinal Cord 36: 18–20.
38. Hutchinson PJ, O'Connell MT, Al-Rawi PG, Kett-White CR, Gupta AK, et al. (2002) Increases in GABA concentrations during cerebral ischaemia: a microdialysis study of extracellular amino acids. J Neurol Neurosurg Psychiatry 72: 99–105.
39. Kanthan R, Shuaib A, Griebel R, Miyashita H (1995) Intracerebral human microdialysis. In vivo study of an acute focal ischemic model of the human brain. Stroke 26: 870–873.
40. Voit EO (2000) Computational analysis of biochemical systems : a practical guide for biochemists and molecular biologists. Cambridge, U.K.: Cambridge University Press. xii, 531 p. p.
41. Voit EO (2013) Biochemical Systems Theory: A Review. Int Scholarly Res Network (ISRN – Biomathematics): 1–53.
42. Torres NV, Voit EO (2002) Pathway Analysis and Optimization in Metabolic Engineering. Cambridge, U.K.: Cambridge University Press. xiv + 305 pp p.
43. Savageau MA (1976) Biochemical Systems Analysis: A Study of Function and Design in Molecular Biology Reading, MA: Addison-Wesley. 199 p. p.
44. Qi Z, Miller GW, Voit EO (2010) The internal state of medium spiny neurons varies in response to different input signals. BMC Syst Biol 4: 26.
45. Qi Z, Miller GW, Voit EO (2008) Computational systems analysis of dopamine metabolism. PLoS One 3: e2444.
46. Qi Z, Miller GM, Voit EO (2012) Mathematical Models of Dopàmine Metabolism in Parkinson's Disease. In: Wellstead P, Cloutier M, editors. Systems Biology of Parkinson's Disease. New York: Springer Science + Business Media, LLC.
47. Carboni S, Isola R, Gessa GL, Rossetti ZL (1993) Ethanol prevents the glutamate release induced by N-methyl-D-aspartate in the rat striatum. Neurosci Lett 152: 133–136.
48. Sano H, Suzuki Y, Ohara K, Yazaki R, Ishigaki T, et al. (1992) Circadian variation in plasma homovanillic acid level during and after alcohol withdrawal in alcoholic patients. Alcohol Clin Exp Res 16: 1047–1051.
49. Clements JD (1996) Transmitter timecourse in the synaptic cleft: its role in central synaptic function. Trends Neurosci 19: 163–171.
50. Lieber CS (1991) Hepatic, metabolic and toxic effects of ethanol: 1991 update. Alcohol Clin Exp Res 15: 573–592.
51. Glue P, Nutt D (1990) Overexcitement and disinhibition. Dynamic neurotransmitter interactions in alcohol withdrawal. Br J Psychiatry 157: 491–499.
52. Nutt D, Glue P, Molyneux S, Clark E (1988) Alpha-2-adrenoceptor function in alcohol withdrawal: a pilot study of the effects of iv. clonidine in alcoholics and normals. Alcohol Clin Exp Res 12: 14–18.
53. Goldstein DB (1973) Alcohol withdrawal reactions in mice: effects of drugs that modify neurotransmission. J Pharmacol Exp Ther 186: 1–9.

9

Alcohol Disinhibition of Behaviors in *C. elegans*

Stephen M. Topper, Sara C. Aguilar, Viktoria Y. Topper, Erin Elbel, Jonathan T. Pierce-Shimomura*

Waggoner Center for Alcohol and Addiction Research, Cell & Molecular Biology, Department of Neuroscience, The University of Texas at Austin, Austin, Texas, United States of America

Abstract

Alcohol has a wide variety of effects on physiology and behavior. One of the most well-recognized behavioral effects is disinhibition, where behaviors that are normally suppressed are displayed following intoxication. A large body of evidence has shown that alcohol-induced disinhibition in humans affects attention, verbal, sexual, and locomotor behaviors. Similar behavioral disinhibition is also seen in many animal models of ethanol response, from invertebrates to mammals and primates. Here we describe several examples of disinhibition in the nematode *C. elegans*. The nematode displays distinct behavioral states associated with locomotion (crawling on land and swimming in water) that are mediated by dopamine. On land, animals crawl and feed freely, but these behaviors are inhibited in water. We found that additional behaviors, including a variety of escape responses are also inhibited in water. Whereas alcohol non-specifically impaired locomotion, feeding, and escape responses in worms on land, alcohol specifically disinhibited these behaviors in worms immersed in water. Loss of dopamine signaling relieved disinhibition of feeding behavior, while loss of the D1-like dopamine receptor DOP-4 impaired the ethanol-induced disinhibition of crawling. The powerful genetics and simple nervous system of *C. elegans* may help uncover conserved molecular mechanisms that underlie alcohol-induced disinhibition of behaviors in higher animals.

Editor: Jill C. Bettinger, Virginia Commonwealth University, United States of America

Funding: Funding was provided by National Institutes of Health grants from NIAAA (R01AA020992) and NINDS (R01NS075541), Waggoner Center for Alcohol and Addiction Research (http://www.utexas.edu/research/wcaar/)to JTP as well as a Bruce Jones Fellowship to ST. The funders had no role in study design, data collection and analysis, decision to publish, or preparation of the manuscript.

Competing Interests: The authors have declared that no competing interests exist.

* E-mail: jonps@austin.utexas.edu

Introduction

Ethanol (EtOH) is the most commonly abused drug, in part because of its culturally condoned role in disinhibiting behaviors that are suppressed during states of anxiety. This disinhibiting effect of EtOH results in a euphoric feeling of release, further reinforcing EtOH drinking habits. A variety of behaviors are disinhibited with EtOH consumption. For example, it is known to reduce anxiety [1,2]. Previous work has found that acute EtOH intoxication decreases motor latency in simple "go/no go" trials [3,4,5]. EtOH also disinhibits behaviors critical for social interaction. Studies have shown that intoxication increases verbal expression and social bonding [6,7]. There is also a wealth of research on the interaction between EtOH and sexual behaviors, with intoxicated individuals reporting higher sexual arousal and an increase in risky sexual behaviors [8,9]. Disinhibition is a common, sometimes desired, effect of EtOH consumption in humans.

While the phenomenon of disinhibition by EtOH in humans has been known for some time, studying the neural mechanisms underlying these behaviors relied upon the development of appropriate animal models. To this end, researchers have established a variety of animal models that display disinhibition in response to EtOH. In rodent models, EtOH disinhibits locomotor patterns, often measured through the transient increase in total movement during acute intoxication as well as grooming [10–12]. Stress has also been shown to potentiate disinhibiting effects of EtOH, with stressed animals displaying an increase in EtOH-induced locomotion [12]. Several rodent studies reported relief of stress-induced behavioral inhibition via EtOH. In mice and rats, EtOH relieves stress-induced inhibition of a number of behaviors. Animals exposed to isolation stress displayed anxiety behaviors, assessed as reduced entries and time spent in the open arm in an elevated plus-maze test, which were partially relived by EtOH intoxication [13,14]. Exposure to EtOH also relieves the impairment of social investigation, social preference, and spatial memory, induced by chronic restraint stress [12,15]. Animals bred to prefer EtOH show a high baseline level of anxiety in the elevated plus-maze test, which is reversed by EtOH administration [16,17]. In addition to mammalian models, evidence of EtOH-induced disinhibition has also been noted in the invertebrate model Drosophila. EtOH was shown to disinhibit sexual and locomotor behaviors in flies [18]. In this study, it was shown that repeated EtOH exposure disinhibited male-male courtship, a behavior unseen in normal flies. Thus, disinhibition is a common feature of EtOH intoxication across many different species.

Efforts to uncover the neuromolecular basis of EtOH-induced disinhibition have focused on the dopaminergic pathway. The dopaminergic system has been shown to be a key component of EtOH-induced disinhibition in mammalian and invertebrate models. Two decades ago, EtOH intoxication was shown to increase dopamine levels, measured via microdialysis, in the nucleus accumbens [19,20]. It was later shown that this increase was due to excess dopamine release from the ventral tegmental area [21,22]. Microinjection of dopamine receptor antagonists, including those that target D1 dopamine receptors, into the nucleus accumbens reduced responses to EtOH-paired stimuli, suggesting a role for these receptors in reward [23–25]. Dopamine release in the nucleus accumbens is also associated with locomotor disinhibition [26]. Pretreatment with dopamine reuptake inhibitors or D1 receptor agonists has been shown to sensitize animals to locomotor disinhibition, though this has not been consistently shown [27–29]. A recent study in flies, however, showed a similar role for D1 receptors in locomotor disinhibition [30]. Likewise, dopamine signaling was also shown to be involved in EtOH-induced disinhibition of male-male courtship in Drosophila [19].

In the present study, we examined whether EtOH induces disinhibition in the model nematode *Caenorhabditis elegans* and if the dopaminergic system was similarly implicated in these effects. Many studies have demonstrated the utility of the nematode *C. elegans* as a simple model to examine conserved molecular bases for behavioral responses to EtOH. While *C. elegans* cannot effectively model the full complexities of alcohol addiction in humans, the nematode has been used to model important aspects of EtOH abuse. During acute intoxication, worms exposed to EtOH display a gradual, dose-dependent decline in locomotor activity, similar to the depressive effects of EtOH seen in other animals [31,32]. Importantly, the internal dose of EtOH that elicits this behavioral change is equivalent to that in humans as well as in rodent models of intoxication, suggesting that the underlying molecular targets may be the same. *C. elegans* also displays acute tolerance to EtOH, as evidenced by a recovery of locomotor behaviors after 30 minutes of intoxication [33]. Withdrawal from EtOH alters a number of behaviors. An increase in a social behavior, apparent as animals clumping together, has been observed during withdrawal [34]. Mitchell *et al.*, (2010) catalogued a number of locomotor defects upon withdrawal, including altered posture and an impaired ability to navigate towards food [34]. Thus, *C. elegans* has been shown to display many aspects of EtOH responses.

For this study, we chose a liquid immersion assay because *C. elegans* displays distinct subsets of behaviors on land, which are controlled by dopamine and are inhibited in aquatic environments [35,36]. On land, the worm displays the crawling locomotor gait that is characterized by tight, low frequency bends, as well as a number of associated feeding behaviors. In water, the worm switches to a distinct swimming gait characterized by shallow and high frequency bends, and cessation of crawl-associated feeding behaviors [35,36]. Initiation of crawling is dependent on the D1-like dopamine receptors DOP-1 and DOP-4, as evident by cessation of forward movement following immersion from water in mutant animals that lack these receptors [35]. Likewise, crawl-associated behaviors can be induced during immersion in water in wild-type animals by external application of dopamine or photostimulation of dopamine neurons with optogenetics [35,36]. In the present study, we found that additional crawl-associated behaviors are also inhibited during immersion in water. Application of EtOH to worms in water resulted in disinhibition of crawling and associated behaviors. Disinhibition of several of these behaviors was reliant on dopamine signaling.

Results

Immersion in liquid inhibits a subset of behaviors in *C. elegans*

Before investigating the potential effects of EtOH on disinhibiting behaviors in *C. elegans*, we quantified a collection of behaviors that the worm displays on semi-moist agar plates (hereafter called the "on land" condition for simplicity) versus when immersed in water.

First, we measured the incidence of a behavior called "foraging" that is associated with feeding. Foraging consists of the worm wiggling the anterior-most tip of its head, which contains the sensory organs and mouth, at about 10 Hz [37]. Foraging bends occur in three dimensions and independently from the dorsoventral full-body bends described above for crawling and swimming. Foraging has been proposed to represent a food-seeking behavior, because it occurs most frequently in the presence of food (bacteria) [37]. As in previous reports, we found that worms displayed foraging and pharyngeal pumping on land, but not in water [35,36] (Figure 1 a).

Second, we tested whether the incidence of locomotor behaviors related to dispersion and escape were distinct on land and in water. Many animals, including humans, rodents, flies, and *C. elegans*, display alternating bouts of extended migration and spontaneous reorienting sharp turns that influence efficiency of local search and rates of dispersion. The primary means of reorienting in *C. elegans* is by temporarily moving backwards for 5–10 seconds in a so-called "reversal". As in our previous study [36], we found that worms displayed three spontaneous reversals per minute on land, but rarely exhibited reversals in water (Figure 1 b). *C. elegans* will also perform a reversal in response to mechanical stimuli [38,39]. Animals touched near the midbody with a platinum wire reversed away from the stimulus. We found that on land, this effect was seen in over 90% of animals, while immersion in water reduced this behavior drastically (Figure 1 c). Blue light is another noxious stimulus to worms (~470 nm wavelength) [40]. Animals exposed to blue light rapidly accelerated away from light, increasing their frequency of bending on land, but not in water (Figure 1 d).

Third, we quantified kinematic aspects of forward locomotion that distinguish the crawling and swimming gaits. During crawling, the worm lies on its left or right side while bending its head dorsoventrally at ~0.5 Hz (Figure 1 e). These bends propagate backwards along the body, causing the worm to form a traveling S-shaped posture during crawling (Figure 1 f). By contrast, during swimming, the worm bends its head dorsoventrally at ~1.6 Hz (Figure 1 e). Swimming is also distinguished from crawling by bends that are synchronized to form a C-shaped body posture twice per locomotor cycle – a posture that is never displayed on land during crawling (Figure 1 f).

Ethanol induces disinhibition of specific behaviors in *C. elegans*

After quantitatively characterizing the inhibition of different worm behaviors by immersion in water, we next examined whether EtOH disinhibited any of these behaviors. We compared the responses of wild-type worms immersed in liquid to those immersed in EtOH. Previous work has shown that *C. elegans* exposed to an exogenous concentration of 500-mM EtOH on land displays a gradual decline in locomotion, feeding, and egg-laying behaviors, and eventually becomes immobile over 30 minutes [31]. Intoxication in liquid at the same concentration was found to result in a steady decrease in locomotion over 6 minutes, after which locomotor rate remained constant [41]. While 500-mM EtOH is well above physiologically relevant levels, Alaimo *et al* (2012) demonstrated that this high exogenous dose resulted in an internal EtOH concentration relevant to human consumption and disinhibition in rodents models [1,4–7,18,30,32,41].

We found that animals exposed to EtOH during immersion in liquid displayed disinhibition of several behaviors that are never (or rarely) observed in water. These included foraging, spontaneous reversal, touch response, and blue light response (Figure 2 a–d). To test whether this effect of EtOH on worms in water was distinct from a generic decline in locomotion performance, animals were treated with 1-mM sodium azide. This compound

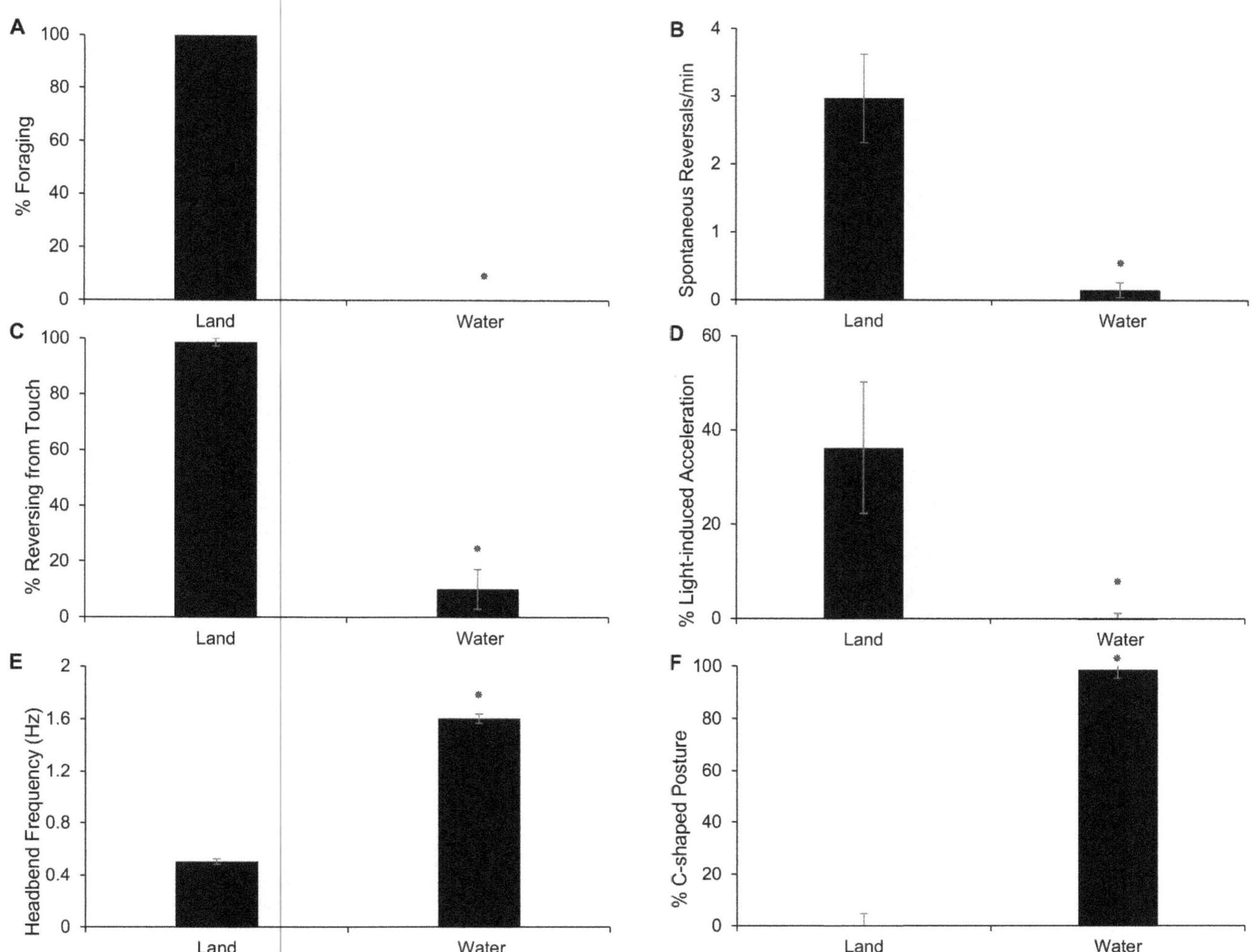

Figure 1. Crawl Behaviors Are Inhibited in Water. Immersion in liquid results in inhibition of many behaviors in wild-type *C. elegans*. Notably, the feeding behavior foraging (A), spontaneous reversals (B), touch response (C), and light response (D) are all inhibited. To assess disinhibition of crawl during immersion in water, headbend frequency (E) and percent body bends with C-shape (F) were assessed. In liquid, worms exhibited only a fast, C-shaped swim. Statistical analyses comparing behaviors on land vs. water were performed using planned unpaired two-tailed t-test. Asterisks indicate $P<0.001$, $n\geq4$ assays, ≥10 worms per assay for all experiments A–C, $n\geq15$ for D–F. Error bars represent standard error of the mean.

inhibits cellular respiration, resulting in a gradual decline of cellular activity [42,43]. Animals treated with sodium azide displayed locomotor decline soon after application. After 7 minutes, head-bend frequencies of sodium azide-treated worms were similar to those of EtOH-treated animals (Figure 2 e). However, despite their lower locomotion rate, these animals did not display significant disinhibition of spontaneous reversals, foraging, touch response, or light response (Figure 2 a–d). In addition, these animals displayed mostly C-shaped body postures characteristic of swim, while animals exposed to EtOH showed significantly fewer C-shaped postures characteristic of swimming (Figure 2 f) and more crawl-like S-shaped postures.

Disinhibition of Foraging is Partially Dependent on D1-like Dopamine Signaling

Our previous work has shown that transition from swimming to crawling is initiated by dopamine release and D1-like dopamine receptor signaling [35]. To investigate the role of the dopaminergic system in the EtOH-induced disinhibition of behaviors, animals deficient in dopamine signaling were evaluated [44–47]. We found that disruption of dopamine synthesis by deletion of the worm tyrosine hydroxylase gene, *cat-2*, partly, but significantly, reduced EtOH-induced disinhibition of foraging behavior (Figure 3 a). Likewise, deletion of D1-like dopamine receptor genes *dop-1* or *dop-4* also reduced disinhibition of foraging (Figure 3 a). We observed the same result for two deletion alleles of *dop-4*, raising the likelihood that this phenotype corresponded with loss of function of the *dop-4* gene. By contrast, deletion of the D2-like receptor genes *dop-2* and *dop-3* in combination had no effect versus WT on disinhibition of foraging (Figure 3 a). Post-hoc statistical analysis of this strain revealed minor differences from WT and similarity to the *dop-1* mutant. As dopamine has been previously shown to activate foraging in water [35], this may point to a partial role for D1-like dopamine signaling in the response to EtOH. Likewise, just as in our previous study [35], more salient effects were found for loss of the DOP-4 receptor versus loss of DOP-1 receptor.

Intriguingly, disruption of dopamine signaling via mutation generally did not alter the level of EtOH-induced disinhibition for other crawl-associated behaviors. This included spontaneous reversals, touch-induced reversals, and acceleration in response

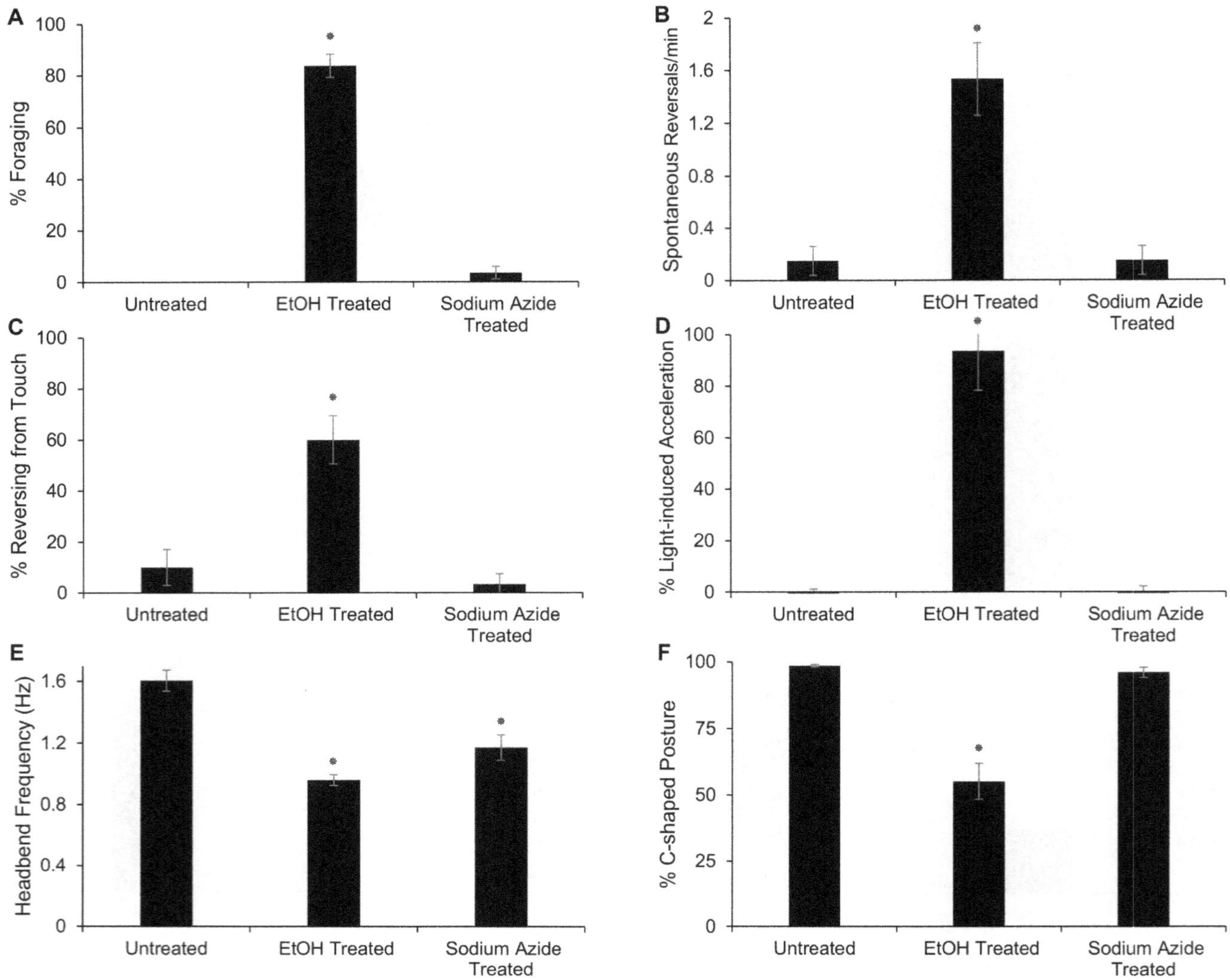

Figure 2. Ethanol Exposure during Immersion in Liquid Results in Disinhibition of Crawl Behaviors. Foraging (A), spontaneous reversals (B), touch response (C), and light response (D), as well as crawling kinematics (E,F) were disinhibited by EtOH. To ensure that such disinhibition was not the result of a decline in cellular function, worms treated with sodium azide were also assessed. No disinhibition was observed in these animals. EtOH treatment resulted in a reduction of bending frequency and a loss of C-shaped body posture. Animals treated with sodium azide experienced a similar decline in bending frequency, but no reduction in C-shape body posture. Statistical analyses comparing EtOH-, azide-, and untreated worms were performed using one-way ANOVA and Tukey's HSD post-hoc test or Kruskal-Wallis and Steel-Dwass-Critchlow-Fligner post-hoc test. Asterisks indicate significance in relation to untreated controls with $P<0.001$, $n\geq4$ assays, ≥10 worms per assay for all experiments A–C, $n\geq15$ for D–F. Error bars represent standard error of the mean.

to blue light (Figure 3 b–d). Post-hoc statistical analysis revealed a slightly lower response to touch for the *dop-4* mutant allele *ok1321* (Figure 3c); however, the other *dop-4* allele *tm1392* did not share this phenotype, suggesting it may not be attributed to loss of the *dop-4* gene. Taken together, these data suggest that a pathway other than dopamine influences these additional aspects of EtOH-induced disinhibition.

One possible pathway for EtOH-induced disinhibition is via the BK potassium channel. Two previous genetic screens revealed that the BK channel SLO-1 was a direct target of EtOH and the major modulator of acute depressive responses to EtOH for crawling and egg laying behaviors in *C. elegans* [32]. This channel is widely expressed in the neurons and muscles, and loss of SLO-1 enhances neurotransmitter release [48]. Thus, it is possible that EtOH-induced disinhibition acts through SLO-1, and its loss would decrease the observed EtOH sensitivity. We found, however, that *slo-1* mutant animals displayed a wild-type level of disinhibition for all quantified behaviors (Figure 3 a–d; raw data for % light-induced acceleration found in Table S1). This strongly indicates that disinhibition is not the result of generalized action of EtOH across the nervous system via this central target of intoxication.

Disinhibition of crawling is dependent on the D1-like dopamine receptor DOP-4

We also investigated whether disinhibition of the crawling locomotor gait depended on dopamine and/or BK channel pathways. When immersed in EtOH, animals lacking the DOP-1 receptor exhibited a slightly lower head bending frequency than wild-type animals (Figure 4 a). In addition, we noticed that many EtOH-treated animals only propagated bends partially down the body or would abnormally move their anterior and posterior halves asynchronously. To quantitatively characterize this unco-

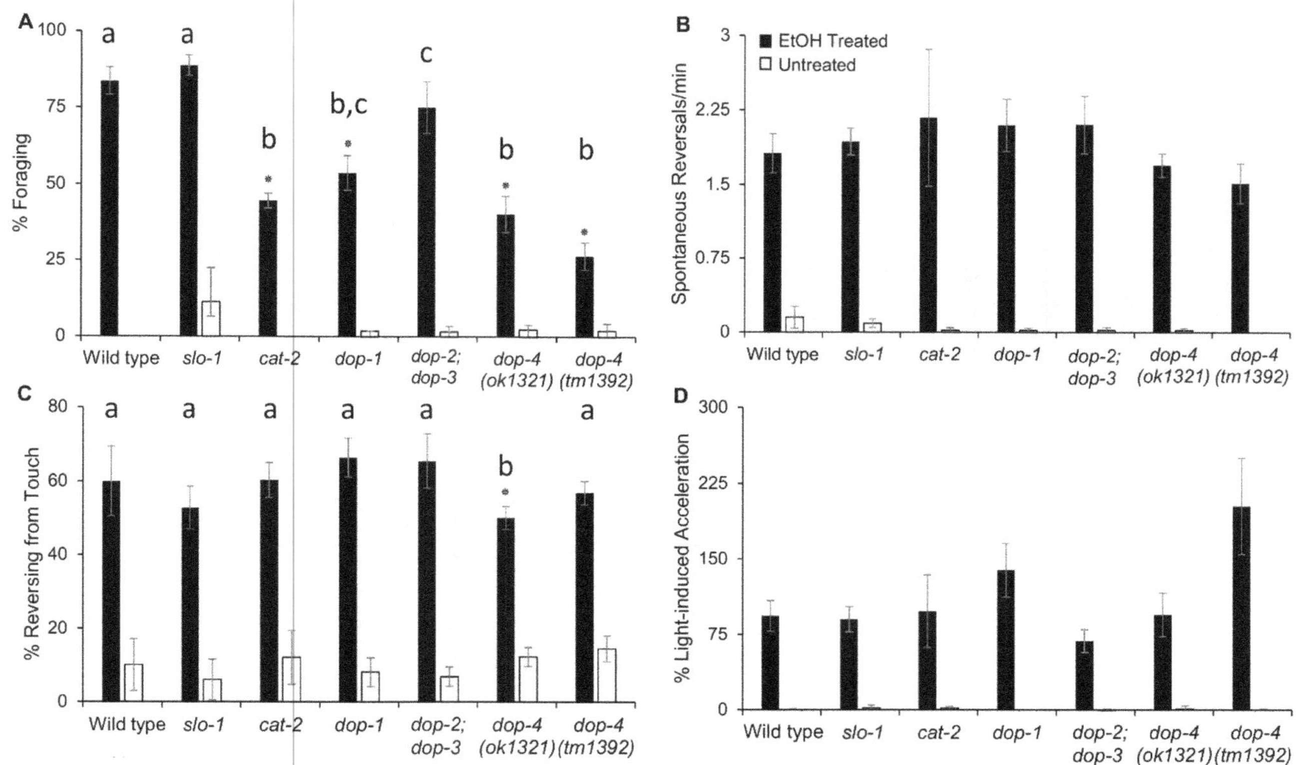

Figure 3. Disinhibition of Foraging Involves Dopamine Signaling. Loss of dopamine synthesis or D1-like dopamine signaling significantly reduced disinhibition of foraging (A). No significant reduction in disinhibition of spontaneous reversals or touch response was observed in animals lacking SLO-1, dopamine synthesis, or dopamine receptors (B,C) except for *dop-4(ok1321)*. Although slightly varied, responses to light did not differ significantly among strains as determined by post-hoc analyses (D). Statistical analyses comparing EtOH-treated mutants to EtOH-treated WT controls were performed using one-way ANOVA and Tukey's HSD post-hoc test or Kruskal-Wallis and Steel-Dwass-Critchlow-Fligner post-hoc test. Letters indicate distinct groupings based on post-hoc statistical comparison among strains. Asterisks indicate significance in relation to WT controls (EtOH-treated or untreated, accordingly) with $P<0.001$, $n\geq4$ assays, ≥10 worms per assay for all experiments. Error bars represent standard error of the mean.

ordinated motion, the percent of bends that fully propagated along the animal body was calculated. This revealed that the majority of head bends were not propagated during EtOH exposure, even in mutant animals lacking SLO-1 (Figure 4 b). This effect was most prominent in mutant strains lacking *dop-4*, which both propagated significantly fewer bends than wild type (Figure 4 b). The phenotype is most likely due to mutation of the *dop-4* gene because an identical phenotype was found in independent alleles of *dop-4* (Figure 4 b). We previously observed a similar failure of the *dop-4* mutant to propagate bends when attempting to transition to crawling following swimming [35]. Thus, the significantly reduced bending observed in *dop-4* mutants may be due to an inability of these animals to transition from swimming to EtOH-induced crawling.

When considering the subset of locomotor cycles with bends that fully propagated down the body, we noticed that only animals lacking *dop-4* displayed significantly more C-shaped posture (Figure 4 c). These data, along with the lower bending propagation seen in *dop-4* mutant animals suggest that DOP-4 is involved in the disinhibition of crawling gait during intoxication. We conclude that *dop-4* mutant animals are unable to engage in EtOH-induced crawling, and thus become either more uncoordinated or display slower C-shaped swim bends when exposed to EtOH. Interestingly, *cat-2* mutant animals, which lack dopamine did not show a similar reduction in crawl disinhibition. Thus, EtOH in worms may act more directly through DOP-4 itself or a downstream pathway for this aspect of EtOH-induced disinhibition.

Discussion

Acute exposure to EtOH is known to disinhibit many behaviors. In humans, this includes social, sexual, and locomotor behaviors [1–5,8,9]. Such disinhibition has also been demonstrated in fly and rodent models [10–12,18,30]. This disinhibition was shown to be reliant on the D1 class of dopamine receptors in flies and rodents. Our present study demonstrated a similar effect in *C. elegans*. First, we have developed a novel paradigm to study EtOH-induced disinhibition of behavior in *C. elegans*. Second, we have shown that some disinhibitory effects are dependent in part on dopamine signaling. Third, we found evidence that EtOH may act directly on a D1-like dopamine receptor or downstream pathway. Together, these findings provide an excellent model to study disinhibition and provide evidence for a role of dopamine in the response to EtOH in *C. elegans*.

C. elegans as a model for EtOH-induced disinhibition of behavior

C. elegans has previously been shown to display many behavioral effects of EtOH seen in other model animals. It was previously described that *C. elegans* displays acute intoxication, acute tolerance, EtOH preference, and withdrawal [31–34,49]. Our

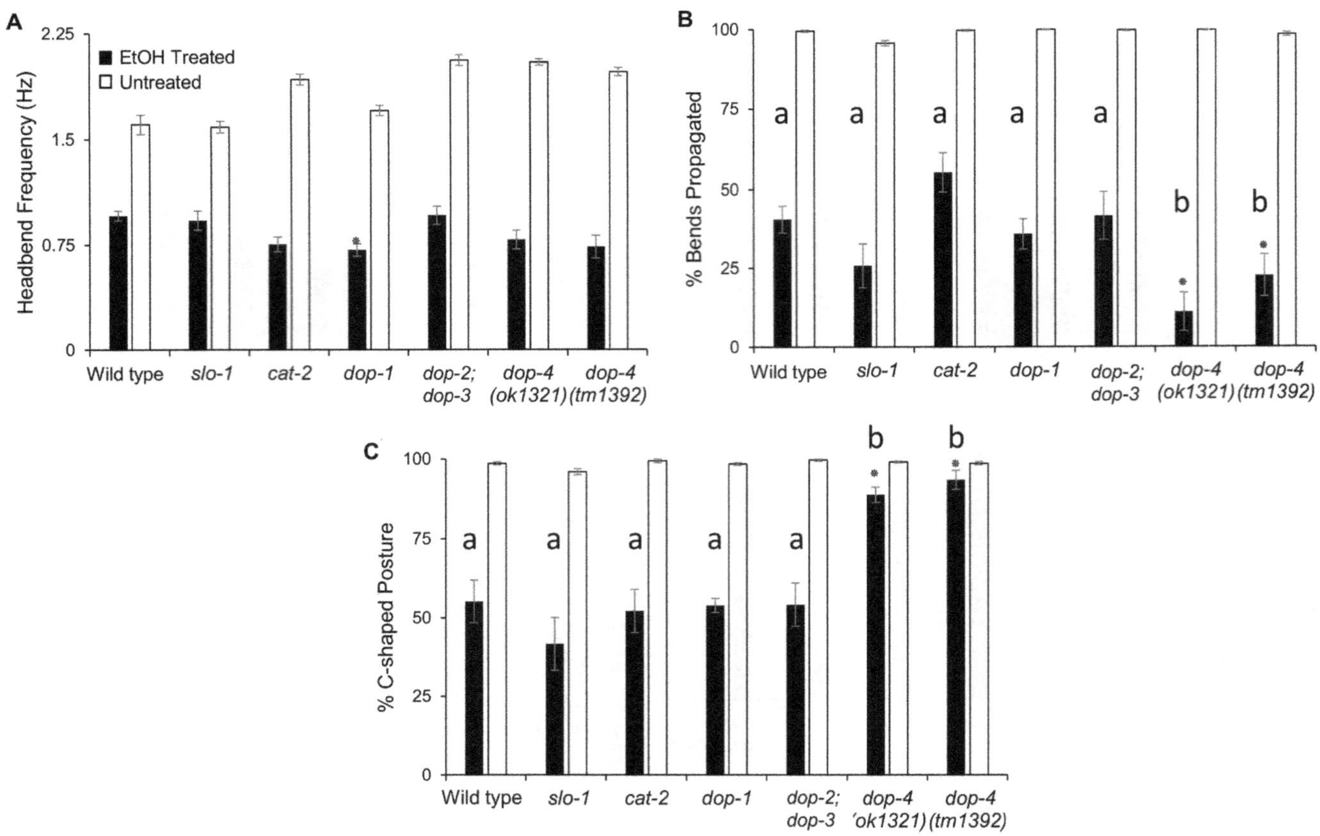

Figure 4. Loss of D1-like Dopamine Receptor DOP-4 Reduces Disinhibition of Crawl. Loss of the D1-like receptor DOP-1 resulted in a slightly lower bending frequency versus WT with EtOH treatment (A). EtOH treatment also caused uncoordination, with significantly fewer bends propagated down the animal. This phenotype was exacerbated in *dop-4* mutant animals (B). Of body bends propagated down the animal, approximately half were C-shaped in most intoxicated animals, indicating disinhibition of crawl. Only animals lacking *dop-4* demonstrated resistance to this effect. Statistical analyses comparing EtOH-treated mutants to EtOH-treated WT controls were performed using one-way ANOVA and Tukey's HSD post-hoc test or Kruskal-Wallis and Steel-Dwass-Critchlow-Fligner post-hoc test. Asterisks indicate significance in relation to WT controls (EtOH-treated or untreated, accordingly) with $P<0.001$, $n\geq10$ worms for all experiments. Letters indicate distinct groupings based on post-hoc statistical comparison among strains. Error bars represent standard error of the mean.

study now adds an important fifth EtOH-induced behavior to this list: disinhibition. This worm model offers many benefits to traditional models of disinhibition, as *C. elegans* quickly matures to genetically identical adults, offers fast generation of transgenic animals, and has a completely described nervous system. In addition, the effects of EtOH on *C. elegans* are robust and easily quantifiable.

Previous studies have shown that several behaviors, including foraging, spontaneous reversal, and crawl are inhibited in water. We further demonstrate that escape responses to blue light and touch are also inhibited in liquid. Upon exposure to EtOH while immersed in liquid, all of these behaviors are disinhibited. This disinhibition was not a result of generalized locomotor or behavioral decline, as disinhibition was not observed in the animals treated with sodium azide. A straight-forward inhibition of swimming would be expected to cause a non-specific decline in locomotor patterns. Instead, we observed that EtOH induced bouts of crawling and a subset of crawl-associated behaviors (e.g. foraging and reversals) that all require coordinated motion. From these results, we conclude that EtOH should be viewed as specifically disinhibiting crawl behaviors rather than inhibiting swimming.

Dopamine is required for disinhibition of foraging in *C. elegans*

Dopamine has been shown to be a key component of acute EtOH intoxication. In mammals, a large body of evidence has demonstrated that dopamine and D1-like dopamine receptors play an important role in EtOH-induced disinhibition of locomotion. The increase in dopamine release following EtOH intoxication is correlated with locomotor disinhibition in rodents [26]. Several studies have shown a sensitization to the disinhibitory effects of EtOH following pretreatment with dopamine reuptake inhibitors or D1 receptor agonists, though this effect is not consistent amongst all rodent models [27–29]. However, recent work in *Drosophila* has also demonstrated a role for dopamine and the D1 dopamine receptors in EtOH-induced disinhibition. Loss of dopamine signaling reduced EtOH disinhibition of male-male courtship [18], while loss of D1 dopamine receptors reduced EtOH disinhibition of locomotion [30].

Previously, the only known interaction between dopamine and EtOH in *C. elegans* was the requirement for dopamine in EtOH preference [50]. We found that EtOH showed potent disinhibition of crawling, spontaneous reversals, and touch and light response in worms immersed in liquid. Disinhibition was not modulated by the SLO-1 potassium channel, the major target of EtOH in *C. elegans* [31], indicating disinhibition is distinct from SLO-1-mediated acute intoxication and is instead mediated by other targets. Interestingly, dopamine signaling did not appear to play a role in disinhibition of spontaneous reversals or response to touch and light. Thus, these behaviors may not be induced by the same dopamine signal as the transition to crawl. As EtOH affects a wide variety of targets, including nicotinic and glutamate receptors, this result is not surprising [50,51]. In addition, a major neuron responsible for harsh touch transduction, PVD, expresses both such receptor subtypes [52–55]. We found that dopamine signaling is important in the induction of foraging in immersed *C. elegans*. Previously, it was shown that both dopamine and D1-like receptors are required for initiation of crawling [35], and foraging can be induced in animals immersed in liquid through application of dopamine [36]. Complementing this result, we found that animals lacking dopamine synthesis or D1-like dopamine receptors display significantly less disinhibition of foraging. This points toward a potentially conserved mechanism for disinhibition in *C. elegans* and higher animals.

Ethanol may act directly on a D1-like dopamine receptor pathway

Unexpectedly, we found evidence that EtOH may act directly on the D1-like dopamine receptor DOP-4 or through its downstream signaling. Disinhibition of crawling, as assessed by presence of C-shaped posture, was only seen in animals lacking DOP-4 and not in animals lacking dopamine or SLO-1. Previous research in mice found extensive evidence for a role of D1-like dopamine receptors in locomotor disinhibition via EtOH. While there are many links between D1-like dopamine receptors and EtOH-induced disinhibition, these have been attributed to the increase in dopamine observed following acute intoxication. Many papers have pointed towards a role for D1-like receptors in the disinhibition of locomotion and EtOH-seeking behaviors [23–25,27–29]. We are not aware of any papers demonstrating any direct interaction of EtOH on dopamine receptors. Thus, this work demonstrates a potential novel effect of EtOH on D1-like receptors that is independent of dopamine release.

Experimental Procedures

Animals

C. elegans were grown on nematode growth media (NGM) agar plates seeded with OP50 bacteria at 20°C as previously described [56]. Mutant strains were obtained from the Caenorhabditis Genetic Center and the *C. elegans* Gene Knockout Consortium. The following strains were used: WT N2, *cat-2(e112)*II, *dop-1(vs101)*X, *dop-1(vs100)*X, *dop-4(ok1321)*X, *dop-4(tm1392)*X, *dop-2(vs105)V;dop-3(vs106)*X, and *slo-1(js118)*V.

Pharmacological Assays

Each EtOH assay was conducted on 10–15, never-starved, young adult worms. Worms were cleaned of bacteria by allowing them to crawl on an empty plate for 2 minutes before each experiment. Assays were performed on plates containing 500-mM EtOH in the agar medium. 10–15 animals were picked into a 6-μL drop of 500-mM EtOH (200 proof; Sigma-Aldrich, St. Louis MO). EtOH solution was prepared by adding 200-proof EtOH to standard nematode growth medium (NGM). As osmolarity is known to affect intoxication, NGM was tested prior to experiments to ensure a constant 180 mOsm. Worm behavior was recorded for 30 minutes continuously. Additional 6-μL drops of 500-mM EtOH were added every 2–3 minutes, when the boundary of the drop began to recede. Worms maintain swimming and suppress crawling behaviors as long as the depth of the drop is greater than the width of the worm [35]. Control assays were performed in the same manner, except EtOH was not added to NGM media. Previously reported internal EtOH concentrations after 10 minutes of 500-mM EtOH exposure ranged from 17.5–67.5 mM for animals on land [41]. This correlates well to disinhibiting doses seen in rodent and human disinhibition studies [4–7,18,30]. Internal EtOH concentration may be lower than those previously reported given that immersion in water inhibits ingestion by pharyngeal pumping [35]. Movie recordings were made at 30 frames/s, 344 pixels/mm using a Flea2 camera (Point Grey Research, Richmond, Canada) and StreamPix software (NorPix, Montreal, Canada). Sodium azide assays were performed by placing a 6-μL drop of 1-mM sodium azide (Sigma-Aldrich) onto a thin pad of agarose. 10–12 worms were then placed inside the drop and their activity was recorded for 30 minutes. Additional 6-μL drops of 1-mM sodium azide were added as needed.

To quantify different behaviors, groups of animals were analyzed for a 1-minute time window after 7 minutes of EtOH exposure at the beginning of the 30-minute recording. Foraging: Foraging was assessed by presence of ~5–10 Hz bending of the tip of the nose for each worm. Percent animals foraging was quantified by number of animals in a group displaying foraging behavior over one minute divided by total number of animals. Bending frequency: Head-bend duration was defined as the time the head traveled from its maximal dorsal flexure to maximal ventral flexure and vice versa. Head bends that did not change from ventral to dorsal flexure (or vice versa) were not counted, nor were bends that did not propagate down the body. Bend Propagation: Bending propagation was quantified by dividing number of bends initiated at the head of an animal divided by bends propagated to the tail. Posture: To characterize body posture, at the apex of each bend a line was drawn from nose to tail. If this line did not intersect the body at any point, then the animal was considered C-shaped. Only bends propagated down the body were analyzed for posture. Reversals: Reversals were defined as a backward movement spanning a distance greater than the pharynx of the animal. Touch Response: Touch response assays were also performed after 7 minutes of intoxication in a 6-μL drop of EtOH. The head of each animal was gently prodded with a platinum wire and a touch response was considered positive if the animal initiated a reversal after prodding. Light Response: To assay blue light response, animal behavior was recorded for 1 minute. The animal was then exposed to 1.6 mW/mm^2 420-nM wavelength blue light from a Prior Lumen200 fluorescent light system for 30 seconds. Head-bending frequencies were counted before and after illumination and the percent increase for each animal was determined.

Statistical Analyses

Statistical analyses were performed using JMP 11.0.0 SAS Software (SAS Institute, Cary, NC, USA). Results are presented as the mean ± standard error. Crawl behavior inhibition in water (Figure 1) was tested by unpaired two-tailed t-test. The statistical significance of differences between EtOH-, azide-treated, and untreated worms (Figure 2), ethanol-treated mutant populations vs. ethanol-treated wild-type worms, and untreated mutant populations vs. untreated wild-type worms (Figures 3 and 4) was demonstrated by a one-way analysis of variance (ANOVA), with Tukey's honest significant difference (HSD) multiple comparison post-hoc tests. If the data did not meet the assumptions for ANOVA test, data were analyzed using a Kruskal-Wallis test followed by a Steel-Dwass-Critchlow-Fligner multiple comparison test between each group. All differences were considered significant at P<0.001 (see Figures 1, 2, 3, 4).

Supporting Information

Table S1 Raw data broken into groups of genotype and treatment used to calculate percentage acceleration in response to blue light for Figure 3D. Paired values represent number of head bends observed in two 60 second time windows before and after blue light for different individual worms. Each worm was recorded and exposed to blue light only once.

Acknowledgments

We thank L. Young for technical assistance; S. Iyer and anonymous reviewers for comments on manuscript. Many worm strains were kindly provided by the *Caenorhabditis* Genetics Center, which is funded by the National Institutes of Health (NIH) National Center for Research Resources; the *C. elegans* Gene Knockout Project at the Oklahoma Medical Research Foundation, which is part of the International *C. elegans* Gene Knockout Consortium; and the National BioResource Project in Japan.

Author Contributions

Conceived and designed the experiments: ST JTP. Performed the experiments: ST SCA EE. Analyzed the data: ST VT JTP. Contributed reagents/materials/analysis tools: ST SCA. Wrote the paper: ST VT JTP.

References

1. Moberg CA, Curtin JJ (2009) Alcohol selectively reduces anxiety but not fear: startle response during unpredictable versus predictable threat. J Abnorm Psychol 118: 335–47.
2. de Boer MC, Schippers GM, van der Staak CP (1993) Alcohol and social anxiety in women and men: pharmacological and expectancy effects. Addict Behav 18: 117–26.
3. Rose AK, Duka T (2007) The influence of alcohol on basic motoric and cognitive disinhibition. Alcohol Alcohol 42: 544–51.
4. Weafer J, Fillmore MT (2012) Comparison of alcohol impairment of behavioral and attentional inhibition. Drug Alcohol Depend 126: 176–82.
5. Marinkovic K, Halgren E, Klopp J, Maltzman I (2000) Alcohol effects on movement-related potentials: a measure of impulsivity? J Stud Alcohol 61: 24–31.
6. Babor TF, Berglas S, Mendelson JH, Ellingboe J, Miller K (1982) Alcohol, affect, and the disinhibition of verbal behavior. Psychopharmacology Berl 80: 53–60.
7. Sayette MA, Creswell KG, Dimoff JD, Fairbairn CE, Cohn JF, et al. (2012) Alcohol and group formation: a multimodal investigation of the effects of alcohol on emotion and social bonding. Psychol Sci 23: 869–78.
8. Prause N, Staley C, Finn P (2011) The Effects of Acute Ethanol Consumption on Sexual Response and Sexual Risk-Taking Intent. Archives of Sexual Behavior 40: 373–384.
9. Stoner S, George WH, Peters LM, Norris J (2007) Liquid Courage: Alcohol Fosters Risky Sexual Decision-Making in Individuals with Sexual Fears. AIDS and Behavior 11: 227–237.
10. Ahlenius S, Brown R, Engel J, Svensson TH, Waldeck B (1974) Short communication. Antagonism by nialamide of the ethanol-induced locomotor stimulation in mice. J Neural Transm 35: 175–8.
11. Imperato A, Di Chiara G (1986) Preferential stimulation of dopamine release in the nucleus accumbens of freely moving rats by ethanol. J Pharmacol Exp Ther 239: 219–28.
12. Varlinskaya EI, Spear LP (2012) Increases in anxiety-like behavior induced by acute stress are reversed by ethanol in adolescent but not adult rats Pharmacol Biochem Behav 100: 440–450.
13. Pisu MG, Mostallino MC, Dore R, Maciocco E, Secci PP, et al. (2011) Effects of voluntary ethanol consumption on emotional state and stress responsiveness in socially isolated rats. Eur Neuropsychopharmacol 21: 414–425.
14. Pohorecky LA (2008) Psychosocial stress and chronic ethanol ingestion in male rats: effects on elevated plus maze behavior and ultrasonic vocalizations. Physiol Behav 94: 432–447.
15. Gomez JL, Lewis MJ, Luine VN (2012) The interaction of chronic restraint stress and voluntary alcohol intake: effects on spatial memory in male rats. Alcohol 46: 499–504.
16. Colombo G, Agabio R, Lobina C, Reali R, Zocchi A, et al. (1995) Sardinian alcohol-preferring rats: a genetic animal model of anxiety. Physiol Behav 57: 1181–1185.
17. Pandey SC, Zhang H, Roy A, Xu TJ (2005) Deficits in amygdaloid cAMP-responsive element-binding protein signaling play a role in genetic predisposition to anxiety and alcoholism. Clin Invest 115: 2762–2773.
18. Lee HG, Kim YC, Dunning JS, Han KA (2008) Recurring ethanol exposure induces disinhibited courtship in Drosophila. PLoS ONE 3: e1391.
19. Weiss F, Lorang MT, Bloom FE, Koob GF (1993) Oral alcohol self-administration stimulates dopamine release in the rat nucleus accumbens: genetic and motivational determinants. J Pharmacol Exp Ther 267: 250–258.
20. Imperato A, Di Chiara G (1986). Preferential stimulation of dopamine release in the nucleus accumbens of freely moving rats by ethanol. J Pharmacol Exp Ther 239: 219–228.
21. Yim HJ, Gonzales RA (2000) Ethanol-induced increases in dopamine extracellular concentration in rat nucleus accumbens are accounted for by increased release and not uptake inhibition. Alcohol 22: 107–115.
22. Gonzales RA, Job MO, Doyon WM (2004) The role of mesolimbic dopamine in the development and maintenance of ethanol reinforcement. Pharmacol Ther 103: 121–146.
23. Hodge CW, Samson HH, Chappelle AM (1997) Alcohol self administration: further examination of the role of dopamine receptors in the nucleus accumbens. Alcohol Clin Exp Res 21: 1083–1091.
24. Rassnick S, Pulvirenti L, Koob GF (1992) Oral ethanol self administration in rats is reduced by the administration of dopamine and glutamate receptor antagonists into the nucleus accumbens. Psychopharmacol 109: 92–98.
25. Samson HH, Hodge CW, Tolliver GA, Haraguchi M (1993) Effect of dopamine agonists and antagonists on ethanol-reinforced behavior: the involvement of the nucleus accumbens. Brain Res Bull 30: 133–141.
26. Melendez RI, Rodd-Henricks ZA, Engleman EA, Li TK, McBride WJ, et al. (2002) Microdialysis of dopamine in the nucleus accumbens of alcohol-preferring (P) rats during anticipation and operant self-administration of ethanol. Alcohol Clin Exp Res 26: 318–325.
27. Abrahao KP, Quadros IM, Souza-Formigoni ML (2011) Nucleus accumbens dopamine D_1 receptors regulate the expression of ethanol-induced behavioural sensitization. Int J Neuropsychopharmacol 14: 175–185.
28. Broadbent J, Kampmueller K, Koonse SA (2005) Role of dopamine in behavioral sensitization to ethanol in DBA/2J mice. Alcohol 45:137–148.
29. Bahi A, Dreyer JL (2012) Involvement of tissue plasminogen activator "tPA" in ethanol-induced locomotor sensitization and conditioned-place preference. Behav Brain Res 226: 250–258.
30. Kong EC, Woo K, Li H, Lebestky T, Mayer N, et al. (2010) A pair of dopamine neurons target the D1-like dopamine receptor DopR in the central complex to promote ethanol-stimulated locomotion in Drosophila. PLoS ONE 5: e9954.
31. Davies AG, Pierce-Shimomura JT, Kim H, VanHoven MK, Thiele TR, et al. (2003) A central role of the BK potassium channel in behavioral responses to ethanol in *C. elegans*. Cell 115: 655–666.
32. Mitchell PH, Bull K, Glautier S, Hopper NA, Holden-Dye L, et al. (2007) The concentration-dependent effects of ethanol on *Caenorhabditis elegans* behaviour. J Pharmacogenomics 7: 411–417.
33. Davies AG, Bettinger JC, Thiele TR, Judy ME, McIntire SL (2004) Natural variation in the *npr-1* gene modifies ethanol responses of wild strains of *C. elegans*. Neuron 42: 731–743.
34. Mitchell P, Mould R, Dillon J, Glautier S, Andrianakis I, et al. (2010) A differential role for neuropeptides in acute and chronic adaptive responses to alcohol: behavioural and genetic analysis in *Caenorhabditis elegans*. PLoS ONE. 5: e10422.
35. Vidal-Gadea A, Topper S, Young L, Crisp A, Kressin L, et al. (2011) *Caenorhabditis elegans* selects distinct crawling and swimming gaits via dopamine and serotonin. Proc Natl Acad Sci 108: 17504–17509.
36. Vidal-Gadea AG, Davis S, Becker L, Pierce-Shimomura JT (2012) Coordination of behavioral hierarchies during environmental transitions in *Caenorhabditis elegans*. Worm 1: 5–11.
37. De Bono, Bargmann CI (1998) Natural variation in a neuropeptide Y receptor homolog modifies social behavior and food response in *C. elegans*. Cell 94: 679–689.
38. Way JC, Chalfie M (1989) The *mec-3* gene of *Caenorhabditis elegans* requires its own product for maintained expression and is expressed in three neuronal cell types. Genes Dev 3: 1823–1833.
39. Sulston J, Dew M, Brenner S (1975). Dopaminergic neurons in the nematode *Caenorhabditis elegans*. J Comp Neurol 163: 215–226.
40. Edwards SL, Charlie NK, Milfort MC, Brown BS, Gravlin CN, et al. (2008) A novel molecular solution for ultraviolet light detection in *Caenorhabditis elegans*. PLoS Biol 6: e198.
41. Alaimo JT, Davis SJ, Song SS, Burnette CR, Grotewiel M, et al. (2012) Ethanol metabolism and osmolarity modify behavioral responses to ethanol in *C. elegans*. Alcohol Clin Exp Res 36: 1840–1850.
42. Herweijer MA, Berden JA, Kemp A, Slater EC (1985) Inhibition of energy-transducing reactions by 8-nitreno-ATP covalently bound to bovine heart submitochondrial particles: direct interaction between ATPase and redox enzymes. Biochim Biophys Acta 809: 81–89.

43. Duncan HM, Mackler B (1966) Electron transport systems of yeast. 3. Preparation and properties of cytochrome oxidase. J Biol Chem 241: 1694–1697.
44. Suo S, Sasagawa N, Ishiura S (2002) Identification of a dopamine receptor from *Caenorhabditis elegans*. Neurosci Lett 319: 13–16.
45. Chase DL, Pepper JS, Koelle MR (2004) Mechanism of extrasynaptic dopamine signaling in *Caenorhabditis elegans*. Nat Neurosci 10: 1096–1103.
46. Sugiura M, Fuke S, Suo S, Sasagawa N, Van Tol HH, et al. (2012) Characterization of a novel D2-like dopamine receptor with a truncated splice variant and a D1-like dopamine receptor unique to invertebrates from *Caenorhabditis elegans*. J Neurochem 94: 1146–57.
47. Suo S, Sasagawa N, Ishiura S (2003) Cloning and characterization of a *Caenorhabditis elegans* D2-like dopamine receptor. J Neurochem 86: 869–878.
48. Wang ZW, Saifee O, Nonet ML, Salkoff L (2001) SLO-1 potassium channels control quantal content of neurotransmitter release at the *C. elegans* neuromuscular junction. Neuron 32: 867–881.
49. Yang X, Criswell HE, Breese GR (1999) Action of ethanol on responses to nicotine from cerebellar interneurons and medial septal neurons: relationship to methyllycaconitine inhibition of nicotine responses. Alcohol Clin Exp Res 23: 983–990.
50. Lee J, Jee C, McIntire SL (2009) Ethanol preference in *C. elegans*. Genes Brain Behav 8: 578–585.
51. Weight FF, Aguayo LG, White G, Lovinger, D M., Peoples, R W (1992) GABA- and glutamate-gated ion channels as molecular sites of alcohol and anesthetic action. Adv Biochem Psychopharmacol 47: 335–347.
52. Mongan NP, Jones AK, Smith GR, Sansom MSP, Sattelle DB (2002) Novel α7-like nicotinic acetylcholine receptor subunits in the nematode *Caenorhabditis elegans*. Protein Sci 11: 1162–1171.
53. Yassin L, Gillo B, Kahan T, Halevi S, Eshel M, et al. (2001) Characterization of the DEG-3/DES-2 receptor: A nicotinic acetylcholine receptor that mutates to cause neuronal degeneration. Mol Cell Neurosci 17: 589–1599.
54. Sprengel R, Aronoff R, Völkner M, Schmitt B, Mosbach R, Kuner T (2001) Glutamate receptor channel signatures. Trends Pharmacol Sci 22: 7–10.
55. Wintle RF, Van Tol HH (2001) Dopamine signaling in *Caenorhabditis elegans*-potential for parkinsonism research. Parkinsonism Relat Disord 7: 177–183.
56. Brenner S (1974) The genetics of *Caenorhabditis elegans*. Genetics 77: 71–94.

10

A Comprehensive Approach to Identify Reliable Reference Gene Candidates to Investigate the Link between Alcoholism and Endocrinology in Sprague-Dawley Rats

Faten A. Taki[1], Abdel A. Abdel-Rahman[2], Baohong Zhang[1]*

1 Department of Biology, East Carolina University, Greenville, North Carolina, United States of America, 2 Department of Pharmacology, East Carolina University, Greenville, North Carolina, United States of America

Abstract

Gender and hormonal differences are often correlated with alcohol dependence and related complications like addiction and breast cancer. Estrogen (E2) is an important sex hormone because it serves as a key protein involved in organism level signaling pathways. Alcoholism has been reported to affect estrogen receptor signaling; however, identifying the players involved in such multi-faceted syndrome is complex and requires an interdisciplinary approach. In many situations, preliminary investigations included a straight forward, yet informative biotechniques such as gene expression analyses using quantitative real time PCR (qRT-PCR). The validity of qRT-PCR-based conclusions is affected by the choice of reliable internal controls. With this in mind, we compiled a list of 15 commonly used housekeeping genes (HKGs) as potential reference gene candidates in rat biological models. A comprehensive comparison among 5 statistical approaches (geNorm, dCt method, NormFinder, BestKeeper, and RefFinder) was performed to identify the minimal number as well the most stable reference genes required for reliable normalization in experimental rat groups that comprised sham operated (SO), ovariectomized rats in the absence (OVX) or presence of E2 (OVXE2). These rat groups were subdivided into subgroups that received alcohol in liquid diet or isocalroic control liquid diet for 12 weeks. Our results showed that U87, 5S rRNA, GAPDH, and U5a were the most reliable gene candidates for reference genes in heart and brain tissue. However, different gene stability ranking was specific for each tissue input combination. The present preliminary findings highlight the variability in reference gene rankings across different experimental conditions and analytic methods and constitute a fundamental step for gene expression assays.

Editor: Turgay Unver, Cankiri Karatekin University, Turkey

Funding: These studies were partly supported by NIH grant 2R01 AA014441 (Abdel-Rahman). The funders had no role in study design, data collection and analysis, decision to publish, or preparation of the manuscript.

* E-mail: zhangb@ecu.edu

Introduction

Alcoholism is linked to many different health problems including cardiovascular and neurological impairments and increased cancer risks [1]. It is hard to dissect the mechanism of action of alcohol abuse because it depends on many factors, such as gender, developmental stage, dose, and duration of alcohol consumption [2]. A link between hormones and alcohol dependence was also previously proposed [3]. Studies show that alcohol altered the hormone levels (i.e. progesterone, estrogen) in pre- and post-menopausal females [4] and in ovariectomized monkeys [5].

The significance of endocrinology in the etiology and mechanism of alcohol dependence and addiction has long been discussed [3,6]. Transient and permanent hormonal changes might be key players in alcohol-associated pathologies such as breast cancer [7–10] and neuro-remodeling phenomena like addiction [6]. These alcoholism-related diseases are promoted by fluctuations in gene expressions of some signaling pathways like estrogen and thyroid hormone receptors [9–11]. Researchers utilized different model systems, which include mice [12], rats [13], nematodes [14], fruit flies [15] to investigate the pathways involved in mediating alcohol's impact on the body. Despite the number of studies on ethanol-associated symptoms, many questions remain unanswered and require further investigations on the behavioral, genetic, and biochemical levels.

Quantitative real-time PCR (qRT-PCR) is a gold-standard biotechnique for gene expression analyses. Despite the emergence of the next generation deep sequencing technology, qRT-PCR remains the validation tool of choice. Even though qRT-PCR is a mature biotechnique, it is greatly affected by RNA integrity, purity, and concentration, primer and enzyme efficiencies, genomic DNA contamination, pipetting errors, as well as the choice of proper internal controls (reference genes) [16]. Molecular analyses necessitate reliable normalization to avoid false positive results, which introduce data misinterpretations and imprecise conclusions. An ideal reference gene should have a stable basal expression in different tissues, genders, developmental stages, and experimental conditions and should have similar expression levels to the target genes of interest [17]. So far, there is no one gene whose expression fulfills these criteria [18] although housekeeping genes (HKGs) were widely used as reference genes. The expression levels of HKGs are affected by various experimental conditions [19,20]. Thus, the identification of suitable reference genes is crucial and should precede gene expression analyses [17]. With this in mind, several statistical approaches have been designed to identify relatively more stable reference genes in response to specific experimental conditions. In this study, we evaluate the stability of 15 commonly used housekeeping genes using 5 statistical methods, which included geNorm [21], delta-Ct (dCt) method [22], NormFinder [23], and BestKeeper [24]. For more accurate ranking of the reference gene candidates, RefFinder was designed to provide a comprehensive ranking [25]. These programs ranked gene candidates based on pairwise comparisons (geNorm, dCt method, BestKeeper) as well as model-based approaches (NormFinder) to determine the most suitable genes.

Alcohol consumption is associated with adverse effects on the cardiovascular and neural systems. Based on the emergent roles of the hormone system in mediating alcohol-induced anomalies, we were interested in understanding the link between alcoholism and estrogen signaling in the heart and brain tissue of Sprague-Dawley rats. For that, we investigated the effect of chronic ethanol treatment on the stability of the expression levels of 15 housekeeping genes in rat heart and brain tissue for identifying most reliable genes as reference genes for gene expression analysis. To perform this study, we treated Sprague-Dawley rats with ethanol (ETOH). The effect of ethanol on the stability of 15 reference gene candidates (Table 1) was investigated using rats with different hormonal backgrounds. The study was based on 6 rat groups. Untreated female (SHAM) and male rats were used as controls. One group of rats underwent ovariectomy (OVX). The last group of rats was ovariectomized and then treated with estrogen hormone (OVXE2). Rats belonging to those two groups were divided into two subgroups. Half of OVX as well as OVXE2 rats served as control (no ETOH treatment), while the remaining rats received ETOH.

Materials and Methods

Animal Handling and Treatment

Animal use and handling protocols were pre-approved and complied with East Carolina University Animal Use and Care Committee guideline. Female and male Sprague-Dawley (SD) rats (9–10 weeks old; Harlan, Indianapolis, UN, USA) were used. Male rats served as control. Female rats were divided into ovariectomized without (OVX) or with and estrogen supplementation (OVXE2) and sham-operated (SO) groups. Ethanol treatment and tissue collection following euthanasia were performed as in our previous studies [26,27]. Tissue isolation quickly followed. Tissue was flash frozen by liquid nitrogen and then stored at −80°C for subsequent molecular assays.

Sample Collection and RNA Extractions

Total RNA extraction was performed for heart and brain tissue weighing about 100–200 mg according to protocol using mirVana miRNA Isolation Kit (Life Technologies, CA, USA). Briefly, lysis buffer was added to each sample. The sample was kept on ice while being thoroughly homogenized. Then, an acid-phenol extraction separated RNAs from DNA and proteins. After adding 100% ethanol, the sample-ethanol mixture was passed through a glass-filter by centrifugation. Several washes preceded the elution of the RNA with DNase/RNase-free water. RNA was quantified and its purity was assessed using the NanoDrop ND-1000 Micro-Volume UVVis Spectrophotometer (NanoDrop Technologies, Wilmington, DE).

Reverse Transcription and qRT-PCR

Reverse transcription was performed using TaqMan microRNA Reverse Transcription kit (Applied Biosystems, Foster City, CA). Poly(T) was used to reverse transcribe the protein coding genes, while specific RT primers were used for the non-coding genes. A total of 1000 ng RNA were used for each RT reaction. RT-PCR was performed in the thermal cycle at 16°C for 30 min followed by 42°C for 30 min, 85°C for 5 min and were finally held at 4°C. For subsequent qRT-PCR, 100 uL DNase/RNase-free water was added to each RT product.

ViiA^{TM} Real-Time PCR System (Applied Biosystem) was used to quantify the expression levels of 15 reference gene candidates on a 384-well-plate. SYBR Green PCR master mix was from SuperArray Bioscience Corp. (Frederick, MD). Specific reverse and forward primers were used (Table 1). Briefly, 5.5 μL DNase/RNase free water, 7.5 μL SYBR Green master mix, 1 μL cDNA (1 ug), 1 μL primer mix were added to each well for a final 15 uL reaction. Four biological replicates were used. Initially, the reaction was set at 95°C for 10 min for enzyme activation and was followed by 40 two-step-cycles of denaturation for 15 sec at 95°C and an annealing/extension step for 60 sec at 60°C.

Data Analysis

Ct values were exported to an excel file. Descriptive statistics were performed in SPSS (20) and excel. More sophisticated analyses were performed using five statistical approaches: geNorm [21], delta-Ct (dCt) method [22], NormFinder [23], BestKeeper [24] and RefFinder [25].

To prepare geNorm [21] input, the minimal Ct value was used for normalization of all Ct values for each gene across all samples ($Ct_{original}-Ct_{min}$). Hence, the lowest value was zero. The difference was then transformed ($2^{-(Ctoriginal-Ctmin)}$). Data was structured such that the gene and sample symbols were in the first row and column, respectively. It was then used as input for geNorm applet. To determine the most stable gene pair, geNorm performs pairwise variation analyses (SD value) for each gene pair across all samples. The software assumes that the genes are not co-regulated and that the transformed expression values of an ideal gene pair are identical across all samples. Then, the geometric mean of the SD values for each gene-related pair combinations is used to compute an M-value. A lower M-value reflects higher gene stability. What follows is a step-wise exclusion of the gene pairs with the highest M-values to reach the most stable gene pair. A beneficial feature of geNorm output is the V-value that reflects the minimal number of genes required for reliable normalization. Such is based on calculating a normalization factor ratio starting with the most stable genes. The program follows a step-wise inclusion process (V_n/V_{n+1}) for more genes until there is no significant change in the normalization factor.

Delta-Ct (dCt) method [22] depends on a concept similar to that of geNorm. However, it does not require a program specialist and can be performed using an excel sheet. This method was designed to overcome limitations associated with small samples like difficulties in using the same standardized mRNA concentrations due to possible protein contaminations. Such technical problems are relieved as genes within one sample are compared to each other by calculating the dCt value. Sensibly, the gene pair with the same dCt value (smallest SD) across all samples is considered to be stable and vice versa. The average of all SD values for each gene set of pairwise combinations is used to rank the gene stability. Genes with lower average SD are more stable than others.

Table 1. A summary of the 15 HKG (housekeeping genes) considered as reference gene candidates in SD rats.

Gene symbol	Locus tag	Gene description	Forward primer (5′→3′)	Reverse primer (5′→3′)
18S rRNA	X01117	18S ribosomal RNA	ACTCAACACGGGAAACCTCA	TCTTAGTTGGTGGAGCGATT
5S rRNA	K01594	5S ribosomal RNA	ATCTCGTCTGATCTCGGAA	TCTCCCATCCAAGTACTAACC
B2m	NM_012512	beta-2 microglobulin	AGTAGGAGGTGCTCGATGAAG	TCCTGTAGAGCCAGCAACAGG
BACT	NM_031144	actin, beta	ACTCTGTGTGGATTGGTGGC	CGCAGCTCAGTAACAGTCCG
GADD45AF	NM_024127	growth arrest and DNA-damage-inducible, alpha	TACACTGTGTGCTGGTGACG	ATCACCGTTCGGGGAATCAC
GAPDH	NM_017008	glyceraldehyde-3-phosphate dehydrogenase	TGACAACTTTGGCATCGTGG	GGGCCATCCACAGTCTTCTG
HPRT	NM_012583	hypoxanthine phosphoribosyltransferase 1	GCCTAAAAGACAGCGGCAAG	GGCTGCCTACAGGCTCATAG
TBP	NM_001004198	TATA box binding protein	ACCTTATGCTCAGGGCTTGG	GTGCCGTAAGGCATCATTGG
TNKS	NM_001106084	TRF1-interacting ankyrin-related ADP-ribose polymerase	CCTACTCCTAGCACATGGCG	AGGTAGGTAAGGCCTCAGGG
U2	K00781	small nuclear RNA	ATCTGATACGTCCTCTATCC	GTGGACGGAGCAAGCTCCTA
U5a	K00783	small nuclear RNA	ACTCTGGTTTCTCTTCAGATCG	CAGAGTTGTTCCTCTCCA
U6	K00784	small nuclear RNA	TTGGAACGATACAGAGAAG	TTTGCGTGTCATCCTTGC
U87	AF272707	small nucleolar RNA	ACAATGATGACTTATGTTTTTG	GCTCAGTCTTAAGATTCTC
UBC	NM_017314	ubiquitin C	CTCGTACCTTTCTCACCACAGT	GACACCTCCCCATCAAACCC
Z39	NR_002705	small nucleolar RNA	GTACATGTGATGAAGCAAATC	TACATCAGAAAGCGTTTACAG

NormFinder [23] is unique as it takes into consideration not only the overall intergroup variation (i.e. control vs. treatment), but also, the intragroup variation (i.e. experimental group replicates). Sample subgroups are taken into account to calculate the most stable gene candidate. Their model adds the two sources of variation to determine the systematic error introduced by the investigated gene. Therefore, this approach is less sensitive to misleading expression patterns for coregulated genes. Meanwhile, the approach takes into account the candidates with less intergroup variations, which might be mistakenly disregarded in the pairwise approaches.

BestKeeper [24] determines the stability of the gene candidates based on the SD of the gene expression levels across samples. Then, genes with least variable Ct values are used for subsequent pairwise comparisons, while those with SD>1 are excluded. The geometric mean of the Ct values of the most highly correlated genes is used to calculate a BestKeeper index. Then, the software calculates Pearson correlation coefficient [r] with a P-value to determine the similarity in the expression levels among the candidates. Thus, genes with least SDs and highest correlation with the index are ranked as the most stable genes. This excel-based applet allows the comparison of only 10 gene candidates. Therefore, we excluded the genes (18S, B2m, BACT, GADD45AF, and TBP) ranked as the least stable using geNorm, dCt method and NormFinder.

RefFinder [25] is another web-based interface that was used to deduce the most stable gene candidates among all methods. For each gene, RefFinder calculates the geometric mean of the ranks calculated by each of the previous approaches. Genes with the lowest rank geometric mean are considered as most stable.

Results

Comparing Gene Stabilities by Descriptive Statistics

We calculated the mean and the standard derivation (SD) of the Ct values for heart and brain samples together, heart samples alone, and brain samples alone. In all combinations, GADD45A, TBP, BACT, 18S rRNA, and HPRT had the most variable expression levels reflected in their high SD values. On the other hand, TBP ($Ct_{avg} = 33.86$), TNKS ($Ct_{avg} = 31.60$), GADD45A ($Ct_{avg} = 29.69$), B2m ($Ct_{avg} = 28.53$), and HPRT ($Ct_{avg} = 26.12$) had the highest Ct values and were therefore the least expressed among the gene candidates in the heart and brain (Figure 1; Tables 2 and 3). Thus, TBP, GADD45A, and HPRT are less likely to be good candidates for normalization.

Regardless of sample combination, the genes with highest expression levels were the same, which included Z39 ($Ct_{avg} = 20.38$), GAPDH ($Ct_{avg} = 20.32$), U6 ($Ct_{avg} = 12.69$), U5a ($Ct_{avg} = 10.69$), and 5S rRNA ($Ct_{avg} = 7.77$). However, Z39, U6, 5S rRNA, U5a, and U87 had the least variation in their expression in heart and in brain, respectively. When considering the Ct values from both tissue, Z39, U2, GAPDH, 5S rRNA, and U87 had the lowest SD (Figure 1; Tables 2 and 3). Thus, U87, Z39, and 5S rRNA genes are more stable across groups and in all combinations. With this in mind, we can conclude that Z39 and 5S rRNA are likely to be used for normalization. However, a gene that is more highly abundant than the target genes of interest might mask true changes in expression if used for normalization. On the other hand, we can't evaluate others like U87 solely based on basic statistics because even though its expression was the least variable, there is still ambiguity in evaluating its relative expression level. Thus, more sophisticated statistical approaches should be employed to evaluate a candidate reference gene.

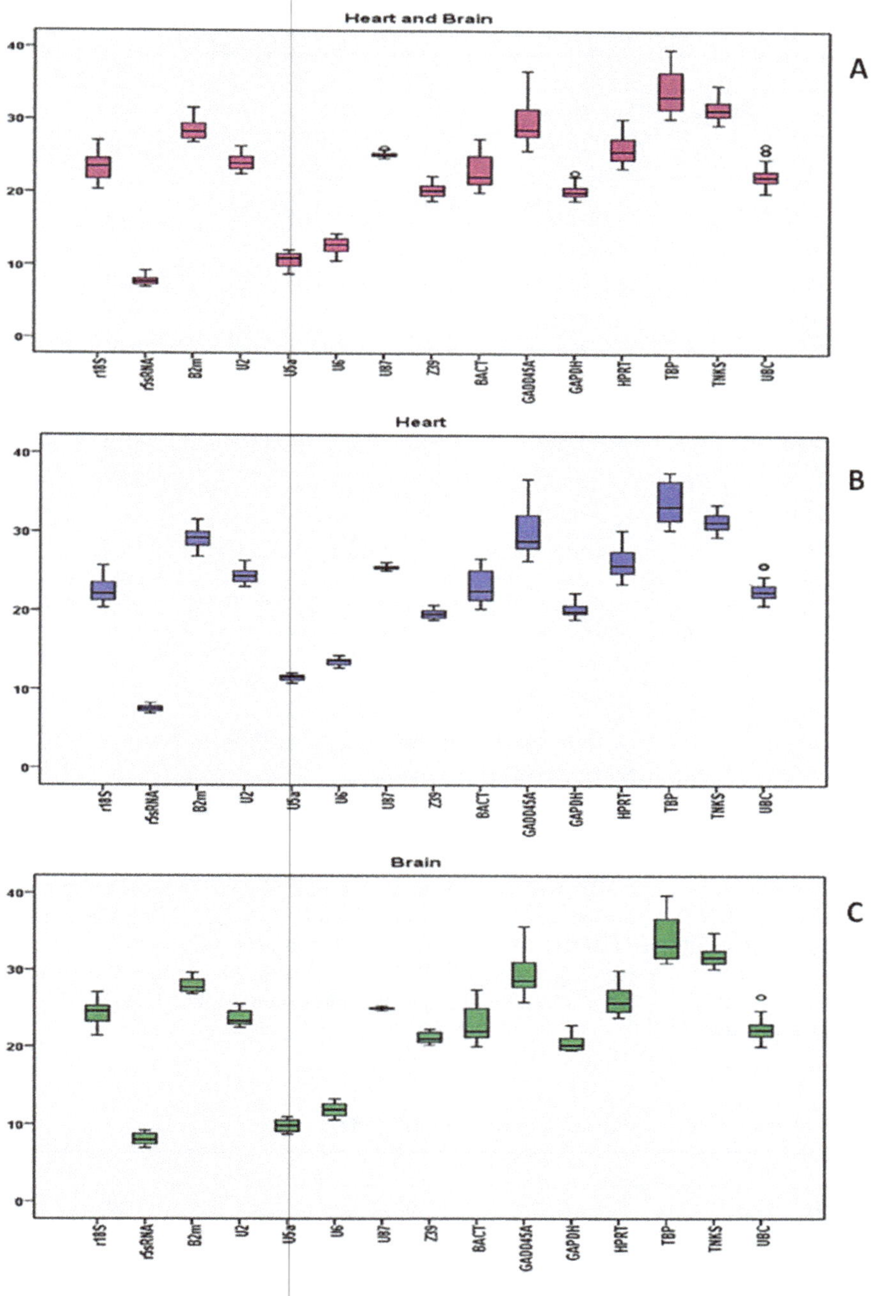

Figure 1. Descriptive statistics of Ct values for heart and brain samples. (A) 48 samples divided into 12 groups for heart and brain tissue combined. (B) 24 samples for 6 groups for heart tissue. (C) 24 samples for 6 groups for brain tissue. Mean Ct values calculated from raw qRT-PCR output for the 15 candidate genes in 6 experimental groups of SD rats (as described in methods). 50% of the values are included in the box. The median is represented by the line in the box. The interquartile range is bordered by the upper and lower edges, which indicate the 75th and 25th percentiles, respectively. The whiskers are inclusive of the maximal and minimal values, but exclusive of the outliers, represented as circles.

Quantitative Analysis of Reference Candidates Based on GeNorm

To determine the minimal number of genes required for normalization, we computed the V-value by geNorm. Starting with 2 genes, the software sequentially adds another gene and recalculates the normalization factor ratio. If the added gene does not increase the normalization factor ratio above the cutoff value (0.15), then the original pair of genes is enough for normalization. However, if the new ratio is above 0.15, then more genes should be included. We combined the heart and brain tissue for input in geNorm. The first V-value<0.15 was after V7/8 (Figure 2B). This means that 6 additional genes were required for reliable normalization. The analysis started with a gene pair (i.e. 2 reference genes) and therefore the total would be 8 HKGs for normalization. That accounted for more than 50% of the gene list.

In the following paragraphs, we analyzed the rankings based on 5 statistical methods using the input for combined Ct values from heart and brain tissue. For a higher stringency measure, we only considered the first 6 ranked genes (<50%) for further analyses.

Table 2. The mean Ct values for each of the 15 gene candidates in descending order.

H+B	Mean	H	Mean	B	Mean
TBP	33.86	TBP	33.81	TBP	33.90
TNKS	31.60	TNKS	31.35	TNKS	31.84
GADD45A	29.69	GADD45A	29.97	GADD45A	29.42
B2m	28.53	B2m	29.10	B2m	27.95
HPRT	26.12	HPRT	26.16	HPRT	26.07
U87	25.23	U87	25.46	U87	24.99
U2	24.02	U2	24.32	r18S	24.31
r18S	23.39	BACT	23.01	U2	23.72
BACT	22.95	UBC	22.65	BACT	22.89
UBC	22.47	r18S	22.47	UBC	22.29
Z39	20.38	GAPDH	20.17	Z39	21.16
GAPDH	20.32	Z39	19.60	GAPDH	20.47
U6	12.69	U6	13.49	U6	11.90
U5a	10.69	U5a	11.51	U5a	9.87
r5sRNA	7.77	r5sRNA	7.51	r5sRNA	8.03

The values for each input case are shown separately.

Determining Best Reference Candidates Based on GeNorm in Both Tissues

GeNorm bases its ranking on the geometric mean of the SD of each transformed gene set of pair combinations (M-value). The lower the M-value is, the higher the ranking. U5a and U6 were co-ranked as most stable genes (M = 0.24). In decreasing order, the third stable gene was U87 (M = 0.69) followed by 5S rRNA (M = 0.85), GAPDH (M = 1.05) and U2 (M = 1.15). The highest M-values ranged between M = 1.32 for UBC and M = 1.83 for GADD45A. Based on M-value, the other genes (HPRT, BACT, 18S rRNA, and TBP) were considered as the least stable genes with M-value between 1.15 to 1.32 (Figure 2A).

Determining Best Reference Candidates Based on dCt Method in Both Tissues

Gene ranking using the dCt method relies on relative pairwise comparisons. Using raw Ct values, the average SD of each gene set is inversely proportional to gene stability. As shown in Tables 4 and 5, U87 (1.48) was the top-ranked gene. 5s rRNA (1.55) was ranked second and was followed by GAPDH (1.56), UBC (1.59), TNKS (1.64) and U6 (1.69). Oppositely, GADD45A (2.43) 18S rRNA (2.37), and TBP (2.37) were ranked last, while B2m, BACT, and Z39 and were among the less stable genes (1.94–1.78).

Table 3. The standard deviations (SD) for each of the 15 gene candidates in descending order.

H+B	SD	H	SD	B	SD
GADD45A	2.67	GADD45A	2.94	TBP	2.73
TBP	2.58	TBP	2.48	GADD45A	2.41
BACT	2.07	BACT	2.05	BACT	2.13
r18S	1.80	HPRT	1.81	HPRT	1.71
HPRT	1.74	r18S	1.51	r18S	1.60
UBC	1.35	UBC	1.30	UBC	1.41
B2m	1.25	B2m	1.28	TNKS	1.28
TNKS	1.22	TNKS	1.14	U2	1.01
U6	1.05	GAPDH	0.90	GAPDH	0.94
U5a	1.02	U2	0.84	B2m	0.93
Z39	1.01	Z39	0.54	U6	0.85
U2	0.97	U6	0.45	U5a	0.76
GAPDH	0.93	r5sRNA	0.41	r5sRNA	0.75
r5sRNA	0.65	U5a	0.37	Z39	0.71
U87	0.32	U87	0.27	U87	0.14

The values for each input case are shown separately.

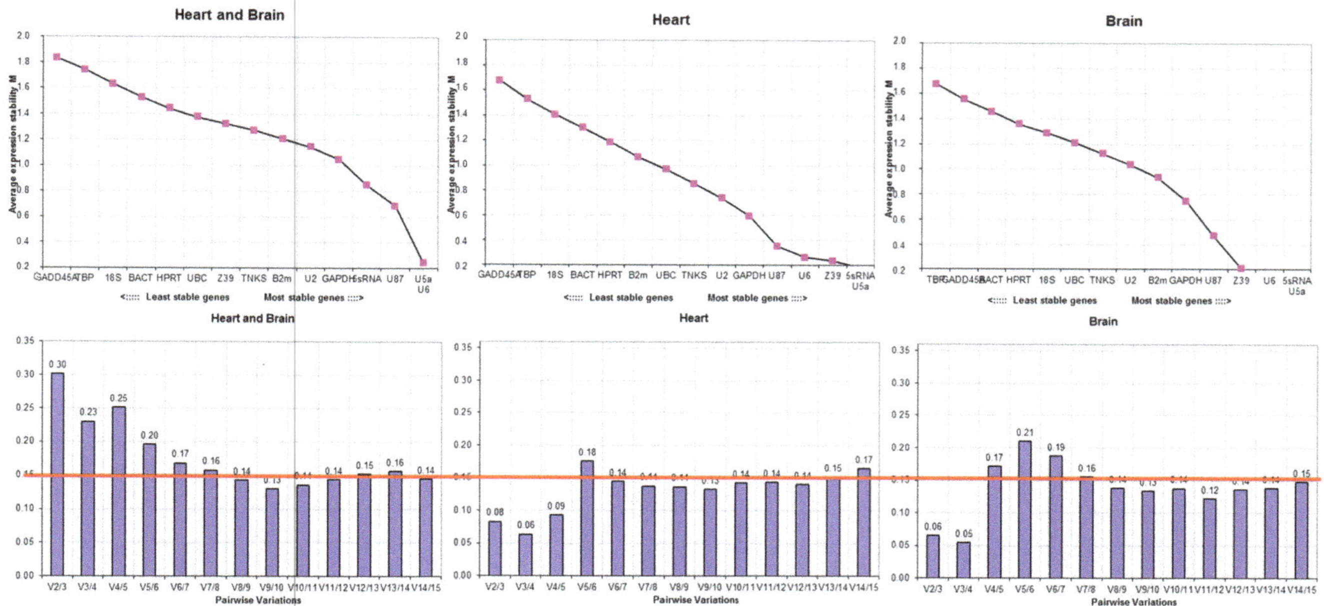

Figure 2. Quantitative and qualitative analysis based on geNorm. (A) Ranking of the 15 gene candidates based on the M-value. Three inputs were used for analysis: Heart and brain combined (48 samples/12 groups), heart alone (24 samples/6 groups), and brain alone (24 samples/6 groups). (B) Determination of the minimal number of reference genes based on V-value for the 3 input combinations. Y-axis represents the ratio of (V_n/V_{n+1}) where 0.15 is the cutoff value. X-axis: $V_{i/j}$ where "i" starts with 2 genes and "j" starts with 3. geNorm starts by a gene pair, and tests whether the inclusion of a 3rd gene adds significant variation. This process is repeated to cover all the genes in the list.

Determining Best Reference Candidates Based on NormFinder in Both Tissues

Complimentary to the pairwise comparisons, NormFinder tests the stability of genes within each sample group as well as between groups. When considering both heart and brain tissue, the total number of sample groups was 12, each having 4 biological replicates. U87 (0.76) was the gene with the least inter and intra-variation in expression levels; thus, U87 would be the most reliable reference gene. The stability values ranged from 0.82 to 1.11 for the other 5 candidate genes (UBC, GAPDH, 5S rRNA, TNKS, and HPRT) (Table 5). Interestingly, based on geNorm, UBC and HPRT were among the least stable genes. This result is based on low intragroup, yet similar intergroup variation. Recalling the model-based approach, NormFinder prevents the exclusion of genes which might have consistent intergroup expression levels. Not necessarily 'similar', these genes have 'minimal' intergroup as well as intragroup variation. Nevertheless, a drawback in NormFinder is the requirement of a minimum of 8 samples/group. For many gene expression studies including our own, it is challenging to have such a large sample size. Taken together, the differences in methodologies might be a reason behind the inclusion of these two genes among the most stable candidates.

Determining Best Reference Candidates Based on BestKeeper in Both Tissues

Due to the input size limitation, BestKeeper only analyzed 10 genes, which were ranked the most stable based on other three programs (geNorm, dCt method, and Normfinder). BestKeeper provided a two-way ranking, which separated the correlation of expression among the genes from the overall variations in expression levels (SD). From each approach, we considered the top 3 genes. Those computed to be highly correlated with p-values <0.05 were UBC ([r] = 0.71), U6 ([r] = 0.70), and HRPT ([r] = 0.67) at p = 0.001. On the other hand, based on BestKeeper, U87 (SD = 0.26), 5S rRNA (SD = 0.53), and GAPDH (SD = 0.74) had the least variable expression levels across all heart and brain samples. 5S rRNA was fairly but significantly correlated with the other genes ([r] = 0.47, p = 0.001), while the weaker correlation of U87 and GAPDH was not statistically significant (Table 6). Statistically speaking, this trend is sensible. When the homogeneity of a group increases, the variance (SD) decreases as in the case of U87, 5S rRNA, GAPDH, and Z39 and [r] tends to zero [28]. In fact, BestKeeper calculated the least SD values for these 4 genes. Thus, these genes will share less variation with the others in pairwise variation and will therefore have the least correlation coefficient. That does not render them unsuitable as reference genes candidates and stresses on the importance of taking both criteria ([r] and SD) to choose the best candidate(s). The inclusion of the top three from the [r]-based and SD-based ranking was consistent with 4 out of 6 best ranked genes in geNorm, and 5 out of 6 top genes in dCt-method and NormFinder (Table 5). In addition, consistent with NormFinder, UBC and HPRT were also ranked among the top 6 by BestKeeper (Table 6). Comparing among the different methodologies helped remove the doubt in NormFinder's result which might have aroused from its requirement of a larger sample size.

Comprehensive Ranking of Best Reference Genes Using RefFinder in Both Tissues

Based on the geometric mean (GM) of the rankings obtained from 4 complementary statistical approaches, U87 was the preferred candidate (GM = 1.32). The remaining highly ranked candidates were 5S rRNA, GAPDH, U6, U5a, and UBC with GM values ranging from 2.83 to 5.18, respectively. On the other hand, B2m, BACT, 18S rRNA, TBP, and GADD45A all had GM values higher than 10 (Table 5). These 5 candidates had the lowest ranking and less likely to serve as reliable reference genes for normalizing gene expression.

Table 4. Summary of mean and SD values of gene pairwise comparison using the dCt method for 15 reference gene candidates.

		Pair 1	Pair 2	Pair 3	Pair 4	Pair5	Pair 6	Pair 7	Pair 8	Pair 9	Pair 10	Pair 11	Pair 12	Pair 13	Pair 14	Avg SD
18S rRNA	Mean	15.6	−5.1	−0.6	12.7	10.7	−1.8	3.0	0.4	−6.3	3.1	−2.7	−10.5	−8.2	0.9	
	SD	1.4	2.6	2.5	2.2	2.1	2.0	1.3	2.9	3.5	2.1	2.8	3.3	2.3	2.3	2.38
5S rRNA	Mean	−15.6	−20.8	−16.3	−2.9	−4.9	−17.5	−12.6	−15.2	−21.9	−12.6	−18.3	−26.1	−23.8	−14.7	
	SD	1.4	1.8	1.6	1.1	1.1	0.8	0.6	2.1	2.7	1.2	1.8	2.6	1.5	1.4	1.55
U2	Mean	0.6	16.3	−4.5	13.3	11.3	−1.2	3.6	1.1	−5.7	3.7	−2.1	−9.8	−7.6	1.5	
	SD	2.5	1.6	0.7	1.5	1.6	0.9	1.8	2.3	2.9	1.1	1.9	2.8	1.5	1.8	1.78
U5a	Mean	−12.7	2.9	−17.8	−13.3	−2.0	−14.5	−9.7	−12.3	−19.0	−9.6	−15.4	−23.2	−20.9	−11.8	
	SD	2.2	1.1	1.6	1.5	0.2	0.9	1.6	2.2	2.7	1.6	2.0	2.7	1.8	1.5	1.69
U6	Mean	−10.7	4.9	−15.8	−11.3	2.0	−12.5	−7.7	−10.3	−17.0	−7.6	−13.4	−21.2	−18.9	−9.8	
	SD	2.1	1.1	1.6	1.6	0.2	0.9	1.6	2.2	2.7	1.6	2.0	2.7	1.8	1.5	1.69
U87	Mean	1.8	17.5	−3.3	1.2	14.5	12.5	4.8	2.3	−4.5	4.9	−0.9	−8.6	−6.4	2.8	
	SD	2.0	0.8	1.1	0.9	0.9	0.9	1.2	2.1	2.7	1.0	1.8	2.6	1.3	1.4	1.48
Z39	Mean	−3.0	12.6	−8.1	−3.6	9.7	7.7	−4.8	−2.6	−9.3	0.1	−5.7	−13.5	−11.2	−2.1	
	SD	1.3	0.6	2.1	1.8	1.6	1.6	1.2	2.3	2.9	1.4	2.0	2.7	1.6	1.7	1.77
B2m	Mean	5.1	20.8	4.5	17.8	15.8	3.3	8.1	5.6	−1.2	8.2	2.4	−5.3	−3.1	6.1	
	SD	2.6	1.8	0.7	1.6	1.6	1.1	2.1	2.5	3.0	1.4	2.1	3.0	1.7	2.0	1.94
BACT	Mean	−0.4	15.2	−5.6	−1.1	12.3	10.3	−2.3	2.6	−6.7	2.6	−3.2	−10.9	−8.6	0.5	
	SD	2.9	2.1	2.5	2.3	2.2	2.2	2.1	2.3	1.4	1.8	1.0	1.0	1.6	1.2	1.90
GADD45A	Mean	6.3	21.9	1.2	5.7	19.0	17.0	4.5	9.3	6.7	9.4	3.6	−4.2	−1.9	7.2	
	SD	3.5	2.7	3.0	2.9	2.7	2.7	2.7	2.9	1.4	2.5	1.4	1.9	2.3	1.5	2.44
GAPDH	Mean	−3.1	12.6	−8.2	−3.7	9.6	7.6	−4.9	−0.1	−2.6	−9.4	−5.8	−13.5	−11.3	−2.1	
	SD	2.1	1.2	1.4	1.1	1.6	1.6	1.0	1.4	1.8	2.5	1.4	2.3	0.8	1.5	1.55
HPRT	Mean	2.7	18.3	−2.4	2.1	15.4	13.4	0.9	5.7	3.2	−3.6	5.8	−7.7	−5.5	3.6	
	SD	2.8	1.8	2.1	1.9	2.0	2.0	1.8	2.0	1.0	1.4	1.4	1.5	1.2	1.1	1.71
TBP	Mean	10.5	26.1	5.3	9.8	23.2	21.2	8.6	13.5	10.9	4.2	13.5	7.7	2.3	11.4	
	SD	3.3	2.6	3.0	2.8	2.7	2.7	2.6	2.7	1.0	1.9	2.3	1.5	2.1	1.9	2.36
TNKS	Mean	8.2	23.8	3.1	7.6	20.9	18.9	6.4	11.2	8.6	1.9	11.3	5.5	−2.3	9.1	
	SD	2.3	1.5	1.7	1.5	1.8	1.8	1.3	1.6	1.6	2.3	0.8	1.2	2.1	1.5	1.64
UBC	Mean	−0.9	14.7	−6.1	−1.5	11.8	9.8	−2.8	2.1	−0.5	−7.2	2.1	−3.6	−11.4	−9.1	
	SD	2.3	1.4	2.0	1.8	1.5	1.5	1.4	1.7	1.2	1.5	1.5	1.1	1.9	1.5	1.59

Table 5. A summary of ranking for reference gene candidates using 5 different statistical approaches.

RefFinder		dCt method		NormFinder		geNorm		BestKeeper			
								Ranking			
Genes	**GM**	**Genes**	**SV**	**Gene name**	**SV**	**Gene name**	**SV**	**[r]**			**SD**
U87	1.32	U87	1.48	U87	0.76	U5a | U6	0.241	UBC	0.71	U87	0.26
5sRNA	2.83	5sRNA	1.55	UBC	0.82	U87	0.688	U6	0.70	5sRNA	0.53
GAPDH	3.41	GAPDH	1.56	GAPDH	0.83	5sRNA	0.85	HPRT	0.67	GAPDH	0.74
U6	4.14	UBC	1.59	5sRNA	0.89	GAPDH	1.05	U5a	0.65	Z39	0.82
U5a	4.28	TNKS	1.64	TNKS	0.94	U2	1.146	5sRNA	0.47	U2	0.84
UBC	5.18	U6	1.69	HPRT	1.11	B2m	1.207	U2	−0.35	U5a	0.86
TNKS	6.32	U5a	1.7	U6	1.16	TNKS	1.273	TNKS	0.31	U6	0.87
U2	7.21	HPRT	1.72	U5a	1.17	Z39	1.323	GAPDH	0.21	TNKS	0.97
Z39	7.54	U2	1.77	Z39	1.28	UBC	1.375	U87	0.20	UBC	1.01
HPRT	8.73	Z39	1.78	U2	1.28	HPRT	1.441	Z39	0.10	HPRT	1.43
B2m	10.02	BACT	1.91	BACT	1.44	BACT	1.526				
BACT	11.72	B2m	1.94	B2m	1.53	18S	1.63				
18S	13.22	TBP	2.37	TBP	2.06	TBP	1.741				
TBP	13.73	18S	2.37	18S	2.06	GADD45A	1.833				
GADD45A	14.74	GADD45A	2.43	GADD45A	2.14						

48 samples were combined from heart and brain experimental groups as input.
Geometric mean (GM); Stability Value (SV); Pearson's correlation coefficient ([r]); Standard Deviation (SD).

Table 6. Ranking of 10 reference gene candidates based on BestKeeper.

	n	GM [Ct]	AM [Ct]	min [Ct]	max [Ct]	SD [± Ct]	CV [% Ct]	[r]	p-value	Ranking	
										[r]	SD
5sRNA	48	7.74	7.77	6.91	9.20	0.53	6.77	0.47	0.001	UBC	U87
U2	48	24.00	24.02	22.48	26.30	0.84	3.48	−0.35	0.015	U6	5sRNA
U5a	48	10.64	10.69	8.71	12.06	0.86	8.05	0.65	0.001	HPRT	GAPDH
U6	48	12.65	12.69	10.57	14.30	0.87	6.85	0.70	0.001	U5a	Z39
U87	48	25.22	25.23	24.68	26.10	0.26	1.03	0.20	0.177	5sRNA	U2
Z39	48	20.36	20.38	18.83	22.26	0.82	4.02	0.10	0.487	U2	U5a
GAPDH	48	20.30	20.32	18.90	22.78	0.74	3.66	0.21	0.151	TNKS	U6
HPRT	48	26.06	26.12	23.40	30.22	1.43	5.46	0.67	0.001	GAPDH	TNKS
TNKS	48	31.57	31.60	29.43	34.77	0.97	3.07	0.31	0.034	U87	UBC
UBC	48	22.43	22.47	19.99	26.52	1.01	4.48	0.71	0.001	Z39	HPRT

Two criteria are considered: Pearson's correlation coefficient and BestKeeper computed SD values. The stability of a gene is directly proportional to the [r] value, while it is inversely proportional to the SD value.
Note: Total sample number (n), Geometric Mean (GM), AM (Arithmetic Mean), Standard Deviation (SD), Coefficient of Varience % (CV), Pearson's correlation coefficient [r], P<0.05.

RefFinder Ranking of Gene Candidates for Heart Hand Brain Tissue

The first analysis was performed for all samples together to identify a common reliable reference gene. Then, we also analyzed brain and heart samples separately to see whether or not there was a difference between tissues.

Based on RefFinder, the 6 most reliable reference genes were the same for brain or heart samples. However, their ranks were a little different between heart and brain. For heart tissue, the order of best reference genes was as follows: U87 (GM = 1.97), U5a (GM = 2.45), 5S rRNA (GM = 3.03), U6 (GM = 3.36), GAPDH (GM = 3.81) and Z39 (GM-5.18) (Table 7). However, 5s rRNA (GM-1.73) was the top ranked gene when using samples from the brain tissue; the following best candidates were Z39 (GM = 2.00), U87 (GM = 2.66), U5a (GM = 2.78), U6 (GM 4.36), and GAPDH (GM = 6.48) (Table 8).

Unlike the results from combined tissue, the first V-value<0.15 was at V2/3 (Figure 2). Thus, only 2 stable reference genes were needed for gene expression analysis in heart or brain tissue. A closer look at the data in Figure 2, the average of V-values for combined heart and brain tissue was 0.18. Individually, the average V-value for the heart and brain were 0.13 and 0.14, respectively. Thus, the gene candidates were merely more stably expressed in the heart tissue than in the brain tissues. However, though the genes' expressions were consistent and stable within each tissue, it was different between the heart and brain. This can be inferred from the dramatic increase in the V-value average when both tissues were combined for analysis.

The top six most stable reference gene candidates were same for heart and brain tissues. The choice of the gene pair depends on the estimated expression levels of the targeted genes of interest. If the expression profiles of the genes of interest is unknown, then choosing reference candidates from the low and high extremes would be recommended such as U87 and 5S rRNA.

Discussion

Housekeeping genes are commonly used for normalizing gene expression because they are thought to be consistently expressed cross different tissues and among different treatment. However, this was challenged recently. Current studies show no one gene remains stable throughout all experimental conditions. Ideal reference genes vary with different species, strains, developmental stage, tissue and even different sampling times [29]. To maintain the integrity of qRT-PCR as a powerful "discovery" and "validation" biotechnique, the choice and the number of reference genes used should be customized to every experiment setting. Thus, the first task is to identify reference gene candidates from either systematic gene expression studies like microarrays or by compiling a gene list from previous studies with similar experimental conditions. Subsequently, their relative stability is compared using statistical approaches. In our study, we followed the same workflow to determine reliable reference genes in SD rats. Normalizing to the top-ranked genes will reveal possible roles of hormonal/gender differences, mainly estrogen levels, in alcoholism. Below, we highlight the significance of our study by discussing some shortcomings associated with employing single statistical approaches in reference gene identification. In the end, we show the advantages of our combinatorial approach and present recommendations of control gene candidates to use or to avoid in similar experimental settings.

Table 7. A summary of ranking for reference gene candidates using 5 different statistical approaches.

RefFinder		dCt method		NormFinder		geNorm		BestKeeper			
								Ranking			
Genes	GM	Genes	SV	Gene name	SV	Gene name	SV		[r]		SD
U87	1.97	U87	1.3	GAPDH	0.64	5sRNA | U5a	0.18	HPRT	0.82	U87	0.21
U5a	2.45	U6	1.33	TNKS	0.66	Z39	0.24	UBC	0.73	U5a	0.32
5sRNA	3.03	U5a	1.34	U87	0.68	U6	0.26	TNKS	0.62	5sRNA	0.34
U6	3.36	5sRNA	1.35	U6	0.78	U87	0.35	U6	0.54	U6	0.37
GAPDH	3.81	GAPDH	1.39	UBC	0.79	GAPDH	0.59	GAPDH	0.49	Z39	0.46
Z39	5.18	Z39	1.43	U5a	0.82	U2	0.74	5sRNA	0.40	U2	0.70
TNKS	5.47	TNKS	1.44	5sRNA	0.85	TNKS	0.86	U5a	0.39	GAPDH	0.70
UBC	7.54	UBC	1.51	Z39	0.99	UBC	0.97	Z39	0.30	TNKS	0.90
U2	7.64	U2	1.54	U2	1.02	B2m	1.07	U87	0.27	UBC	0.97
HPRT	10.72	HPRT	1.72	HPRT	1.21	HPRT	1.19	U2	−0.22	HPRT	1.44
B2m	10.95	BACT	1.85	BACT	1.46	BACT	1.30				
BACT	11.72	B2m	1.86	B2m	1.50	18S	1.407				
18S	12.94	TBP	2.22	TBP	1.96	TBP	1.53				
TBP	13.49	18S	2.23	18S	2.01	GADD45A	1.68				
GADD45A	15	GADD45A	2.64	GADD45A	2.46						

24 samples were combined from heart experimental groups as input.
Geometric mean (GM); Stability Value (SV); Pearson's correlation coefficient ([r]); Standard Deviation (SD).

Table 8. A summary of ranking for reference gene candidates using 5 different statistical approaches.

RefFinder		**dCt**		**NormFinder**		**Genorm**		**BestKeeper**			
								Ranking			
Genes	**GM**	**Genes**	**SV**	**Gene name**	**SV**	**Gene name**	**SV**		**[r]**		**SD**
5sRNA	1.73	5sRNA	1.34	Z39	0.82	5sRNA | U5a	0.11	5sRNA	0.82	U87	0.11
Z39	2.00	Z39	1.35	U87	0.83	U6	0.17	Z39	0.80	Z39	0.61
U87	2.66	U5a	1.37	5sRNA	0.84	Z39	0.21	U6	0.79	5sRNA	0.64
U5a	2.78	U6	1.4	UBC	0.86	U87	0.47	U5a	0.79	U5a	0.65
U6	4.36	U87	1.41	U5a	0.89	GAPDH	0.75	UBC	0.71	U6	0.70
GAPDH	6.48	UBC	1.53	U6	0.93	B2m	0.93	U2	−0.69	GAPDH	0.76
UBC	7.00	GAPDH	1.54	GAPDH	0.96	U2	1.04	HPRT	0.64	U2	0.87
B2m	8.37	HPRT	1.62	HPRT	1.04	TNKS	1.13	U87	−0.59	TNKS	0.98
TNKS	9.00	TNKS	1.65	TNKS	1.10	UBC	1.21	TNKS	0.28	UBC	1.02
U2	9.59	B2m	1.75	B2m	1.38	18S	1.29	GAPDH	0.16	HPRT	1.41
HPRT	9.80	U2	1.82	BACT	1.47	HPRT	1.36				
18S	11.72	18S	1.87	U2	1.48	BACT	1.46				
BACT	12.47	BACT	1.88	18S	1.54	GADD45A	1.55				
GADD45A	14.00	GADD45A	2.13	GADD45A	1.81	TBP	1.67				
TBP	15.00	TBP	2.45	TBP	2.20						

48 samples were combined from heart and brain experimental groups as input.
Geometric mean (GM); Stability Value (SV); Pearson's correlation coefficient ([r]); Standard Deviation (SD).

Comparing RefFinder Results Across Tissue Combinations

The top 6 most stable reference candidates in the bi-tissue input were U87, 5S rRNA, GAPDH, U6, U5a, and UBC. In the single-tissue input, the top 6 were similar and only with a slight difference in the order. Results for the combined and separate inputs differed by only one reference gene 'Z39'. This means that Z39 was stable within each tissue (SD<1), but its expression differed between heart ($Ct_{avg} = 19.6 \pm 0.5$) and brain ($Ct_{avg} = 21.16 \pm 0.7$). Moreover, U5a ($\Delta Ct_{avg} = 1.64$) and U6 ($\Delta Ct_{avg} = 1.59$) also had the highest Ct_{avg} difference between heart and brain tissue (Table 2). Even though the SD for Z39, U5a, and U6 was <1 in heart or brain tissue, their expression varied between heart and brain. Due to the inter-tissue variation, using Z39, U5a, and U6 in combined gene expression analysis is not recommended. In all input combinations, 18S rRNA, TBP, GADD45A, and BACT were the least stable among the 15 tested genes. These genes might cause inaccurate conclusions in gene expression normalizations for heart and/or brain tissue and therefore should not be used as reference genes.

Comparing Among Different Methods and Tissue

When considering all brain and heart tissue samples together, U87, 5S rRNA, and GAPDH were commonly ranked among the top 6 most stable reference genes in all 5 statistical approaches. On the other hand, only 'U87 and U5a', and 'U87, U5a, U6, and Z39' were ubiquitously ranked among the top 6 across 5 methods in each of the heart tissue, and brain tissue, respectively. As shown in Figure 3, seniority of U87 was common to all statistical methods and all tissue combinations. If the targeted genes of interest are expressed at a lower level, we recommend the use of U87 with GAPDH for the two tissues. If the targeted genes are expressed at a higher level, then 5S rRNA and U87 would be better for normalization. U87 and U5a were commonly ranked among the best in each of heart and brain tissue. Thus, for gene expression analysis concerned with heart tissue or brain tissue, U87 and U5a would serve as better reference genes.

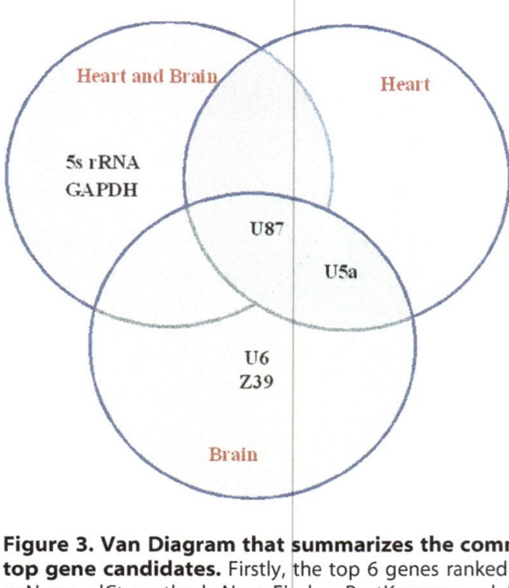

Figure 3. Van Diagram that summarizes the commonly ranked top gene candidates. Firstly, the top 6 genes ranked by each of the geNorm, dCt method, NormFinder, BestKeeper, and RefFinder were compared for each input: Heart+brain, heart, and brain samples. Only genes common for all 5 methods were chosen for each input. Those genes were then compared among all input combinations and presented in the diagram above.

Fallibility of Normalizations to Single Commonly Used HKGs

There is a wealth of resourceful studies that identified experiment-specific reference genes for normalization. We summarized some of the results for investigations that employed similar experimental conditions (i.e. rats, estrogen, and alcohol). Table 9 shows different HKGs as better reference genes for different tissue, treatments, treatment times, strains, species, and statistical methods. This suggests the necessity of conducting preliminary studies to use reference genes adapted for particular experimental conditions. In our study, U87, 5S rRNA, GAPDH and U5a were ranked as the top gene candidates using a combination of 5 statistical approaches. Even though, 5S rRNA was stable in rat liver treated with hepatotoxins [30], both U87 and 5S rRNA were among the least stable in SD rats suffering from oxygen-induced retinopathy [31]. While some studies reported GAPDH to be a relatively stable housekeeping gene in heart and brain tissue [29,32–34], its expression was nevertheless affected by treatments such as MB in rat brain [35], estrogen in ovariectomized C57BL6 mice [36], male and female fathead minnow fish [37], and RARAW 264.7, ATDCDC5 and HFLS cells [38].

On the contrary, 18S rRNA was among the least stable gene candidates in our settings. This is in agreement with other studies using carotid body from different SD strains under different oxygenation levels [39], oligodendrocyte cells from age-asynchronized Winstar rats treated with LXR agonist [40], male flinder rat hippocampus treated with MB [35], and liver of hypophysectomized male and female SD rats [41]. However, 18S rRNA was considered a good reference gene in Winstar rat livers treated with hepatotoxins [30], human livers with alcoholic liver disease [42], the uterus of ovarietomized C57BL6 mice treated with estradiol [36], and in liver and gonads of male and female fathead minnow fish [37]. We also showed that TBP was unstable and that was supported by another study on heart tissue of young and adult SD rats subjected to PHDI treatments under different oxygen pressures [33]. However, that was not the case in the heart of Zucker obese rats under different glycemic states [43], nor in the hippocampus of SD rats with TBI [34]. TBP was also considered stable in response to estrogen in multiple tissue of the fathead minnow fish [37].

The Importance of Using More than One Statistical Approach

No one statistical approach can cover all variables associated with gene expression studies. Therefore basing conclusions on one method can be associated with false positive results and misleading conclusions. In our study, we followed a round-about approach to determine good reference candidates for reliable normalization of gene expression data in Sprague-Dawley rats. This allowed us to correct for some inaccurate ranking such as geNorm's raking of UBC, which was corrected by NormFinder. Also, based on the systematic interpretation, we were able to get a clearer picture on the minimal number of reference genes required for reliable normalization. After removing Z39, U5a and U6, only 3 genes are enough to serve as reference genes for analysis on heart and brain tissue combined. This makes the study more practical (8 vs. 3 control genes) and reliable at the same time.

In conclusion, it is difficult to ascertain whether the inconsistency or variability in the stability of the housekeeping genes arises from the employment of different statistical methodologies or different treatments. For example, in two studies concerned with rat liver, GAPDH was stable after TCDD treatment based on

Table 9. A minireview of the reference gene candidates ranked as top or least stable in different experimental settings using higher organisms.

Model system	Experimental condition	Statistical method	Genes Ranked		Reference
			Top	Least	
Young adult male Sprague-Dawley (SD) rats, New Zealand White (NZW) rabbits	Intervertebral disc (IVD)	geNorm, NormFinder, BestKeeper	HPRT1, CYCA		PMC 3118343 [45]
Fischer 344 (F344, resistant to OIR) and Sprague-Dawley rats (SD, susceptible to OIR) (both albino inbred)	Oxygen-induced retinopathy, Different strains, Different development stage	Basic Statistics	U6, MIR-16	U87, 5S, 4.5S	PMID 23441123, PMC 3580969 [31]
Timed-pregnant Sprague-Dawley rats;	Dissected carotid body; Norm/ hyper/hypo-oxial; Different developmental timing; Different strains	geNorm, NormFinder BestKeeper		18S, Actin	PMID 22023793[39]
Adult Sprague-Dawley rats	Surgically isolated 8 different liver cells at different times of liver regeneration	geNorm	ACTB, B2M, UBC	GAPDH	PMID 20339955[44]
TCDD-sensitive inbred Long-Evans rats	TCDD, Liver spleen hypothalamus	Basic Statistics	PGK1, GAPDH		PMID 16466705[32]
Sprague–Dawley (SD) neonatal + adult rat	Heart, PHDI treatment, Normoxia; hypoxia	geNorm, NormFinder	GAPDH, ACTB, B2M	TBP	PMC 3294216[33]
Wistar Rat brain cells: astrocytes and OLG cultures; OLG from mature + neonatal rats	No treatment, LXR agonist	geNorm; NormFinder	CYCA, PGK1, PRPL13A, YWHAZ, CYCA, PGK1, PRPL13A	GAPDH, 18S, HMBS, GAPDH, 18S	PMID 20036692[40]
Obese Zucker rats	Heart	geNor	SDHA, TBP, HPRT1		PMID 22493144[43]
Obese Zucker rats	Kidney	geNor	TBP, GAPDH, ACTB		PMID 22493144[43]
Obese Zucker rats	Pulmonary	geNor	ACTB, YWHAG, SDHA		PMID 22493144[43]
Male flinders rats	Hippocampus, Methylene Blue	NormFinder; geNorm	YWHAZ, CYCA, RPL13A, HPRT1	GAPDH, ACTB, 18S	PMID 18241047 [35]
Male and female Sprague-Dawley rats	Liver, Hypophysectomy	Basic Statistics		Tubulin, G3DPH, Bactin, TAT, Cyclophilin, 18S	PMID 16724986[41]
Adult male Sprague-Dawley	Collagenase-intracerebral hemorrhage in RBG and LBG, 5 hr and 24 hrs	geNorm	GAPDH, HPRT, B2MG, GUSB		PMID 20089183[29]
Adult Male Wistar rats	Liver, Acetaminophen (AA), Carbon tetrachloride (CT), D-galactosamine (GA), Thioacetamide (TA)	geNorm; NormFinder; BestKeeper	MIR-16, 5S, B2M, 18S		PMID 22563491[30]
Adult male Sprague-Dawley rats	3 days following traumatic brain injury (TBI), Cerebral cortex, Hippocampus	geNorm	HPRT, SDHA, GUSB, B2MG, TBP, GAPDH		PMID 18711751[34]
RARAW 264.7 (Mouse leukaemic monocyte macrophage), ATDCDC5 (chondrogenic) and HFLS (Human Fibroblast-Like Synoviocytes)	Estrogen			GAPDH	PMID 21472208[38]
Humans	Alcoholic liver disease	Basic statistics	18S, SFRS4	Bactin, GAPDH	PMID 21913943[42]

Table 9. Cont.

Model system	Experimental condition	Statistical method	Genes Ranked		Reference
			Top	Least	
C57BL6 mice	Ovariectomized, Uterus, Estradiol	Basic Statistics	RPL13A, 18S	GAPDH, HPRT1, PPIA, B2M, GUSB, ACTB, HSP90AB1	PMID: 19219570[36]
Male and female fathead minnow fish	Estrogen, Liver, Gonad	Basic Statistics	18S, RPL8, HPRT1,TBP	EF1A, G6PD, Bactin, GAPDH	PMID 17288598[37]

Basic Statistics: bi/multivariable; parametric/non-parametric hypothesis testing (e.g. t-test, ANOVA) and clustering methods.

geNorm [44], but it was not when using other statistical methods in liver cells under different conditions [32]. What is noteworthy is that the ranking of the reference genes is always relative and that can change simply by changing a few candidates in the gene list. Therefore, despite the superfluous publications, research concerned with the determination of reference remains juvenile. With more efforts being dedicated to tackle this issue, a meta-analysis would help reveal patterns that might redirect and standardize our normalization methods for more accurate interpretation of results.

Acknowledgments

We greatly appreciate Ms. Kun Sun for conducting the animal studies and for tissue preparation.

Author Contributions

Conceived and designed the experiments: FAT AAA BZ. Performed the experiments: FAT AAA BZ. Analyzed the data: FAT AAA BZ. Contributed reagents/materials/analysis tools: FAT AAA BZ. Wrote the paper: FAT AAA BZ.

References

1. CDC CfDCaP (2012) Fact Sheets- Alcohol Use and Health. Retrieved from http://www.cdc.gov/alcohol/fact-sheets/alcohol-use.htm on May.14.2013.
2. Oscar-Berman M, Marinkovic K (2004) Alcoholism and the Brain: An Overview. NIAAA. Retrieved online from http://pubs.niaaa.nih.gov/publications/arh27-2/125-133.htm on May.15.2013.
3. Ruusa J, Bergman B (1996) Sex hormones and alcohol withdrawal: does a good supply of testosterone prevent serious symptoms during detoxification? Alcohol 13: 139–145.
4. Gill J (2000) The effects of moderate alcohol consumption on female hormone levels and reproductive function. Alcohol Alcohol 35: 417–423.
5. Mello N, Mendelson J, Bree M, Skupny A (1988) Alcohol effects on LH and FSH in recently ovariectomized female monkeys. NIDA Res Monogr 81: 122–128.
6. Lenz B, Muller CP, Stoessel C, Sperling W, Biermann T, et al. (2012) Sex hormone activity in alcohol addiction: integrating organizational and activational effects. Prog Neurobiol 96: 136–163.
7. Purohit V (1998) Moderate alcohol consumption and estrogen levels in postmenopausal women: a review. Alcohol Clin Exp Res 22: 994–997.
8. Onland-Moret NC, Peeters PH, van der Schouw YT, Grobbee DE, van Gils CH (2005) Alcohol and endogenous sex steroid levels in postmenopausal women: a cross-sectional study. J Clin Endocrinol Metab 90: 1414–1419.
9. Wong AW, Dunlap SM, Holcomb VB, Nunez NP (2012) Alcohol promotes mammary tumor development via the estrogen pathway in estrogen receptor alpha-negative HER2/neu mice. Alcohol Clin Exp Res 36: 577–587.
10. Fan S, Meng Q, Gao B, Grossman J, Yadegari M, et al. (2000) Alcohol stimulates estrogen receptor signaling in human breast cancer cell lines. Cancer Res 60: 5635–5639.
11. Scott HC, Sun GY, Zoeller RT (1998) Prenatal ethanol exposure selectively reduces the mRNA encoding alpha-1 thyroid hormone receptor in fetal rat brain. Alcohol Clin Exp Res 22: 2111–2117.
12. Bennett B, Downing C, Parker C, Johnson TE (2006) Mouse genetic models in alcohol research. Trends Genet 22: 367–374.
13. Tabakoff B, Hoffman PL (2000) Animal Models in Alcohol Research. NIAAA Retrieved from http://pubsniaaanihgov/publications/arh24-2/77-84pdf on May152013 24.
14. Lee J, Jee C, McIntire SL (2009) Ethanol preference in C. elegans. Genes Brain Behav 8: 578–585.
15. Guarnieri DJ, Heberlein U (2003) Drosophila melanogaster, a genetic model system for alcohol research. Int Rev Neurobiol 54: 199–228.
16. Nolan T, Hands RE, Bustin SA (2006) Quantification of mRNA using real-time RT-PCR. Nat Protoc 1: 1559–1582.
17. Cappelli K, Felicetti M, Capomaccio S, Spinsanti G, Silvestrelli M, et al. (2008) Exercise induced stress in horses: selection of the most stable reference genes for quantitative RT-PCR normalization. BMC Mol Biol 9: 49.
18. Gutierrez L, Mauriat M, Guenin S, Pelloux J, Lefebvre JF, et al. (2008) The lack of a systematic validation of reference genes: a serious pitfall undervalued in reverse transcription-polymerase chain reaction (RT-PCR) analysis in plants. Plant Biotechnol J 6: 609–618.
19. Thellin O, Zorzi W, Lakaye B, De Borman B, Coumans B, et al. (1999) Housekeeping genes as internal standards: use and limits. J Biotechnol 75: 291–295.
20. Suzuki T, Higgins PJ, Crawford DR (2000) Control selection for RNA quantitation. Biotechniques 29: 332-+.
21. Vandesompele J, De Preter K, Pattyn F, Poppe B, Van Roy N, et al. (2002) Accurate normalization of real-time quantitative RT-PCR data by geometric averaging of multiple internal control genes. Genome Biol 3: RESEARCH0034.
22. Silver N, Best S, Jiang J, Thein SL (2006) Selection of housekeeping genes for gene expression studies in human reticulocytes using real-time PCR. BMC Mol Biol 7: 33.
23. Andersen CL, Jensen JL, Orntoft TF (2004) Normalization of real-time quantitative reverse transcription-PCR data: a model-based variance estimation approach to identify genes suited for normalization, applied to bladder and colon cancer data sets. Cancer Res 64: 5245–5250.
24. Pfaffl MW, Tichopad A, Prgomet C, Neuvians TP (2004) Determination of stable housekeeping genes, differentially regulated target genes and sample integrity: BestKeeper-Excel-based tool using pair-wise correlations. Biotechnol Lett 26: 509–515.
25. Xie F, Xiao P, Chen D, Xu L, Zhang B (2012) miRDeepFinder: a miRNA analysis tool for deep sequencing of plant small RNAs. Plant Mol Biol.
26. Mohamed M, Abdel-Rahman A (2000) Effect of long-term ovariectomy and estrogen replacement on the expression of estrogen receptor gene in female rats. European Journal of Endocrinology 142: 307–314.
27. El-Mas MM, Abdel-Rahman AA (2004) Effects of long-term ovariectomy and estrogen replacement on clonidine-evoked reductions in blood pressure and hemodynamic variability. Journal of Cardiovascular Pharmacology 43: 607–615.
28. Calkins KG (2005) Applied Statistics: Correlation Coefficients.Andrews University. Retrieved on June.5.2013online from http://www.andrews.edu/~calkins/math/edrm611/edrm05.htm.
29. Cook NL, Kleinig TJ, van den Heuvel C, Vink R (2010) Reference genes for normalising gene expression data in collagenase-induced rat intracerebral haemorrhage. BMC Mol Biol 11: 7.

30. Lardizabal MN, Nocito AL, Daniele SM, Ornella LA, Palatnik JF, et al. (2012) Reference genes for real-time PCR quantification of microRNAs and messenger RNAs in rat models of hepatotoxicity. PLoS One 7: e36323.
31. Tea M, Michael MZ, Brereton HM, Williams KA (2013) Stability of small non-coding RNA reference gene expression in the rat retina during exposure to cyclic hyperoxia. Mol Vis 19: 501–508.
32. Pohjanvirta R, Niittynen M, Linden J, Boutros PC, Moffat ID, et al. (2006) Evaluation of various housekeeping genes for their applicability for normalization of mRNA expression in dioxin-treated rats. Chem Biol Interact 160: 134–149.
33. Caldani M, Batailler M, Thiery JC, Dubois MP (1988) LHRH-immunoreactive structures in the sheep brain. Histochemistry 89: 129–139.
34. Cook NL, Vink R, Donkin JJ, van den Heuvel C (2009) Validation of reference genes for normalization of real-time quantitative RT-PCR data in traumatic brain injury. J Neurosci Res 87: 34–41.
35. Bonefeld BE, Elfving B, Wegener G (2008) Reference genes for normalization: a study of rat brain tissue. Synapse 62: 302–309.
36. Schroder AL, Pelch KE, Nagel SC (2009) Estrogen modulates expression of putative housekeeping genes in the mouse uterus. Endocrine 35: 211–219.
37. Filby AL, Tyler CR (2007) Appropriate 'housekeeping' genes for use in expression profiling the effects of environmental estrogens in fish. BMC Mol Biol 8: 10.
38. Galal N, El-Beialy W, Deyama Y, Yoshimura Y, Tei K, et al. (2010) Up-regulation of the G3PDH 'housekeeping' gene by estrogen. Mol Med Rep 3: 111–113.
39. Kim I, Yang D, Tang X, Carroll JL (2011) Reference gene validation for qPCR in rat carotid body during postnatal development. BMC Res Notes 4: 440.
40. Nelissen K, Smeets K, Mulder M, Hendriks JJ, Ameloot M (2010) Selection of reference genes for gene expression studies in rat oligodendrocytes using quantitative real time PCR. J Neurosci Methods 187: 78–83.
41. Verma AS, Shapiro BH (2006) Sex-dependent expression of seven housekeeping genes in rat liver. J Gastroenterol Hepatol 21: 1004–1008.
42. Boujedidi H, Bouchet-Delbos L, Cassard-Doulcier AM, Njike-Nakseu M, Maitre S, et al. (2012) Housekeeping gene variability in the liver of alcoholic patients. Alcohol Clin Exp Res 36: 258–266.
43. Cabiati M, Raucci S, Caselli C, Guzzardi MA, D'Amico A, et al. (2012) Tissue-specific selection of stable reference genes for real-time PCR normalization in an obese rat model. J Mol Endocrinol 48: 251–260.
44. Wang GP, Xu CS (2010) Reference gene selection for real-time RT-PCR in eight kinds of rat regenerating hepatic cells. Mol Biotechnol 46: 49–57.
45. Di Pasquale C (1986) [Economics of oral health and socio-economic development]. Odontostomatol Trop 9: 175–181.

11

Acute Binge Drinking Increases Serum Endotoxin and Bacterial DNA Levels in Healthy Individuals

Shashi Bala[⁹], **Miguel Marcos**[⁹], **Arijeet Gattu, Donna Catalano, Gyongyi Szabo***

Department of Medicine, University of Massachusetts Medical School, Worcester, Massachusetts, United States of America

Abstract

Binge drinking, the most common form of alcohol consumption, is associated with increased mortality and morbidity; yet, its biological consequences are poorly defined. Previous studies demonstrated that chronic alcohol use results in increased gut permeability and increased serum endotoxin levels that contribute to many of the biological effects of chronic alcohol, including alcoholic liver disease. In this study, we evaluated the effects of acute binge drinking in healthy adults on serum endotoxin levels. We found that acute alcohol binge resulted in a rapid increase in serum endotoxin and 16S rDNA, a marker of bacterial translocation from the gut. Compared to men, women had higher blood alcohol and circulating endotoxin levels. In addition, alcohol binge caused a prolonged increase in acute phase protein levels in the systemic circulation. The biological significance of the in vivo endotoxin elevation was underscored by increased levels of inflammatory cytokines, TNFα and IL-6, and chemokine, MCP-1, measured in total blood after in vitro lipopolysaccharide stimulation. Our findings indicate that even a single alcohol binge results in increased serum endotoxin levels likely due to translocation of gut bacterial products and disturbs innate immune responses that can contribute to the deleterious effects of binge drinking.

Editor: Wenke Feng, University of Louisville School of Medicine, United States of America

Funding: This work was supported by NIH grant AA 011576. The funders had no role in study design, data collection and analysis, decision to publish, or preparation of the manuscript.

Competing Interests: The authors have declared that no competing interests exist.

* E-mail: gyongyi.szabo@umassmed.edu

⁹ These authors contributed equally to this work.

Introduction

Alcohol binge drinking defined as more than 4 drinks consumed is the most frequent form of alcohol consumption worldwide. This drinking pattern is popular among underage drinkers and young adults leading to increased mortality and morbidity [1–3]. While the behavioral consequences of binge drinking are well characterized, little is known about its systemic effects on various organs and on immune responses. On immune cells, acute alcohol intake has immunosuppressive and anti-inflammatory effects, it reduces antiviral immunity and in the liver it causes liver injury and steatosis [4,5].

Animal models of chronic alcohol administration and human studies indicate that alcoholic liver disease is associated with increased endotoxin (lipopolysaccharide; LPS) levels in the portal and systemic circulation and that endotoxin contributes to alcoholic steatohepatitis [3,6], however, interplay between endotoxin and binge drinking is not well understood. LPS is a Toll-like Receptor 4 ligand that triggers inflammatory cytokine activation in immune cells and has a broad range of effects on various cell types in different organs [6]. Increased serum LPS is the result of increased gut permeability and it is associated with a low-grade inflammation in various conditions such as alcoholic hepatitis, cirrhosis, HIV and HCV infection [7]. Impaired gut barrier function, bacterial translocation and alterations in the gut microbiome are found in animal models of chronic alcohol consumption [8,9]. An alteration in colonic microbiome was also reported in chronic alcoholics [10]. In this study, we tested the effects of acute binge drinking on serum endotoxin and bacterial 16S rDNA in normal human adults.

Materials and Methods

Human studies

Healthy individuals (11 males and 14 females, age range 21–56) with no history of alcohol use disorder were enrolled in the study after informed consent was obtained. All participants signed written consent and the study was approved by Institutional Review Board for the Protection of Human subjects in research at the University of Massachusetts Medical School. Written consent files are kept in locked cabinets and samples were de-identified. Alcohol use habits were determined by a questionnaire that incorporated the Alcohol Use Disorders Identification Test and CAGE tests as described [11]. To qualify for the study, males had alcohol use of fewer than 12 drinks/wk, females fewer than 9 drinks/wk, and all abstained from alcohol for at least 48 hours before participation [11]. Alcohol was given @ 2 ml vodka 40% v/v ethanol/kg body weight in a total volume of 300 ml orange/strawberry juice in the Clinical Research Center (CRC). Blood was drawn at baseline and after every 30 minutes for the first 4 hours and again after 24 hours post alcohol consumption in serum separating tubes (BD Biosciences) as indicated in figures. Average body mass index (BMI) ± standard error of men and women was 29.3±1.1 and 28.8±1.38 respectively. For control subjects, blood samples were collected from alcohol-abstinent

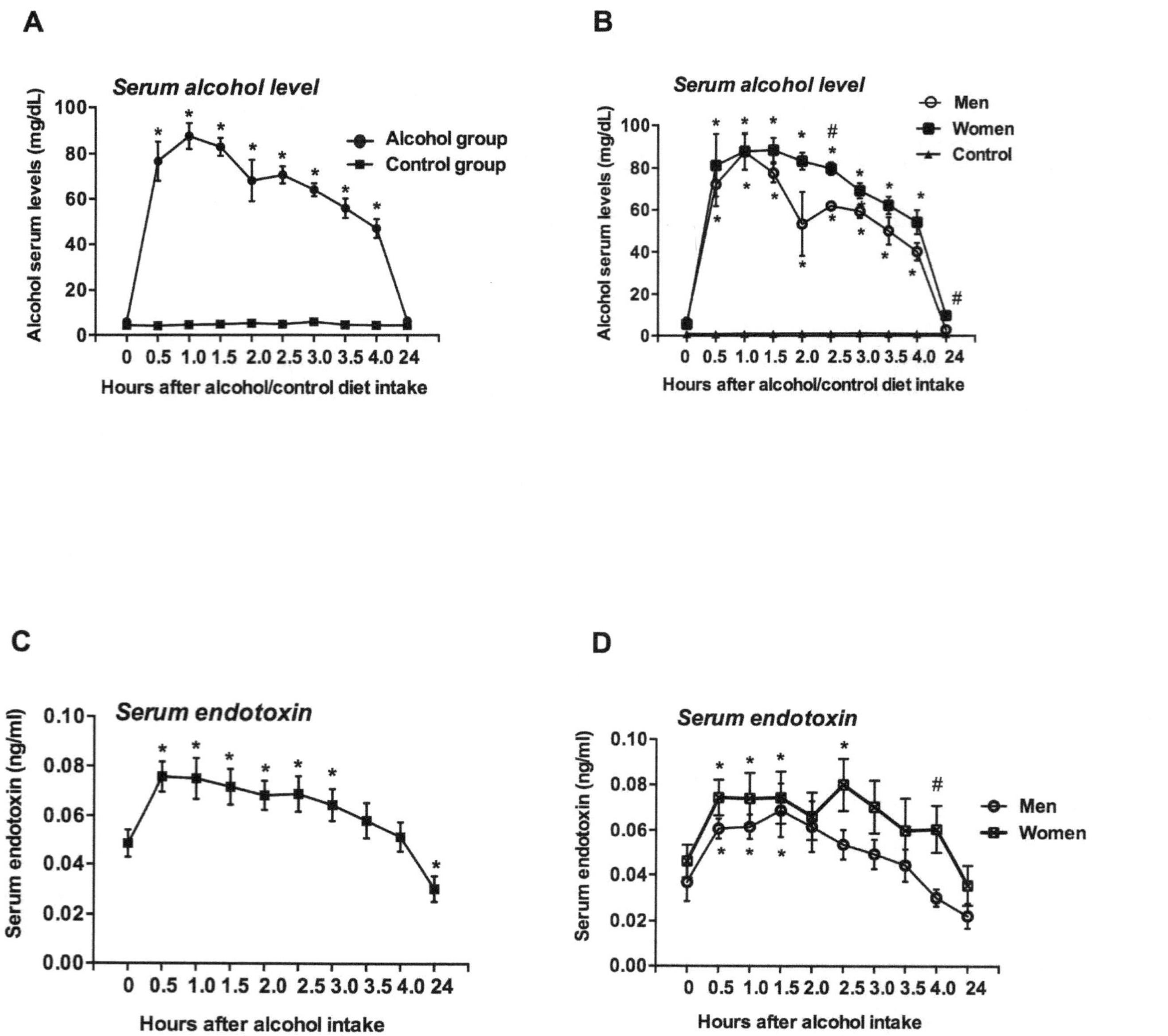

Figure 1. Induction of blood alcohol content and serum endotoxin after an acute binge drink in healthy humans. A–D. Serum alcohol (A and B, n = 8) and endotoxin (C and D, n = 16) levels were measured as described in methods. The data for serum alcohol (B) and endotoxin (D) was presented separately for men and women. Data is presented as mean ± S.E., and depending upon the data distribution, statistical analysis was performed either with Mann-Whitney *U* test or Student's two-tailed test. *$p<0.05$. *represents comparison between baseline and treatment groups. # represents comparison between men and women.

individuals (age- and gender-matched) receiving equal volume of orange juice.

Alcohol concentration and Endotoxin Assay

The amount of alcohol in the serum samples was measured by an Analox Alcohol Analyzer. Serum endotoxin was measured using Endotoxin kit (Capecod Inc, USA) as per manufacturer instructions.

Measurement of LBP and sCD14

LBP and sCD14 were measured from the serum using ELISA kits from Lonza (Lonza, USA).

Bacterial DNA isolation and identification

DNA was isolated from equal volume of serum samples using QIAamp mini kit (Qiagen, USA) in endotoxin free conditions. PCR reaction was performed with universal 16S primer [12], and the product was analyzed on 1% agarose gel. *Escherichia coli DNA* was used as a positive control and "reaction mix alone" was used as a negative control to avoid any false positive amplification. PCR was performed using primer sequence, forward 5′-TCCTACGG-GAGGCAGCAGT-3′ and the reverse 5′-GACTACCAGGG-TATCTAATCCTGTT-3′, and an amplicon of 466 bp was detected. The fold change was calculated compared to baseline samples of the same individual. Experiment was performed in a bacterial free chamber.

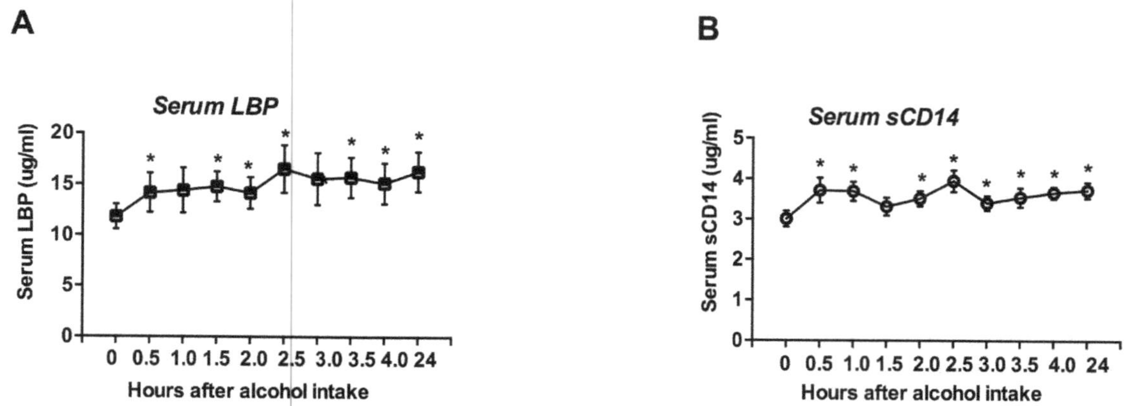

Figure 2. Induction of acute phase proteins after an acute binge drink in healthy humans. A–B. Serum LBP (A, n = 21) and serum sCD14 (B, n = 21) were measured as described in methods. Data is presented as mean ± S.E., and depending upon the data distribution, statistical analysis was performed either with Mann-Whitney *U* test or Student's two-tailed test. *p<0.05.

LPS treatment of whole blood samples

For blood cytokines, whole blood was diluted 1:1 with warm RPMI in a polypropylene tube with the cap loose. Samples were either stimulated or not with LPS (100 pg/ml), then placed on a rocker platform in a CO2 chamber for 18 h. The next day tubes were centrifuged at 3000RPM for 10 minutes and clear plasma was collected and stored at −80°C for cytokine measurements.

Measurement of cytokines

Plasma collected from LPS treated whole blood samples was used to measure TNFα, IL-6 and MCP1 using ELISA kits (Thermo Scientific, USA [TNFα] and BD Biosciences, USA [IL-6 and MCP1]).

Statistical analysis

Depending upon the data distribution, statistical analysis was performed either with Mann-Whitney *U* test or Student's two-tailed test.

Results

Increased blood alcohol content and serum endotoxin after an acute binge drink in healthy humans

Alcohol intake increases blood alcohol level (BAL) in the circulation. In normal volunteers, acute alcohol binge resulted in maximum BAL at 60 minutes after alcohol consumption with a gradual decline thereafter (Fig. 1A). Compared to men, women showed a slower decrease in BAL and even 24 h after the alcohol binge BALs were higher in women than that in men (Fig. 1B). There was no detectable blood alcohol level (BAL) before alcohol intake in any of the individuals. Parallel to BAL levels, serum endotoxin levels rapidly increased by 30 minutes, remained elevated for 3 hours and returned to lower than baseline levels by 24 hours after alcohol intake (Fig. 1C). Serum endotoxin levels were also higher in women after alcohol intake and a significant difference in endotoxin level was observed at 4 h between men and women (Fig. 1D). Blood alcohol and serum endotoxin levels remained constant in control individuals who received no alcohol.

Induction of acute phase proteins after an acute binge drink

Circulating endotoxin induces elevations in acute phase proteins [13]. We found that acute alcohol consumption also induced rapid and prolonged increases in serum lipoprotein binding protein (LBP) (Fig. 2A) and soluble CD14 (sCD14) (Fig. 2B) while there was no change in controls who received no alcohol (data not shown).

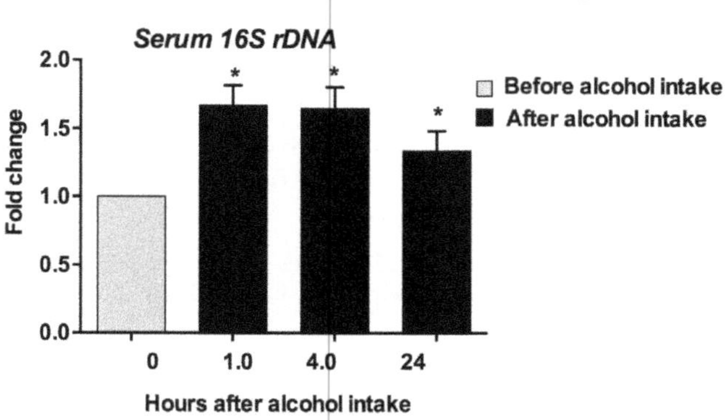

Figure 3. Induction of bacterial DNA after an acute binge drink in healthy humans. DNA was isolated from the serum (n = 22) using QIAamp mini kit (Qiagen) and 16S rDNA was amplified using 16S universal primers. The fold change was calculated compared to baseline samples of the same individual. Data is presented as mean ± S.E. *p< 0.05.

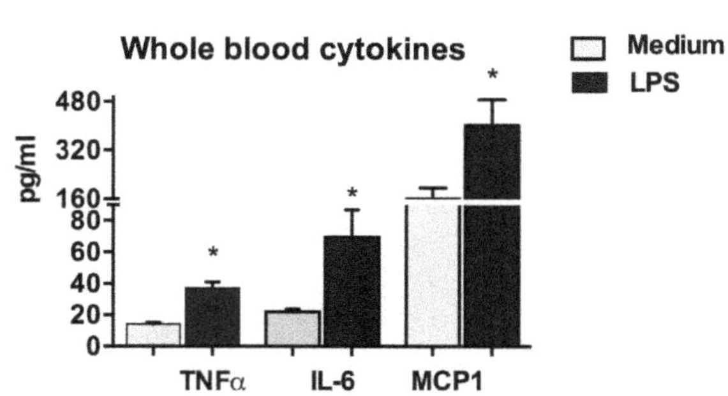

Figure 4. Physiological dose of LPS induces immune response in whole blood plasma of normal individuals. The amount of TNFα, IL-6 and MCP1 was measured by ELISA from the whole blood plasma collected after 18 h of LPS (100 pg/ml) treatment (n = 4). Data is presented as mean ± S.E. *p<0.05.

Induction of bacterial DNA after an acute binge drink in healthy humans

LPS is a component of Gram-negative bacteria and increased serum LPS is thought to be a result of microbial translocation from the gut [14]. Because LPS represents only some enteric bacterial microbiota (Gram negative) we further determined the levels of the well-conserved 16S rRNA subunit (16S rDNA), which is common to most bacteria. We found a significant increase in serum 16S bacterial rDNA levels at 1, 4 and even 24 hours after binge drinking (Fig. 3) and not in controls (data not shown).

"Physiological" dose of LPS induces immune response in whole blood of normal individuals

To evaluate the biological significance of the serum endotoxin increase found in vivo after acute alcohol binge, we evaluated the effect of the biologically comparable concentrations of LPS in whole blood of normal volunteers. We found that the concentrations of endotoxin observed in the serum after acute binge had significant biological activity. In vitro treatment of whole blood samples with a "physiological" dose of LPS (100 pg/ml for 18 h) resulted in a significant induction of inflammatory cytokines, tumor necrosis factorα (TNFα), IL-6 and MCP1 in normal subjects (Fig. 4).

Discussion

Our novel data demonstrate that a single alcohol binge in normal subjects resulted in a rapid and transient increase in serum endotoxin levels and that even this modest increase in serum LPS had substantial biological effects in modulating TNFα, IL-6 and MCP1. Endotoxin, LPS, is a potent trigger of the inflammatory cascade via activation of the TLR4 complex [6]. Recent studies in mice indicate that in addition to its effects on innate immunity, LPS administration also contributes to alcohol dependence and promotes prolonged increase of alcohol intake in mice [15]. Mutant mice lacking genes related to immune function exhibit decreased alcohol consumption indicating immune signaling promotes alcohol consumption [16]. Thus, it is tempting to speculate that LPS increase in the systemic circulation after an acute alcohol binge could promote the desire for alcohol consumption. This speculation merits further investigation. Consistent with our data, acute ethanol exposure in rodents (rats) is shown to increase circulating endotoxin levels [17]. The systemic biologic activity of the increased LPS after alcohol binge was associated with increased serum LBP and soluble CD14 levels. LBP and sCD14 are both LPS-inducible protective molecules and are considered as "acute phase reactants" [18]. Increases in LBP and sCD14 have the biologic function of binding circulating LPS thereby preventing activation of the TLR4 complex [18]. In chronic alcohol use activation of the inflammatory cascade is a major component of organ damage in the brain and liver. Alcohol binge can cause altered immune functions that can also contribute to immunosuppression and reduced immune-mediated host defense to pathogens [3]. Despite similar BMI between men and women in our study, women showed higher levels of blood alcohol and circulating endotoxin levels. This could be due to the fact that the volume of distribution in women is less than that in men and gender differences in the effects of binge drinking deserve additional investigation.

Our study also demonstrated the elevation of other bacterial products such as 16S rDNA levels after acute binge drinking indicating transient gut-derived microbial translocation as a likely mechanism for the serum LPS increase. It is noteworthy that increase in circulating bacterial components after acute binge not only included Gram-negative bacteria (LPS) but extended to other enteric bacterial elements such as 16S rDNA. The significance of increased bacterial DNA in alcohol binge model deserves further investigation as it may represent a danger signal that is different from LPS. The persistent increase in bacterial components including 16S rDNA after repeated binge drinking might result in immune activation thereby resulting in inflammation and initiation of alcoholic liver disease. Increase in bacterial translocation and 16S rRNA was found in chronic alcohol mouse model [19]. In other pathological conditions such as in HIV infection, plasma levels of bacterial DNA have been shown to correlate with immune activation [20] and translocation of microbial elements is also observed in inflammatory bowel disease [21].

It is possible that LPS along with bacterial DNA activates the immune system during binge drinking. The pro-inflammatory effects of chronic alcohol are associated with increased serum LPS and this is thought to be due to alcohol-induced impairment of the gut barrier function [8]. To our best knowledge, we show for the first time that acute alcohol binge causes 16S rDNA translocation (conserved bacterial genetic component) into the systemic circulation in otherwise healthy adults. The mechanism of alcohol-induced gut barrier dysfunction is likely multifactorial. Decrease in tight junction proteins, occludin and zonulin-1 were found after chronic alcohol use and this was mechanistically linked to increased expression of miRNA-212 in mice [22]. Expression levels of defensins that have protective effects in the gut are also decreased in chronic alcohol feeding in mice although the effects of acute alcohol binge on these proteins are yet to be explored [19].

In summary, our study demonstrates that acute alcohol binge increased serum levels of bacterial products (endotoxin and bacterial 16S rDNA) which might contribute to innate immune responses and potentially to the behavioral effects of alcohol binge drinking. These results suggest that acute binge drinking has significant adverse health effects even in healthy individuals.

Acknowledgments

The authors thank the UMMS Clinical Trials Unit and Bernadette White, RN for the assistance with the study

Author Contributions

Wrote the paper: GS SB MM AG DC. Study concept and design: GS SB MM. Acquisition, analysis and interpretation of data: GS SB MM AG DC.

References

1. NIAAA website. Available: http://pubs.niaaa.nih.gov/publications/aa68/aa68.htm. Accessed 2014 Jan 10.
2. Mathurin P, Deltenre P (2009) Effect of binge drinking on the liver: An alarming public health issue? Gut 58: 613–617.
3. Shukla SD, Pruett SB, Szabo G, Arteel GE (2013) Binge ethanol and liver: New molecular developments. Alcohol Clin Exp Res 37: 550–557.
4. Bala S, Tang A, Catalano D, Petrasek J, Taha O, et al. (2012) Induction of bcl-3 by acute binge alcohol results in toll-like receptor 4/LPS tolerance. J Leukoc Biol 92: 611–620.
5. Massey VL, Arteel GE (2012) Acute alcohol-induced liver injury. Front Physiol 3: 193.
6. Szabo G, Bala S, Petrasek J, Gattu A (2010) Gut-liver axis and sensing microbes. Dig Dis 28: 737–744.
7. Szabo G, Wands JR, Eken A, Osna NA, Weinman SA, et al. (2010) Alcohol and hepatitis C virus—interactions in immune dysfunctions and liver damage. Alcohol Clin Exp Res 34: 1675–1686.
8. Keshavarzian A, Farhadi A, Forsyth CB, Rangan J, Jakate S, et al. (2009) Evidence that chronic alcohol exposure promotes intestinal oxidative stress,

intestinal hyperpermeability and endotoxemia prior to development of alcoholic steatohepatitis in rats. J Hepatol 50: 538–547.
9. Hartmann P, Chen WC, Schnabl B (2012) The intestinal microbiome and the leaky gut as therapeutic targets in alcoholic liver disease. Front Physiol 3: 402.
10. Mutlu EA, Gillevet PM, Rangwala H, Sikaroodi M, Naqvi A, et al. (2012) Colonic microbiome is altered in alcoholism. Am J Physiol Gastrointest Liver Physiol 302: G966–78.
11. Norkina O, Dolganiuc A, Catalano D, Kodys K, Mandrekar P, et al. (2008) Acute alcohol intake induces SOCS1 and SOCS3 and inhibits cytokine-induced STAT1 and STAT3 signaling in human monocytes. Alcohol Clin Exp Res 32: 1565–1573.
12. Horz HP, Vianna ME, Gomes BP, Conrads G (2005) Evaluation of universal probes and primer sets for assessing total bacterial load in clinical samples: General implications and practical use in endodontic antimicrobial therapy. J Clin Microbiol 43: 5332–5337.
13. Levy O, Teixeira-Pinto A, White ML, Carroll SF, Lehmann L, et al. (2003) Endotoxemia and elevation of lipopolysaccharide-binding protein after hematopoietic stem cell transplantation. Pediatr Infect Dis J 22: 978–981.
14. Schnabl B (2013) Linking intestinal homeostasis and liver disease. Curr Opin Gastroenterol 29: 264–270.
15. Blednov YA, Benavidez JM, Geil C, Perra S, Morikawa H, et al. (2011) Activation of inflammatory signaling by lipopolysaccharide produces a prolonged increase of voluntary alcohol intake in mice. Brain Behav Immun 25 Suppl 1: S92–S105.
16. Blednov YA, Ponomarev I, Geil C, Bergeson S, Koob GF, et al. (2012) Neuroimmune regulation of alcohol consumption: Behavioral validation of genes obtained from genomic studies. Addict Biol 17: 108–120.
17. Rivera CA, Bradford BU, Seabra V, Thurman RG (1998) Role of endotoxin in the hypermetabolic state after acute ethanol exposure. Am J Physiol 275: G1252–8.
18. Hamann L, Alexander C, Stamme C, Zahringer U, Schumann RR (2005) Acute-phase concentrations of lipopolysaccharide (LPS)-binding protein inhibit innate immune cell activation by different LPS chemotypes via different mechanisms. Infect Immun 73: 193–200.
19. Yan AW, Fouts DE, Brandl J, Starkel P, Torralba M, et al. (2011) Enteric dysbiosis associated with a mouse model of alcoholic liver disease. Hepatology 53: 96–105.
20. Jiang W, Lederman MM, Hunt P, Sieg SF, Haley K, et al. (2009) Plasma levels of bacterial DNA correlate with immune activation and the magnitude of immune restoration in persons with antiretroviral-treated HIV infection. J Infect Dis 199: 1177–1185.
21. Caradonna L, Amati L, Magrone T, Pellegrino NM, Jirillo E, et al. (2000) Enteric bacteria, lipopolysaccharides and related cytokines in inflammatory bowel disease: Biological and clinical significance. J Endotoxin Res 6: 205–214.
22. Tang Y, Banan A, Forsyth CB, Fields JZ, Lau CK, et al. (2008) Effect of alcohol on miR-212 expression in intestinal epithelial cells and its potential role in alcoholic liver disease. Alcohol Clin Exp Res 32: 355–364.

12

Alcohol Consumption and Breast Cancer Risk among Women in Three Sub-Saharan African Countries

Frank Qian[1]✉, Temidayo Ogundiran[2]✉, Ningqi Hou[3], Paul Ndom[4], Antony Gakwaya[5], Johashaphat Jombwe[5], Imran Morhason-Bello[6], Clement Adebamowo[7], Adeyinka Ademola[2], Oladosu Ojengbede[6], Olufunmilayo I. Olopade[1], Dezheng Huo[3]*

1 Center for Clinical Cancer Genetics and Global Health, Department of Medicine, University of Chicago, Chicago, Illinois, United States of America, **2** Department of Surgery, College of Medicine, University of Ibadan, Ibadan, Nigeria, **3** Department of Health Studies, University of Chicago, Chicago, Illinois, United States of America, **4** Medical Oncology Service, Yaoundé General Hospital, Yaoundé, Cameroon, **5** Mulago Hospital, Makerere University, Kampala, Uganda, **6** Center for Population and Reproductive Health, University College Hospital, Ibadan, Nigeria, **7** Department of Epidemiology and Public Health, University of Maryland, Baltimore, Maryland, United States of America

Abstract

Background: Alcohol drinking is linked to the development of breast cancer. However, there is little knowledge about the impact of alcohol consumption on breast cancer risk among African women.

Methods: We conducted a case-control study among 2,138 women with invasive breast cancer and 2,589 controls in Nigeria, Cameroon, and Uganda from 1998 to 2013. A structured questionnaire was used to collect information on alcohol consumption, defined as consuming alcoholic beverages at least once a week for six months or more. Logistic regression was used to estimate adjusted odds ratio (aOR) and 95% confidence interval (CI).

Results: Among healthy controls, the overall alcohol consumption prevalence was 10.4%, and the prevalence in Nigeria, Cameroon, and Uganda were 5.0%, 34.6%, and 50.0%, respectively. Cases were more likely to have consumed alcohol (aOR = 1.62, 95% CI: 1.33–1.97). Both past (aOR = 1.54; 95% CI: 1.19–2.00) and current drinking (aOR = 1.71; 95% CI: 1.30–2.23) were associated with breast cancer risk. A dose-response relationship was observed for duration of alcohol drinking (*P*-trend <0.001), with 10-year increase of drinking associated with a 54% increased risk (95% CI: 1.29–1.84).

Conclusion: We found a positive relationship between alcohol consumption and breast cancer risk, suggesting that this modifiable risk factor should be addressed in breast cancer prevention programs in Africa.

Editor: Olivia Fletcher, The Institute of Cancer Research, United Kingdom

Funding: The study was supported by grants from the National Cancer Institute of National Institutes of Health (CA-RO1 89085-01A and P50 CA125183), the Dr. Ralph and Marian Falk Medical Research Trust, and Avon Foundation for Women (URL: http://www.avonfoundation.org/). The funders had no role in study design, data collection and analysis, decision to publish, or preparation of the manuscript.

Competing Interests: The authors have declared that no competing interests exist.

* Email: dhuo@uchicago.edu

✉ These authors contributed equally to this work.

Introduction

Breast cancer is a leading cause of cancer morbidity and mortality for women world-wide [1,2,3,4,5,6]. In recent decades, breast cancer incidence has seen a steady increase in many developing countries while it reached a plateau in developed nations [6,7,8]. Alcohol consumption has been considered a plausible risk factor for breast cancer. This relationship has been confirmed in some studies [9,10,11,12,13,14,15], but not in others [16,17,18,19]. However, the majority of these studies were conducted among women in high income countries [9,18,20,21,22], with few in developing countries [19,23,24]. To our knowledge, there is no large study on alcohol intake and breast cancer conducted in Africa. Studies of the relationship between alcohol consumption and breast cancer risk among African Americans have found inconclusive results [16,25,26,27,28]. The extent of alcohol drinking's effect on breast cancer risk may vary across races, possibly due to different drinking habits, metabolism and genetic factors. In general, alcohol drinking is less common among African women than their counterparts in North America and Europe [29], but the prevalence rates vary by country in Africa: ever drinking prevalence ranges from <1% to over 40% and current drinking prevalence ranges from none to nearly 30% [29,30,31]. The general trend among African women is towards greater prevalence of alcohol consumption [29,32].

Most studies of alcohol and breast cancer have assessed alcohol use in terms of ever-drinking versus nondrinking or the average daily dose [33]. Other patterns of alcohol use such as duration of alcohol consumption or age when first started drinking and their relationship to breast cancer risk are less well understood [12]. We conducted a case-control study of alcohol consumption patterns and breast cancer risk among women in three sub-Saharan African countries: Nigeria, Cameroon, and Uganda.

Materials and Methods

Study population

The African Breast Cancer Study was originally started in Nigeria in 1998 and was expanded to Uganda and Cameroon in 2011 using the same questionnaire and protocol. The study protocol was reviewed by the institutional review boards of the three sites and the University of Chicago (University of Chicago Biological Sciences Division Institutional Review Board (13304B and 10-023-B), University of Ibadan/University College Hospital Ethics Committee (UI/IRC/02/0003), Cameroon National Ethics Committee (N141/CNE/SE/2010), and Makerere University College of Health Sciences Ethics Committee (2011-023)). The study setting and design at the Nigeria site are described in detail elsewhere [34,35,36]. Briefly, cases were identified through University College Hospital (UCH), University of Ibadan, in Ibadan, Nigeria. Serving a population of more than 3 million people, UCH is a referral center for other hospitals and thus treat the majority of breast cancer cases in the region. All consecutive females who were 18 years or older, black of African descent, capable of providing informed consent, and had a histologic or clinical diagnosis of invasive breast cancer were recruited through the surgical oncology and radiotherapy units of the UCH. Controls were females aged 18 years or older, absent of breast cancer, and able to give informed consent. During the period of case enrollment, several communities were randomly selected by ballot from the list of all the communities in catchment area of UCH and considered to be stable, socio-economically and ethnically diverse, and represent UCH patients. Field interviewers randomly approached households in these communities and invited eligible women to visit community centers for the study. We also enrolled clinical controls through general outpatient and ophthalmology clinics in the UCH, matched for age and ethnicity. Women were enrolled during their waiting in clinics and they are unselected for their medical conditions. As the characteristics of hospital-based and community controls were similar, they were pooled in the further analysis. In Uganda, cases were identified at the breast and endocrine unit in department of surgery of the Mulago Hospital, Makerere University in Kampala. Mulago Hospital is a national referral hospital in Uganda and serves the 1.3 million residents in Kampala. Controls were randomly recruited from the general outpatient clinics and surgical ward admissions at Mulago Hospital, matched to cases for age and ethnicity. In Cameroon, breast cancer cases were enrolled at the department of medical oncology of Yaoundé General Hospital, Yaoundé University I in Yaoundé. Yaoundé General Hospital serves a population of 2.5 million people. Controls were randomly recruited from the clinics of general medicine and obstetrics and gynecology departments at the same hospital, matched to cases for age and ethnicity. At the Kampala and Yaoundé sites, hospital controls were unselected for their medical conditions. All study participants provided written informed consent prior to their interview. During the recruitment, both patients and controls were enthusiastic to participate in the study, with a response rate of > 90%.

Data collection and measures

Trained interviewers at the three sites performed structured questionnaire interviews, measured height and weight, and obtained blood samples. The questionnaire included questions about demographics, family history of breast cancer and history of benign breast disease, lifestyle factors, menstrual and reproductive history, and alcohol consumption patterns.

Before 2006, alcohol consumption was asked in Nigeria in terms of average volume of alcohol consumed per week (among 1,492 women). After 2006, the measurement was changed to average number of drinks per week. In Uganda and Cameroon, the alcohol consumption was asked in terms of average number of drinks per week. To convert the amount of alcohol into a common unit, the following conversion criteria were used: 350 mL bottle of beer (5% alcohol volume) ≈150 mL glass of wine (including local wine such as tonto or ajon in Uganda, 15% alcohol) ≈50 mL shot of spirits (including local spirits such as waragi or enguli in Uganda, 40% alcohol) ≈18 mL pure ethanol, which is equivalent to one standard drink. We then summed the amount of pure ethanol the participant consumed irrespective of the type of drink. We subsequently converted the volume of pure ethanol to gram: 1 mL = 0.8 gram. Each standard drink is hence equivalent to about 14.4 grams of pure ethanol. We also constructed a new variable called the life-time alcohol consumption, which was defined as gram-years: the average daily amount of alcohol in grams was multiplied by the subject's duration of alcohol consumption in years.

We defined alcohol drinking as having ever consumed alcoholic beverages at least once a week for continuous six months or more. In addition, we measured other alcohol drinking patterns: status of drinking (never drank, past drank, and current drinking; current drinking is defined as consuming alcohol at least once a week up until one year before breast cancer diagnosis or interview date), age at first drink, duration of alcohol drinking, and average amount of alcohol consumed daily. Duration of alcohol drinking was grouped into four categories: never drank, 1–9, 10–19, and ≥ 20 years. Average amount of alcohol consumed daily was also grouped into four categories: never drank, 0.1–4.9, 5.0–9.9, and ≥ 10.0 grams. Age at first drink had five categories: never drank, ≤ 18, 19–24, 25–29, and ≥30 years. Life-time alcohol consumption was also categorized into five groups: never drank, 0.1–29.9, 30.0–79.9, 80.0–159.9, and ≥160.0 gram-years.

Statistical analyses

Demographic factors and potential confounding factors for breast cancer were compared between cases and controls using student t-test or Wilcoxon rank-sum test for continuous variables and χ^2 test or Fisher's exact test for categorical variables. All P-values reported are two-sided. We calculated the percentages of control women who were currently consuming alcohol by the age groups of 18–34, 35–44, 45–54, and ≥55 years.

Multiple logistic regression models were used to examine the association between breast cancer and various patterns of alcohol consumption while adjusting for study site and other potential confounders listed below. These confounders were adjusted for in every multivariable logistic regression model and were defined as follows: age at diagnosis or interview (5-year interval categories), ethnicity (Yoruba, Ibo, Hausa, Baganda, Bantous, Semi-Bantous, others), education (none, elementary, secondary, some college or above, and vocational), age at menarche (≤14, 15–16, 17–18, ≥ 19 year), family history of breast cancer (yes, no), history of benign breast disease (yes, no), hormonal contraceptive use (ever, never), fertility drugs (ever, never), height, body mass index (BMI, kg/m^2), menopausal status (premenopausal, natural postmenopausal,

Table 1. Demographics of women with invasive breast cancer (cases) and those without (controls) in Nigeria, Cameroon and Uganda, 1998–2013.

Demographics	Nigeria	Cameroon		Uganda			Total	
	Case (N = 1756)	Control[a] (N = 2217)	Case (N = 192)	Control[a] (N = 182)	Case (N = 190)	Control[a] (N = 190)	Case (N = 2138)	Control[a] (N = 2589)
Age, year (mean ± SD)	47.6 ± 11.7	42.5 ± 13.0	47.6 ± 11.4	47.5 ± 11.7	46.6 ± 12.7	46.3 ± 12.2	47.5 ± 11.8	43.1 ± 13.0
***P*-value**		<0.001		0.94		0.80		<0.001
Ethnicity, n (%)								
Yoruba	1,288 (73.4)	1,816 (81.2)					1,288 (60.2)	1,816 (68.3)
Ibo	226 (12.9)	101 (5.0)					226 (10.6)	101 (4.2)
Hausa	22 (1.3)	171 (8.0)					22 (1.0)	171 (6.8)
Baganda					83 (43.7)	84 (44.2)	83 (3.9)	84 (3.4)
Bantous			101 (52.6)	94 (53.3)			101 (4.7)	94 (4.4)
Semi-Bantous			74 (38.5)	85 (45.1)			74 (3.5)	85 (4.3)
Other (Cameroon)			17 (8.9)	3 (1.5)			17 (0.8)	3 (0.1)
Other (Nigeria)	220 (12.5)	129 (5.8)					220 (10.3)	129 (4.9)
Other (Uganda)					107 (56.3)	106 (55.8)	107 (5.0)	106 (4.4)
***P*-value**		<0.001		0.02		0.99		<0.001
Education, n (%)								
No formal	354 (20.2)	315 (14.0)	8 (4.2)	2 (0.7)	21 (11.1)	11 (6.9)	383 (17.9)	328 (12.3)
Elementary	415 (23.6)	481 (22.2)	58 (30.2)	46 (22.8)	76 (40.0)	90 (46.3)	549 (25.7)	617 (24.4)
Secondary	354 (20.2)	534 (22.8)	84 (43.8)	101 (57.9)	59 (31.1)	46 (22.5)	497 (23.3)	681 (25.7)
Some college or above	418 (23.8)	607 (28.3)	33 (17.2)	23 (12.3)	18 (9.5)	15 (6.4)	469 (21.9)	645 (25.2)
Vocational/technical	215 (12.2)	280 (12.6)	9 (4.7)	10 (6.4)	16 (8.4)	28 (17.9)	240 (11.2)	318 (12.5)
***P*-value**		0.30		0.14		0.16		0.21
Family history of breast cancer, n (%)								
Yes	107 (6.1)	77 (3.3)	45 (23.4)	15 (8.5)	7 (3.7)	10 (4.2)	159 (7.4)	102 (3.8)
No	1,649 (93.9)	2,140 (96.7)	147 (76.6)	167 (91.5)	183 (96.3)	180 (95.8)	1,979 (92.6)	2,487 (96.2)
***P*-value**		<0.001		<0.001		0.68		<0.001
Benign breast disease, n (%)								
Yes	173 (9.9)	149 (7.4)	20 (10.4)	9 (5.3)	16 (8.4)	8 (2.7)	209 (9.8)	166 (6.9)
No	1,583 (90.1)	2,068 (92.6)	172 (89.6)	173 (94.7)	174 (91.6)	182 (97.3)	1,929 (90.2)	2,423 (93.1)
***P*-value**		0.004		0.04		0.01		<0.001
Menopause status								
Premenopausal	925 (52.7)	1,545 (69.0)	131 (68.2)	123 (71.6)	110 (57.9)	114 (62.9)	1,166 (54.5)	1,782 (68.7)
Postmenopausal, artificial	94 (5.3)	64 (3.2)	19 (9.9)	8 (4.5)	11 (5.8)	5 (3.1)	124 (5.8)	77 (3.3)
Postmenopausal, natural	737 (42.0)	608 (27.8)	42 (21.9)	51 (23.9)	69 (36.3)	71 (33.9)	848 (39.7)	730 (28.0)
***P*-value**		<0.001		0.06		0.34		<0.001

Table 1. Cont.

Demographics	Nigeria	Cameroon		Uganda			Total	
	Case (N = 1756)	Control[a] (N = 2217)	Case (N = 192)	Control[a] (N = 182)	Case (N = 190)	Control[a] (N = 190)	Case (N = 2138)	Control[a] (N = 2589)
Age at natural menopause (mean ± SD)	48.8±5.3	49.0±5.1	48.1±4.4	48.4±4.5	47.5±4.6	48.3±5.6	48.7±5.2	48.9±5.1
P-value		0.54		0.70		0.09		0.31
Hormonal contraceptives, n (%)								
Yes	495 (28.2)	706 (35.0)	51 (26.6)	77 (43.4)	83 (43.7)	88 (45.3)	629 (29.4)	871 (36.6)
No	1,261 (71.8)	1,511 (65.0)	141 (73.4)	105 (56.6)	107 (56.3)	102 (54.8)	1,509 (70.6)	1,718 (63.4)
P-value		0.002		0.001		0.84		<0.001
Fertility drugs, n (%)								
Yes	102 (10.1)	137 (11.3)	28 (14.7)	29 (17.7)	7 (3.8)	1 (0.9)	137 (9.9)	167 (10.8)
No	909 (89.9)	1,295 (88.7)	162 (85.3)	153 (82.3)	177 (96.2)	188 (99.1)	1,248 (90.1)	1,636 (89.2)
P-value		0.59		0.71		0.13		0.83
Age at menarche, year (mean ± SD)	15.3±2.1	15.3±2.2	14.2±1.6	14.2±1.7	14.7±1.6	14.7±1.6	15.1±2.0	15.1±2.1
P-value		0.23		0.97		0.75		0.16
Height, cm (mean ± SD)	161.1±7.7	159.0±6.5	164.4±6.2	163.9±6.4	161.0±8.5	162.5±9.9	161.4±7.7	159.6±6.9
P-value		<0.001		0.27		0.13		<0.001
BMI, kg/m^2 (mean ± SD)	25.8±6.0	27.0±5.7	27.1±5.4	28.2±4.5	24.2±4.9	25.8±5.1	25.8±5.9	27.0±5.6
P-value		<0.001		0.07		0.03		<0.001
Radiation exposure, n (%)								
Yes	11 (1.1)	187 (13.8)	46 (24.0)	5 (2.7)	20 (10.5)	15 (6.7)	77 (5.5)	207 (11.9)
No	1,006 (98.9)	1,252 (86.2)	146 (76.0)	177 (97.3)	170 (89.5)	175 (93.3)	1,322 (94.5)	1,604 (88.1)
P-value		<0.001		<0.001		0.37		<0.001
Parity, n (%)								
0	159 (9.1)	254 (5.0)	21 (10.9)	15 (7.5)	29 (15.3)	11 (5.0)	209 (9.8)	280 (5.3)
1–2	308 (17.5)	474 (17.7)	45 (23.4)	52 (28.3)	40 (21.1)	47 (22.3)	393 (18.4)	573 (18.7)
3–4	543 (30.9)	708 (37.1)	60 (31.3)	44 (26.6)	33 (17.4)	47 (26.5)	636 (29.8)	799 (35.4)
5–6	498 (28.4)	524 (27.6)	32 (16.7)	41 (23.8)	49 (25.8)	40 (23.9)	579 (27.1)	605 (27.0)
≥7	248 (14.1)	257 (12.6)	34 (17.7)	30 (13.8)	39 (20.5)	45 (22.2)	321 (15.0)	332 (13.7)
P-value		<0.001		0.24		0.01		<0.001
Age at first live birth, year (mean ± SD)[b]	23.3±4.9	23.4±4.8	21.3±4.9	21.5±5.6	20.4±4.4	20.8±4.7	22.9±4.9	23.0±4.9
P-value		0.77		0.62		0.56		0.92
Ever breast feed, n (%)								
Yes	1,581 (90.8)	1,950 (94.9)	167 (87.0)	160 (88.6)	154 (82.4)	177 (95.6)	1,902 (89.7)	2,287 (94.4)
No	161 (9.2)	254 (5.1)	25 (13.0)	22 (11.4)	33 (17.7)	11 (4.4)	219 (10.3)	287 (5.6)

Table 1. Cont.

Demographics	Nigeria		Cameroon		Uganda		Total	
	Case (N = 1756)	Control[a] (N = 2217)	Case (N = 192)	Control[a] (N = 182)	Case (N = 190)	Control[a] (N = 190)	Case (N = 2138)	Control[a] (N = 2589)
P-value		<0.001		0.84		<0.001		<0.001
Lifetime duration of breastfeeding, month, n (%)								
≤24	417 (23.9)	599 (18.2)	68 (35.4)	71 (37.9)	62 (33.2)	46 (22.6)	547 (25.8)	716 (20.1)
25–48	387 (22.2)	476 (23.2)	46 (24.0)	36 (21.9)	24 (12.8)	25 (12.1)	457 (21.6)	537 (22.2)
49–72	374 (21.5)	492 (26.6)	36 (18.8)	32 (18.9)	26 (13.9)	36 (20.1)	436 (20.6)	560 (25.5)
73–96	241 (13.8)	264 (13.6)	22 (11.5)	14 (7.8)	19 (10.2)	21 (12.1)	282 (13.3)	299 (13.0)
>96	323 (18.5)	373 (18.4)	20 (10.4)	29 (13.6)	56 (30.0)	60 (33.2)	399 (18.8)	462 (19.2)
P-value		<0.001		0.30		0.42		<0.001

Note: Numbers in parentheses are proportions (%). SD: standard deviation.
[a]Proportions or means for the controls are adjusted values based on the age distribution of cases; *P*-values were also age-adjusted in logistic regressions.
[b]Among parous women.

artificial postmenopausal), age at first live birth (<20, 20–24, 25–29, ≥30 years), and parity (0, 1–2, 3–4, 5–6, ≥7). Adjusted odds ratio (aOR) and 95% confidence interval (CI) were computed from the logistic regression models. Ever drank, status of drinking, and type of alcohol consumed (never drank, beer, wine, spirits) were included in the models solely as categorical variables. Age at first drink, duration of alcohol drinking, average amount of alcohol consumed daily, and life-time alcohol consumption were analyzed as both categorical variables and continuous variables. Stratified analyses were also performed to compare the breast cancer risk between ever-drinkers vs. never-drinkers across different strata of demographic and reproductive variables, such as premenopausal vs. post-menopausal women. Potential confounding variables were adjusted for in these analyses.

There were missing data for age at first drink, duration of alcohol drinking, average volume of drinking, and other important covariates. To use all available information and avoid bias due to list-wise deletion in the multivariable analysis, we conducted multiple imputations via chained equations approach for imputation [37,38]. All covariates and outcome variable (case-control status) were included in the imputation model. We ran 100 imputations to improve statistical efficiency of the imputation estimates to be over 99.5%. The logistic regression models described above were fitted using each of the imputed data sets. Results across the multiply imputed datasets were combined according to Rubin's rules [39]. Multiple imputation approach assumes missing at random. Older women tended to forget how much alcohol they consumed in the past. By including age in the multiple imputation models, it is reasonable to believe that the probability of missing alcohol data was at random. As a sensitivity analysis, we conducted the analysis using data without missing value in any of the covariates in the models (i.e. complete case analysis). All statistical analyses, including the imputation (*ice* module), were conducted with STATA 13.0 (StataCorp, College Station, TX, USA).

Results

A total of 2,138 breast cancer cases and 2,589 controls (women without breast cancer) were enrolled in the study between March 1998 and July 2013, including 1,756 cases and 2,217 controls in Nigeria, 192 cases and 182 controls in Cameroon, and 190 cases and 190 controls in Uganda. Table 1 shows selected demographic and reproductive characteristics of study participants. Since Nigeria comprises the largest proportion of the study population, demographic differences between cases and controls in the Nigerian population will influence the difference in the overall population. Cases in Nigeria were 5.1 years older than controls on average; there was no difference in age between cases and controls in Cameroon or Uganda. Most participants in Nigeria were Yoruba, and over half of the participants in Uganda were Baganda and in Cameroon were Bantous. In all study participants, about 40% had less than a secondary education. About 75% of women had ≥3 live births. There were no differences between cases and controls in terms of their average age at menarche and use of fertility drugs in the crude analysis. In the Nigerian population, cases were taller than controls, on average. Cases were more likely to have a family history of breast cancer and a history of benign breast disease in Nigeria and Cameroon. Similarly, controls were more likely to have ever used hormonal contraceptives. In the Cameroon population, the proportion of cases who had a family history of breast cancer (23.4%) was considerably larger than the controls (8.2%). This difference was less pronounced in Nigeria

Table 2. Patterns of alcohol consumption among women in Nigeria, Cameroon and Uganda, 1998–2013

Variable	Nigeria		Cameroon		Uganda		Total	
	No. of Cases, n (%)	No. of Controls, n (%)	No. of Cases, n (%)	No. of Controls, n (%)	No. of Cases, n (%)	No. of Controls, n (%)	No. of Cases, n (%)	No. of Controls, n (%)
Ever drank alcohol								
No	1,546 (88.0)	2,106 (95.0)	94 (49.0)	119 (65.4)	90 (47.4)	95 (50.0)	1,730 (80.9)	2,320 (89.6)
Yes	210 (12.0)	111 (5.0)	98 (51.0)	63 (34.6)	100 (52.6)	95 (50.0)	408 (19.1)	269 (10.4)
Status of drinking								
Never	1,546 (89.3)	2,106 (95.4)	94 (49.2)	119 (65.8)	90 (48.1)	95 (51.1)	1,730 (82.0)	2,320 (90.1)
Past	117 (6.8)	55 (2.5)	17 (8.9)	19 (10.5)	59 (31.6)	51 (27.4)	193 (9.2)	125 (4.9)
Current	68 (3.9)	46 (2.1)	80 (41.9)	43 (23.8)	38 (20.3)	40 (21.5)	186 (8.8)	129 (5.0)
Age at first drink, year								
Never	1,546 (88.8)	2,106 (95.2)	94 (49.0)	119 (65.8)	90 (50.0)	95 (51.4)	1,730 (81.9)	2,320 (90.0)
drank								
≤18	26 (1.5)	13 (0.6)	16 (8.3)	14 (7.7)	25 (13.9)	23 (12.4)	67 (5.2)	50 (1.9)
19–24	64 (3.7)	32 (1.5)	36 (18.8)	22 (12.2)	26 (14.4)	26 (14.1)	126 (6.0)	80 (3.1)
25–29	42 (2.4)	28 (1.3)	27 (14.1)	8 (4.4)	12 (6.7)	13 (7.0)	81 (3.8)	49 (1.9)
≥30	63 (3.6)	34 (1.5)	19 (9.9)	18 (9.9)	27 (15.0)	28 (15.1)	109 (5.2)	80 (3.1)
Mean ± SD	26.7±9.3	26.3±7.8	24.0±6.6	23.9±8.2	24.3±8.5	24.0±9.4	25.5±8.6	24.9±8.6
P-value		0.72		0.93		0.85		0.45
Duration of alcohol drinking, year								
Never drank	1,546 (89.0)	2,106 (95.1)	94 (50.3)	119 (73.0)	90 (55.6)	95 (62.1)	1,730 (82.9)	2,320 (91.7)
1–9	63 (3.6)	59 (2.7)	17 (9.2)	9 (5.5)	30 (18.5)	24 (15.7)	110 (5.3)	92 (3.6)
10–19	69 (4.0)	32 (1.5)	27 (14.6)	12 (7.4)	18 (11.1)	13 (8.5)	114 (5.5)	57 (2.3)
≥ 20	60 (3.5)	17 (0.8)	48 (26.0)	23 (14.1)	24 (14.8)	21 (13.7)	132 (6.3)	61 (2.4)
Mean ± SD[†]	15.0±10.3	10.3±9.1	21.1±11.8	20.0±12.7	17.2±12.8	14.8±12.6	17.0±11.6	14.2±11.9
P-value		<0.001		0.57		0.18		0.002
Average amount of alcohol consumed daily, gram								
Never	1,546 (90.5)	2,106 (96.2)	94 (49.2)	119 (65.8)	90 (71.4)	95 (69.9)	1,730 (85.4)	2,320 (92.5)
Drank	51 (3.0)	18 (0.8)	42 (22.0)	19 (10.5)	20 (15.9)	24 (17.7)	113 (5.6)	61 (2.4)
5.0–9.9	66 (3.9)	35 (1.6)	28 (14.7)	22 (12.2)	7 (5.6)	13 (9.6)	101 (5.0)	70 (2.8)
≥10	46 (2.7)	31 (1.4)	27 (14.1)	21 (11.6)	9 (7.1)	4 (2.9)	82 (4.1)	56 (2.2)
Mean ± SD[†]	10.1±28.7	13.2±39.4	11.9±29.9	8.8±7.6	10.1±15.6	9.3±13.0	10.6±26.4	10.8±26.7
P-value		0.43		0.42		0.69		0.92
Life-time alcohol consumption, gram-years								
Never	1,546 (90.9)	2,106 (96.2)	94 (50.3)	119 (73.0)	90 (70.9)	95 (73.1)	1,730 (86.0)	2,320 (93.3)
Drank	43 (2.4)	36 (1.6)	12 (5.5)	5 (3.1)	6 (5.1)	9 (6.9)	56 (2.8)	52 (2.0)

Table 2. Cont.

Variable	Nigeria		Cameroon		Uganda		Total	
	No. of Cases, n (%)	No. of Controls, n (%)	No. of Cases, n (%)	No. of Controls, n (%)	No. of Cases, n (%)	No. of Controls, n (%)	No. of Cases, n (%)	No. of Controls, n (%)
30.0–79.9	47 (2.8)	20 (0.8)	29 (13.7)	9 (5.5)	6 (5.1)	11 (8.5)	78 (3.9)	39 (1.5)
80.0–159.9	42 (2.1)	12 (0.7)	17 (12.6)	11 (6.7)	9 (7.7)	10 (7.7)	68 (3.4)	32 (1.5)
≥160.0	23 (1.9)	15 (0.7)	33 (18.0)	19 (11.7)	13 (11.1)	5 (3.9)	78 (3.9)	39 (1.7)
Mean ± SD†	144.0±370.1	238.1±888.5	319.1±1211.4	186.2±182.0	179.0±211.6	84.3±66.9	205.1±748.8	190.8±644.6
***P*-value**		0.25		0.47		0.01		0.84
Type of alcohol‡								
Never drank	1,546 (88.0)	2,106 (95.0)	94 (49.0)	119 (65.4)	90 (47.4)	95 (50.0)	1,730 (80.9)	2,320 (89.6)
Beer	166 (9.5)	93 (4.2)	84 (43.8)	61 (33.5)	20 (10.5)	28 (14.7)	270 (12.6)	182 (7.0)
Wine	35 (2.0)	16 (0.7)	29 (15.1)	25 (13.7)	19 (10.0)	16 (8.4)	83 (3.9)	57 (2.2)
Spirits	27 (1.5)	16 (0.7)	22 (11.5)	15 (8.2)	17 (9.0)	13 (6.8)	66 (3.1)	44 (1.7)

†Among drinkers.
‡Includes drinkers who drink a combination of alcoholic beverages, percentages may not add up to 100%.

and Uganda, though the difference was still statistically significant in Nigeria.

Overall, there were 1,311 (1.7%) missing values across 16 variables in Tables 1 and 2 (excluding derivative variables). Complete information was available for ethnicity, ever drink alcohol, menopausal status, and site of study. About 5% of participants had a missing value for age at menarche, and 3% of them had missing values for height and weight. Data were occasionally missing for other variables as well. One hundred data sets were generated by multiple imputation such that the efficiency of estimating OR was greater than 99.5% for the fraction of missing information up to 0.08.

Among healthy controls, 10.4% were alcohol drinkers, and the percentage of ever drinkers in Cameroon, Nigeria, and Uganda were 34.6%, 5.0%, and 50.0%, respectively. Figure 1 shows the percentages of current alcohol drinking among women by age group. Women in Cameroon and Uganda were more likely to be current drinkers than those in Nigeria. Among women in Cameroon and Nigeria, current drinking was proportionately more common in middle-aged women (aged 35–44 and 45–54 years) than younger or older women, while in Uganda, young women (aged 18–34) had the highest prevalence of current drinking.

Table 2 presents the alcohol drinking patterns among cases and controls. There was no statistical difference in the mean age at first drink and mean amount of alcohol consumed daily in the overall data. In terms of duration of alcohol consumption, cases were found to drink for 2.8 years longer on average than in controls. In the overall population, 86.4% of drinkers consumed ≤1 drink per day (1 drink = 14.4 g of pure ethanol), 8.8% of drinkers consumed 1–2 drinks per day, 2.8% of drinkers consumed 2–3 drinks per day, and 2.1% of drinkers consumed more than 3 drinks per day. In drinkers, there was no considerable difference in amount of alcohol drinking among the three countries.

Table 3 presents the relationship of the alcohol drinking patterns to breast cancer risk with calculated odds ratio and 95% CI using imputed data. Among the whole study sample, cases were more likely than controls to have ever consumed alcohol (aOR: 1.62, 95% CI: 1.33–1.97). Both past drinking (aOR: 1.54; 95% CI: 1.19–2.00) or current drinking (aOR: 1.71; 95% CI: 1.30–2.23) were associated with increased breast cancer risk. Breast cancer risk was relatively consistent regardless of when the women first started drinking. Compared with non-drinkers, women who had drunk for <10 years had 41% higher odds of having breast cancer (aOR: 1.41; 95% CI: 1.04–1.91), and those who had drunk for 10–19 years had 71% (aOR: 1.71; 95% CI: 1.23–2.39) and those for ≥20 years had 82% (aOR: 1.82; 95% CI: 1.30–2.54) higher odds of having breast cancer. Every 10-year increase in the duration of drinking was associated with a 54% increase in breast cancer risk (aOR: 1.54; 95% CI: 1.29–1.84; *P*-trend: <0.001). We also found that alcohol consumption was associated with breast cancer risk, regardless of alcohol amount; breast cancer risk increase was shown even in the category of women who consume 0.1–4.9 g/day (aOR: 1.82, 95% CI: 1.31–2.54). In the variable life-time alcohol consumption, increased breast cancer risk was observed for subjects who consume at least 30 gram-years or more of alcohol (aOR: 1.85, 95% CI: 1.26–2.72). We also found a statistically significant trend, with each 100 gram-years contributing a 29% increase in breast cancer risk (aOR: 1.29; 95% CI: 1.12–1.51; *P*-trend = 0.001). The complete case analysis, in which subjects with missing values in any of the variables in the models were dropped, showed similar study findings (Table S1).

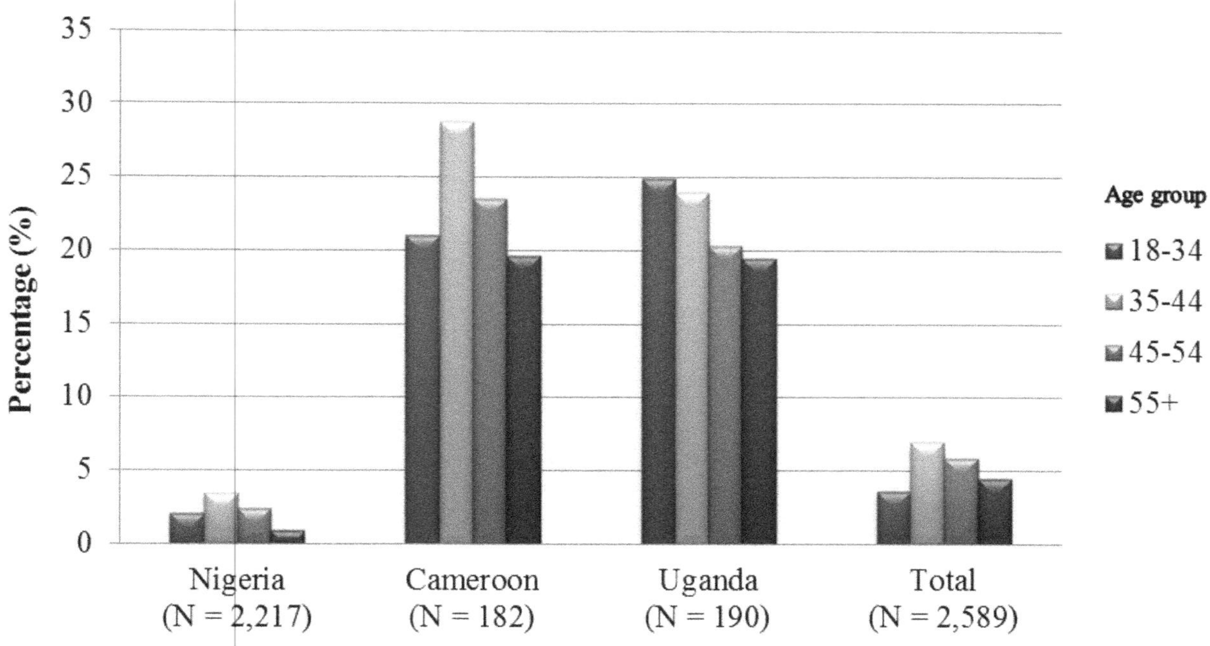

Figure 1. Percentage of healthy controls who were current drinkers by age group in the three African countries.

Table 4 shows the relationship between ever-drinking and breast cancer risk by strata of age at interview or diagnosis, ethnicity, height and other demographic and reproductive variables. When the interactions between the stratified variables and ever drinking alcohol were tested, parity and BMI were found to have a statistically significant interaction with alcohol drinking ($P = 0.03$ for both tests). In parous women, the association between drinking alcohol and breast cancer was weaker (aOR: 1.55; 95% CI: 1.26–1.91) than that in nulliparous women (aOR: 2.81; 95% CI: 1.24–6.35). There was no statistically significant association between alcohol consumption and breast cancer among women with BMI ≤25 kg/m^2 (aOR: 1.09; 95% CI: 0.79–1.50), while among women with BMI >25 kg/m^2, ever-drinkers had nearly twice the odds for breast cancer than never-drinkers (aOR: 2.06, 95% CI: 1.59–2.68). For other stratification variables, drinkers had similarly elevated risks for breast cancer compared to non-drinkers across the strata of these variables.

Discussion

Our case-control study of 4,727 African women from Nigeria, Cameroon, and Uganda showed a positive relationship between breast cancer and alcohol drinking. Overall, the odds of having breast cancer were 62% higher among women who ever consumed alcohol than among no-drinkers. This finding was in general agreement with literature. The current evidence on the relationship between alcohol consumption and female breast cancer risk is largely based on studies conducted in Caucasian populations [40,41], and the observed evidence in African American women was inconsistent [17,18,42,43]. Numerous reasons may explain for the racial difference, including drinking habits, metabolism and genetic factors. For example, there are racial differences in distributions of genetic polymorphisms related to ethanol metabolism [44,45]. Traditionally, alcohol consumption among African women is less common compared with those in developed countries. However, as women in Africa are increasingly influenced by western cultures and begin to change their lifestyle and as the populations in African countries are becoming more affluent, more and more women may be exposed to alcohol [29,46,47]. Few studies have investigated this relationship among African women [1]. Our study is the first multi-country study using a large African women sample. The incidence of breast cancer is anticipated to increase in African countries such as in Nigeria [48].

Our study also found that women who were past drinkers (54% increase) had almost the same elevated risk as women who were current drinkers (71% increase). Our study showed a dose-response relationship between duration of alcohol drinking and breast cancer risk; women who drank for 20 years or longer had almost twice the odds of being cancer cases compared with non-drinkers. This relationship was confirmed in some studies [12,49] but not in others [12,43]. We did not find dose-response relationship between amount of alcohol intake and breast cancer risk, possibly because there were few heavy drinkers in our study population. Studies have suggested that a moderate level of alcohol consumption (e.g., 5–10 g/day) may be sufficient for increasing breast cancer risk [50,51,52], while other studies did not show that low-level consumption of alcohol increases breast cancer risk in premenopausal women [53].

The effect of alcohol drinking among nulliparous women was significantly elevated compared to that among parous women. This result is consistent with prior studies which suggests that the carcinogenic effect of alcohol consumption is strongest between menarche and the first full term pregnancy and could be implicated in both increased risk of breast cancer and benign breast disease [54,55,56]. Starting to drink at a young reproductive age (<30 year, particularly during 25–29 years) was associated with an increased risk of breast cancer in our study sample. This finding is consistent with other studies [43,57,58,59].

In addition, alcohol drinking among women with BMI >25 kg/m^2, clinically defined as overweight or obese, had a greater risk of developing breast cancer. This suggests that obesity and alcohol drinking may have joint effects on risk of breast cancer among women. Being overweight or obese has been shown to be a risk factor for postmenopausal breast cancer [60,61]. The proposed mechanism in both animal models and humans of the mediating

Table 3. Multivariable logistic regression analyses of alcohol consumption and breast cancer risk among women in Nigeria, Cameroon and Uganda, 1998–2013, using data after multiple imputation (N = 4727).

Variable	Nigeria	Cameroon	Uganda	Overall
	Adjusted OR (95% CI)†	Adjusted OR (95% CI)†	Adjusted OR (95% CI)†	Adjusted OR (95% CI)‡
Ever drank alcohol				
No	1.0 (ref.)	1.0 (ref.)	1.0 (ref.)	1.0 (ref.)
Yes	1.80 (1.38–2.35)	1.80 (1.11–2.92)	1.00 (0.62–1.62)	1.62 (1.33–1.97)
Status of drinking				
Never	1.0 (ref.)	1.0 (ref.)	1.0 (ref.)	1.0 (ref.)
Past	1.88 (1.33–2.67)	1.00 (0.45–2.23)	0.99 (0.57–1.75)	1.54 (1.19–2.00)
Current	1.70 (1.13–2.55)	2.17 (1.28-3.69)	1.01 (0.55–1.85)	1.71 (1.30–2.23)
Age at first drink, year				
Never drank	1.0 (ref.)	1.0 (ref.)	1.0 (ref.)	1.0 (ref.)
≤18	2.34 (1.14–4.80)	1.21 (0.49–2.96)	1.09 (0.53–2.23)	1.68 (1.11–2.54)
19–24	1.94 (1.20–3.14)	1.59 (0.80–3.16)	0.95 (0.46–1.93)	1.74 (1.26–2.41)
25–29	1.53 (0.91–2.56)	4.09 (1.63–10.2)	0.81 (0.31–2.11)	1.77 (1.20–2.61)
≥30	1.72 (1.10–2.69)	1.47 (0.67–3.21)	1.09 (0.53–2.24)	1.39 (1.01–1.91)
P-value for trend	<0.001	0.08	0.99	<0.001
Duration of alcohol drinking, year				
Never	1.0 (ref.)	1.0 (ref.)	1.0 (ref.)	1.0 (ref.)
Drank	1.35 (0.92–1.99)	1.25 (0.51 3.05)	0.94 (0.49–1.80)	1.41 (1.04–1.91)
10–19	1.90 (1.22–2.97)	1.63 (0.75–2.74)	1.16 (0.52–2.57)	1.71 (1.23–2.39)
≥ 20	2.97 (1.66–5.31)	2.30 (1.19–4.45)	0.99 (0.49–2.00)	1.82 (1.30–2.54)
P-value for trend	<0.001	0.002	0.85	<0.001
Per 10-year increase	1.84 (1.43–2.37)	1.85 (1.24–2.75)	1.04 (0.68–1.60)	1.54 (1.29–1.84)
Average amount of alcohol consumed daily, gram				
Never drank	1.0 (ref.)	1.0 (ref.)	1.0 (ref.)	1.0 (ref.)
0.1–4.9	2.27 (1.33–3.87)	2.62 (1.31–5.20)	0.99 (0.53–1.87)	1.82 (1.31–2.54)
5.0–9.9	1.91 (1.23–2.96)	1.31 (0.65–2.64)	0.72 (0.31–1.69)	1.52 (1.10–2.11)
≥10	1.37 (0.85–2.22)	1.61 (0.77–3.35)	1.48 (0.58–3.80)	1.50 (1.04–2.18)
P-value for trend	0.03	0.13	0.57	0.007
Per 10g increase	1.43 (1.05–1.96)	1.50 (0.89–2.52)	1.20 (0.63–2.28)	1.39 (1.09–1.76)
Life-time alcohol consumption, gram-years				
Never	1.0 (ref.)	1.0 (ref.)	1.0 (ref.)	1.0 (ref.)
Drank	1.24 (0.79–1.94)	1.24 (0.38–4.04)	0.90 (0.44–1.83)	1.29 (0.91–1.83)
30.0–79.9	2.61 (1.49–4.58)	2.21 (0.96–5.11)	0.76 (0.32–1.82)	1.85 (1.26–2.72)
80.0–159.9	2.11 (1.13–3.93)	1.96 (0.88–4.41)	0.81 (0.33–1.98)	1.73 (1.15–2.60)
≥160.0	1.87 (1.01–3.45)	1.67 (0.83–3.36)	1.98 (0.75–5.26)	1.76 (1.17–2.64)
P-value for trend	0.001	0.06	0.19	0.001
Per 100 gram-year increase	1.45 (1.16–1.81)	1.29 (0.99–1.70)	1.26 (0.89–1.77)	1.29 (1.12–1.51)
Type of alcohol⇮				
Never drank	1.0 (ref.)	1.0 (ref.)	1.0 (ref.)	1.0 (ref.)
Beer	1.80 (1.35–2.40)	1.51 (0.92–2.46)	0.88 (0.48–1.61)	1.53 (1.22–1.91)
Wine	2.32 (1.20–4.50)	1.01 (0.52–1.98)	1.11 (0.58–2.13)	1.32 (0.91–1.92)
Spirits	1.76 (0.89–3.48)	1.31 (0.58–2.95)	1.30 (0.64–2.67)	1.52 (0.99–2.32)

†Adjusted for age at diagnosis or interview (categorical), ethnicity, education (categorical), age at menarche (categorical), number of live births (categorical), age at first live birth (categorical), menopausal status, family history of breast cancer, benign breast disease, hormonal contraceptive use, BMI (continuous), and height (continuous);
‡Adjusted for the above variables and study site.
⇮Includes drinkers who drink a combination of alcoholic beverages.

effect of alcohol as well as adiposity's effect on serum estradiol and insulin levels may account for the interaction effect observed between BMI and alcohol consumption [62,63].

Heterogeneity in the level of alcohol consumption was observed among women in three African countries. Using a definition of alcohol drinking as having at least one drink every week for a continuous 6 months or more, the percentage of ever drinkers in Nigeria, Cameroon, and Uganda were 5.0%, 34.6%, and 50.0%, respectively. This is in line with previous surveys of alcohol consumption in the three countries, although it is not straightforward to directly compare with previous studies due to different definition of alcohol drinking. According to the WHO country surveys conducted from 2003 to 2005, the percent of women who are lifetime abstainers in Nigeria, Cameroon, and Uganda were 50.9%, 39.8%, 36.7%, respectively [64,65,66]. Heterogeneity in the relationship between alcohol drinking and breast cancer was also observed across the three countries. In Nigeria and Cameroon, women who drank alcohol had a moderate increased risk of breast cancer compared to never-drinkers, whereas in Uganda there was only a marginal increase in risk. A small sample size (n = 380) may explain for these non-significant findings in Uganda. A previous study found that a larger proportion of Nigerian women who drank alcohol regularly tended to be heavy drinkers compared to Ugandan women [29], which may also account for the weak correlation between alcohol consumption and breast cancer risk for women in Uganda. Larger sample size in Uganda and Cameroon are desirable to confirm these study findings.

Although some studies have suggested that recall bias only had minor effects on alcohol reporting and on the estimation of risk for breast cancer [67], we could not exclude the possibility of recall bias in reporting alcohol consumption in our study. Due to the retrospective nature of the study, participants might have difficulty in recalling alcohol consumption patterns, especially if the patterns changed over time for older women. In addition, cultural stigmas against alcohol use among women might also have resulted in

Table 4. Stratified analyses of alcohol consumption and breast cancer risk among women in Nigeria, Cameroon, and Uganda using data after multiple imputation, 1998–2013.

Stratified variable	Number of participants	Number and prevalence of ever-drinkers, n (%)	Adjusted OR for being ever-drinkers vs. non-drinkers (95% CI)*	*P*-value for interaction
Age at interview or diagnosis, year				
<50	3,047	384 (12.6)	1.64 (1.28–2.11)	
≥50	1,680	293 (17.4)	1.97 (1.42–2.73)	0.49
Menopausal status				
Premenopausal	2,948	376 (12.8)	1.64 (1.26–2.12)	
Post-menopausal	1,779	301 (16.9)	1.82 (1.32–2.52)	0.14
Parity				
Nulliparous	489	68 (13.9)	2.81 (1.24–6.35)	
Parous	4,238	609 (14.4)	1.55 (1.26–1.91)	0.03
Family history of breast cancer				
Yes	261	85 (32.6)	2.66 (1.08–6.57)	
No	4,466	592 (13.3)	1.59 (1.29–1.96)	0.67
Benign breast disease				
Yes	375	86 (22.9)	2.43 (1.25–4.75)	
No	4,352	591 (13.6)	1.56 (1.26–1.93)	0.11
Ever use of hormonal contraceptives				
Yes	1,500	294 (19.6)	1.48 (1.09–2.02)	
No	3,227	383 (11.9)	1.73 (1.32–2.27)	0.58
Body mass index, kg/m^2				
≤25	2,209	292 (13.2)	1.09 (0.79–1.50)	
>25	2,518	385 (15.3)	2.06 (1.59–2.68)	0.03
Height, cm				
≤160	2,510	286 (11.4)	1.64 (1.23–2.20)	
>160	2,217	391 (17.6)	1.72 (1.29–2.29)	0.11
Age at menarche, year				
≤15	2,943	442 (15.0)	1.71 (1.33–2.20)	
>15	1,784	235 (13.2)	1.55 (1.09–2.21)	0.86
Ethnicity				
Yoruba	3,104	217 (7.0)	1.51 (1.12–2.04)	
Other	1,623	460 (28.3)	1.62 (1.27–2.07)	0.81

*Adjusted for all other variables listed in this table as well as age at first live birth and study site.

under-reporting of alcohol consumption [68,69,70]. Nigerian women might tend to under-report alcohol consumption, as it is often considered culturally inappropriate for them to drink alcohol outside of religious settings [70]. The majority of subjects in the study were considered to be light drinkers whereas there were few moderate and heavy drinkers. This observation could also account for the lack of a dose-response relationship with respect to the amount of alcohol consumed. Our study did not assess alcohol consumption at each stage of a woman's life, and therefore, it was assumed that alcohol consumption was constant over a subject's lifetime. Since ethanol and its primary metabolite, acetaldehyde, can affect estrogen levels and are involved in carcinogenic pathways [71], alcohol consumption later in life may further accelerate genetic mutations.

In conclusion, our study found a positive relationship between alcohol consumption and breast cancer risk among sub-Saharan African women. The adoption of a Western lifestyle and erosion of many traditional customs that prohibited alcohol drinking has led to drastic changes in alcohol consumption patterns, including greater drinking among young people and women [72,73,74]. According to the 2011 WHO data, 25.3% of the population in Africa is displaying an increase in five-year trends for recorded adult per capita alcohol consumption [75]. Surveys from 2005 also show that in Nigeria and Uganda, total adult (defined as 15 years or older) per capita alcohol consumption (10.00–12.49 liters) has already exceeded the per capita alcohol consumption in the United States (7.50–9.99) [75]. If we assumed a common odds ratio of 1.62 and observed alcohol prevalence in the three countries, 4.6%, 19.5%, and 20.1% of breast cancer cases can be attributed to alcohol drinking in Nigeria, Cameroon, and Uganda, respectively. As breast cancer incidence is increasing in African countries and alcohol drinking is increasingly popular among African women [29,30,31,32,46,47], public health programs in Africa should take proactive measures to prevent breast cancer through addressing the modifiable risk factor of alcohol consumption, including providing current information on the risk of alcohol consumption among women and advocating proper regulation of alcohol sale through more effective alcohol policies [76,77,78].

Author Contributions

Conceived and designed the experiments: NH OIO DH. Performed the experiments: TO NH PN AG JJ IMB CA AA OO OIO DH. Analyzed the data: FQ NH DH. Contributed reagents/materials/analysis tools: FQ NH CA OIO DH. Contributed to the writing of the manuscript: FQ TO NH PN AG JJ IMB CA AA OO OIO DH.

References

1. Adebamowo CA, Adekunle OO (1999) Case-controlled study of the epidemiological risk factors for breast cancer in Nigeria. Br J Surg 86: 665–668.
2. Adebamowo CA, Ajayi OO (2000) Breast cancer in Nigeria. West Afr J Med 19: 179–191.
3. Hutchinson L (2010) Breast cancer: challenges, controversies, breakthroughs. Nat Rev Clin Oncol 7: 669–670.
4. Anothaisintawee T, Wiratkapun C, Lerdsitthichai P, Kasamesup V, Wongwaisayawan S, et al. (2013) Risk factors of breast cancer: a systematic review and meta-analysis. Asia Pac J Public Health 25: 368–387.
5. Warner E (2011) Clinical practice. Breast-cancer screening. N Engl J Med 365: 1025–1032.
6. Jemal A, Ward E, Thun MJ (2007) Recent trends in breast cancer incidence rates by age and tumor characteristics among U.S. women. Breast Cancer Res 9: R28.
7. Parkin DM, Sitas F, Chirenje M, Stein L, Abratt R, et al. (2008) Part I: Cancer in Indigenous Africans—burden, distribution, and trends. Lancet Oncol 9: 683–692.
8. Sitas F, Parkin DM, Chirenje M, Stein L, Abratt R, et al. (2008) Part II: Cancer in Indigenous Africans—causes and control. Lancet Oncol 9: 786–795.
9. Suzuki R, Orsini N, Mignone L, Saji S, Wolk A (2008) Alcohol intake and risk of breast cancer defined by estrogen and progesterone receptor status—a meta-analysis of epidemiological studies. Int J Cancer 122: 1832–1841.
10. Hamajima N, Hirose K, Tajima K, Rohan T, Calle EE, et al. (2002) Alcohol, tobacco and breast cancer—collaborative reanalysis of individual data from 53 epidemiological studies, including 58,515 women with breast cancer and 95,067 women without the disease. Br J Cancer 87: 1234–1245.
11. Key J, Hodgson S, Omar RZ, Jensen TK, Thompson SG, et al. (2006) Meta-analysis of studies of alcohol and breast cancer with consideration of the methodological issues. Cancer Causes Control 17: 759–770.
12. Bowlin SJ, Leske MC, Varma A, Nasca P, Weinstein A, et al. (1997) Breast cancer risk and alcohol consumption: results from a large case-control study. Int J Epidemiol 26: 915–923.
13. Bagnardi V, Blangiardo M, La Vecchia C, Corrao G (2001) A meta-analysis of alcohol drinking and cancer risk. Br J Cancer 85: 1700–1705.
14. Nasca PC, Baptiste MS, Field NA, Metzger BB, Black M, et al. (1990) An epidemiological case-control study of breast cancer and alcohol consumption. Int J Epidemiol 19: 532–538.
15. Thun MJ, Peto R, Lopez AD, Monaco JH, Henley SJ, et al. (1997) Alcohol consumption and mortality among middle-aged and elderly U.S. adults. N Engl J Med 337: 1705–1714.
16. Kinney AY, Millikan RC, Lin YH, Moorman PG, Newman B (2000) Alcohol consumption and breast cancer among black and white women in North Carolina (United States). Cancer Causes Control 11: 345–357.
17. Llanos AA, Makambi KH, Tucker CA, Shields PG, Adams-Campbell LL (2012) Alcohol, anthropometrics, and breast cancer risk in African American women. Breast J 18: 394–395.
18. Chandran U, Zirpoli G, Ciupak G, McCann SE, Gong Z, et al. (2013) Does alcohol increase breast cancer risk in African-American women? Findings from a case–control study. British Journal of Cancer.
19. Zhang M, Holman CD (2011) Low-to-moderate alcohol intake and breast cancer risk in Chinese women. Br J Cancer 105: 1089–1095.
20. Baumgartner KB, Annegers JF, McPherson RS, Frankowski RF, Gilliland FD, et al. (2002) Is alcohol intake associated with breast cancer in Hispanic women? The New Mexico Women's Health Study. Ethn Dis 12: 460–469.
21. Yoo KY, Tajima K, Miura S, Takeuchi T, Hirose K, et al. (1997) Breast cancer risk factors according to combined estrogen and progesterone receptor status: a case-control analysis. Am J Epidemiol 146: 307–314.
22. McDonald JA, Mandel MG, Marchbanks PA, Folger SG, Daling JR, et al. (2004) Alcohol exposure and breast cancer: results of the women's contraceptive and reproductive experiences study. Cancer Epidemiol Biomarkers Prev 13: 2106–2116.
23. Bao PP, Shu XO, Gao YT, Zheng Y, Cai H, et al. (2011) Association of hormone-related characteristics and breast cancer risk by estrogen receptor/progesterone receptor status in the shanghai breast cancer study. Am J Epidemiol 174: 661–671.
24. Nichols HB, Trentham-Dietz A, Love RR, Hampton JM, Hoang Anh PT, et al. (2005) Differences in breast cancer risk factors by tumor marker subtypes among premenopausal Vietnamese and Chinese women. Cancer Epidemiol Biomarkers Prev 14: 41–47.
25. Hiatt RA, Bawol RD (1984) Alcoholic beverage consumption and breast cancer incidence. Am J Epidemiol 120: 676–683.
26. Hiatt RA, Klatsky AL, Armstrong MA (1988) Alcohol consumption and the risk of breast cancer in a prepaid health plan. Cancer Res 48: 2284–2287.
27. Brinton LA, Benichou J, Gammon MD, Brogan DR, Coates R, et al. (1997) Ethnicity and variation in breast cancer incidence. Int J Cancer 73: 349–355.
28. Zhu K, Davidson NE, Hunter S, Yang X, Payne-Wilks K, et al. (2003) Methyl-group dietary intake and risk of breast cancer among African-American women: a case-control study by methylation status of the estrogen receptor alpha genes. Cancer Causes Control 14: 827–836.
29. Martinez P, Roislien J, Naidoo N, Clausen T (2011) Alcohol abstinence and drinking among African women: data from the World Health Surveys. BMC Public Health 11: 160.
30. Ibanga A, Adetula AV, Dagona Z, Karick H, Ojiji O (2005) The contexts of alcohol consumption by men and women in Nigeria. In: Obot I, Room R, editors. Alcohol, Gender and Drinking Problems: perspectives from low and middle income countries. 1st ed. Geneva: World Health Organization. pp. 143–166.

31. Tumwesigye NM, Kasirye R (2005) Gender and the major consequences of alcohol consumption in Uganda. In: Obot I, Room R, editors. Alcohol, Gender and Drinking Problems: perspectives from low and middle income countries. 1st ed. Geneva: World Health Organization. pp. 189–208.
32. Mamman LS, Brieger WR, Oshiname FO (2002) Alcohol consumption pattern among women in a rural Yoruba community in Nigeria. Subst Use Misuse 37: 579–597.
33. Smith-Warner SA, Spiegelman D, Yaun SS, van den Brandt PA, Folsom AR, et al. (1998) Alcohol and breast cancer in women: a pooled analysis of cohort studies. JAMA 279: 535–540.
34. Huo D, Kim H-J, Adebamowo CA, Ogundiran TO, Akang EE, et al. (2007) Genetic polymorphisms in uridine diphospho-glucuronosyltransferase 1A1 and breast cancer risk in Africans. Breast Cancer Research and Treatment 110: 367–376.
35. Huo D, Adebamowo CA, Ogundiran TO, Akang EE, Campbell O, et al. (2008) Parity and breastfeeding are protective against breast cancer in Nigerian women. British Journal of Cancer 98: 992–996.
36. Hou N, Ogundiran T, Ojengbede O, Morhason-Bello I, Zheng Y, et al. (2013) Risk factors for pregnancy-associated breast cancer: a report from the Nigerian Breast Cancer Study. Ann Epidemiol 23: 551–557.
37. van Buuren S, Boshuizen HC, Knook DL (1999) Multiple imputation of missing blood pressure covariates in survival analysis. Stat Med 18: 681–694.
38. Horton NJ, Kleinman KP (2007) Much ado about nothing: A comparison of missing data methods and software to fit incomplete data regression models. Am Stat 61: 79–90.
39. Rubin DB (1987) Multiple Imputation for Nonresponse in Surveys. New York: John Wiley & Sons, Inc.
40. Seitz HK, Pelucchi C, Bagnardi V, La Vecchia C (2012) Epidemiology and pathophysiology of alcohol and breast cancer: Update 2012. Alcohol Alcohol 47: 204–212.
41. Kushi LH, Doyle C, McCullough M, Rock CL, Demark-Wahnefried W, et al. (2012) American Cancer Society Guidelines on nutrition and physical activity for cancer prevention: reducing the risk of cancer with healthy food choices and physical activity. CA Cancer J Clin 62: 30–67.
42. Chandran U, Hirshfield KM, Bandera EV (2012) The role of anthropometric and nutritional factors on breast cancer risk in African-American women. Public Health Nutr 15: 738–748.
43. Park SY, Kolonel LN, Lim U, White KK, Henderson BE, et al. (2013) Alcohol consumption and breast cancer risk among women from five ethnic groups with light to moderate intakes: The Multiethnic Cohort Study. Int J Cancer.
44. Dumitrescu RG, Shields PG (2005) The etiology of alcohol-induced breast cancer. Alcohol 35: 213–225.
45. McCarver DG, Byun R, Hines RN, Hichme M, Wegenek W (1998) A genetic polymorphism in the regulatory sequences of human CYP2E1: association with increased chlorzoxazone hydroxylation in the presence of obesity and ethanol intake. Toxicol Appl Pharmacol 152: 276–281.
46. Francis JM, Grosskurth H, Changalucha J, Kapiga SH, Weiss HA (2014) Systematic review and meta-analysis: prevalence of alcohol use among young people in eastern Africa. Trop Med Int Health.
47. Peer N, Lombard C, Steyn K, Levitt N (2014) Rising alcohol consumption and a high prevalence of problem drinking in black men and women in Cape Town: the CRIBSA study. J Epidemiol Community Health.
48. Akarolo-Anthony SN, Ogundiran TO, Adebamowo CA (2010) Emerging breast cancer epidemic: evidence from Africa. Breast Cancer Res 12 Suppl 4: S8.
49. Wu AH, Vigen C, Razavi P, Tseng CC, Stancyzk FZ (2012) Alcohol and breast cancer risk among Asian-American women in Los Angeles County. Breast Cancer Res 14: R151.
50. Willett WC, Stampfer MJ, Colditz GA, Rosner BA, Hennekens CH, et al. (1987) Moderate alcohol consumption and the risk of breast cancer. N Engl J Med 316: 1174–1180.
51. Chen WY, Rosner B, Hankinson SE, Colditz GA, Willett WC (2011) Moderate alcohol consumption during adult life, drinking patterns, and breast cancer risk. JAMA 306: 1884–1890.
52. Longnecker MP, Newcomb PA, Mittendorf R, Greenberg ER, Clapp RW, et al. (1995) Risk of breast cancer in relation to lifetime alcohol consumption. J Natl Cancer Inst 87: 923–929.
53. Garland M, Hunter DJ, Colditz GA, Spiegelman DL, Manson JE, et al. (1999) Alcohol consumption in relation to breast cancer risk in a cohort of United States women 25–42 years of age. Cancer Epidemiol Biomarkers Prev 8: 1017–1021.
54. Colditz GA, Frazier AL (1995) Models of breast cancer show that risk is set by events of early life: prevention efforts must shift focus. Cancer Epidemiol Biomarkers Prev 4: 567–571.
55. Liu Y, Colditz GA, Rosner B, Berkey CS, Collins LC, et al. (2013) Alcohol intake between menarche and first pregnancy: a prospective study of breast cancer risk. J Natl Cancer Inst 105: 1571–1578.
56. Liu Y, Tamimi RM, Berkey CS, Willett WC, Collins LC, et al. (2012) Intakes of alcohol and folate during adolescence and risk of proliferative benign breast disease. Pediatrics 129: e1192–1198.
57. Harvey EB, Schairer C, Brinton LA, Hoover RN, Fraumeni JF Jr. (1987) Alcohol consumption and breast cancer. J Natl Cancer Inst 78: 657–661.
58. Schatzkin A, Jones DY, Hoover RN, Taylor PR, Brinton LA, et al. (1987) Alcohol consumption and breast cancer in the epidemiologic follow-up study of the first National Health and Nutrition Examination Survey. N Engl J Med 316: 1169–1173.
59. Young TB (1989) A case-control study of breast cancer and alcohol consumption habits. Cancer 64: 552–558.
60. Key TJ, Appleby PN, Reeves GK, Roddam A, Dorgan JF, et al. (2003) Body mass index, serum sex hormones, and breast cancer risk in postmenopausal women. J Natl Cancer Inst 95: 1218–1226.
61. Rinaldi S, Key TJ, Peeters PH, Lahmann PH, Lukanova A, et al. (2006) Anthropometric measures, endogenous sex steroids and breast cancer risk in postmenopausal women: a study within the EPIC cohort. Int J Cancer 118: 2832–2839.
62. Hong J, Holcomb VB, Dang F, Porampornpilas K, Nunez NP (2010) Alcohol consumption, obesity, estrogen treatment and breast cancer. Anticancer Res 30: 1–8.
63. Hvidtfeldt UA, Gunter MJ, Lange T, Chlebowski RT, Lane D, et al. (2012) Quantifying mediating effects of endogenous estrogen and insulin in the relation between obesity, alcohol consumption, and breast cancer. Cancer Epidemiol Biomarkers Prev 21: 1203–1212.
64. WHO (2005) World Health Organization Global Status Report on Alcohol 2004. Country Profiles, Africa - Uganda. WHO.
65. WHO (2005) World Health Organization Global Status Report on Alcohol 2004. Country Profiles, Africa - Nigeria. WHO.
66. WHO (2005) World Health Organization Global Status Report on Alcohol 2004. Country Profiles, Africa - Cameroon. WHO.
67. Giovannucci E, Stampfer MJ, Colditz GA, Manson JE, Rosner BA, et al. (1993) Recall and selection bias in reporting past alcohol consumption among breast cancer cases. Cancer Causes Control 4: 441–448.
68. Stockwell T, Donath S, Cooper-Stanbury M, Chikritzhs T, Catalano P, et al. (2004) Under-reporting of alcohol consumption in household surveys: a comparison of quantity-frequency, graduated-frequency and recent recall. Addiction 99: 1024–1033.
69. Ernhart CB, Morrow-Tlucak M, Sokol RJ, Martier S (1988) Underreporting of alcohol use in pregnancy. Alcohol Clin Exp Res 12: 506–511.
70. Ikuesan BA (1994) Drinking problems and the position of women in Nigeria. Addiction 89: 941–944; discussion 951–960.
71. Seitz HK, Maurer B (2007) The relationship between alcohol metabolism, estrogen levels, and breast cancer risk. Alcohol Res Health 30: 42–43.
72. Dumbili E (2013) Changing patterns of alcohol consumption in Nigeria: an exploration of responsible factors and consequences. Medical Sociology Online 7: 20–33.
73. Chikere EI, Mayowa MO (2011) Prevalence and perceived health effect of alcohol use among male undergraduate students in Owerri, South-East Nigeria: a descriptive cross-sectional study. BMC Public Health 11: 118.
74. Ramsoomar L, Morojele NK (2012) Trends in alcohol prevalence, age of initiation and association with alcohol-related harm among South African youth: implications for policy. S Afr Med J 102: 609–612.
75. WHO (2011) Global status report on alcohol and health. Geneva: WHO. 1–286 p.
76. Adebamowo CA, Akarolo-Anthony S (2009) Cancer in Africa: opportunities for collaborative research and training. Afr J Med Med Sci 38 Suppl 2: 5–13.
77. Lawhon M, Herrick C (2013) Alcohol control in the news: the politics of media representations of alcohol policy in South Africa. J Health Polit Policy Law 38: 987–1021.
78. Parry C, Burnhams NH, London L (2012) A total ban on alcohol advertising: presenting the public health case. S Afr Med J 102: 602–604.

13

Drinking Patterns and Alcohol Use Disorders in São Paulo, Brazil: The Role of Neighborhood Social Deprivation and Socioeconomic Status

Camila Magalhães Silveira[1,2*,☯¶], Erica Rosanna Siu[1☯¶], James C. Anthony[3], Luis Paulo Saito[1], Arthur Guerra de Andrade[2], Andressa Kutschenko[1], Maria Carmen Viana[1], Yuan-Pang Wang[1], Silvia S. Martins[4], Laura Helena Andrade[1]

1 Section of Psychiatric Epidemiology - LIM 23, Institute of Psychiatry, School of Medicine, University of São Paulo, São Paulo, São Paulo, Brazil, **2** Program of the Interdisciplinary Group of Studies on Alcohol and Drugs (GREA), Department and Institute of Psychiatry, School of Medicine, University of São Paulo, São Paulo, São Paulo, Brazil, **3** Department of Epidemiology and Statistics, Michigan State University, East Lansing, Michigan, United States of America, **4** Department of Epidemiology, Mailman School Of Public Health, Columbia University, New York, New York, United States of America

Abstract

Background: Research conducted in high-income countries has investigated influences of socioeconomic inequalities on drinking outcomes such as alcohol use disorders (AUD), however, associations between area-level neighborhood social deprivation (NSD) and individual socioeconomic status with these outcomes have not been explored in Brazil. Thus, we investigated the role of these factors on drink-related outcomes in a Brazilian population, attending to male-female variations.

Methods: A multi-stage area probability sample of adult household residents in the São Paulo Metropolitan Area was assessed using the WHO Composite International Diagnostic Interview (WMH-CIDI) (n = 5,037). Estimation focused on prevalence and correlates of past-year alcohol disturbances [heavy drinking of lower frequency (HDLF), heavy drinking of higher frequency (HDHF), abuse, dependence, and DMS-5 AUD] among regular users (RU); odds ratio (OR) were obtained.

Results: Higher NSD, measured as an area-level variable with individual level variables held constant, showed an excess odds for most alcohol disturbances analyzed. Prevalence estimates for HDLF and HDHF among RU were 9% and 20%, respectively, with excess odds in higher NSD areas; schooling (inverse association) and low income were associated with male HDLF. The only individual-level association with female HDLF involved employment status. Prevalence estimates for abuse, dependence, and DSM-5 AUD among RU were 8%, 4%, and 8%, respectively, with excess odds of: dependence in higher NSD areas for males; abuse and AUD for females. Among RU, AUD was associated with unemployment, and low education with dependence and AUD.

Conclusions: Regular alcohol users with alcohol-related disturbances are more likely to be found where area-level neighborhood characteristics reflect social disadvantage. Although we cannot draw inferences about causal influence, the associations are strong enough to warrant future longitudinal alcohol studies to explore causal mechanisms related to the heterogeneous patterns of association and male-female variations observed herein. Hopefully, these findings may help guide future directions for public health.

Editor: Svetlana Popova, Centre for Addiction and Mental Health, Canada

Funding: The São Paulo Megacity Mental Health Survey was funded by the State of São Paulo Research Foundation, Brazil (FAPESP Grants 03/00204-3 and 2011/50517-4, URL: http://www.fapesp.br/materia/176/projeto-tematico/projeto-tematico.htm), National Council for Scientific and Technological Development (CNPq - grant 313675/2009-0). Instrument development was supported by the Foundation for Science and Technology of Vitoria, Espírito Santo, Brazil (Fundo de Apoio à Ciência e Tecnologia do Município de Vitória - FACITEC 002/2003). Dr. Martins received research support from National Institute on Drug Abuse (NIDA) grants DA020667 and DA023434 and from National Institute of Child and Human Development (NICHD) grant HD060072, USA while working on this manuscript. Dr. Anthony also had NIDA grants to support his work: R01DA016558, and K05DA015799. The São Paulo Megacity Mental Health Survey is carried out in conjunction with the World Health Organization World Mental Health (WMH) Survey Initiative. The authors thank the WMH staff for assistance with instrumentation, fieldwork, and data analysis. The main coordination center activities, at Harvard University, were supported by the United States National Institutes of Mental Health (R01MH070884), the John D. and Catherine T. MacArthur Foundation, the Pfizer Foundation, the US Public Health Service (R13-MH066849, R01-MH069864, and R01 DA016558), the Fogarty International Center (FIRCA R03-TW006481), the Pan American Health Organization, the Eli Lilly and Company Foundation, Ortho-McNeil Pharmaceutical, Inc., GlaxoSmithKline, Bristol-Myers Squibb, and Shire. The authors declare that the funders of the SPMHS had no role in study design, data collection and analysis, decision to publish, or preparation of the manuscript. The authors also declare that the commercial funders of the Harvard coordination center had no role in study design, data collection and analysis, decision to publish, or preparation of the manuscript. The authors thank the SPMHS staff members, Beatriz Margarita Adler, Marlene Galativicis Teixeira, Indaiá de Santana Bassani, and Fidel Beraldi. Thanks also are due to the WMH staff for assistance with instrumentation, fieldwork, and data analysis. A complete list of WMH publications can be found at http://www.hcp.med.harvard.edu/wmh/.

Competing Interests: The authors have read the journal's policy and have the following conflicts: The main coordination center activities, at Harvard University, were supported by the United States National Institutes of Mental Health (R01MH070884), the John D. and Catherine T. MacArthur Foundation, the Pfizer Foundation, the US Public Health Service (R13-MH066849, R01-MH069864, and R01 DA016558), the Fogarty International Center (FIRCA R03-TW006481), the Pan American Health Organization, the Eli Lilly and Company Foundation, Ortho-McNeil Pharmaceutical, Inc., GlaxoSmithKline, Bristol-Myers Squibb, and Shire.

* Email: camilams@usp.br

These authors contributed equally to this work.

¶ These authors are shared first authors on this work.

Introduction

Alcohol consumption is a leading risk factor for global disability-adjusted life years (DALYs). In 2010, alcohol use was the 5th ranked DALYs determinant at the global level and was in the 1st rank for parts of Latin America, Eastern Europe, and southern sub-Saharan Africa [1]. Moreover, alcohol ranks as a major determinant of non-communicable diseases, especially in middle-income countries [2,3]. In Brazil, the largest middle-income country in Latin America and the site of the São Paulo Megacity Mental Health Survey, alcohol consumption represents a significant burden. In 2004, countries were ranked by size of alcohol-attributable DALYs affecting men: Russia was top-ranked at #1 on the list; Brazil was #2. Among women, the alcohol-attributable DALYs placed Brazil at #3 behind Russia and the USA [4].

The worrisome impact of alcohol use on health outcomes in Brazil might derive from separately identifiable drinking patterns and alcohol-related disturbances such as alcohol use disorders (AUD). These, in turn, are subject to both individual-level and society-level influences, including macro area-level contextual influences [5–7]. For instance, the top 10% of drinkers by volume in Brazil drink about half of all alcohol consumed in the country [8]. An estimated 12% of the adult general population in Brazil meet criteria for lifetime history of AUD [9–11]. Brazil's rather permissive drinking culture is reflected in data showing that most alcohol users initiate alcohol consumption when they are 17 years old [9] or even earlier [10,12,13] and also drink in risky patterns [10,12,14–16]. Furthermore, Brazil ranks well above many other countries on the 5-point harmful drinking score created for the Comparative Risk Assessment module of the Global Burden of Diseases project in an effort to estimate how changes in population health might depend upon harmful drinking. Brazil's summary score value of three out of five is based on its relatively high position on indicators such as frequency of drinking, frequency of heavy drinking occasions, usual quantity of alcohol consumed per occasion, drinking in public settings and during festive events, proportion of drinking events when drinkers get drunk, proportion of drinkers who drink daily or nearly daily, and only drinking with meals [17–19].

As for male-female variations, as is true in many countries, Brazilian women are more likely to abstain from alcohol. Other research has shown that males in the total population (including abstainers) are more than twice as likely as women to be heavy drinkers or to meet criteria for AUD [15,16,20–23]. Distinctive and innovative features of this study include diversity of neighborhoods within the megacity and the study team's attempt to shed light on male-female variations in the associations between alcohol outcomes with individual-level facets of socioeconomic status (SES), such as income, employment and educational attainment [22,24–27], within the context of a conceptual model that holds constant macro area-level neighborhood social deprivation (NSD) using source of data that are external and not reliant on the responses of the survey participants [28]. For the first time in Brazil, and for males and for females separately, we have estimated associations linking alcohol outcomes with independently derived area-level NSD scores, within a conceptual model that holds constant potentially influential individual-level variables.

We are not the first to study SES in relation to drinking outcomes, and our study has the character of an initial exploratory step in Brazil, with a primary focus on whether there might be statistically robust associations linking higher NSD with greater occurrence of heavy drinking and other alcohol-related disturbances (such as AUD) among drinkers who have consumed at least 12 drinks in the past year. In prior studies, from other countries, there is evidence that social position is associated with alcohol use and related problems [29–33], but alcohol consumption does not seem to follow the conventional pattern of lower socioeconomic groups having worse health than those at higher SES [31,34]. Previous research in North America found that household income, education, and employment status were positively associated with current and frequent drinking, but were negatively associated with heavy drinking and AUD (e.g. [34,35]). Hemmingsson's research group [36] found comparatively more diversity among suspected causal influences for alcohol dependence among lower SES and unemployed individuals. Conversely, research from low-middle income countries and from countries in transition such as Russia found higher SES to be positively associated with AUD and problem drinking [37].

Attempts to integrate lines of sex differences research with lines of SES research add some complexity. In higher income countries, well-educated professional women sometimes have been found with equal or greater occurrence of heavy drinking and alcohol problems as compared to men [38,39]. Adding more complexity, research conducted in high-income countries recently discloses evidence of potential neighborhood-level deprivation effects on drinking patterns and AUD, which might vary across the sexes [40,41]. Nonetheless, in general, living in less deprived neighborhoods has been associated with being an alcohol drinker [42,43] and regularly using alcohol [44], while living in more deprived areas has been associated with abstinence from alcohol [45], heavy drinking [45,46], and alcohol-related problems [45,47].

We designed this project with a focus on investigating male-female variations in associations linking various alcohol outcomes with neighborhood social deprivation measured as a macro characteristic of areas of residence, with an emphasis on active alcohol-related disturbances (heavy drinking through AUD) among adults with at least 12 drinks in the past year. We also offer estimates for prevalence of alcohol outcomes in Brazil, in an exploration of those more basic epidemiological topics. To clarify which NSD-alcohol associations might be strong enough to warrant future prospective or longitudinal research to build upon this initial foundation of cross-sectional data, our modeling of these outcomes allows for statistical control of individual-level covariates (e.g., SES) when estimating the NSD associations. We understand that the cross-sectional character of the data from Brazil means that we can draw no firm causal inferences, but what is most interesting to us is whether there is a consistently observed and sufficiently large association linking area-level NSD with alcohol-related disturbances among recently active drinkers, even with individual-level covariates held constant. If there is no robust NSD association with these alcohol outcomes, then research planning should be directed toward other facets of neighborhood context beyond the boundaries set for the area-level NSD construct as studied in this project.

Table 1. Estimated subgroup-specific prevalence proportions for recently active alcohol use, drinking patterns and related disturbances.

Characteristics	N	Past-year use (n = 2180)			Regular use[1] (n = 1513)			Among Regular Drinkers									Abuse[2] (n = 125)			Dependence[2] (n = 59)			DSM-5 AUD[2] (n = 132)		
								Non-heavy drinking[2] (n = 1105)			Heavy drinking of lower frequency[2] (n = 111)			Heavy drinking of higher frequency[2] (n = 297)											
		n	% (SE)	P (χ2)	n	% (SE)	P (χ2)	n	% (SE)	P (χ2)	n	% (SE)	P (χ2)	n	% (SE)	P (χ2)	n	% (SE)	P (χ2)	n	% (SE)	P (χ2)	n	% (SE)	P (χ2)
Age. years				<0.0001			0.5676			<0.0001			<0.0001			<0.0001			<0.0001			0.7892			0.0939
18–34	1841	879	49.8 (1.2)		579	69.7 (2.1)		378	61.9 (2.4)		77	14.2 (1.3)		142	24.0 (2.0)		59	9.5 (1.5)		22	4.0 (1.1)		54	8.8 (1.6)	
35–54	2160	966	46.6 (1.9)		676	72.4 (2.1)		511	75.5 (2.2)		29	4.3 (1.2)		136	20.3 (2.4)		60	8.2 (1.4)		33	4.0 (0.8)		70	8.9 (1.3)	
55+	1036	335	32.6 (2.2)		240	72.9 (3.8)		216	92.0 (2.4)		5	1.3 (0.6)		19	6.7 (2.0)		6	1.2 (0.6)		4	2.4 (1.8)		8	3.2 (1.9)	
Sex				<0.0001			<0.0001			0.0884			0.9111			0.0185			0.0927			0.0948			0.0708
Men	2187	1330	61.8 (1.2)		1040	78.6 (1.5)		744	69.1 (1.9)		77	8.7 (1.0)		219	22.2 (1.5)		102	6.3 (1.2)		45	4.4 (.7)		108	9.1 (1.0)	
Women	2850	850	31.3 (1.1)		473	58.1 (2.2)		361	75.6 (2.5)		34	8.4 (2.0)		78	15.9 (2.1)		23	1.7 (1.4)		14	2.5 (.6)		24	5.9 (1.4)	
Marital status				0.0343			0.7217			0.0271			0.0172			0.3287			0.3282			0.8687			0.2073
Married/ cohabiting	3250	1397	45.0 (1.1)		981	72.0 (1.4)		736	74.8 (2.0)		61	6.2 (1.0)		184	19.0 (1.6)		74	7.1 (1.2)		37	3.5 (.7)		78	7.1 (1.1)	
Previously married	894	353	42.0 (1.8)		238	70.2 (4.6)		179	73.4 (2.7)		13	7.3 (2.9)		46	19.4 (2.5)		18	7.0 (1.7)		11	4.2 (1.4)		20	7.1 (1.6)	
Never married	893	430	49.3 (1.4)		294	69.9 (2.5)		190	61.7 (3.4)		37	14.6 (2.3)		67	23.7 (2.8)		33	10.2 (2.0)		11	4.2 (1.6)		34	10.8 (1.9)	
Education				<0.0001			0.9946			0.5539			<.0001			0.7751			0.6995			0.1088			0.0634
Low	1344	453	34.9 (1.8)		314	71.0 (2.8)		239	74.4 (3.8)		11	3.4 (1.2)		64	22.2 (4.4)		32	8.6 (1.6)		25	7.8 (1.8)		42	11.4 (2.4)	
Low-average	1262	546	45.8 (1.4)		387	71.0 (1.8)		289	72.4 (3.5)		23	6.0 (1.5)		75	21.6 (3.4)		34	8.9 (2.2)		14	3.4 (1.4)		39	9.8 (2.2)	
High-average+High	2431	1181	49.9 (0.9)		812	71.3 (2.0)		577	69.5 (1.4)		77	11.2 (1.1)		158	19.3 (1.5)		59	7.4 (1.3)		20	2.8 (0.8)		51	6.5 (1.1)	
Income				0.0002			0.0018			0.1709			0.3603			0.5537			0.0949			0.1066			0.1612
Low	1200	443	39.4 (2.2)		302	69.6 (2.4)		204	65.5 (2.9)		28	11.0 (1.9)		70	23.5 (3.1)		35	11.8 (2.3)		16	4.1 (1.2)		38	11.4 (2.1)	
Low-average	1367	557	42.5 (1.8)		399	72.7 (2.4)		283	70.6 (2.7)		31	8.5 (1.7)		85	20.9 (2.4)		41	9.6 (1.7)		23	6.4 (1.4)		42	9.9 (1.9)	
High-average	1212	525	47.6 (1.7)		345	65.3 (2.0)		266	71.3 (3.9)		23	9.2 (2.0)		56	19.5 (3.5)		21	5.1 (1.5)		12	3.0 (1.2)		23	5.2 (1.4)	

Table 1. Cont.

Characteristics	N	Past-year use (n = 2180)			Regular use[1] (n = 1513)			Among Regular Drinkers: Non-heavy drinking[2] (n = 1105)			Among Regular Drinkers: Heavy drinking of lower frequency[2] (n = 111)			Among Regular Drinkers: Heavy drinking of higher frequency[2] (n = 297)			Abuse[2] (n = 125)			Dependence[2] (n = 59)			DSM-5 AUD[2] (n = 132)		
		n	% (SE)	P (χ2)	n	% (SE)	P (χ2)	n	% (SE)	P (χ2)	n	% (SE)	P (χ2)	n	% (SE)	P (χ2)	n	% (SE)	P (χ2)	n	% (SE)	P (χ2)	n	% (SE)	P (χ2)
High	1258	655	52.5 (1.4)		467	75.9 (2.3)		352	74.6 (2.1)		29	6.8 (1.4)		86	18.6 (1.8)		28	6.3 (1.2)		8	2.1 (0.9)		29	6.8 (1.8)	
Employment status				<0.0001			<0.0001			0.0031			0.0001			0.0553			0.002			0.072			0.0060
Working (including student)	3086	1539	51.0 (1.1)		1095	72.7 (1.4)		791	70.7 (1.6)		87	9.1 (1.0)		217	20.2 (1.5)		80	6.7 (0.8)		33	2.7 (0.5)		84	6.8 (0.9)	
Retired and homemaker	1330	364	28.4 (1.2)		214	57.0 (3.4)		180	84.8 (3.8)		8	2.4 (0.9)		26	12.8 (3.7)		8	3.3 (1.6)		6	2.0 (0.7)		8	3.2 (1.4)	
Unemployed	621	277	47.2 (2.6)		204	76.8 (2.8)		134	63.1 (4.1)		16	10.6 (2.9)		54	26.3 (3.0)		37	17.6 (3.7)		20	10.4 (2.9)		40	18.0 (3.6)	
Neighborhood Social Deprivation level				0.0079			0.6253			<0.0001			0.0571			<0.0001			0.0443			0.016			0.0450
No+Low	1369	675	49.6 (1.3)		478	70.5 (3.1)		389	80.9 (1.5)		28	5.7 (1.2)		61	13.4 (1.7)		30	5.7 (1.3)		11	1.9 (0.6)		31	5.8 (1.2)	
Medium-low+ Medium	1878	775	45.0 (1.3)		547	72.7 (1.2)		379	64.4 (2.5)		42	10.1 (1.8)		126	25.5 (2.5)		42	6.6 (1.6)		27	4.8 (0.9)		49	8.2 (1.5)	
High+Very-high	1729	709	42.5 (1.7)		477	70.5 (2.8)		328	67.4 (2.5)		41	10.4 (1.5)		108	22.2 (1.8)		53	12.5 (2.3)		21	4.9 (1.1)		52	10.9 (1.7)	
Total	5037	2180	45.6 (0.72)		1513	71.2 (1.5)		1105	71.0 (1.2)		111	8.6 (0.9)		297	20.3 (1.3)		125	7.9 (1.0)		59	3.8 (0.5)		132	8.1 (0.9)	

Data from the São Paulo Megacity Mental Health Survey (SPMHS), Brazil, 2005–2007 (n = 5037).
[1]Among past-year users.
[2]Among regular users.

Table 2. Comparison of non-heavy drinkers, heavy drinkers of lower frequency and heavy drinkers of higher frequency in terms of quantity and frequency of alcohol consumption, by sex, in the São Paulo Megacity Mental Health Survey (SPMHS).

Quantity and frequency of alcohol consumption	Non-heavy drinkers (n = 1105)		Heavy drinkers of lower frequency, HDLF (n = 111)		Heavy drinkers of higher frequency, HDHF (n = 297)	
	Men	Women	Men	Women	Men	Women
Modal frequency of consumption	1–3 days per month	1–3 days per month	1–2 days per week	1–2 days per week	1–2 days per week	1–2 days per week
Modal doses on a typical drinking day	2	1	5	6	5	6
Median number of doses on a typical drinking day	2	2	6	6	7	6

Materials and Methods

Survey characteristics and study population

The "São Paulo Megacity Mental Health Survey" (SPMHS) is part of the World Mental Health Survey Initiative (WMHS), which was launched by WHO in 2000 and has been carried out in 28 countries with similar methodology. The present study assessed a probabilistic sample of household residents aged 18 years or older in the São Paulo Metropolitan Area (SPMA), which is composed by 38 municipalities and the city of São Paulo, Brazil. A detailed overview of the survey, including aims, design, sampling procedures and field implementation, has been reported elsewhere [48].

Eligible respondents were selected from a stratified multistage-clustered area probability sample of households. In all strata, the primary sampling units (PSUs) were 2,000 census count areas, according to updated geographical definitions of the Instituto Brasileiro de Geografia e Estatística (IBGE – Brazilian Institute of Geography and Statistics) [49]. The 38 municipalities composed 60% of the total sample, with municipalities being self-representative and contributing to the total sample size proportional to their population density. In complement, the city of São Paulo, formed by five regions with 96 PSUs, contributed to 40% of the total sample. Within each sampled household, one respondent per dwelling was sampled by a Kish selection table [50].

The total observed sample consisted of 5,037 individuals, with a summary participation level of 81%. Before fieldwork, lay-interviewers received a 7-day standardized training by the Principal Investigators (LHA and MCV). For all respondents, face-to-face interviews were conducted between May/2005 and April/2007, after signing a written informed consent.

Ethics Statements

The SPMHS procedures for recruitment, obtaining informed consent, and protecting human subjects during field procedures were approved by the Research and Ethics Committee of the University of São Paulo Medical School. Respondents were interviewed only after informed written consent was obtained, and total confidentiality was assured. Eligible respondents were those who were 18 or older, Portuguese-speaking, and without any disability or handicap that would otherwise impair their ability to participate in the interview.

Assessment procedures

The WMH version of the Composite International Diagnostic Interview 3.0 (WMH-CIDI 3.0) was translated and adapted to the Brazilian-Portuguese language [48]. The WMH-CIDI 3.0 is a fully structured diagnostic interview that generates psychiatric diagnoses according to both ICD-10 (International Statistical Classification of Diseases and Related Health Problems, 10th revision) and DSM-IV criteria [51,52].

The WMH-CIDI has clinical and non-clinical modules distributed across Part 1 and Part 2 sections, with 'core' psychiatric disturbances assessed in Part 1. Part 1 is administered to all WMH respondents. Based on Part 1 responses, those who meet criteria for lifetime history of core disturbances, plus a 25% random sample of all others, are asked to complete Part 2 modules, which include non-clinical modules and non-core diagnostic assessments.

The alcohol module of WMH-CIDI 3.0 is in Part 1 so that all participants answered questions regarding alcohol use, drinking patterns, and related disturbances. Those who consumed at least one drink in the previous year are termed 'past-year users'. Across a broad range from the most frequent alcohol consumers to those who consumed at least 12 drinks in the previous 12 months, we have a heterogeneous subgroup of past year drinkers, distinguished with the somewhat arbitrary term 'regular user' (RU) [9,53–55]. Within this RU subgroup, three mutually exclusive subgroups were formed to distinguish between (1) heavy drinkers of lower frequency (HDLF, sometimes termed 'heavy episodic drinkers') who have consumed five or more drinks in a row for men and four or more drinks in a row for women, but no more often than two times per month; (2) heavy drinkers of higher frequency for whom heavy drinking occurs at least three times per month (HDHF). Alcohol use disorders qualify as separate alcohol-related disturbances among regular users, and were identified via the WMH-CIDI and its diagnostic algorithm's application of both DSM-IV (abuse and dependence), independently assessed via the 'ungated' approach described in prior papers [9,56]) and DSM-5 criteria (for AUD: alcohol use disorders) diagnoses.

Many of this study's prevalence analyses are 'conditional' in that they restrict the denominator of each proportion to 'past-year drinkers', while other analyses are 'conditional' because the denominator is restricted to individuals who had consumed at least 12 drinks in the past year (RU); all others are assumed to be effectively not at risk for being an active heavy drinker or for qualifying as a case of a DSM-IV or DSM-5 alcohol disorder in the past year.

An alternative approach is used when the goal is to produce total population estimates for alcohol outcomes that are directly comparable to total population estimates for some other condition (e.g., cannabis outcomes), in which case the denominator for the proportion is the total population, and the resulting estimates can be used to derive an estimated count of cases in the population

Table 3. Total sample: Estimated odds ratios (OR) linking alcohol outcomes with Neighborhood Social Deprivation and other suspected determinants.

Characteristics	Past-year use[a]	Regular use[b]	Heavy drinking of lower frequency (HDLF)[c]	Heavy drinking of higher frequency (HDHF)[c]	Abuse[d]	Dependence[e]	DSM-5 AUD[f]
	AOR (95% CI)	AOR (95% CI)	AOR (95% CI)	AOR (95% CI)	AOR (95% CI)	AOR (95% CI)	AOR (95% CI)
Sex							
Men	3.5 (2.9–4.2)‡	2.5 (1.9–3.4)‡	1.3 (0.6–2.5)	1.6 (1.1–2.5)*	1.7 (0.8–3.6)	1.6 (0.7–3.6)	1.5 (0.8–2.8)
Women	1.0	1.0	1.0	1.0	1.0	1.0	1.0
Age, years							
18–34	2.0 (1.6–2.6)‡	0.7 (0.5–1.1)	7.3 (2.7–19.9)†	5.9 (2.1–17.0)†	7.0 (2.4–20.0)†	2.0 (0.5–9.0)	2.3 (0.7–7.0)
35–54	1.7 (1.2–2.3)†	0.8 (0.5–1.2)	2.5 (0.8–7.1)	4.1 (1.4–12.7)*	6.8 (2.6–17.7)‡	1.9 (0.4–8.7)	2.8 (0.9–9.1)
55+	1.0	1.0	1.0	1.0	1.0	1.0	1.0
Marital status							
Previously married	1.4 (1.1–1.8)†	1.1 (0.7–1.8)	1.1 (0.5–2.5)	1.1 (0.8–1.5)	1.0 (0.5–2.2)	1.2 (0.5–3.1)	1.0 (0.5–2.0)
Never married	0.9 (0.7–1.1)	0.9 (0.6–1.2)	1.3 (0.7–2.4)	1.2 (0.8–1.8)	1.3 (0.7–2.5)	1.2 (0.4–3.3)	1.9 (1.0–3.4)*
Married/cohabiting	1.0	1.0	1.0	1.0	1.0	1.0	1.0
Education							
Low	0.8 (0.6–1.0)	0.9 (0.7–1.3)	0.4 (0.2–0.8)†	1.4 (0.7–2.6)	1.3 (0.7–2.5)	3.0 (1.2–7.5)*	2.2 (1.0–5.0)*
Low-average	1.0 (0.8–1.2)	1.0 (0.7–1.3)	0.5 (0.2–1.0)	1.1 (0.6–1.9)	1.1 (0.5–2.4)	1.1 (0.3–3.3)	1.6 (0.8–3.3)
High-average+High	1.0	1.0	1.0	1.0	1.0	1.0	1.0
Income							
Low	0.6 (0.4–0.9)†	0.8 (0.5–1.0)	1.8 (0.8–3.9)	0.9 (0.5–1.5)	1.0 (0.5–2.0)	0.9 (0.2–4.0)	0.9 (0.4–2.3)
Low-average	0.6 (0.5–0.8)†	0.8 (0.6–1.0)	1.1 (0.6–1.9)	0.8 (0.5–1.2)	0.9 (0.5–1.7)	1.8 (0.6–5.5)	0.9 (0.3–2.2)
High-average	0.8 (0.6–1.0)*	0.5 (0.4–0.7)‡	1.2 (0.6–2.4)	0.8 (0.5–1.4)	0.6 (0.3–1.2)	1.0 (0.2–4.0)	0.5 (0.2–1.2)
High	1.0	1.0	1.0	1.0	1.0	1.0	1.0
Employment status							
Working (including student)	1.3 (1.1–1.5)‡	1.6 (1.2–2.1)†	1.8 (0.7–4.5)	0.8 (0.4–1.7)	0.9 (0.3–3.0)	0.9 (0.3–2.6)	1.3 (0.4–3.8)
Unemployed	1.3 (1.0–1.8)*	2.2 (1.4–3.5)†	1.7 (0.4–6.5)	1.8 (0.7–4.5)	2.5 (1.0–6.8)	3.5 (0.7–16.2)	3.5 (1.1–11.3)*
Retired and homemaker	1.0	1.0	1.0	1.0	1.0	1.0	1.0
Neighborhood Social Deprivation level							
No+Low	1.0	1.0	1.0	1.0	1.0	1.0	1.0
Medium-low+Medium	0.8 (0.7–0.9)†	1.1 (0.8–1.4)	2.0 (1.1–3.8)*	2.1 (1.4–3.1)†	0.9 (0.4–2.1)	1.7 (0.8–3.9)	1.1 (0.5–2.2)

Table 3. Cont.

Characteristics	Past-year use[a]	Regular use[b]	Heavy drinking of lower frequency (HDLF)[c]	Heavy drinking of higher frequency (HDHF)[c]	Abuse[d]	Dependence[e]	DSM-5 AUD[f]
	AOR (95% CI)	AOR (95% CI)	AOR (95% CI)	AOR (95% CI)	AOR (95% CI)	AOR (95% CI)	AOR (95% CI)
High+Very-high	0.7 (0.5–1.0)	1.0 (0.6–1.5)	2.1 (1.1–3.8)*	1.7 (1.2–2.3)†	1.6 (0.7–3.6)	1.5 (0.7–3.4)	1.3 (0.7–2.7)

Data from the São Paulo Megacity Mental Health Survey (SPMHS), Brazil, 2005–2007 (n = 5037).
Reference categories: a) non-past year users; b) non-regular users; c) non-heavy drinkers; d) regular users who did not fulfill criteria for abuse; e) regular users who did not fulfill criteria for dependence; f) regular users who did not fulfill criteria for DSM-5 AUD.
AOR, adjusted odds-ratio; CI, confidence interval.
All OR were adjusted for sex and age.
*$p<0.05$;
†$p<0.01$;
‡$p<0.001$.

who might need alcohol treatment services or cannabis treatment services. Here, we have restricted some denominators to 'past year drinkers' and to 'regular drinkers' so as to understand the relative occurrence and patterns of association of alcohol outcomes among the recently active users, as explained in footnotes to the tables. For example, for the 'conditional prevalence' of RU among past-year drinkers, the denominator excludes lifelong abstainers as well as those who drank in past years but have not had a drink in the past year. Further in 'conditional prevalence' analyses restricted to regular users, the interpretation of the estimates involves thinking about how many of the current regular users now qualify as cases of heavy drinking, or DSM-IV abuse, dependence or DSM-5 AUD.

Covariates

The key covariate focus is on the macro area-level NSD values related to alcohol outcomes, with individual-level SES held constant via terms for education, employment status, and income. Regression models also held constant age (18–34, 35–54, 55 years or more) and marital status (never married; previously married; married or cohabiting); for total sample (men and women combined), sex was held constant as well. For women with DSM-IV abuse, dependence or DSM-5 AUD age strata were divided into two subgroups of 18–34, 34–54 because no woman over the age of 55 years filled criteria for these diagnoses.

Education was coded by years of schooling: 0–4 (low); 5–8 (low-average); and 9+ (high-average and high). Employment status was coded as (1) workers paid outside the household and students, (2) unemployed, and (3) retired or working as a homemaker in one's own household.

For income, the standard international labor economics method was used [57], with per capita income calculated by dividing total household income by the number of household members. Income levels were defined according to the per capita income in comparison with the Brazilian median per capita income (7,050 dollars/year): low (less than half the Brazilian median), low-average (more than half of the Brazilian median up to the median), high-average (above the Brazilian median up to three times the median), and high (above three times the Brazilian median).

The area-level NSD variable was developed by the Center of Metropolitan Studies (http://www.centrodametropole.org.br) and assigned to each census unit, to reflect social conditions in the SPMA geographical space using data from the 2000 Census. This index, derived from external census sources, combines socioeconomic deprivation indicators (income, level of education, family size, and percentage of families headed by a woman with low educational level) and the population's age structure. The NSD index ranges from 1 (no social deprivation) to 8 (high social deprivation). These eight levels were summarized in 3 indicators: no-low (combined index of 1, 2, and 3 NSD level), medium-low/medium (6 and 4), and high/very high NSD (5, 7, and 8).

Data analysis

Since data were obtained from a complex stratified sample design, sample weights and design variables that account for sample clustering were applied. Prior to analysis, all respondents received a pre-stratification weight to adjust for within household and PSU probabilities of selection, and a post-stratification weight to adjust for the known age and sex structure of the SPMA population and non-response [48].

The analysis weight for the World Mental Health Surveys initiative, for this study's prevalence estimates, and for this study's regression analyses is based on (a) the inverse of the probability of selection into the sample, and (b) a post-stratification adjustment

Table 4. Males: Estimated odds ratios (OR) linking alcohol outcomes with Neighborhood Social Deprivation and other suspected determinants.

Characteristics	Past-year use[a] (n = 1330)	Regular use[b] (n = 1040)	Heavy drinking of lower frequency, HDLF[c] (n = 77)	Heavy drinking of higher frequency, HDHF[c] (n = 219)	Abuse[d] (n = 102)	Dependence[e] (n = 45)	DSM-5 AUD[f] (n = 108)
	AOR (95% CI)	AOR (95% CI)	AOR (95% CI)	AOR (95% CI)	AOR (95% CI)	AOR (95% CI)	AOR (95% CI)
Age, years							
18–34	1.3 (0.9–2.0)	0.7 (0.4–1.2)	40.0 (3.6–449.9)†	4.9 (1.6–15.2)†	12.9 (3.7–45.0)‡	2.0 (0.4–9.3)	2.4 (0.8–6.7)
35–54	1.2 (0.8–1.9)	07 (0.4–1.3)	9.9 (1.0–99.6)	2.7 (0.8–8.7)	8.2 (2.9–23.4)‡	1.5 (0.3–8.0)	2.0 (0.6–6.7)
55+	1.0	1.0	1.0	1.0	1.0	1.0	1.0
Marital status							
Previously married	1.3 (0.8–2.1)	1.1 (0.5–2.1)	0.3 (0.1–1.3)	1.0 (0.7–1.6)	1.4 (0.7–2.7)	1.3 (0.5–3.2)	1.3 (0.7–2.5)
Never married	0.8 (0.6–1.2)	0.7 (0.5–1.0)	1.4 (0.6–3.7)	1.2 (0.7–2.0)	0.8 (0.4–1.8)	1.1 (0.3–4.4)	1.3 (0.6–3.0)
Married/cohabiting	1.0	1.0	1.0	1.0	1.0	1.0	1.0
Education							
Low	1.0 (0.7–1.3)	1.1 (0.7–1.7)	0.2 (0.1–0.6)†	1.2 (0.7–2.3)	1.3 (0.6–2.6)	2.6 (0.9–7.3)	2.3 (0.9–6.0)
Low-average	0.9 (0.8–1.1)	1.4 (0.9–2.1)	0.6 (0.2–1.4)	1.1 (0.7–1.9)	1.1 (0.5–2.2)	0.9 (0.3–2.8)	1.6 (0.9–3.0)
High-average+High	1.0	1.0	1.0	1.0	1.0	1.0	1.0
Income							
Low	0.5 (0.3–0.7)†	0.5 (0.2–1.0)	2.1 (1.0–4.5)*	0.8 (0.4–1.6)	1.2 (0.6–2.4)	0.9 (0.1–5.6)	1.0 (0.4–2.9)
Low-average	0.6 (0.5–0.9)†	0.7 (0.5–1.1)	1.0 (0.5–2.2)	0.6 (0.4–1.0)	0.9 (0.5–1.6)	1.5 (0.4–5.0)	0.8 (0.3–2.2)
High-average	0.9 (0.7–1.3)	0.4 (0.3–0.7)*	1.5 (0.6–3.4)	0.9 (0.5–1.6)	0.5 (00.2–1.1)	0.6 (0.1–2.7)	0.5 (0.2–1.3)
High	1.0	1.0	1.0	1.0	1.0	1.0	1.0
Employment status							
Working (including student)	2.0 (1.4–2.8)‡	1.7 (0.9–3.3)	0.3 (0.03–2.4)	1.3 (0.4–4.3)	0.3 (0.1–1.2)	0.8 (0.1–5.7)	1.6 (0.3–8.6)
Unemployed	2.4 (1.6–3.6)‡	2.8 (1.2–6.2)*	0.2 (0.02–1.3)	1.5 (0.5–4.7)	1.0 (0.2–4.6)	3.1 (0.2–40.7)	4.3 (0.6–30.4)
Retired and homemaker	1.0	1.0	1.0	1.0	1.0	1.0	1.0
Neighborhood Social Deprivation level							
No+Low	1.0	1.0	1.0	1.0	1.0	1.0	1.0
Medium-low+Medium	1.0 (0.7–1.4)	1.0 (0.7–1.6)	1.6 (0.8–3.3)	2.1 (1.3–3.3)†	0.8 (0.3–2.3)	2.4 (1.2–4.9)*	1.1 (0.5–2.5)
High+Very-high	0.8 (0.6–1.2)	1.2 (0.6–2.1)	1.6 (0.5–5.0)	1.5 (0.9–2.5)	1.3 (0.6–3.1)	1.5 (0.5–4.0)	1.1 (0.6–2.2)

Data from the São Paulo Megacity Mental Health Survey (SPMHS), Brazil, 2005–2007 (n = 2187).

Reference categories: a) non-past year users; b) non-regular users; c) non-heavy drinkers; d) regular users who did not fulfill criteria for abuse; e) regular users who did not fulfill criteria for dependence; f) regular users who did not fulfill criteria for DSM-5 AUD.

AOR, adjusted odds-ratio; CI, confidence interval.

All OR were adjusted for age.

*$p<0.05$;

†$p<0.01$;

‡$p<0.001$.

Table 5. Females: Estimated odds ratios (OR) linking alcohol outcomes with Neighborhood Social Deprivation and other suspected determinants.

Characteristics	Past-year use[a] (n = 850)	Regular use[b] (n = 473)	Heavy drinking of lower frequency, HDLF[c] (n = 34)	Heavy drinking of higher frequency, HDHF[c] (n = 78)	Abuse[d] (n = 23)	Dependence[e] (n = 14)	DSM-5 AUD[f] (n = 24)
	AOR (95% CI)	AOR (95% CI)	AOR (95% CI)	AOR (95% CI)	AOR (95% CI)	AOR (95% CI)	AOR (95% CI)
Age, years							
18–34	3.0 (1.8–4.8)‡	0.8 (0.5–1.5)	2.3 (0.4–12.0)	15.6 (3.1–78.1)‡	0.3 (0.1–1.2)	07 (0.2–3.4)	0.3 (0.1–1.2)
35–54	2.1 (1.3–3.4)‡	0.9 (0.5–1.5)	1.7 (0.4–8.1)	21.7 (4.3–111.2)‡	1.0	1.0	1.0
55+	1.0	1.0	1.0	1.0			
Marital status							
Previously married	1.6 (1.2–2.2)†	1.2 (0.7–2.0)	1.8 (0.5–5.8)	1.0 (0.5–1.9)	0.7 (0.1–3.3)	1.0 (0.3–3.5)	0.9 (0.3–3.0)
Never married	1.0 (0.8–1.4)	1.1 (0.6–1.9)	1.1 (0.3–4.1)	1.3 (0.5–3.5)	5.0 (1.2–21.0)*	1.8 (0.5–7.0)	6.3 (1.6–25.2)†
Married/cohabiting	1.0	1.0	1.0	1.0	1.0	1.0	1.0
Education							
Low	0.7 (0.4–0.9)‡	0.8 (0.5–1.2)	1.1 (0.3–4.2)	2.2 (0.7–7.0)	1.3 (0.3–6.3)	6.4 (1.3–31.4)*	1.9 (0.4–8.5)
Low-average	1.1 (0.8–1.4)	0.7 (0.4–1.1)	0.4 (0.1–1.8)	0.9 (0.2–3.5)	1.7 (0.1–18.1)	2.2 (0.3–17.8)	2.2 (0.2–20.3)
High-average+High	1.0	1.0	1.0	1.0	1.0	1.0	1.0
Income							
Low	0.8 (0.5–1.2)	1.1 (0.6–1.9)	1.1 (0.3–5.1)	1.2 (0.3–4.2)	0.7 (0.1–3.4)	0.4 (0.1–2.4)	0.7 (0.1–3.2)
Low-average	0.6 (0.4–0.8)*	0.8 (0.5–1.2)	1.2 (0.3–4.9)	1.8 (0.6–4.9)	1.3 (0.3–5.1)	1.5 (0.2–13.4)	1.6 (0.4–6.6)
High-average	0.7 (0.4–1.0)	0.7 (0.4–1.0)	0.8 (0.2–3.0)	0.7 (0.2–2.8)	0.9 (0.2–3.4)	1.0	0.8 (0.2–3.4)
High	1.0	1.0	1.0	1.0	1.0	1.0	1.0
Employment status							
Working (including student)	1.1 (0.9–1.4)	1.5 (1.0–2.2)*	3.1 (1.3–7.5)*	0.8 (0.3–2.0)	1.6 (0.2–10.6)	1.8 (0.5–5.9)	1.2 (0.3–6.0)
Unemployed	1.1 (0.7–1.6)	1.9 (1.1–3.1)*	6.1 (1.5–23.8)*	1.7 (0.5–5.9)	4.8 (0.9–26.8)	6.9 (0.7–66.5)	4.4 (0.9–22.3)
Retired and homemaker	1.0	1.0	1.0	1.0	1.0	1.0	1.0
Neighborhood Social Deprivation level							
No+Low	1.0	1.0	1.0	1.0	1.0	1.0	1.0
Medium-low+Medium	0.6 (0.4–0.8)‡	1.1 (0.8–1.5)	4.9 (0.9–25.6)	2.3 (1.0–5.2)*	1.4 (0.3–5.7)	0.4 (0.1–3.2)	1.4 (0.4–5.4)
High+Very-high	0.6 (0.4–0.9)‡	0.8 (0.5–1.4)	5.8 (1.0–33.9)*	2.4 (1.1–5.3)*	3.7 (1.0–13.6)*	2.6 (0.6–10.3)	3.2 (0.9–11.6)

Data from the São Paulo Megacity Mental Health Survey (SPMHS), Brazil, 2005–2007 (n = 2850).

Reference categories: a) non-past year users; b) non-regular users; c) non-heavy drinkers; d) regular users who did not fulfill criteria for abuse; e) regular users who did not fulfill criteria for dependence; f) regular users who did not fulfill criteria for DSM-5 AUD.

AOR, adjusted odds-ratio; CI, confidence interval.

All OR were adjusted for age.

$*p<0.05$;

†$p<0.01$;

‡$p<0.001$.

factor such that, after weighting, the survey-based estimates for basic demographic distributions (e.g., age, sex) serve well as population projections for the São Paulo Megacity Mental Health Survey population (as best they are known from the most recent corresponding census distributions for the São Paulo Metropolitan Area that was surveyed). The application of these analysis weights in the survey analyses, via SAS procedures, are as described in Chapter 4 of a recently published textbook authored by WMHS collaborators [58].

Data analyses were conducted using the SAS software version 9.1 (SAS, 2004) and SUDAAN (Research Triangle Institute, 2004). Cross-tabulations were used to estimate overall prevalence of recently active (past-year) drinking, as well as 'conditional prevalences' for the other alcohol outcomes. Male-female variations in associations were estimated via stratified analyses.

Quantity and frequency of alcohol consumption in the last 12 months were determined for non-heavy drinkers, heavy drinkers of lower frequency and heavy drinkers of higher frequency by sex.

Bivariate analyses and multiple logistic regression were used to estimate area-level NSD associations with alcohol outcomes, and then to explore associations with covariates, with secondary focus on the SES indicators, holding area-level NSD constant and vice versa. For HDLF and HDHF, polychotomous logistic regression was performed with non-heavy drinking as the reference category.

Odds ratios (OR) were estimated for NSD and the other covariates, first in unadjusted form with Wald tests [59]. Thereafter, OR estimation was with covariate adjustment to obtain a final multivariate model. For total sample analysis, models were adjusted for both age and sex; while for male-female stratified analyses were adjusted for age. Significance testing, standard errors (SE) and 95% confidence intervals (95% CI) were estimated using Taylor series linearization methods for complex sample data [60], as implemented in SUDAAN (Research Triangle Institute, 2004). Multivariate significance tests were conducted with Wald χ^2 tests using Taylor series design-based coefficient variance-covariance matrices. All significance tests were based on two-sided tests at a 0.05 significance level.

Results

Study Sample

Socio-demographic characteristics of the study sample have been described elsewhere [48]. Briefly, there were more women (57%) than men in the sample, and it was a relatively young sample: 60% of the subjects aged less or equal to 45 years old; 71% of the men and 60% of the women were married. Approximately half of the subjects had low/low-average education and around 60% were employed (76% of men, 50% of women). Table S1 provides the full distribution of the NSD variable based on unweighted sample statistics, a distribution based on application of the analysis weights, (i) for the sample as a whole, and (ii) for males and for females, separately.

Prevalences of alcohol use and outcomes: unconditional and conditional

Table 1, bottom half, shows unconditional prevalence of recently active (past-year) drinking, as well as the estimated conditional prevalence for all recently active alcohol outcomes. Overall, an estimated 46% of the São Paulo adult population had consumed alcohol in the past year. Among past year drinkers, overall, 71% qualified as 'regular users', having consumed at least 12 drinks in the past year.

When we examined HDLF and HDHF outcomes among the past-year regular users (RU), about 9% qualified as recent 'heavy drinkers of lower frequency' and about 20% qualified as 'heavy drinkers of higher frequency' (versus the complement of 71% non-HDLF/HDHF). Also conditioned on past-year RU, about 4%–8% qualified for these recently active DSM conditions: DSM-IV abuse (7.9%); DSM-IV dependence (3.8%); DSM-5 AUD (8.1%). In basic cross-tabulations, males were more likely than females to be past-year users, RU, and HDHF drinkers (all $p<0.05$), but were not more likely to qualify for DSM conditions (among RU).

Regarding the main focus on area-level NSD, with two exceptions (RU and HDLF), all alcohol outcomes were associated with NSD ($p<0.05$). NSD inverse associations were seen for past-year use and for non-heavy drinking among RU. Positive NSD associations were seen with higher frequency heavy drinking (HDHF) and with all three DSM conditions.

Among men who reported drinking in the past 12 months (62%), nearly 80% drank regularly. For women, 30% reported alcohol use in the previous year and among those around 60% consumed alcohol in a regular basis. There were also more men than women with heavy and frequent drinking patterns among regular users. Unexpectedly, such sex differences were no longer observed for non-heavy drinkers and heavy drinkers, DSM-IV abuse, DSM-IV dependence, and DSM-5 AUD.

For RU, there was a higher prevalence of heavy drinking patterns in younger cohorts than in the oldest cohort (55 years old and more). For example, about 25% of those aged 18–34 years drank in the HDHF pattern, whereas around 7% of those aged 55 or more engaged in those drinking patterns.

In Table 2, we compared men and women in terms of quantity and frequency of alcohol consumption, by drinking patterns. We note that men and women had the same modal frequency of consumption per week within each drinking pattern category (1–3 days a month for non-heavy drinkers, and 1–2 days a week for HDLF and HDHF). However, women surpassed men in the modal number of doses on a typical drinking day when drinking in heavy drinking patterns. For both HDLF men and women, and HDHF women, the median number of doses on a typical drinking day was 6. When drinking in the heavy and frequent pattern, men had the modal number of doses of 7.

Correlates of recently active alcohol use, drinking patterns, and AUD for total sample, males and females

Neighborhood social deprivation level. The bottom part of Table 3 shows covariate-adjusted NSD associations with past-year drinking and both forms of heavy drinking ($p<0.05$). Individuals in mid NSD neighborhoods are less likely to be past-year drinkers ($p<0.05$). Among RU, those in the mid to higher level NSD neighborhoods are more considerably likely to drink heavily ($p<0.05$). When we hold constant age and neighborhood social deprivation, the inverse association with low income that stands out such that regular drinkers of low education are under-represented among heavier drinkers at the low frequency level, and, under the same constraints, these drinkers with low education are neither over- nor under-represented among heavier frequent drinkers ($p>0.05$) (Table 3).

Table 4, bottom part, indicates the association for men with respect to NSD. It is possible to see statistically robust, but not exceptionally strong, covariate-adjusted NSD associations with DSM-IV alcohol dependence and with heavy drinking at high frequency. The pattern of estimates is such that the excess odds of these outcomes are found when the RU lives in a mid-range NSD neighborhood ($p<0.05$).

Table 5, bottom part, shows no covariate-adjusted NSD-dependence association for women, but it is noteworthy that women living in areas with lower NSD level are more likely to be past-year drinkers ($p<0.05$). For 'regular drinking' outcome among women, no association was observed for NSD ($p>0.05$). Nevertheless, among RU, women in the higher level NSD neighborhoods are more substantially likely to qualify as cases of both forms of heavy drinking ($p<0.05$). In addition, when the RU lives in a mid NSD neighborhood, there also are excess odds of HFD ($p<0.05$). As for DSM-IV abuse, the covariate adjusted excess odds are seen for female RU living in the neighborhoods with higher levels of neighborhood social deprivation ($p<0.05$).

Income. Study of Tables 3, 4 and 5, column by column, discloses statistically independent inverse associations of past-year drinking with low to high-average income among total sample, with low-average income among both men and women, and with low income among men (but not women), where high income is the reference category ($p<0.05$).

The only other statistically robust associations with income are seen in Tables 3′s and 4′s column on regular use among total sample and male past-year users and heavy drinking among male regular users, and in Table 5′s column on female past-year drinking. Here, it is the high-average income male drinkers who are less likely than the high income drinkers to be recently active regular users ($p<0.05$) and low income male regular users being more likely to drink heavily in a low frequency ($p<0.05$). As compared to high income women, the covariate-adjusted odds ratio shows that low-average income women are less likely to be past-year drinkers ($p<0.05$).

Education. Educational attainment is another individual-level SES indicator that shows no general strength as a correlate of alcohol outcomes with few exceptions. In the covariate-adjusted model for past-year drinking among women, it is the least well educated women who are under-represented, as compared to their better educated peers ($p<0.05$). Among women RU, low education is associated with excess odds of being an active alcohol dependence case ($p<0.05$). This is also observed for the total sample, which shows 2–3-fold excess odds of alcohol dependence and DSM-5 AUD among regular users with low education attainment as compared to their peers with higher education levels.

Education is not associated with past-year drinking among men, but it is associated with HDLF status among male RU. In Table 4 the most educated male RU have excess odds of low frequency heavy drinking (HDLF) ($p<0.05$). This last finding is also valid for the total sample (Table 3).

Employment status. Our third individual-level SES indicator is employment status, which seems to have more to do with the lower levels of drinking status [past-year drinking (total sample and male), RU among past-year drinkers (total sample, male and female), and HDLF among RU (female)]. The first column of Table 4 shows a 2-fold excess odds of past-year drinking among unemployed (and among currently employed) males, as compared to the formerly employed ($p<0.05$). The 2nd and third columns of Table 5 also highlight excess odds of alcohol outcomes among unemployed, here in comparison with the formerly employed and unpaid homemakers in the household: (1) among female past-year users, RU is associated with being unemployed (and also with being employed); (2) among female RU, these same employment status values are associated with our alcohol outcome called 'heavy drinking of lower frequency' ($p<0.05$). The only statistically robust employment status association involves DSM-5 AUD among total RU, which can be seen in the last column of Table 3, where there is an estimated 4-fold excess odds of AUD among RU who are unemployed as compared to formerly employed ($p<0.05$).

Marital status. As for marital status, there are no noteworthy associations with alcohol outcomes among males (Table 4). Among women and total sample, in a comparison with those who are married or cohabiting, it is the previously married who are modestly more likely to be past-year drinkers ($p<0.05$; Table 5, first column). Among the female RU, the never married are more likely to be cases of the alcohol-related disturbances in the form of DSM-IV abuse and DSM-5 AUD.

Discussion

With all the strengths of a transversal epidemiological survey of a representative sample of the adult general population living in the São Paulo Metropolitan Area, Brazil, this is the first Brazilian study to explore alcohol outcomes such as DSM-5 AUD in relation to suspected influences measured at both individual and neighborhood area levels and the associations of these outcomes with social position and possible socioeconomic inequalities. Overall, the main finding of note may be that regular alcohol users showing alcohol-related disturbances are generally more often found where area-level neighborhood characteristics reflect social disadvantage, even when important individual-level covariates have been held constant. More specifically, living in less deprived neighborhoods was associated with being a past-year alcohol drinker, while living in more deprived areas was associated with heavy drinking and some alcohol-related disturbances. As noted below, we would rather not offer a causal interpretation of this main finding. Nonetheless, it may be pertinent that those living in disadvantaged neighborhoods, with social exclusion and deprivation, might be most exposed to stress, less coping resources, high density of alcohol outlets. As such, the disadvantages experienced by residents of these neighborhoods extend beyond the indicators captured in our NSD assessment, which may influence heavy drinking [46] and the occurrence of alcohol related problems [45,47,61–63].

Other findings deserve to be highlighted as well, starting with a secondary focal point – namely, the individual-level SES indicators. Unemployed individuals often showed excess odds of alcohol-related disturbance (DSM-5 AUD), as compared to formerly employed or homemakers. In sex-specific analyses, female regular drinkers in the workforce were more likely to qualify for one of the forms of heavy drinking. Education associations also were noted, although not always with a consistently interpretable pattern.

As for our tertiary focal points, marital status was generally unrelated to alcohol outcomes among men, but among women, it was the previously married women who were more likely to be past-year drinkers; it was the never married women who were more likely to qualify as active cases of DSM-IV alcohol abuse and for DSM-5 AUD. It should not be surprising that adults age 18–34 were found to be over-represented among past-year drinkers. Among these young adults with at least 12 drinks in the past year, both forms of heavy drinking showed excess odds, relative to older RU, as did DSM-IV alcohol abuse (but not alcohol dependence nor DSM-5 AUD).

The results on prevalence estimates also may be of interest. These estimates reveal that although half of the sample is abstinent, nearly 30% of the past-year regular users drink in a heavy drinking pattern. It is particularly worrisome that, among heavy drinkers, two-thirds reports drinking in this pattern frequently - three or more times in a month period. Another important finding is the male-female convergence in the prevalence of heavy drinking pattern, reinforced by the observation that women are surpassing men in terms of estimated modal doses of alcohol consumption and women have reached men in terms of modal frequency of consumption in both heavy drinking patterns.

The phenomenon of convergence in Brazil seems to be more due to an increase in female consumption than a reduction in male drinking [64]. For past-year use and regular use, the male/female ratio is similar to what has usually being found in the literature, with men surpassing a group of high educated women who work outside home [65–67]. When considering only those who were past-year regular users the sex-specific prevalence estimates for drinking patterns and AUD did not differ appreciably.

We note that heavy drinking was a common drinking pattern, similar to what has been found in other recent Brazilian surveys [10,16,68–70]. This pattern is specifically frequent in young adults aged between 18–34 years, which exposes them to a range of risk behaviors with adverse short- and long-term consequences, from social and physical problems - such as hangovers or medical illnesses, unprotected sexual activity, alcohol-related car crashes and other unintentional injuries - to increased risk for AUD [16,20,71,72].

The 12-month prevalence of any DSM-IV AUD (alcohol abuse or dependence) among regular drinkers was 9.1%, which is slightly lower than reports from nationwide Brazilian studies probably due to methodological and sample differences [10,11] and greater than a national survey conducted in Australia with similar methods as ours (6%) [73]. Conversely, when the DSM-5 AUD criteria were considered, we found a prevalence of 8.1%, which is lower than other two recent studies examining the impact of the new DSM-5 criteria on the prevalence of AUD: 12.3% in US (among alcohol lifetime users) [74] and 9.7% in Australia (among regular users) [73]. It is possible to hypothesize that the changes in the constructs required for DSM-5 AUD diagnoses - namely the inclusion of craving and exclusion of legal problem's criterion - could have reflected in the prevalence of AUD differentially across countries and cultures, for SPMA and US the impact was lighter than the one observed for Australia. Moreover, the new AUD DSM-5 criteria may have led the AUD prevalence to a more consistent estimate in our sample, considering that 15% of the positive cases for both DSM-IV AUD had concurrent onsets of abuse and dependence as showed in a previous SPMHS report [9].

In Brazil, public health campaigns mainly target drinking driving and AUD. However, specific preventive strategies might be more targeted in relation to subgroups showing higher prevalence of "at risk" drinking, and those living in social disadvantageous situations. Other considerations note studied here are the current living circumstances and social support network of the individuals with harmful drinking practices. Of course, counter-balancing enthusiasm for these targeted interventions is evidence that often it is interventions working at both the individual and population levels (alcohol taxation, restrictions on alcohol availability) that prove to be the most effective policy options [3,75].

Study strengths and limitations

Our study has three important strengths. First of all, this project is based on data from a large, representative sample of adults residing in the metropolitan area of São Paulo. Secondly, it examines distinct alcohol outcomes using conditional prevalences and studies both the DSM-5 AUD and DSM-IV abuse and dependence, which were independently assessed by using the ungated approach described elsewhere. Thirdly, this study contributes to the recent theoretical discussion about effects on drinking patterns due to individual SES and neighborhood level deprivation.

In spite of these strengths, some limitations should be considered. Despite the representativeness of our sample, it is restricted to residents of a large urbanized area, which precludes generalization of our findings to the general population living in rural settings of Brazil. Moreover, there was insufficient information to take race or ethnicity into account as covariate in the models because in the CIDI version questionnaire used herein the question about ethnicity was only asked for respondents who self-identified as minorities (n = 156). Thus, this study cannot shed much light on sources of causal variation in drinking outcomes in Brazil as might involve linkages of race or ethnicity with neighborhood social deprivation and SES. Our survey measurements were not perfect and did not include constructs that belong in conceptual models of linkages between SES and alcohol outcomes (e.g., stress; social support buffers; access, availability, and cost of alcohol). As another aspect of measurement, lay interviewers with five days of training may not have the ability to make a refined assessment of alcohol related problems, although we note the generally favorable results on validity of the alcohol and other drug use disorders diagnoses, as assessed using clinical reappraisal study designs since the mid-1980s [51,76,77].

With a transversal epidemiological survey design, this project has a major limitation that tempers interpretation of its main finding on NSD and alcohol outcomes. As has been recognized for more than 80 years, individuals with alcohol problems may have selective migration toward neighborhoods at the higher NSD levels. Alternately, it is possible for these cases to be left behind as others without problems migrate upwardly and out to neighborhoods with lower NSD levels. Moreover, we cannot state whether these cases occurred as a consequence of disadvantageous social conditions (a social causation hypothesis) or whether the alcohol outcomes caused neglect and a worsening of social conditions (a social selection hypothesis), which are alternatives that have been most thoroughly discussed in psychiatric epidemiology and allied social sciences [74,78,79].

Future research of a prospective and longitudinal character can explore what might prove to be causal mechanisms that account for the otherwise heterogeneous patterns of association and male-female variations observed across alcohol outcomes in this study. For example, among RU, the AUD-unemployment association is possibly strong enough to rule out the possibility of a spurious association, but even so, the unemployment might cause AUD or it might be caused by AUD, among various alternative mechanisms. In future studies, it also should be possible to examine in detail the potential roles of social exclusion and deprivation as part of the underlying causal mechanisms.

Conclusions

In this study, we found an association between neighborhood socioeconomic deprivation with heavy drinking patterns and AUD. This project brings important contributions to the study of alcohol use patterns in Brazil where it is the first study to investigate area-level neighborhood socioeconomic deprivation (independent of household income and other SES indicators) in an effort to build evidence for public health alcohol policy development in this country. As noted above, access to alcohol may be a neglected component of NSD in the Brazilian area-level scaling approach, and we may find that higher NSD are those in which alcohol outlets are largely concentrated (as has been found elsewhere; [80–82]). If this also is the case in Brazil, one important policy measure would be reduce the number of outlets that sell alcohol in these neighborhoods; another measure might be an increase in taxes on alcohol, with revenues directed toward future project to improve alcohol prevention and treatment in our country. The implementation of such policies has proved successful on other countries [3,75], and we are hopeful that these epidemiological findings may help guide future directions for public health work along these lines, not only in Brazil but also more globally.

Author Contributions

Conceived and designed the experiments: CMS ERS LHA. Performed the experiments: CMS ERS LPS AK LHA. Analyzed the data: CMS ERS JCA LPS SSM LHA. Wrote the paper: CMS ERS JCA LPS AGA YPW SSM LHA. Created databank: LHA MCV.

References

1. Lim SS, Vos T, Flaxman AD, Danaei G, Shibuya K, et al. (2012) A comparative risk assessment of burden of disease and injury attributable to 67 risk factors and risk factor clusters in 21 regions, 1990–2010: a systematic analysis for the Global Burden of Disease Study 2010. Lancet 380: 2224–2260.
2. UN (2011) Prevention and control of non-communicable diseases - Report of the Secretary-General A/66/83. United Nations.
3. WHO (2010) Global strategy to reduce the harmful use of alcohol. Geneve: World Health Organization.
4. Rehm J, Mathers C, Popova S, Thavorncharoensap M, Teerawattananon Y, et al. (2009) Global burden of disease and injury and economic cost attributable to alcohol use and alcohol-use disorders. Lancet 373: 2223–2233.
5. Rehm J, Room R, Monteiro M, Gmel G, Graham K, et al. (2004) Alcohol use. In: M Ezzati AL, A Rodgers, CJL Murray, editor. Comparative quantification of health risks Global and regional burden of disease attributable to selected major risk factors. Geneva: WHO. 959–1108.
6. Shield KD, Rylett M, Gmel G, Kehoe-Chan TA, Rehm J (2013) Global alcohol exposure estimates by country, territory and region for 2005–a contribution to the Comparative Risk Assessment for the 2010 Global Burden of Disease Study. Addiction 108: 912–922.
7. Rehm J, Monteiro M (2005) Alcohol consumption and burden of disease in the Americas: implications for alcohol policy. Rev Panam Salud Publica 18: 241–248.
8. Caetano R, Mills B, Pinsky I, Zaleski M, Laranjeira R (2012) The distribution of alcohol consumption and the prevention paradox in Brazil. Addiction 107: 60–68.
9. Silveira CM, Viana MC, Siu ER, de Andrade AG, Anthony JC, et al. (2011) Sociodemographic correlates of transitions from alcohol use to disorders and remission in the Sao Paulo megacity mental health survey, Brazil. Alcohol Alcohol 46: 324–332.
10. Laranjeira R, Pinsky I, Sanches M, Zaleski M, Caetano R (2010) Alcohol use patterns among Brazilian adults. Rev Bras Psiquiatr 32: 231–241.
11. Fonseca AM, Galduróz JCF, Noto AR, Carlini ELA (2010) Comparison between two household surveys on psychotropic drug use in Brazil: 2001 and 2004. Ciência & Saúde Coletiva 15: 663–670.
12. Sanchez ZM, Santos MG, Pereira AP, Nappo SA, Carlini EA, et al. (2013) Childhood Alcohol Use May Predict Adolescent Binge Drinking: A Multivariate Analysis among Adolescents in Brazil. J Pediatr 163: 363–368.
13. Galduroz JC, Carlini EA (2007) Use of alcohol among the inhabitants of the 107 largest cities in Brazil–2001. Braz J Med Biol Res 40: 367–375.
14. Kerr-Correa F, Tucci AM, Hegedus AM, Trinca LA, de Oliveira JB, et al. (2008) Drinking patterns between men and women in two distinct Brazilian communities. Rev Bras Psiquiatr 30: 235–242.
15. Kerr-Correa F, Hegedus AM, Sanches AF, Trinca LA, Kerr-Pontes LRS, et al. (2005) Differences in drinking patterns between men and women in Brazil. In: Room ISOR, editor. Alcohol, gender and drinking problems: perspectives from low and middle income countries. Geneva: World Health Organization. pp. 49–68.
16. Silveira CM, Wang YP, Andrade AG, Andrade LH (2007) Heavy episodic drinking in the Sao Paulo epidemiologic catchment area study in Brazil: gender and sociodemographic correlates. J Stud Alcohol Drugs 68: 18–27.
17. Rehm J, Baliunas D, Borges GL, Graham K, Irving H, et al. (2010) The relation between different dimensions of alcohol consumption and burden of disease: an overview. Addiction 105: 817–843.
18. Rehm J, Klotsche J, Patra J (2007) Comparative quantification of alcohol exposure as risk factor for global burden of disease. Int J Methods Psychiatr Res 16: 66–76.
19. WHO (2011) Global status report on alcohol and health. Geneve: World Health Organization.
20. Silveira CM, Siu ER, Wang YP, Viana MC, Andrade AG, et al. (2012) Gender differences in drinking patterns and alcohol-related problems in a community sample in Sao Paulo, Brazil. Clinics (Sao Paulo) 67: 205–212.
21. Almeida-Filho N, Lessa I, Magalh es L, Araujo MJ, Aquino E, et al. (2004) Alcohol drinking patterns by gender, ethnicity, and social class in Bahia, Brazil. Rev Saude Publica 38: 45–54.
22. Barros MB, Botega NJ, Dalgalarrondo P, Marin-Leon L, de Oliveira HB (2007) Prevalence of alcohol abuse and associated factors in a population-based study. Rev Saude Publica 41: 502–509.
23. Castro DS, Sanchez ZM, Zaleski M, Alves HN, Pinsky I, et al. (2012) Sociodemographic characteristics associated with binge drinking among Brazilians. Drug Alcohol Depend 126: 272–276.
24. Mendoza-Sassi RA, Beria JU (2003) Prevalence of alcohol use disorders and associated factors: a population-based study using AUDIT in southern Brazil. Addiction 98: 799–804.
25. Moreira LB, Fuchs FD, Moraes RS, Bredemeier M, Cardozo S, et al. (1996) Alcoholic beverage consumption and associated factors in Porto Alegre, a southern Brazilian city: a population-based survey. J Stud Alcohol 57: 253–259.
26. Primo NLNP, Stein AT (2004) Prevalência do abuso e da dependência de álcool em Rio Grande (RS): um estudo transversal de base populacional. Rev Psiquiatr Rio Gd Sul 26: 280–286.
27. Almeida-Filho N, Lessa I, Magalhaes L, Araujo MJ, Aquino E, et al. (2005) Social inequality and alcohol consumption-abuse in Bahia, Brazil– interactions of gender, ethnicity and social class. Soc Psychiatry Psychiatr Epidemiol 40: 214–222.
28. Luo Z, Breslau J, Gardiner JC, Chen Q, Breslau N (2013) Assessing interchangeability at cluster levels with multiple-informant data. Stat Med.
29. Hosseinpoor AR, Bergen N, Kunst A, Harper S, Guthold R, et al. (2012) Socioeconomic inequalities in risk factors for non communicable diseases in low-income and middle-income countries: results from the World Health Survey. BMC Public Health 12: 912.
30. Grittner U, Kuntsche S, Gmel G, Bloomfield K (2013) Alcohol consumption and social inequality at the individual and country levels–results from an international study. Eur J Public Health 23: 332–339.
31. Bloomfield K, Grittner U, Kramer S, Gmel G (2006) Social inequalities in alcohol consumption and alcohol-related problems in the study countries of the EU concerted action 'Gender, Culture and Alcohol Problems: a Multi-national Study'. Alcohol Alcohol Suppl 41: i26–36.
32. Room R (2005) Stigma, social inequality and alcohol and drug use. Drug Alcohol Rev 24: 143–155.
33. Dzurova D, Spilkova J, Pikhart H (2010) Social inequalities in alcohol consumption in the Czech Republic: a multilevel analysis. Health Place 16: 590–597.
34. Greenfield TK, Midanik LT, Rogers JD (2000) A 10-year national trend study of alcohol consumption, 1984–1995: is the period of declining drinking over? Am J Public Health 90: 47–52.
35. Midanik LT, Clark WB (1994) The demographic distribution of US drinking patterns in 1990: description and trends from 1984. Am J Public Health 84: 1218–1222.
36. Hemmingsson T, Lundberg I, Diderichsen F, Allebeck P (1998) Explanations of social class differences in alcoholism among young men. Soc Sci Med 47: 1399–1405.
37. Malyutina S, Bobak M, Kurilovitch S, Nikitin Y, Marmot M (2004) Trends in alcohol intake by education and marital status in urban population in Russia between the mid 1980s and the mid 1990s. Alcohol Alcohol 39: 64–69.
38. Marmot M (1997) Inequality, deprivation and alcohol use. Addiction 92 Suppl 1: S13–20.
39. Bloomfield K (2000) Alcohol Consumption and Alcohol Problems Among Women in European Countries. Subst Abus 21: 223–229.
40. Matheson FI, White HL, Moineddin R, Dunn JR, Glazier RH (2012) Drinking in context: the influence of gender and neighbourhood deprivation on alcohol consumption. J Epidemiol Community Health 66: e4.
41. Mulia N, Karriker-Jaffe KJ (2012) Interactive influences of neighborhood and individual socioeconomic status on alcohol consumption and problems. Alcohol Alcohol 47: 178–186.
42. Galea S, Ahern J, Tracy M, Rudenstine S, Vlahov D (2007) Education inequality and use of cigarettes, alcohol, and marijuana. Drug Alcohol Depend 90 Suppl 1: S4–15.

43. Galea S, Ahern J, Tracy M, Vlahov D (2007) Neighborhood income and income distribution and the use of cigarettes, alcohol, and marijuana. Am J Prev Med 32: S195–202.
44. Pollack CE, Cubbin C, Ahn D, Winkleby M (2005) Neighbourhood deprivation and alcohol consumption: does the availability of alcohol play a role? Int J Epidemiol 34: 772–780.
45. Karriker-Jaffe KJ, Zemore SE, Mulia N, Jones-Webb R, Bond J, et al. (2012) Neighborhood disadvantage and adult alcohol outcomes: differential risk by race and gender. J Stud Alcohol Drugs 73: 865–873.
46. Stimpson JP, Ju H, Raji MA, Eschbach K (2007) Neighborhood deprivation and health risk behaviors in NHANES III. Am J Health Behav 31: 215–222.
47. Jones-Webb R, Snowden L, Herd D, Short B, Hannan P (1997) Alcohol-related problems among black, Hispanic and white men: the contribution of neighborhood poverty. J Stud Alcohol 58: 539–545.
48. Viana MC, Teixeira MG, Beraldi F, Bassani Ide S, Andrade LH (2009) Sao Paulo Megacity Mental Health Survey - a population-based epidemiological study of psychiatric morbidity in the Sao Paulo metropolitan area: aims, design and field implementation. Rev Bras Psiquiatr 31: 375–386.
49. IBGE (2001) Censo demográfico populacional do ano 2000. Instituto Brasileiro de Geografia e Estatística.
50. Kish L, Frankel MR (1970) Balanced Repeated Replications for Standard Errors. J Amer Stat Assoc 65: 1071–1094.
51. Haro JM, Arbabzadeh-Bouchez S, Brugha TS, de Girolamo G, Guyer ME, et al. (2006) Concordance of the Composite International Diagnostic Interview Version 3.0 (CIDI 3.0) with standardized clinical assessments in the WHO World Mental Health surveys. Int J Methods Psychiatr Res 15: 167–180.
52. Kessler RC, Ustun TB (2004) The World Mental Health (WMH) Survey Initiative Version of the World Health Organization (WHO) Composite International Diagnostic Interview (CIDI). Int J Methods Psychiatr Res 13: 93–121.
53. Esan O, Makanjuola V, Oladeji B, Gureje O (2013) Determinants of transition across the spectrum of alcohol use and misuse in Nigeria. Alcohol 47: 249–255.
54. Abdin E, Subramaniam M, Vaingankar JA, Chong SA (2014) The role of sociodemographic factors in the risk of transition from alcohol use to disorders and remission in singapore. Alcohol Alcohol 49: 103–108.
55. Tuithof M, ten Have M, van den Brink W, Vollebergh W, de Graaf R (2012) The role of conduct disorder in the association between ADHD and alcohol use (disorder). Results from the Netherlands Mental Health Survey and Incidence Study-2. Drug Alcohol Depend 123: 115–121.
56. Degenhardt L, Bohnert KM, Anthony JC (2007) Case ascertainment of alcohol dependence in general population surveys: 'gated' versus 'ungated' approaches. Int J Methods Psychiatr Res 16: 111–123.
57. Degenhardt L, Chiu WT, Sampson N, Kessler RC, Anthony JC, et al. (2008) Toward a global view of alcohol, tobacco, cannabis, and cocaine use: findings from the WHO World Mental Health Surveys. PLoS Med 5: e141.
58. Heeringa SG, West BT, Berglund PA (2010) Preparation for complex sample survey data analysis. Applied Survey Data Analysis. 91–116.
59. Harrel Jr FE (2001) Regression Modeling Strategies. With Applications to Linear Models, Logistic Regression, and Survival Analysis. New York: Springer-Verlag.
60. Wolter KM (1985) Introduction to variance estimation. New York, NY: Springer-Verlag.
61. Chuang YC, Li YS, Wu YH, Chao HJ (2007) A multilevel analysis of neighborhood and individual effects on individual smoking and drinking in Taiwan. BMC Public Health 7: 151.
62. Elliott M (2000) The stress process in neighborhood context. Health Place 6: 287–299.
63. Romley JA, Cohen D, Ringel J, Sturm R (2007) Alcohol and environmental justice: the density of liquor stores and bars in urban neighborhoods in the United States. J Stud Alcohol Drugs 68: 48–55.
64. WHO (2005) Alcohol, gender and drinking problems: perspectives from low and middle income countries. Geneve: World Health Organization.
65. Neve RJ, Drop MJ, Lemmens PH, Swinkels H (1996) Gender differences in drinking behaviour in the Netherlands: convergence or stability? Addiction 91: 357–373.
66. Holmila M, Raitasalo K (2005) Gender differences in drinking: why do they still exist? Addiction 100: 1763–1769.
67. Wilsnack SC (2005) Honouring Ludek Kubicka: an introduction to the symposium. Addiction 100: 1760–1762.
68. Lima MC, Kerr-Correa F, Rehm J (2013) [Alcohol consumption pattern and Coronary Heart Disease risk in Metropolitan Sao Paulo: analyses of GENACIS Project]. Rev Bras Epidemiol 16: 49–57.
69. Lima MC, Kerr-Corrêa F, Tucci AM, Simão MO, Oliveira JB, et al. (2007) Gender difference in heavy alcohol use: a general population survey (The Genacis Project) of São Paulo City, Brazil. Contemp Drug Problems 34: 427–444.
70. Guimarães VV, Florindo AA, Stopa SR, César CLG, Barros MBA, et al. (2010) Consumo abusivo e dependência de álcool em população adulta no Estado de São Paulo, Brasil. Revista Brasileira de Epidemiologia 13: 314–325.
71. Bromet EJ, Gluzman SF, Paniotto VI, Webb CP, Tintle NL, et al. (2005) Epidemiology of psychiatric and alcohol disorders in Ukraine: findings from the Ukraine World Mental Health survey. Soc Psychiatry Psychiatr Epidemiol 40: 681–690.
72. Kim JH, Lee S, Chow J, Lau J, Tsang A, et al. (2008) Prevalence and the factors associated with binge drinking, alcohol abuse, and alcohol dependence: a population-based study of Chinese adults in Hong Kong. Alcohol Alcohol 43: 360–370.
73. Mewton L, Slade T, McBride O, Grove R, Teesson M (2011) An evaluation of the proposed DSM-5 alcohol use disorder criteria using Australian national data. Addiction 106: 941–950.
74. Agrawal A, Heath AC, Lynskey MT (2011) DSM-IV to DSM-5: the impact of proposed revisions on diagnosis of alcohol use disorders. Addiction 106: 1935–1943.
75. Anderson P, Chisholm D, Fuhr DC (2009) Effectiveness and cost-effectiveness of policies and programmes to reduce the harm caused by alcohol. Lancet 373: 2234–2246.
76. Anthony JC, Folstein M, Romanoski AJ, Von Korff MR, Nestadt GR, et al. (1985) Comparison of the lay Diagnostic Interview Schedule and a standardized psychiatric diagnosis. Experience in eastern Baltimore. Arch Gen Psychiatry 42: 667–675.
77. Wittchen HU (1994) Reliability and validity studies of the WHO–Composite International Diagnostic Interview (CIDI): a critical review. J Psychiatr Res 28: 57–84.
78. Johnson JG, Cohen P, Dohrenwend BP, Link BG, Brook JS (1999) A longitudinal investigation of social causation and social selection processes involved in the association between socioeconomic status and psychiatric disorders. J Abnorm Psychol 108: 490–499.
79. Dohrenwend BP, Levav I, Shrout PE, Schwartz S, Naveh G, et al. (1992) Socioeconomic status and psychiatric disorders: the causation-selection issue. Science 255: 946–952.
80. Gruenewald PJ (2007) The spatial ecology of alcohol problems: niche theory and assortative drinking. Addiction 102: 870–878.
81. Mair C, Gruenewald PJ, Ponicki WR, Remer L (2013) Varying impacts of alcohol outlet densities on violent assaults: explaining differences across neighborhoods. J Stud Alcohol Drugs 74: 50–58.
82. Toomey TL, Erickson DJ, Carlin BP, Lenk KM, Quick HS, et al. (2012) The association between density of alcohol establishments and violent crime within urban neighborhoods. Alcohol Clin Exp Res 36: 1468–1473.

14

LAT Software Induced Savings on Medical Costs of Alcohol Addicts' Care - Results from a Matched-Pairs Case-Control Study

Mihajlo Jakovljevic[1]*, Mirjana Jovanovic[2], Nemanja Rancic[3], Benjamin Vyssoki[4], Natasa Djordjevic[5]

1 Department of Pharmacology and Toxicology; The Faculty of Medical Sciences, University of Kragujevac, Kragujevac, Serbia, **2** Department of Psychiatry; The Faculty of Medical Sciences, University of Kragujevac, Kragujevac, Serbia, **3** Centre for Clinical Pharmacology; Medical Faculty Military Medical Academy, University of Defense, Belgrade, Serbia, **4** Department of Psychiatry and Psychotherapy; Medical University of Vienna, Vienna, Austria, **5** Department of Pharmacology and Toxicology; The Faculty of Medical Sciences, University of Kragujevac, Kragujevac, Serbia

Abstract

Lesch Alcoholism Typology (LAT) is one of the most widely used clinical typologies of alcohol addiction. Study tested whether introduction of LAT software in clinical practice leaded to improved outcomes and reduced costs. Retrospective matched-pairs case-control cost comparison study was conducted at the Regional Addiction Center of the University Clinic in Serbia involving 250 patients during the four-year period. Mean relapse frequency followed by outpatient detoxification was 0.42±0.90 vs. 0.70±1.66 (LAT/non-LAT; p = 0.267). Adding relapses after inpatient treatment total mean-number of relapses per patient was 0.70±1.74 vs. 0.97±1.89 (LAT/non-LAT; p = 0.201). However, these relapse frequency differentials were not statistically significant. Total hospital costs of Psychiatry clinic based non-LAT addicts' care (€54,660) were significantly reduced to €36,569 after initiation of LAT. Mean total cost per patient was reduced almost by half after initiation of LAT based treatment: €331±381 vs. €626±795 (LAT/non-LAT; p = 0.001). Mean cost of single psychiatry clinic admission among non-LAT treatment group was €320±330 (CI 95% 262–378) and among LAT €197±165 (CI 95% 168–226) (p = 0.019). Mean LAT software induced net savings on psychiatric care costs were €144 per patient. Total net savings on hospital care including F10 associated somatic co-morbidities amounted to €295 per patient. More sensitive diagnostic assessment and sub-type specific pharmacotherapy and psychotherapy following implementation of LAT software lead to significant savings on costs of hospital care.

Editor: Helge Bruns, University Hospital Oldenburg, Germany

Funding: The Ministry of Education, Science and Technological Development of the Republic of Serbia through OI Grant N° 175014, has fully financed this study. The funder had no role in study design, data collection and analysis, decision to publish, or preparation of the manuscript.

Competing Interests: The authors have declared that no competing interests exist.

* Email: jakovljevicm@medf.kg.ac.rs

Introduction

Due to its high prevalence [1] and chronic clinical course [2], alcohol dependence represents a heavy burden for health care systems across the globe [3]. National health budgets are becoming increasingly constrained and therefore effortis put into assessment of cost-effectiveness of specificmedical treatment strategies, such as addiction specific psychotherapy techniques [4,5] or anticraving medication for relapse prevention [6–8]. Theseresults contributed to more efficient care and evidence based allocation of resources [9]. However, the impactof distinct medical typologies that contain clinical practice guidelines on medical costs have not been researched thoroughly [10–13]. There are several typologies of alcohol dependence [14–16] which are widely adopted in the published literature.

Through the course of past century over a dozen of distinct clinical typologies of alcoholic dependence have been developed with Cloninger, Jellinek's, Babor's, LAT being only some of the most famous and broadly adopted. Lesch Alcoholism Typology (LAT), introduced in 1991, is regarded particularly helpful in terms of providing treatment recommendations grounded in patient's age of onset, family history, co-morbidity, and alcohol-related disabilities. The LAT typology is applied in clinical practice as a clinician's oriented software. It has been translated in 12 languages and validated in many countries, offering essential recommendations for pharmacological treatment of withdrawal and relapse prevention [17–21]. As to our best knowledge, so far there have been no attempts to assess the impact of clinical typologies implementation to the overall costs of alcohol addicts' medical care in a clinical trial. In this study we therefore want to evaluate the impact of a newly introduced sub-type specific treatment program, the LAT, on the cost of medical treatment in alcohol dependent patients.

Materials and Methods

Ethics Statement

The study was conducted according to Helsinki Declaration; current positive legislature on good clinical practice and guidelines on retrospective database analysis. Ethical committee approval was granted by the Ethical Committee of University Clinical Center Kragujevac, Serbia – Submission N° 01/11639 date 30. October 2013; Decision reached on 18. November 2013; N° 01-12299. Patient data were handled anonymously during the study. Patient records/information was anonymized and de-identified prior to analysis.

Setting

Since January 2012, LAT typology and software, translated and administered in Serbian language, was introduced to the clinical practice in seven regional addiction centers throughout Serbia [22,23]. The Regional Addiction Center Kragujevac provides services for up to 400 alcohol dependent patients per year and belongs to the Psychiatry Clinic of the single largest tertiary care university hospital in Central Serbia region with 1300 beds capacity (www.kc-kg.rs). Southeastern European country of Serbia has an upper middle income post-socialist transitional economy [9]. It's healthcare system is marked with typical strengths and weaknesses familiar to the most Eastern European economies including post-2004 EU members [22,23]. Therefore, Serbia can be regarded representative of a wider regional setting. Its substantial national deficit of budget allocation to combat huge alcohol dependency burden emphasizes urgent need for effective resource allocation in this field [24]. So far, health economics principles were not part of routine policy making on reimbursement of antic raving medicines, detoxification procedures or psychotherapy techniques indicated in alcohol addiction treatment [25].

Data

Study sample was selected out of 813 alcohol dependent cases being either outpatients or inpatients within the institutional framework of the Regional Addiction Center of the University Clinical Center Kragujevac, Serbia during the period 2010–2013. One hundred and twenty five case-control pairs were selected based on their clinically confirmed diagnosis of alcohol dependence according to ICD-10 and DSM-IV-TR, age and gender. There were no other grounds for patient selection except the possibility of close clinical matching so this was the maximum of available patient couples for comparison. LAT patients' medical services utilization was observed during 2012–2013 period, while non-LAT processed alcohol addicts were observedin2010–2011 period. Economic data on resource use and costs were extracted out of the University Clinical Center electronic registry of discharge invoices. Observed clinical setting was state owned not-for-profit hospital which is generally charging governmental budget subsidized prices to the citizens. Therefore this database presents reliable insight into the actual costs of care. Although individual periods while these costs accrued slightly varied, complete symmetry was obeyed in duration of the observation among cases coupled. That means that medical and resource use history for each single case was extracted either for one or for two years (depending on his/her actual physician visits and admissions) duration while his/her counterpart from control pool, was observed during equally long period of time (either one or two years). Clinical outcomes data accessible was individual frequency of relapse events followed by either outpatient detoxification or hospital admission. According to availability these relapses were evidenced for 2012–2013 observation time, in equal duration between patient pairs. Resource use and costs accrued due to alcohol dependence diagnostics, treatment and rehabilitation were observed separately within institutional frameworks of Psychiatry Clinic, Internal Medicine Clinic and Neurology Clinic for each case.

Analysis

It is rather difficult to assess trends in clinical decision making and resource use patterns among alcohol addicts due to high clinical heterogeneity of patient's backgrounds [26]. Therefore, in the present study, matched-pairs case control retrospective study design was employed in a cost comparison analysis framework [27]. This approach, previously applied in clinical trials on addiction disorders [26–29], allows reliable elimination of statistical bias impact to the study results. Grounds for choosing such methodology was lying in the fact that medical services utilization patterns and associated costs otherwise might have been affected with differences between groups in clinical background, disease course and treatment response [30].

Costs were converted from national currency – Republic of Serbian Dinar (RSD) to Euro (€) in line with mean official exchange rates of the National Bank of Serbia in the respective years (www.nbs.rs). This way the effect of slight devaluation of domestic currency was avoided. There were no sudden swifts in pricing policy or significant changes in medical service charges related to alcoholism treatment during this period of time. Therefore chronological gap between experimental and control group (before and after LAT intervention) had rather minor impact to the price levels 2010–2013. Foreign currency (€) based prices remained stable.

Statistics

Complete statistical analysis was carried out using Statistical Software PASW Statistics 18 and Microsoft Office Excel 2007. Cases and controls were matched according to sex, age and diagnosis. After pairing patients, cost analysis has done, during one-year or two-year period, between controls observed before and cases observed after implementation of LAT software - guidelines. Categorical variables were presented as frequencies of certain categories, while statistical significance of differences was tested using Chi-square test. Continuous variables were summarized as mean, standard deviation, range and 95% confidence interval. Continuous variables were compared using the Student's *t* test for independent samples and the Mann-Whitney U test, while nonparametric Kruskal Wallis H test was used to test the statistical significance among continuous variables with three or more categories. Analysis of money spending was done by nonparametric tests (the large standard deviations). Multiple regression analysis was performed on both LAT and non-LAT patients, while dependent variable were total hospital costs. Two models (LAT and non-LAT) were developed indicating key predictors of costs of care. All the analyses were estimated at $p<0.05$ level of the statistical significance.

Results

Number of relapses

Mean number of relapses followed by outpatient detoxification was 0.42 ± 0.90 vs. 0.70 ± 1.66 (LAT/non-LAT) ($p=0.267$) (see Table 1). Frequency of relapses followed by hospital admission was 0.28 ± 1.10 vs. 0.26 ± 0.58 (LAT/non-LAT) ($p=0.339$). Thus we come to the average rate of total relapses of 0.70 ± 1.74 vs. 0.97 ± 1.89 (LAT/non-LAT) while this difference was not statistically significant ($p=0.201$).

Inpatient and outpatient care

Total number of Psychiatry Clinic hospital admissions was 155 vs. 156 while there were 6 vs. 26 Internal Medicine Clinic admissions (Chi square test; $p=0.0016$) and 5 vs. 6 Neurology Clinic admissions (Chi square test; $p=0.8415$) (LAT/non-LAT)

Table 1. Demography and resource use patterns among alcohol dependent matched patient pairs, LAT vs. non-LAT comparison.

	LAT (n = 125)	Non-LAT (n = 125)	p value**
ICD-10 codes#	F.10.0–F10.9	F.10.0–F10.9	N/A
Age (M ± SD)	48.26±10.51	48.20±10.49	p = 0.966
Gender (male/female)	120/5	120/5	N/A
Relapses followed by hospital admission	0.28±1.10	0.26±0.58	p = 0.339
Relapses followed by outpatient detoxification	0.42±0.90	0.70±1.66	p = 0.267
Total relapse rates (2012–2013)	0.70±1.74	0.97±1.89	p = 0.201
Outpatient physician consultations	10.45±9.09	10.29±12.50	**p = 0.050***
Inpatient physician consultations	7.19±57.81	2.95±9.37	p = 0.777
Mean N° Hospital admissions per patient - Psychiatry Clinic	1.24±1.42	1.25±1.42	p = 0.986
Hospital admissions N° - Internal Medicine Clinic (due to F10)	0.05±0.31	0.21±0.65	**p = 0.008***
Hospital admissions N° - Neurology clinic (due to F10)	0.04±0.20	0.05±0.33	p = 0.491
Mean admissions N° (Internal + Neurology)	1.44±1.73	1.59±1.54	p = 0.151
Mean N° of all hospital admissions (M ± SD)	0.94±1.27	0.92±0.74	p = 0.855
Duration of Hospital admissions (M ± SD)	12.49±14.77	10.80±11.52	p = 0.315
Total hospital admissions – Psychiatry	155	156	N/A
Total N° of all hospital admissions – Internal Clinic	6	26	**p = 0.0016***
Total N° of all hospital admissions – Neurology Clinic	5	6	p = 0.8415
Total joint Internal Medicine Clinic and Neurology Clinic hospital admissions	11	32	**p = 0.0047***
Typology according to Lesch (type I/II/III/IV)	10/27/57/31	N/A	N/A

#All resource use at the Internal Medicine Clinic and Neurology Clinic were accounted exclusively for medical services consumed in relation to alcohol dependence diagnostics, treatment and rehabilitation (ICD-10 F10 diagnostic code group); p value- statistical signifiance of difference;
**- Mann-Whitney U test; !- Chi square test;
*- p<0.05; M ± SD- mean ± standard deviation.

(see Table 1). Total joint Internal Medicine Clinic and Neurology Clinic hospital admissions frequency was 11 vs. 32 (LAT/non-LAT) (Chi square test; p = 0.0047). Mean Internal Medicine Clinic admissions frequency was significantly higher in non-LAT group 0.05±0.31 vs. 0.21±0.65 (p = 0.008).

Mean hospital costs per patient due to joint Internal Medicine Clinic and Neurology Clinic admissions were higher among non-LAT patients €38±238 vs. €189±623 (LAT/non-LAT; p = 0.102) (see Table 2). Total costs of hospital care in all clinics were substantially lower in LAT group, €41,331 compared to €78,226 in non-LAT patients (p = 0.001) (see Table 2 and Fig. 1). Average net savings on direct medical costs of psychiatric hospital care highly likely attributable to the LAT software implementation were €144 per patient. Average net savings in total costs of hospital care for F10 associated mental and somatic disorders across all clinics were €295 per patient.

Mean number of hospital admissions per patient to the Psychiatry Clinic, during the examined time period was 1.24±1.42/1.25±1.42 (LAT/non-LAT) (p = 0.986). Mean total duration of hospital admissions was 12.49±14.77/10.80±11.52 days (LAT/non-LAT) (p = 0.315). Attending psychiatrists delivered on average 10.69±9.06/12.81±16.06 sessions of social therapy, including implementation of psychotherapeutic techniques (LAT/non-LAT) (p = 0.200). Total Psychiatry Clinic hospital costs of non-LAT addicts' care amounted to €54,660, which were significantly reduced (€36,569, p = 0.008) after initiation of LAT (see Fig. 1). Mean cost of psychiatric care per patient decreased after initiation of LAT based treatment (€293±308 (CI 95%- 239-347) *vs.* €437±415 (CI 95%- 364-510) €), and the decrease was significant (p = 0.008). Mean per patient values of all cost domains in the non-LAT controls were higher than among LAT cases but only some of these findings were statistically significant (see Table 2; Fig. 2).

Lesch Alcoholism Typology- Subtypes

Mean costs of care per LAT subtypes differed significantly (Kruskal Wallis H test; p = 0.005) and amounted to: LAT I – €326±88 (CI 95% 271–380) €, LAT II – €256±304 (CI 95% 141–370) €, LAT III – €256±295 (CI 95% 180–333) € and LAT IV – €381±368 (CI 95% 251–511) € among LAT classified patients. Mean cost of single hospital admission among non-LAT treatment group was €320±330 (CI 95% 262–378) € and among LAT €197±165 (CI 95% 168–226) € (Mann-Whitney U test; p = 0.019).

Multiple regression analysis was conducted using value of total hospital cost as dependent variable. It showed that model developed for LAT treated patients significantly better explaines costs variance compared to non-LAT ($R^2 = 0.517$ vs. $R^2 = 0.132$) (see Table 3 and Table 4). Variables exposing strongest impact to total cost of care among LAT cases were: age, duration of hospital admissions and outpatient physician consultations, while among non-LAT controls there were no such predictors with significant impact to the total cost of care.

Discussion

The impact of good clinical practice guidelines implementation to the clinicians' prescription patterns and their economic awareness was previously assessed and reported in recent studies [24]. Our study is the first to evaluate the impact of a newly introduced, sub-type specific alcohol dependency classification system on economic and clinical outcomes.

Table 2. Costs of hospital medical care; LAT vs. non-LAT comparison (€).

Cost domain (total values per group)#	LAT (n = 125)	Non-LAT (n = 125)	p value**
Psychiatry Clinic			
Outpatient Care	11,113	12,598	p = 0.773
Inpatient Care	25,456	42,062	**p = 0.008***
Total costs of hospital care	36,569	54,660	**p = 0.008***
Main Cost Domains			
Physician Consultations	6,132	7,942	p = 0.966
Outpatient physician consultations	5,074	4,785	p = 0.382
Inpatient physician consultations	1,058	3,157	p = 0.757
Psychotherapeutic Interventions	5,726	7,235	p = 0.720
Hospital admission	18,604	18,765	p = 0.430
General Medical Care	929	5,438	**p<0.001***
Laboratory Analysis	2,044	6,794	**p<0.001***
Imaging Diagnostics	887	2,976	**p = 0.044***
Pharmaceuticals	2,246	5,510	p = 0.081
Other Clinics			
Internal Medicine Clinic	3,562	20,161	**p = 0.008***
Neurology clinic	1,200	3,405	p = 0.497
Total somatic ward costs (Internal + Neurology Clinic)	4,762	23,566	p = 0.102
Total Hospital costs	**41,331**	**78,226**	**p = 0.001***
Mean cost per patient – Psychiatry (M ± SD)	293±308	437±415	**p = 0.008***
Mean cost per patient - Somatic wards/clinics (M ± SD)	38±238	189±623	p = 0.102
Mean total hospital costs per patient (M ± SD)	**331±381**	**626±795**	**p = 0.001***

#All admission costs to the Internal Medicine Clinic and Neurology Clinic were accounted exclusively for medical services consumed in relation to alcohol dependence diagnostics, treatment and rehabilitation (ICD-10 F10 diagnostic code group); p value- statistical signifiance of difference;
**- Mann-Whitney U test;
*- p<0.05; M ± SD- mean ± standard deviation.

LAT cases exposed statistically significantly higher demand for outpatient physician consultations. On the opposite, Internal Medicine Clinic admissions were significantly more frequent among non-LAT controls. All other resource use differentials between the two groups were not statistically significant. With regards to costs of care, statistical significance in favor of LAT cases (substantially lower cost of care) was proved on numerous cost domains: Inpatient Care, Total costs of hospital care and Internal Medicine Clinic costs. Besides these aforementioned domains, LAT cases exhibited significantly lower costs of care

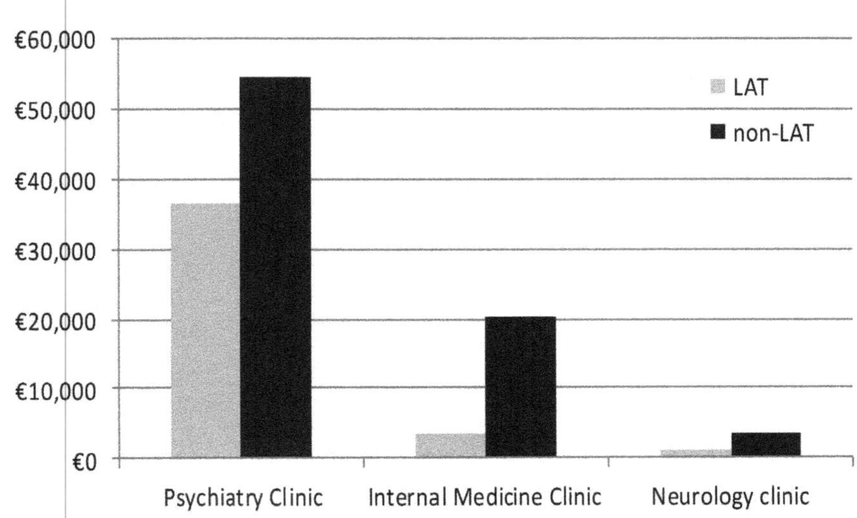

Figure 1. Costs of hospital care, inter-clinic differentials; total amounts per group; comparison LAT vs. non-LAT matched pairs (Y axis presents € values).

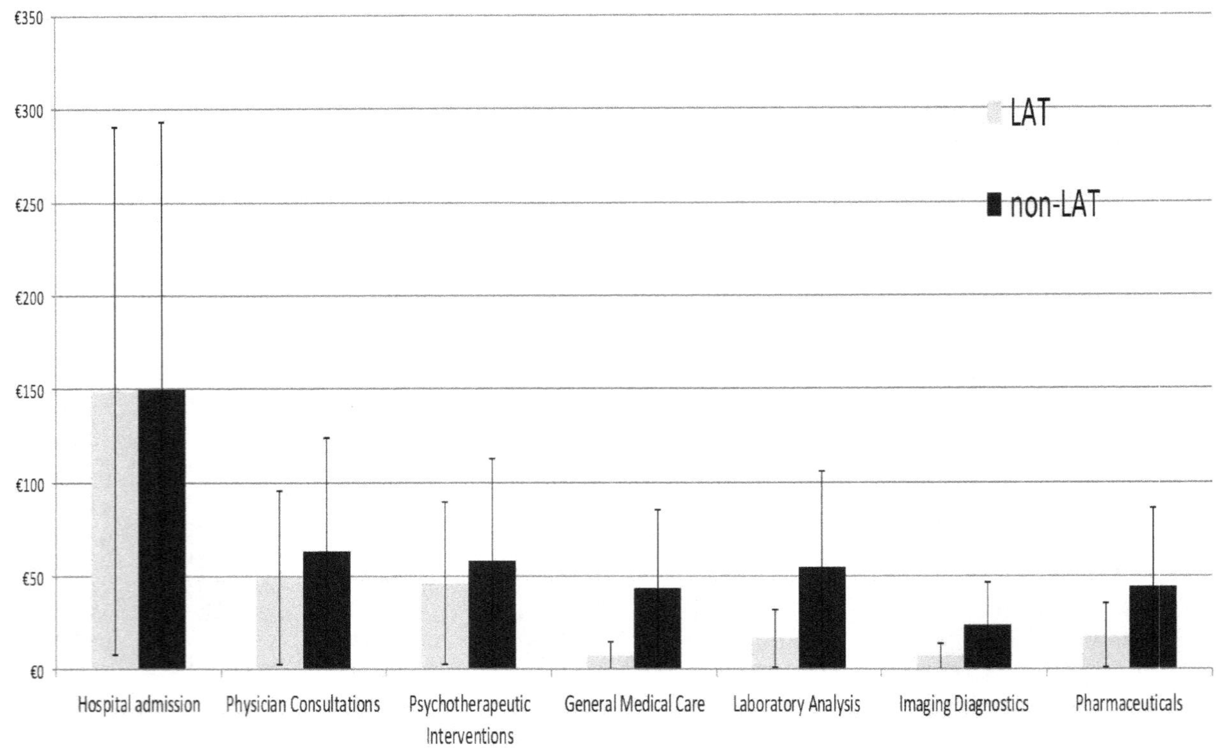

Figure 2. Cost domains; Mean values per patient presented with CI 95% range; comparison LAT vs. non-LAT matched pairs (Y axis presents € values).

compared to non-LAT controls in terms of mean cost per patient treated at Psychiatry Clinic as well as ultimately total hospital costs per patient. Noticed cost saving trend after LAT software and guidelines implementation in clinical practice was also statistically significant in consecutive domains: Laboratory analysis and Imaging diagnostics and General Medical (dominantly nursing) Care. An explanation for this phenomenon was overutilization of CTs and NMR imaging of the brain which was wide spreaded clinicans' practice before LAT introduction. Demands to perform blood tests covering too broad variety of targeted medical conditions (substance addiction, infections etc.) were also more frequent in 2010–2011. Cost savings on nursing care among LAT patients are partly attributable to more frequent outpatient visits to the attending psychiatrists recommended by LAT software acting as substitute for more costly hospital treatment being quite effective in controlling disease.

Resource use patterns exhibited in this trial point to the opportunity of reshaping clinician's behavior with evidence based guidelines [32]. We could observe frequency of outpatient visits to the attending psychiatrist and frequency of hospital admissions as an indirect sign of occasional relapses that these patients commonly experience [25].

LAT patients tended to consume less nursing care, laboratory analysis, imaging diagnostics and pharmaceuticals (see Table 2

Table 3. The impact of independent variables on total hospital cost among non-LAT treated patients (multiple regression analysis).

Model non-LAT	b	SE-b	beta	Pearson r
Constant	58.480	535.195		
Age	5.523	6.812	0.073	0.048
Gender	−15.258	328.707	−0.004	−0.007
Number of hospital admissions	265.450	140.739	0.246	0.316
Duration of hospital admissions	4.429	9.620	0.064	0.296
Outpatient physician consultations	−1.858	5.545	−0.029	−0.016
Inpatient physician consultations	11.342	8.243	0.134	0.211
Relapses followed by hospital admission	65.125	123.029	0.048	0.035
Relapses followed by outpatient detoxification	−9.298	43.931	−0.019	−0.066

Note: The dependent variable was Total hospital cost. $R^2 = 0.132$, Adjusted $R^2 = 0.072$.

Table 4. The impact of independent variables on total hospital cost among LAT treated patients (multiple regression analysis).

Model LAT	b	SE-b	beta	Pearson r
Constant	442.672	213.732		
Age*	−4.862	2.445	**−0.134**	−0.206
Gender	−94.649	130.726	−0.049	−0.109
Number of hospital admissions	66.641	40.408	0.221	0.645
Duration of hospital admissions*	11.905	3.450	**0.461**	0.675
Type of LAT	−16.626	29.024	−0.038	0.036
Outpatient physician consultations*	5.608	2.798	**0.134**	0.138
Inpatient physician consultations	0.233	0.442	0.035	0.159
Relapses followed by hospital admission	28.232	27.235	0.081	0.027
Relapses followed by outpatient detoxification	−26.307	33.150	−0.062	−0.087

Note: The dependent variable was Total hospital cost. $R^2=0.517$, Adjusted $R^2=0.480$; $p<0.05$*.

and Fig. 2). Interestingly, recently published trial testing efficiency of sodium oxibate in maintaining alcohol abstinence among addicts showed that anticraving medicines could prove themselves useful regardless of actual LAT type of patient. This finding might support lack of significant differences between LAT and non-LAT cases in drug acquisition costs [31]. Lower demand for diagnostic services by the attending psychiatrists is attributable to the precise and focused clinical tools provided by interactive LAT software. These are allowing for earlier diagnostic recognition of patient type based on accurate anamnesis and examination criteria.

Statistically significant cost differentials among four stages of alcoholism clinical evolution according to LAT confirms broadly recognized LAT sensitivity for distinct recognition of patients with profoundly different drinking patterns and treatment needs [16–18,21].

Non-LAT cases were more frequently treated at the Internal Clinic (Gastrointestinal and Hepatology wards) and Neurology Clinic due to alcohol related somatic disorders such as liver cirrhosis, polyneuritis and others. These wards demand much more expensive imaging examinations and blood tests compared to Psychiatry clinic [33]. Cost-reduction observed among LAT patients, probably happened due to their less severe somatic complications compared to respective non-LAT couples during the investigated time period consecutively somatic disorders worsened by occasional heavy drinking episodes were rather seldom among LAT cases. Authors believe that patient rambling among specialty Internal Medicine Clinic and Neurology Clinic delayed alcoholism type recognition and was additional underlying reason for their more demanding and expensive hospital care.

The hot issue of cost containment remains high on the agenda of regional health policy makers due to Western Balkan's difficulties in provision of sustainable health care funding, triggered by worldwide economic crisis [22,23]. Cost saving procedures are considered by many experts a trade off with quality of medical services [34,35]. In this particular alcohol addicted population, authors assumed that patients experienced clinical improvement because of more efficient diagnostic algorithm leading to the more targeted, individually adjusted treatment and weaker demand for health care. As a consequence, it appears that they needed less frequent outpatient physician consultations and consumed less resources which is the phenomena well described in literature [30]. Range of costs reported in upper-middle income Serbia is rather modest compared to high-income settings [24,25]. Regardless of some evidenced intra-European differences in LAT sub-type structure across ethnicities [36], LAT associated savings should be expected elsewhere. Observed resource use patterns will likely cause decrease in overall costs of medical care for somatic symptoms, in other countries as well.

Limitations

Matching of patients into couples with highly similar clinical background should have eliminated the potential bias and external validity issues in the study, which might have been affected by medical heterogeneity of samples in other similar clinical trials [26]. Regardless of few minor setbacks in this study design it provides high statistical reliability for generalizations of conclusions [37].

University Clinical Center Kragujevac electronic database of discharge invoices was used as a source of data on medical services utilization costs. Tight internal and external control of accounting offices of respective Clinics is conducted due to the fact that these invoices serve as grounds for negotiations on reimbursement with republican Health Insurance fund representatives. Therefore, these data should be regarded of satisfactory reliability and quality. Sample size is rather modest, due to the fact that authors had no access to other addiction centers throughout the country or abroad. According to authors' opinion this would probably be the core weakness of the study. Nevertheless, matching of patient pairs forms an appropriate control group allowing for the generalizability of conclusions. Deeper insight into indirect costs of lost productivity would be very helpful and would allow for more inclusive insight into the costs of care [38], as, due to adopting payer's perspective, these were rather out of scope of present trial. Clinical background data relied on relapse rates only. In real world clinical setting, there is no efficient way to assess any relapses that did not lead to additional treatment, so frequency of relapses marked as "total relapse rates" in this article, actually presents clinically visible fraction of them. Lack of an in-depth assessment of other clinical outcomes such as abstinence duration, was the another key weakness of this trial. The prospective approach would certainly provide deeper insight into the clinical efficiency of LAT based treatments.

Conclusions

In conclusion, the significant medical savings documented by this matched-pair case-control study are anticipated consequence of more targeted therapeutic approach. Here we explain that noticed cost savings induced by LAT typology, and LAT software introduction the core underlying cost driver was higher rate of hospital admissions to the Internal Medicine wards due to severe somatic symptoms among non-LAT patients. Likely clinical improvements among LAT patients are believed to be achieved due to proper LAT type recognition and decreased need for physicians' consultations, detoxifications, fewer and shorter hospital admissions and lower drug acquisition costs. The present study is one of the pioneering assessments of health economic justifications for systematic relying on common typologies in clinical practice. These are promising signs of delivering more efficient and cost saving care to alcohol addicts based on LAT in Southeastern Europe. Such evidence should be regarded a stimuli for further research on guidelines impact on the costs of addiction disorders medical care. Applied health economics research in increasingly prevalent addiction disorders could bring partial release to the constrained national health care budgets. Finding alternative ways to deliver cost-effective medical care for alcohol dependents bears particularly heavy policy impact among aging nations of northern hemisphere. Vast economic consequences for the community are particularly evident in these disorders affecting young population. Various substance addictions bring huge opportunity cost due to long lasting decreased working ability, absenteeism and premature mortality. Dissemination of good clinical practice guidelines recommending cost-effective diagnostics and treatment options could be highly effective policy tool for the future of addiction medicine.

Author Contributions

Conceived and designed the experiments: M. Jakovljevic BV M. Jovanovic ND NR. Performed the experiments: M. Jakovljevic M. Jovanovic. Analyzed the data: M. Jakovljevic ND NR. Contributed reagents/materials/analysis tools: M. Jakovljevic ND. Wrote the paper: M. Jakovljevic BV M. Jovanovic ND NR.

References

1. Shield KD, Rylett M, Gmel G, Gmel G, Kehoe-Chan TA, et al. (2013) Global alcohol exposure estimates by country, territory and region for 2005–a contribution to the comparative risk assessment for the 2010 Global Burden of Disease Study. Addiction 108: 912–922.
2. Ando B, Rozsa S, Kurgyis E, Szkaliczki A, Demeter I, et al. (2013) Direct and Indirect Symptom Severity Indicators of Alcohol Dependence and the Personality Concept of the Biosocial Model. Subst Use Misuse.
3. Chisholm D, Rehm J, Van Ommeren M, Monteiro M (2004) Reducing the global burden of hazardous alcohol use: a comparative cost-effectiveness analysis. J Stud Alcohol 65: 782–793.
4. Neighbors CJ, Barnett NP, Rohsenow DJ, Colby SM, Monti PM (2010) Cost-effectiveness of a motivational intervention for alcohol-involved youth in a hospital emergency department. J Stud Alcohol Drugs 71: 384–394.
5. Wutzke SE, Shiell A, Gomel MK, Conigrave KM (2001) Cost effectiveness of brief interventions for reducing alcohol consumption. Soc Sci Med 52: 863–870.
6. Palmer AJ, Neeser K, Weiss C, Brandt A, Comte S, et al. (2000) The long-term cost-effectiveness of improving alcohol abstinence with adjuvant acamprosate. Alcohol Alcohol 35: 478–492.
7. Rychlik R, Siedentop H, Pfeil T, Daniel D (2003) Cost-effectiveness of adjuvant treatment with acamprosate in maintaining abstinence in alcohol dependent patients. Eur Addict Res 9: 59–64.
8. Walters D, Connor JP, Feeney GF, Young RM (2009) The cost effectiveness of naltrexone added to cognitive-behavioral therapy in the treatment of alcohol dependence. J Addict Dis 28: 137–144.
9. Jakovljevic M, Jovanovic M, Lazic Z, Jakovljevic V, Djukic A, et al. (2011) Current efforts and proposals to reduce healthcare costs in Serbia. Ser J Exp Clin Res 12: 161–163.
10. Ciaranello AL, Perez F, Engelsmann B, Walensky RP, Mushavi A, et al. (2013) Cost-effectiveness of World Health Organization 2010 guidelines for prevention of mother-to-child HIV transmission in Zimbabwe. Clin Infect Dis 56: 430–446.
11. Drozda JP (2013) Physician specialty society clinical guidelines and bending the cost curve: comment on "Cost consideration in the clinical guidance documents of physician specialty societies in the United States". JAMA Intern Med 173: 1097–1099.
12. French MT, Salome HJ, Sindelar JL, McLellan AT (2002) Benefit-cost analysis of addiction treatment: methodological guidelines and empirical application using the DATCAP and ASI. Health Serv Res 37: 433–455.
13. Picon PD, Beltrame A, Banta D (2013) National guidelines for high-cost drugs in Brazil: achievements and constraints of an innovative national evidence-based public health policy. Int J Technol Assess Health Care 29: 198–206.
14. Babor TF, Dolinsky ZS, Meyer RE, Hesselbrock M, Hofmann M, et al. (1992) Types of alcoholics: concurrent and predictive validity of some common classification schemes. Br J Addict 87: 1415–1431.
15. Cloninger CR, Bohman M, Sigvardsson S (1981) Inheritance of alcohol abuse. Cross-fostering analysis of adopted men. Arch Gen Psychiatry 38: 861–868.
16. Lesch WC, Celuch KG (1991) Females' use of alcoholic beverages: a study in context. J Health Soc Policy 2: 23–38.
17. Lesch OM, Walter H (1996) Subtypes of alcoholism and their role in therapy. Alcohol Alcohol Suppl 1: 63–67.
18. Bleich S, Bayerlein K, Reulbach U, Hillemacher T, Bonsch D, et al. (2004) Homocysteine levels in patients classified according to Lesch's typology. Alcohol Alcohol 39: 493–498.
19. Kiefer F, Helwig H, Tarnaske T, Otte C, Jahn H, et al. (2005) Pharmacological relapse prevention of alcoholism: clinical predictors of outcome. Eur Addict Res 11: 83–91.
20. Leggio L, Kenna GA, Fenton M, Bonenfant E, Swift RM (2009) Typologies of alcohol dependence. From Jellinek to genetics and beyond. Neuropsychol Rev 19: 115–129.
21. Lesch OM, Walter H, Wetschka C, Hesselbrock M, Hesselbrock V (2011) Alcohol and tobacco. Medical and sociological aspects of use, abuse and addiction.Vienna, Austria, Springer-Verlag.
22. Jakovljevic M, Rankovic A, Rancic N, Jovanovic M, Ivanovic M, et al. (2013) Radiology services costs and utilization patterns estimates in Southeastern Europe - a retrospective analysis from Serbia. Value in health regional issues 2: 218–225.
23. Jakovljevic MB (2013) Resource allocation strategies in Southeastern European health policy. Eur J Health Econ 14: 153–159.
24. Jovanovic M, Jakovljevic M (2011) Inpatient detoxification procedure and facilities: financing considerations from an Eastern European perspective. Alcohol Alcohol 46: 364–365.
25. Jakovljevic M, Jovanovic M, Nikic K, Radovanovic A, Pirkovic I, et al. (2011) Inpatient detoxification and law enforcement costs following acute drinking event, in typical eastern European upper – middle income, health care setting. Health Behavior & Public Health 1: 1–7.
26. Pedrero Perez E, Rojo Mota G (2008) [Personality differences between substance addicts and general population. Study of clinical cases with matched controls using Cloninger's TCI-R]. Adicciones 20: 251–261. Spanish.
27. Westermeyer J, Specker S (1999) Social resources and social function in comorbid eating and substance disorder: a matched-pairs study. Am J Addict 8: 332–336.
28. Johnson RS, Tobin JW, Cellucci T (1992) Personality characteristics of cocaine and alcohol abusers: more alike than different. Addict Behav 17: 159–166.
29. Westermeyer J, Peng G (1977) Opium and heroin addicts in Laos. II. A study of matched pairs. J Nerv Ment Dis 164: 351–354.
30. Stockwell T (1998) Towards guidelines for low-risk drinking: quantifying the short- and long-term costs of hazardous alcohol consumption. Alcohol Clin Exp Res 22: 63S–69S.
31. Caputo F, Del Re A, Brambilla R, Grignaschi A, Vignoli T et al. (2014). Sodium oxybate in maintaining alcohol abstinence in alcoholic patients according to Lesch typologies: A pilot study. Journal of Psychopharmacology, 28(1), 23–30.
32. Djordjevic ND, Jankovic SM (2006) Characteristics of decision-making process during prescribing in general practice. Vojnosanit Pregl 63: 279–285.
33. Rankovic A, Rancic N, Jovanovic M, Ivanovic M, Gajovic O, et al. (2013) Impact of imaging diagnostics on the budget-are we spending too much? Vojnosanit Pregl 70: 709–711.
34. Jakovljevic M, Vukovic M, Chia-Ching C, Yamada T, Antunovic M, et al. (2013) Do policy measures impact cost consciousness of healthcare professionals? Value in Health 16: A542, doi:10.1016/j.jval.2013.08.1376.
35. Haas L, Stargardt T, Schreyoegg J, Schlosser R, Klapp BF, et al. (2013) The trade-off between costs and quality of care in the treatment of psychosomatic patients with somatoform pain disorder. Appl Health Econ Health Policy 11: 359–368.
36. Jakovljevic M, Riegler A, Jovanovic M, Djordjevic N, Patek K, et al. (2013) Serbian and Austrian alcohol-dependent patients: a comparison of two samples regarding therapeutically relevant clinical features. Alcohol Alcohol 48: 505–508.
37. Hussey AM, Koch G, Preisser JS, Saville RB (2013) Analysis of matched studies with dichotomous outcomes using nonparametric randomization-based analysis of covariance. Statistics in Biopharmaceutical Research, 5.
38. Zweifel P (2012) The Grossman model after 40 years. Eur J Health Econ 13: 677–682.

15

Adolescent, but not Adult, Binge Ethanol Exposure Leads to Persistent Global Reductions of Choline Acetyltransferase Expressing Neurons in Brain

Ryan P. Vetreno[1]*, Margaret Broadwater[2], Wen Liu[1], Linda P. Spear[2], Fulton T. Crews[1]

1 Bowles Center for Alcohol Studies, School of Medicine, University of North Carolina at Chapel Hill, Chapel Hill, North Carolina, 27599, United States of America, **2** Center for Developmental and Behavioral Neuroscience, Department of Psychology, Binghamton University, Binghamton, New York, 13902, United States of America

Abstract

During the adolescent transition from childhood to adulthood, notable maturational changes occur in brain neurotransmitter systems. The cholinergic system is composed of several distinct nuclei that exert neuromodulatory control over cognition, arousal, and reward. Binge drinking and alcohol abuse are common during this stage, which might alter the developmental trajectory of this system leading to long-term changes in adult neurobiology. In Experiment 1, adolescent intermittent ethanol (AIE; 5.0 g/kg, i.g., 2-day on/2-day off from postnatal day [P] 25 to P55) treatment led to persistent, global reductions of choline acetyltransferase (ChAT) expression. Administration of the Toll-like receptor 4 agonist lipopolysaccharide to young adult rats (P70) produced a reduction in ChAT+IR that mimicked AIE. To determine if the binge ethanol-induced ChAT decline was unique to the adolescent, Experiment 2 examined ChAT+IR in the basal forebrain following adolescent (P28–P48) and adult (P70–P90) binge ethanol exposure. Twenty-five days later, ChAT expression was reduced in adolescent, but not adult, binge ethanol-exposed animals. In Experiment 3, expression of ChAT and vesicular acetylcholine transporter expression was found to be significantly reduced in the alcoholic basal forebrain relative to moderate drinking controls. Together, these data suggest that adolescent binge ethanol decreases adult ChAT expression, possibly through neuroimmune mechanisms, which might impact adult cognition, arousal, or reward sensitivity.

Editor: Yael Abreu-Villaça, Universidade do Estado do Rio de Janeiro, Brazil

Funding: This work was supported in part by the National Institutes of Health, National Institute on Alcoholism and Alcohol Abuse (AA019767, AA11605, AA007573, AA021040, and AA018026), the Neurobiology of Adolescent Drinking in Adulthood (NADIA [AA020023, AA020024, and AA020022]), and the Bowles Center for Alcohol Studies. The NIH, NIAAA, NADIA, and Bowles Center for Alcohol Studies had no further role in the study design, collection, analysis, and interpretation of data, writing of the report, or decision to submit the article for publication.

Competing Interests: The authors have declared that no competing interests exist.

* Email: rvetreno@email.unc.edu

Introduction

Adolescence is a neurodevelopmental period in humans and other mammalian species encompassing the transition from childhood to adulthood, and includes increased social interactions, interest in risky behavior (i.e., novelty- and sensation-seeking), and ethanol consumption [1]. Studies of the adolescent brain indicate that many regions continue to undergo significant morphological maturation and refinement of several neurotransmitter systems [2,3], including the cholinergic system [2]. The cholinergic system is divided into eight nuclei of projection neurons in the basal forebrain and hindbrain (Ch1–Ch8) as well as brain region specific intrinsic interneurons, such as striatal cholinergic interneurons. The basal forebrain consists of the medial septum and vertical limb of the diagonal band (Ch1/2) that project to the hippocampus. The horizontal limb of the diagonal band (Ch3) projects to the olfactory bulbs as well as the piriform and entorhinal cortices. Cholinergic neurons of the nucleus basalis magnocellularis (Ch4) provide major inputs to the entire neocortex and basolateral amygdala, consistent with involvement of the basal forebrain in cognition, executive function, and stress/anxiety states [4–7]. Cholinergic cells of the pedunculopontine (Ch5) and the laterodorsal tegmental nucleus (Ch6) project to the thalamus [7], and regulate cortical arousal and behavioral control [8]. The medial habenula (Ch7) projects to the interpeduncular nucleus [9], and plays a role in avoidance learning and behavioral control [10] as well as possibly contributing to habenular regulation of reward pathways [11]. The parabigeminal nucleus (Ch8), which projects to several subcortical visual centers as well as the amygdala [12], is involved in processing of visual information [13]. Thus, continued maturation of the brain cholinergic system during adolescence likely contributes to maturation of multiple brain functions.

Adolescent risk-taking and sensation-novelty seeking coincide with increased experimentation with alcohol and other drugs of abuse [14]. Recent studies find that by 14 years of age, alcohol use has become normative among youth in the United States, with current statistics indicating that approximately 10% of 13–14 year old 8th graders, 25% of 12th graders, and >40% of college students reporting heavy episodic binge drinking (i.e., >5 consecutive drinks per binge drinking episode) [15]. Adolescence and young adulthood are developmental periods with the greatest risk for the onset of alcohol abuse, and adult alcohol use disorders and other drinking problems are associated with a younger age of drinking onset [16]. Developing neurons are generally more sensitive to alcohol and other drugs of abuse, and hence developmental changes occurring in the adolescent brain may imbue adolescence as a vulnerable period of elevated risk for later addictive and other disorders [17]. The developing cholinergic system may be particularly vulnerable. Studies of nicotine exposure suggest that adolescence is a critical period of risk for the developing cholinergic system [18]. Ehlers and colleagues [19] found that adolescent ethanol vapor-exposed rats exhibited reduced ChAT+IR in the basal forebrain (Ch1–4) in adulthood that correlated with increased "disinhibitory" open field behavior as well as altered adult arousal and affective states. These findings support the hypothesis that adolescent binge ethanol exposure persistently alters expression of ChAT+IR cells throughout the cholinergic nuclei of the brain, which might contribute to long-term dysfunction.

We report here that adolescent intermittent ethanol (AIE) decreased ChAT+IR in the majority of cholinergic projection nuclei as well as striatal cholinergic interneurons. Further, we found reductions of basal forebrain ChAT+IR immediately following the conclusion of AIE (postnatal day [P]56) that persisted into later adulthood (P220). Since AIE has been found to increase brain neuroimmune gene expression and signaling, we induced neuroimmune genes using the TLR4 agonist lipopolysaccharide and found a reduction of ChAT+IR that was similar to AIE. Interestingly, a comparison of ethanol exposure in adolescents with comparable exposure in mature adults found that only adolescents undergo a prolonged loss of ChAT+IR following ethanol exposure. Finally, assessment of cholinergic cell markers in the post-mortem human brain revealed diminished protein expression of vesicular acetylcholine transporter and ChAT in the alcoholic basal forebrain, relative to moderate drinking controls. These data suggest that adolescent cholinergic neurons are uniquely sensitive to binge ethanol exposure. Further, a loss of brain cholinergic neurons could contribute to long-term changes in arousal, sleep patterns, cognition, and a variety of other brain functions observed in alcoholism.

Materials and Methods

Experiment 1

Animals. Young time-mated pregnant female Wistar rats (embryonic day 17; Harlan Sprague-Dawley, Indianapolis, IN) were acclimated to our animal facility prior to birthing at the University of North Carolina at Chapel Hill. On postnatal day (P)1 (24 h after birth), litters were culled to 10 pups. Litters were housed in standard clear plastic tubs with shavings until group housing with same-sex littermates at the time of weaning on P21. All animals were housed in a temperature- (20°C) and humidity-controlled vivarium on a 12 h/12 h light/dark cycle (light onset at 0700 h), and provided *ad libitum* access to food and water. Experimental procedures were approved by the IACUC of the University of North Carolina at Chapel Hill, and conducted in accordance with NIH regulations for the care and use of animals in research.

Adolescent Intermittent Ethanol (AIE) Treatment. On P21, male Wistar rats were randomly assigned to either: (i) AIE or (ii) water control (CON). From P25 to P55, AIE animals received intragastric (i.g.) administration of ethanol (5.0 g/kg, 20% ethanol w/v) and CON subjects received comparable volumes of H_2O on a 2-day on/2-day off schedule. Body weights (g) were measured for the duration of experimentation. Tail blood was collected to assess blood ethanol content (BEC) one h after ethanol administration on P38 and P54, and BECs were calculated using a GM7 Analyzer (Analox; London, UK). On P38 and P54, mean BECs (±SEM) were 189±5 mg/dL and 190±8 mg/dL, respectively, and did not differ across experiments (all p's≥0.2; see Figure 1A insert). For the duration of AIE exposure, subjects evidenced dramatic increases in body weight that did not differ as a function of treatment during AIE exposure (all p's>0.05, P25: CON = 73±1 g, AIE = 73±1 g; P55: CON = 304±6 g, AIE = 286±6 g; P80: 405±8 g, AIE = 389±7 g). However, by P220, AIE-exposed animals weighed significantly less than CON animals (CON = 622±18 g, AIE = 553±17 g [one-way ANOVA: $F = 7.9$, $p<0.05$ (see Figure 1)]).

Lipopolysaccharide (LPS) Administration. On P70, AIE- and CON-exposed animals received a single intraperitoneal (i.p.) injection of 1.0 mg/kg LPS (*E. Coli*, serotype 0111:B4; Sigma-Aldrich, St. Louis, MO). Subjects were monitored for 24 h following LPS administration and sacrificed 10 days later on P80.

Experiment 2

Animals. For the adolescent vs. adult intermittent ethanol experiment, male Sprague-Dawley rats were bred and reared at Binghamton University. On P1, litters were culled to 10 pups. Pups were housed in standard clear plastic tubs with shavings until being pair-housed with a same-sex littermate at the time of weaning on P21. All animals were housed in a temperature- (20°C) and humidity-controlled vivarium on a 12 h/12 h light/dark cycle (light onset at 0700 h), and provided *ad libitum* access to food and water. All experimental procedures were approved by the IACUC of the Binghamton University – State University of New York, and conducted in accordance with NIH regulations for the care and use of animals in research.

AIE Treatment. On P21, male Sprague-Dawley rats were randomly assigned to either: (i) binge ethanol exposure (BINGE) or (ii) CON. All animals were treated i.g. with ethanol (4.0 g/kg, 25% ethanol v/v) or comparable volumes of H_20 every other day either during adolescence (P28 – P48) or young adulthood (P70–P90). After the last exposure day, animals were left undisturbed except for routine animal care and adult Pavlovian fear conditioning, which was previously published [20]. Tissue samples were collected 25 days later for assessment of immunohistochemical assessment of ChAT+IR (see below).

Perfusion, Brain Tissue Preparation, and Immunohistochemistry. At the conclusion of EXPERIMENT 1 and 2, animals were anesthetized with sodium pentobarbital (100 mg/kg, i.p.) and transcardially perfused with 0.1 M phosphate-buffered saline (PBS, pH 7.4), followed by 4.0% paraformaldehyde in PBS. Brains were excised and post-fixed in 4.0% paraformaldehyde for 24 h at 4°C followed by 4 days of fixation in 30% sucrose solution. Coronal sections were cut (40 μm) on a sliding microtome (MICROM HM450; Thermo-Scientific, Austin, TX), and sections were sequentially collected into well plates and stored at −20°C in a cryoprotectant solution (30% glycol/30% ethylene glycol in PBS) for later immunohistochemistry.

Free-floating sections (every 6th section containing the region of interest) were washed in 0.1 M PBS, incubated in 0.3% H_2O_2 to inhibit endogenous peroxidases, and blocked with normal goat serum (MP Biomedicals, Solon, OH). Sections were incubated in goat polyclonal anti-ChAT (catalog #AB144P; Millipore, Temecula, CA) for 24 h at 4°C or goat polyclonal anti-vesicular acetylcholine transporter (VAChT; catalog #ABN100; Millipore). Sections were then washed with PBS, incubated for 1 h in biotinylated secondary antibody (1:200; Vector Laboratories, Burlingame, CA), and incubated for 1 h in avidin-biotin complex solution (Vectastain ABC Kit; Vector Laboratories). The chromagen, nickel-enhanced diaminobenzidine (Sigma-Aldrich, St. Louis,

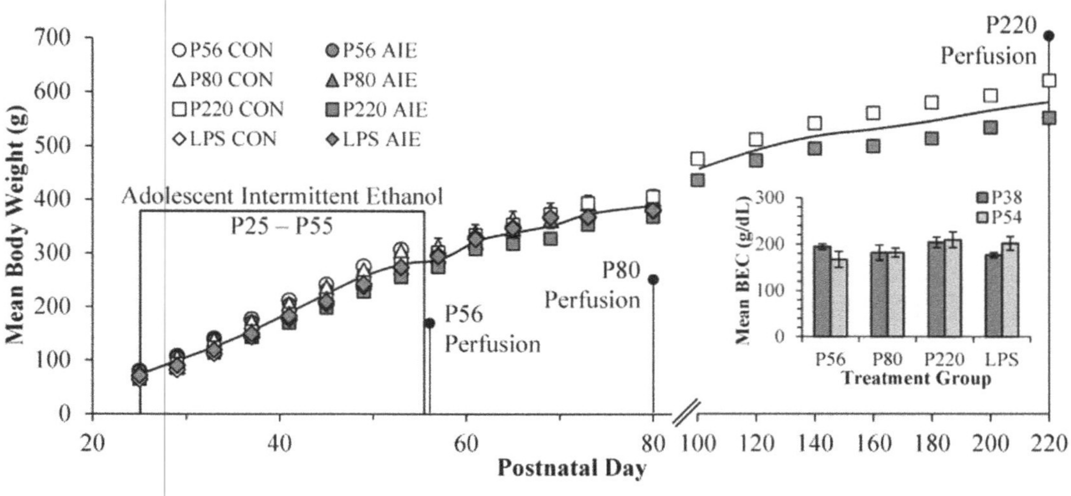

Figure 1. Graphical representation of the adolescent intermittent ethanol (AIE) exposure paradigm. Rats were treated from postnatal day (P) 25 to P55 with either ethanol (5.0 g/kg 20% ethanol v/v, i.g.) or a comparable volume of water on a 2-day on/2-day off administration schedule. Blood ethanol concentration (BEC) was measured one hr after ethanol exposure on P38 and P54. Twenty-four hours, 25 days, and 165 days following the conclusion of AIE, rats were sacrificed for immunohistochemistry.

MO), was used to visualize immunoreactivity. Tissue was mounted onto slides, dehydrated, and coverslipped. Negative control for non-specific binding was conducted on separate sections employing the abovementioned procedures with the exception that the primary antibody was omitted.

Microscopic Quantification and Image Analysis. Across studies, BioQuant Nova Advanced Image Analysis (R&M Biometric, Nashville, TN) was used for image capture and analysis. Images were captured with an Olympus UPlan Fl objective (10×/0.30) using an Olympus BX50 microscope and Sony DXC-390 video camera linked to a computer. For each measure, the microscope, camera, and software were background corrected and normalized to preset light levels to ensure fidelity of data acquisition. Assessment of ChAT+IR was performed in Ch1–Ch8, interpeduncular nucleus, and striatum (see Figure 2) according to the atlas of Paxinos and Watson [21]. The total number of ChAT+IR cells was quantified in a 1:6 series throughout Ch1–Ch6, and striatal tissue samples, and data are expressed as cells per mm^2. Since ChAT expression was densely distributed throughout Ch7, Ch8, and interpeduncular tissue samples making identification of individual neurons difficult, ChAT+IR pixel density was assessed in a 1:6 series and rigorously thresholded to normalize pixel intensity [22]. The threshold for pixel density was determined from the control subjects by calculating the average of the darkest and lightest values from each region of interest (i.e., Ch5 [medial habenula], Ch8 [parabigeminal nucleus], and interpeduncular nucleus), and sections were imaged under identical conditions to avoid non-systematic variations [23]. The outlined regions of interest were determined and staining density calculated by dividing the pixel count by the overall area (mm^2).

Experiment 3

Post-mortem Human Samples. Frozen samples of post-mortem human basal forebrain were obtained from the New South Wales Tissue Resource Centre at the University of Sydney (ethics committee approval number: X11-0107), supported by the National Health and Medical Research Council of Australia-Schizophrenia Research Institute and the National Institute of Alcohol Abuse and Alcoholism (NIH [NIAAA] R24AA012725). Subject information was collected through personal interviews, next-of-kin interviews, and medical records, and is presented in Table 1. Only individuals with alcohol dependence uncomplicated by liver cirrhosis and/or nutritional deficiencies were included. All psychiatric and alcohol use disorder diagnoses were confirmed using the Diagnostic Instrument for Brain Studies that complies with the Diagnostic and Statistical Manual of Mental Disorders [24].

Western Blot Analysis. Approximately 75 mg of frozen basal forebrain tissue was homogenized in 0.8 ml RIPA lysis buffer (Sigma-Aldrich) containing protease inhibitor (1:100; Sigma-Aldrich) and centrifuged at 14,000 rpm at 4°C for 20 min. After centrifugation, protein content in the supernatant was assessed using the Pierce BCA Protein Assay Kit (ThermoScientific, Rockford, IL, Cat # 23227), and 20 μg of protein from each denatured sample was loaded into precast polyacrylamide mini-gel (4–15%; Bio-Rad, Hercules, CA), and blotted onto immunoblot PVDF membranes (Bio-Rad). Immunoblot membranes were blocked in Odyssey blocking buffer (LiCOR Biosciences, Lincoln, NE), and incubated in a primary antibody solution containing either goat anti-ChAT (1:2000; Millipore) and rabbit anti-tubulin (1:1000; Cat # 2128; Cell Signaling Technologies, Danvers, MA), mouse anti-VAChT (1:200; Cat # ab68984; Abcam, Cambridge, MA) and rabbit anti-tubulin (1:1000), or goat anti-acetylcholinesterase (AChE; 1:200; Cat # ab31276; Abcam, Cambridge, MA) and rabbit anti-tubulin (1:1000) for 24 h at 4°C. After washing, the immunoblot membranes were incubated in appropriate fluorescent secondary antibodies (Rockland Immunochemicals, Gilbertsville, PA), and bands were scanned with an Odyssey Infrared Imager (LiCOR Biosciences). Band intensity was quantified using Odyssey Imaging software and normalized to tubulin. All experiments were run in triplicate.

Enzyme-linked Immunoabsorbent Assay (ELISA) Analysis. Frozen basal forebrain tissue samples were homogenized in cold lysis buffer (20 mM Tris, 0.25 M sucrose, 2 mM EDTA, 10 mM EGTA, 1% Triton X-100) containing one tablet of Complete Mini Protease Inhibitor Cocktail (Roche Diagnostics, Indianapolis, IN). Homogenates were centrifuged at 5,000× g for five min, supernatant was collected, and protein levels determined using the Pierce BCA Protein Assay Kit (ThermoScientific). The

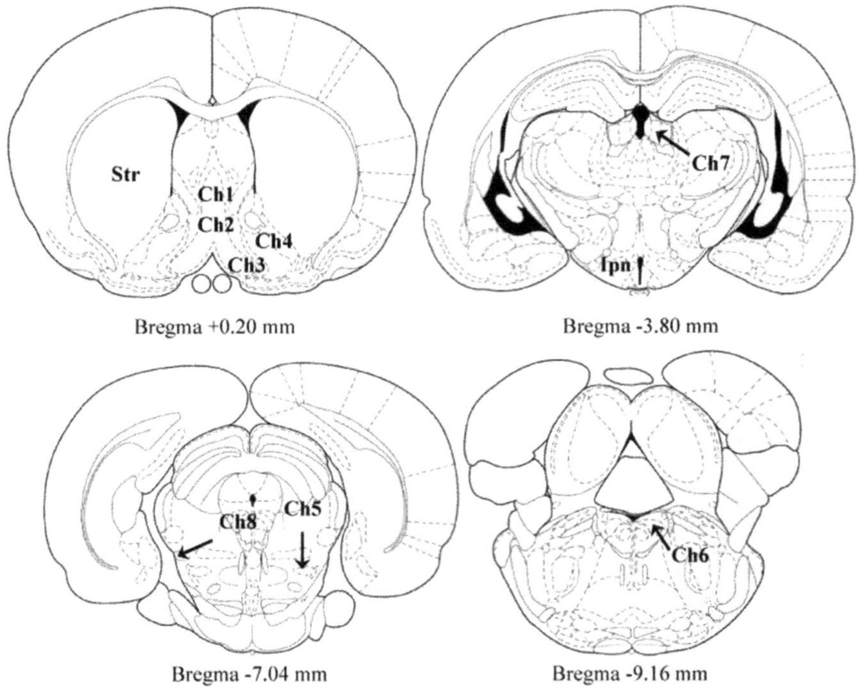

Figure 2. Schematic depicting the location of cholinergic nuclei of the rat brain. Representative micrographs based on the atlas of Paxinos and Watson [21] defining cholinergic brain nuclei assessed for choline acetyltransferase immunoreactivity. Ch1 = medial septum; Ch2 = horizontal limb of the diagonal band; Ch3 = vertical limb of the diagonal band; Ch4 = nucleus basalis magnocellularis; Ch5 = pedunculopontine nuclei; Ch6 = lateral dorsal tegmental nucleus; Ch7 = medial habenula; Ch8 = parabigeminal nuclei; Str = striatum; Ipn = interpeduncular nucleus.

Table 1. Case characteristics of human subjects.

Group	Age at Death	Gender	PMI	Clinical Cause of Death
Control	24	Male	43	Undetermined (Consistent with idiopathic cardiac arrhythmia)
Control	43	Male	66	Aspiration pneumonia
Control	44	Male	50	Ischemic heart disease
Control	46	Male	29	Acute myocardial infarction
Control	50	Male	30	Coronary artery disease
Control	50	Male	40	Haemopericardium
Control	53	Male	16	Dilated cardiomyopathy
Control	60	Male	28	Ischemic heart disease
Control	62	Male	46	Ischemic heart disease
Control	48	Male	24	Ischemic heart disease
Alcoholic	49	Male	16	Coronary artery thrombosis
Alcoholic	45	Male	7	Drowning
Alcoholic	49	Male	44	Ischemic heart disease
Alcoholic	61	Male	59	Myocarditis
Alcoholic	51	Male	27	Gastrointestinal hemorrhage
Alcoholic	61	Male	23	Atherosclerotic cardiovascular disease
Alcoholic	42	Male	41	Combined bromoxynil and alcohol toxicity
Alcoholic	50	Male	17	Ischemic heart disease
Alcoholic	44	Male	15	Ischemic heart disease
Alcoholic	43	Male	43	Carbon monoxide intoxication/Alcohol intoxication

PMI: post-mortem interval.

levels of ChAT in the basal forebrain were measured with a human ELISA kit for ChAT from Mybiosource (MBS2020762; San Diego, CA) according to the manufacturer's instruction.

Statistical Analysis. Statistical analysis was performed using SPSS (Chicago, IL). Analysis of variance (ANOVA) was used to assess BECs, body weights, immunohistochemistry, Western blot, and ELISA data. To ensure normal distribution of data sets, the Shapiro-Wilk Test of Normality was performed, and data sets identified as non-parametric were analyzed with the independent samples Mann-Whitney U Test. Post-hoc analyses were performed using Tukey's HSD when necessary. Outlier tests were run in each experiment, and any subject with a score exceeding 2 standard deviations greater or less than the group mean was removed from further analysis. No more than one animal was removed from any group. All values are reported as mean ± SEM, and significance was defined as $p \leq 0.05$.

Results

Adolescent binge ethanol exposure reduces ChAT+IR throughout brain cholinergic nuclei

Choline acetyltransferase, which provides a measure of cholinergic cell populations [25], was assessed in all major cholinergic brain nuclei following adolescent binge ethanol exposure. We model human adolescent drinking behavior using an intermittent schedule consistent with known patterns of heavy weekend binge drinking, but not daily drinking associated with alcoholism in adulthood. Immunohistochemistry was used to assess ChAT+IR in cholinergic projection neurons of Ch1–Ch8 as well as cholinergic interneurons of the striatum and medial habenular (Ch7) terminal fields in the interpeduncular nucleus 25 days after AIE in young adulthood (P80). In CON and AIE basal forebrain samples, assessment of ChAT+IR cells revealed darkly stained cell bodies and processes, with less cell staining in the AIE-exposed animals. Within the basal forebrain, AIE decreased ChAT+IR cell populations by 29% (±4%) and 36% (±6%) in the medial septum/vertical limb of the diagonal band (Ch1/Ch2; one-way ANOVA: $F_{[1,15]} = 21.1$, $p<0.01$) and the horizontal limb of the diagonal band/nucleus basalis magnocellularis (Ch3/Ch4; one-way ANOVA: $F_{[1,15]} = 20.5$, $p<0.01$ [see Figure 3A]), respectively. Thus, AIE reduced ChAT+IR cells in the young adult basal forebrain.

In the brainstem, ChAT+IR was characterized by large and small darkly stained cell bodies and processes. In the pedunculopontine nucleus (Ch5), adolescent binge ethanol reduced ChAT+IR by approximately 21% (±3%), relative to CON animals (one-way ANOVA: $F_{[1,15]} = 19.4$, $p<0.01$). Similarly, in the laterodorsal tegmental nucleus (Ch6), AIE reduced ChAT expression by 17% (±5%) when compared to CON subjects (one-way ANOVA: $F_{[1,15]} = 4.9$, $p<0.05$ [see Figure 3B]). Thus, similar to the basal forebrain, adolescent binge ethanol exposure reduced ChAT+IR in the young adult brainstem cholinergic nuclei.

Since ChAT expression was reduced in the basal forebrain and brainstem cholinergic nuclei, we also assessed immunoreactivity in the medial habenula (Ch7) and parabigeminal nucleus (Ch8) as well as the interpeduncular nucleus. In the medial habenula (Ch7), ChAT+IR was characterized by well-defined homogenous expression and dense neuropil prompting quantification of ChAT+IR by pixel density. Adolescent binge ethanol exposure reduced ChAT+IR by 34% (±7%) in the medial habenula (Ch7; one-way ANOVA: $F_{[1,15]} = 10.8$, $p<0.01$ [see Figure 3C]), relative to CON animals. The interpeduncular nucleus, a major cholinergic projection site of medial habenula via the fasciculus retroflexus, showed darkly stained ChAT+IR terminal fields in CON- and AIE-exposed animals. Choline acetyltransferase expression was reduced by 27% (±4%) in the AIE animals (one-way ANOVA: $F_{[1,15]} = 28.1$, $p<0.01$ [see Figure 3D]) as compared to CONs. Analysis of ChAT+IR in the parabigeminal nucleus (Ch8) found that AIE did not affect ChAT+IR ($p>0.6$ [data not shown]). In the striatum, ChAT+IR was characterized by darkly stained neurons that were homogenously distributed and ChAT-immunopositive neuron counts were reduced by 20% (±5%) in the AIE animals (one-way ANOVA: $F_{[1,7]} = 9.5$, $p<0.01$ [see Figure 4]), relative to the CONs. Together, these data reveal that binge ethanol exposure during adolescence reduces ChAT+IR in most, but not all, cholinergic brain nuclei in the young adult brain.

To further determine the impact of AIE treatment on cholinergic cells in the young adult basal forebrain, expression of vesicular acetylcholine transporter (VAChT) expression was assessed. VAChT transports cytosolic acetylcholine into synaptic vesicles for storage until release and provides an additional marker for cholinergic cells [26]. In CON and AIE basal forebrain samples, assessment of VAChT+IR cells revealed immunoreactive cell bodies, with less cell staining in the AIE-treated animals. The Shapiro-Wilk Test of Normality was significant for this analysis ($p<0.05$) indicating that the data was not normally distributed. In the young adult basal forebrain, AIE treatment decreased VAChT+IR cell populations by 16% (±1%), relative to CONs (Independent Samples Mann-Whitney U Test: $U[13] = 0.0$, $Z = -3.13$, $p<0.01$; see Figure 5). Thus, AIE treatment reduced VAChT+IR cells in the young adult basal forebrain.

Choline acetyltransferase expression is persistently reduced in the basal forebrain following adolescent binge ethanol exposure

Our finding that adolescent binge ethanol exposure decreased ChAT+IR throughout the young adult brain (P80) prompted us to assess the persistence of the ChAT reductions in the basal forebrain following AIE treatment. Tissue samples were collected from the basal forebrain, and ChAT+IR was assessed in animals sacrificed on P56 (24 h post-AIE treatment), P80 (25 days post-AIE treatment), and P220 (165 days post-AIE treatment). Evaluation of ChAT+IR neurons revealed well defined heterogeneously distributed large and small darkly stained cell bodies and processes in CON and AIE basal forebrain samples (see Figure 6). A 2×3 ANOVA (Treatment [CON vs AIE]×Age [P56 vs P80 vs P220]) found that relative to CON subjects, AIE treatment significantly reduced ChAT+IR in the medial septum/vertical limb of the diagonal band (Ch1/Ch2; main effect of Treatment: $F_{[1,41]} = 25.2$, $p<0.01$; see Figure 6A). Similarly, AIE treatment significantly reduced ChAT expression in the horizontal limb of the diagonal band/nucleus basalis magnocellularis (Ch3/Ch4), relative to CONs (main effect of Treatment: $F_{[1,41]} = 47.4$, $p<0.01$; see Figure 6B). There were no main effects of Age or interactions of Treatment×Age in either analysis. Taken together, these data reveal that adolescent binge ethanol exposure reduces ChAT expression (P56) that persists for long periods (P220), perhaps for the duration of the organism's life.

Lipopolysaccharide exposure mimics adolescent binge ethanol-induced reductions of ChAT+IR cell populations in the basal forebrain

Previous research from our laboratory found that adolescent binge ethanol exposure persistently upregulates innate immune signaling and Toll-like receptor 4 (TLR4) expression that persists in the young adult brain [22,27]. Lipopolysaccharide (LPS) is an endotoxin agonist at TLR4 whose activation leads to proinflam-

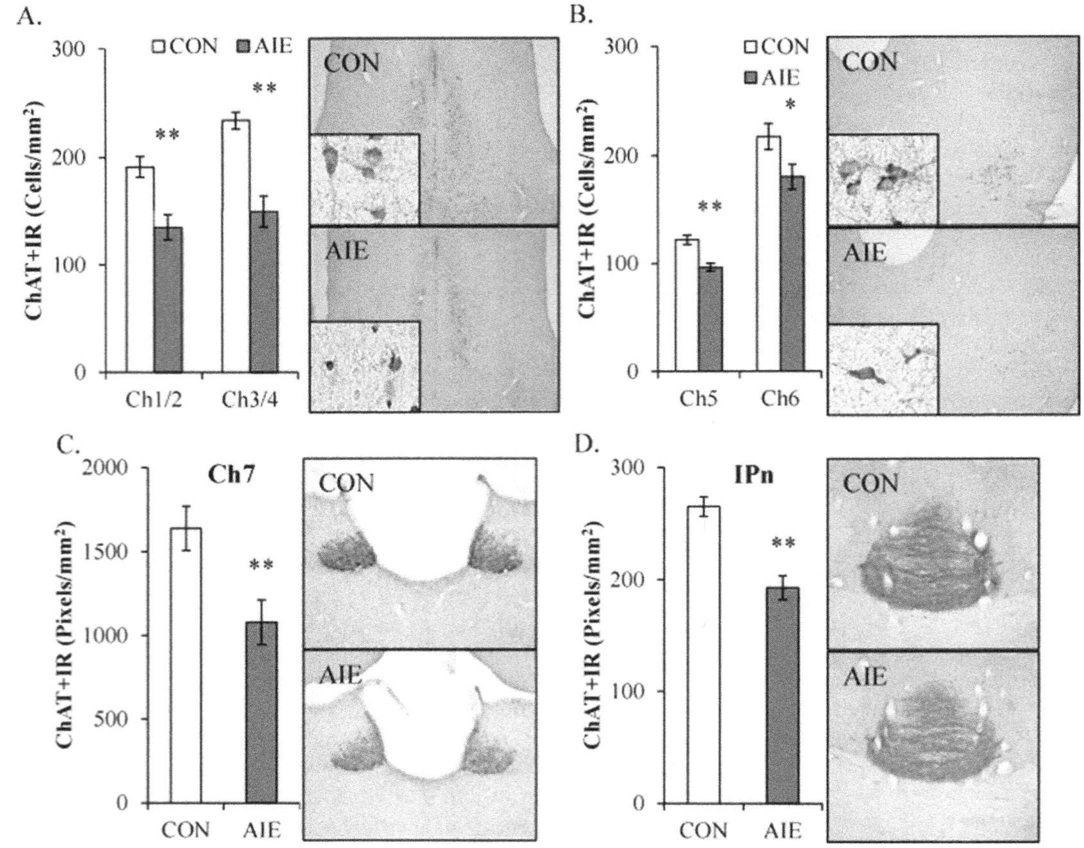

Figure 3. Adolescent intermittent ethanol (AIE) exposure leads to global reductions of choline acetyltransferase (ChAT)-immunopositive cells in the young adult brain. (A) Profile counts revealed that AIE reduced ChAT+IR in the medial septum/vertical limb of the diagonal band (Ch1/Ch2 [29%±4%]) and horizontal limb of the diagonal band/nucleus basalis magnocellularis (Ch3/Ch4 [36%±6%]) of the basal forebrain, relative to controls (CONs). Representative photomicrographs of ChAT+IR cells in Ch1/Ch2 of CON- and AIE-exposed basal forebrain. (B) Profile counts found that AIE reduced ChAT+IR in the pedunculopontine nucleus (Ch5; 21%±3%) and the laterodorsal tegmental nucleus (Ch6; 17%±5%) of the brainstem, relative to CONs. Representative photomicrographs of ChAT+IR cells in Ch5 of the brainstem from CON- and AIE-exposed animals. (C) ChAT pixel density (×1000 pixels/mm^2) was reduced by 34% (±7%) in the medial habenula (Ch7) of AIE-exposed animals, relative to CONs. Representative photomicrographs of ChAT+IR cells in Ch7 from CON- and AIE-exposed animals. (D) AIE reduced ChAT pixel density (×1000 pixels/mm^2) by 27% (±4%) in the interpeduncular nucleus (IPn), relative to CONs. Representative photomicrographs of ChAT immunoreactivity cells in the IPn from CON- and AIE-exposed animals. Data are presented as mean ± SEM. * indicates $p<0.05$ and ** indicates <0.01, relative to CON rats.

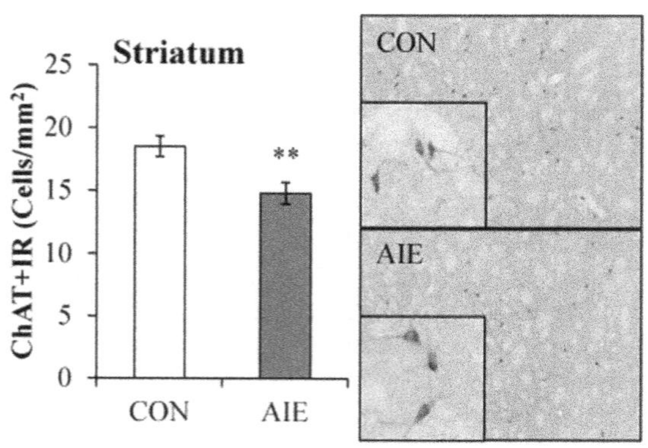

Figure 4. Adolescent intermittent ethanol (AIE) exposure leads to long-term reductions of choline acetyltransferase (ChAT)-immunopositive cells in the young adult striatum. Profile counts of ChAT+IR found a 12% (±3%) reduction of ChAT expression in the striatum of AIE-exposed young adult rats, relative to CONs. Representative photomicrographs of ChAT+IR cells in the striatum from CON- and AIE-exposed animals. Data are presented as mean ± SEM. ** indicates $p<0.01$, relative to CON rats.

matory cytokine and oxidase induction in brain [28]. To determine if neuroimmune activation contributes to the reduction of cholinergic cells, CON- and AIE-exposed animals received a single dose of LPS (1.0 mg/kg, i.p.) on P70, and ChAT+IR was assessed in the basal forebrain on P80. In CONs, immunohistochemistry revealed darkly stained soma and processes throughout the basal forebrain. ChAT-immunopositive cells in the AIE-exposed animals appeared diminished relative to CONs with a similar staining profile observed in the LPS- and AIE+LPS-exposed animals. Expression of ChAT in the medial septum/vertical limb of the diagonal band (Ch1/Ch2) and the horizontal limb of the diagonal band/nucleus basalis magnocellularis (Ch3/Ch4) of the basal forebrain was analyzed using separate 2×2 ANOVAs (Treatment [CON vs AIE]×Drug [LPS vs SAL]). Within the medial septum/vertical limb of the diagonal band (Ch1/Ch2), AIE treatment significantly reduced ChAT+IR, relative to CONs (main effect of Treatment: $F_{[1,28]}=5.6$, $p<0.05$). Although there was no main effect of Drug ($p>0.05$), there was a significant interaction ($F_{[1,28]}=7.2$, $p<0.05$). Post-hoc analysis found that ChAT+IR was reduced following AIE (29% [±6%]; $p<0.01$), CON+LPS (27% [±6%]; $p<0.05$), and AIE+LPS (25% [±6%]; $p<0.05$), relative to CONs (see Figure 7A).

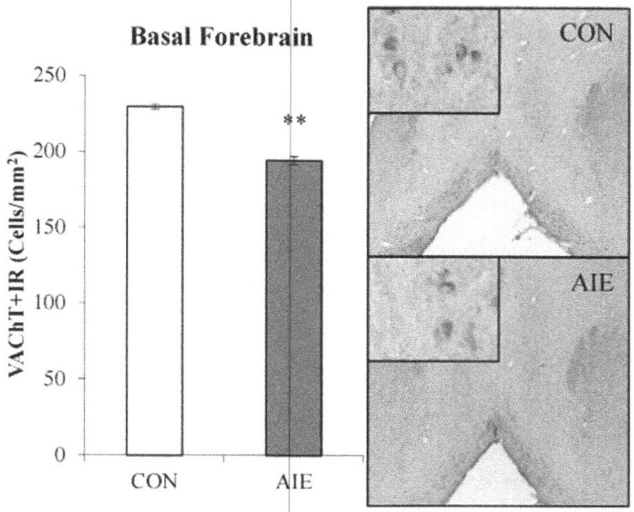

Figure 5. Adolescent intermittent ethanol (AIE) exposure reduces vesicular acetylcholine transporter (VAChT) expression in the young adult basal forebrain. Profile cell counts revealed a 16% (±1%) decrease of VAChT+IR cells in the basal forebrain, relative to controls (CON). Data are presented as mean ± SEM. ** indicates $p<0.01$, relative to CON rats.

Analysis of the horizontal limb of the diagonal band/nucleus basalis magnocellularis (Ch3/Ch4) revealed a significant main effect of Treatment ($F_{[1,28]} = 4.5$, $p<0.05$) and Drug ($F_{[1,28]} = 4.5$, $p<0.05$) as well as a significant interaction ($F_{[1,28]} = 10.2$, $p<0.01$). Post-hoc analysis revealed that AIE (36% [±7%]; $p<0.01$), CON+LPS (36% [±7%]; $p<0.01$), and AIE+LPS (30% [±7%]; $p<0.05$) reduced ChAT+IR, relative to CONs (see Figure 7B). Thus, administration of the TLR4 agonist LPS produced a similar decrease in ChAT+IR neurons in CONs, but did not further reduce ChAT+IR cells in AIE-exposed animals.

Adolescent, but not adult, binge ethanol exposure reduces ChAT+IR neurons in the basal forebrain

Adolescents respond differently to alcohol than adults [3], being particularly sensitive to binge ethanol-induced frontal cortical brain damage [29] and inhibition of neurogenesis [30] while adult neurogenesis is only transiently reduced following binge ethanol exposure [31]. To determine the potential age-associated vulnerability of ChAT+IR cells in the basal forebrain, adolescent (P28–48) and young adult (P70–90) male Sprague-Dawley rats received binge ethanol exposure (4.0 g/kg, 25% ethanol v/v; every other day). In CON- and BINGE-exposed basal forebrain samples, assessment of ChAT+IR cells revealed large and small darkly stained cell bodies and processes in adolescent and young adult animals. Assessment of ChAT+IR in the medial septum/vertical limb of the diagonal band (Ch1/Ch2) with a 2×2 ANOVA (Treatment [CON vs BINGE] ×Age [Adolescent vs Young Adult]) did not reveal any main effects (both p's>0.05), but did find a significant interaction ($F_{[1,24]} = 9.7$, $p<0.01$). Post-hoc analyses found that, relative to adolescent CON subjects, ChAT expression was reduced in adolescent binge-exposed rats (37% [±6%]; $p<0.01$), but not adult subjects in either treatment group (both p's>0.4; see Figure 8A). Analysis of ChAT+IR in the horizontal limb of the diagonal band/nucleus basalis magnocellularis (Ch3/Ch4) did not yield any significant main effects (both p's>0.1), but did reveal a significant interaction ($F_{[1,24]} = 7.3$, $p<0.05$). Post-hoc analyses found that, relative to adolescent CON subjects, ChAT expression was reduced in adolescent BINGE-exposed rats (34% [±10%]; $p<0.05$), but not adult subjects in either group (both p's>0.4; see Figure 8B). Our observation of diminished ChAT expression across rat stains (Wistar and Sprague-Dawley) using different exposure parameters indicates that this effect is a general consequence of adolescent binge ethanol exposure. Thus, these data reveal that cholinergic neurons of the adolescent, but not adult, basal forebrain are uniquely vulnerable to the neurotoxic effects of binge ethanol exposure.

Cholinergic cell marker expression is reduced in the post-mortem human alcoholic basal forebrain

To determine whether cholinergic cell marker expression is altered in the human alcoholic basal forebrain, we first performed Western blot analysis of VAChT, AChE, and ChAT expression in postmortem basal forebrain tissue samples from moderate drinking controls and alcoholic. Analysis of VAChT protein concentrations revealed a significant 30% [±7%] reduction in the postmortem human alcoholic basal forebrain, relative to moderate drinking controls (one-way ANOVA: $F_{[1,16]} = 6.8$, $p<0.05$; see Figure 9A). In contrast, we did not observe a difference in between controls and alcoholics in the amount of AChE expression in the basal forebrain ($p>0.70$). Western blot analysis of ChAT yielded multiple bands at different molecular weights consistent with the presence of multiple slice variants that could not be quantitated reliably prompting us to use ELISA methodologies. ELISA assessment of ChAT protein expression revealed a significant 51% [±11%] reduction in the alcoholic basal forebrain, relative to moderate drinking control subjects (one-way ANOVA: $F_{[1,17]} = 6.0$, $p<0.05$; see Figure 9B). Thus, expression of cholinergic cell marker proteins are reduced in the human alcoholic basal forebrain.

Discussion

We report here for the first time that protein expression of ChAT and VAChT are reduced in the postmortem human alcoholic basal forebrain in comparison to moderate drinking controls. In our animal model, ChAT immunoreactivity is also reduced in the basal forebrain (Ch1–4) of late adolescent rats (P56) that persists into later adulthood (P220) following exposure to a model of adolescent binge drinking. In addition, we found that ChAT+IR is diminished throughout the young adult (P80) midbrain cholinergic system (Ch5–Ch7) and striatum. In addition to the loss of ChAT+IR in the basal forebrain, expression of VAChT was also reduced in the basal forebrain on P80. Our finding of diminished cholinergic cell protein expression in the human basal forebrain and the persistent loss of cholinergic cell markers in adults rats following adolescent binge ethanol exposure may increase the risk for dysfunction and diseases associated with aging, such as Alzheimer's disease, which also involves a loss of ChAT+IR. Adolescent alcohol abuse is associated with an increased risk for lifetime development of alcoholism [32] and alcohol-associated violence [33]. Thus, these data support the hypothesis that adolescent binge ethanol persistently reduces ChAT expression throughout the brain and these cholinergic changes might contribute to the development of adult psychopathology.

Impaired executive functioning is commonly observed in human alcoholics [34], and the basal forebrain cholinergic system is critically involved in cognitive processes. Indeed, De Rosa and colleagues [35] found that impaired cognitive flexibility in human alcoholics was associated with diminished basal forebrain activation as assessed using fMRI. While they did not directly assess the

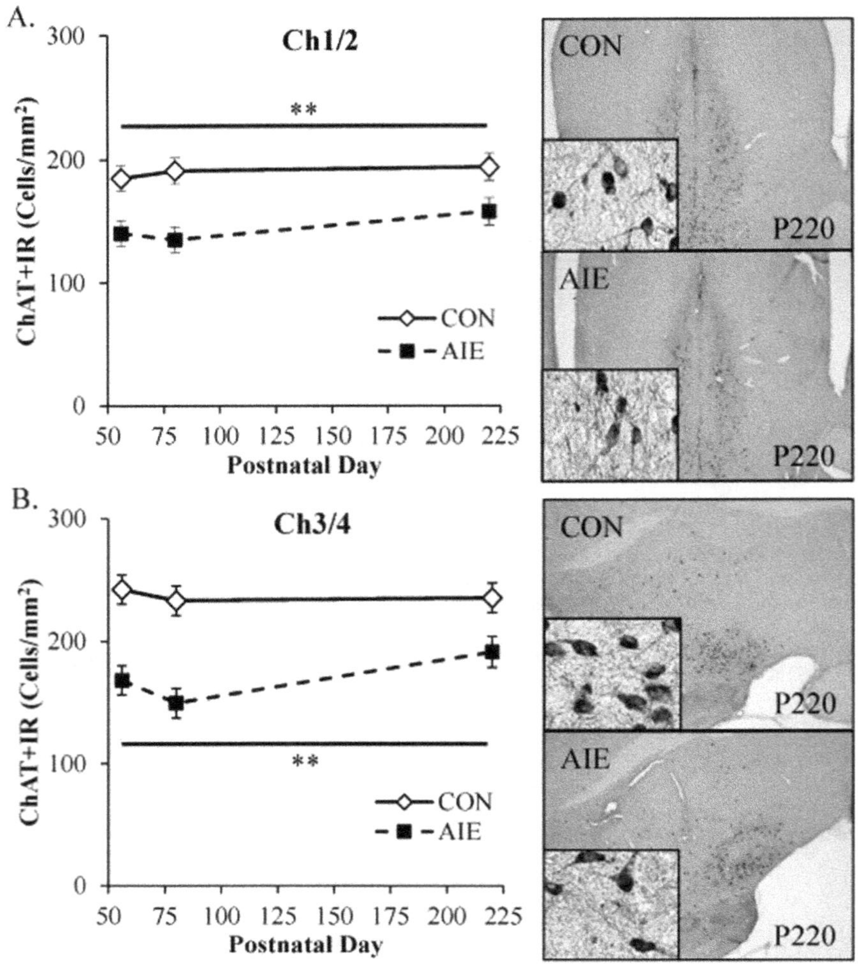

Figure 6. Choline acetyltransferase (ChAT) expression is persistently decreased in the basal forebrain following adolescent intermittent ethanol (AIE) exposure. (A) Profile counts revealed a 24% (±7%) decrease of ChAT+IR cells in the medial septum/vertical limb of the diagonal band (Ch1/Ch2) of adolescent rats (P56) 24 hours following the conclusion of AIE that persisted into adulthood (P220 [19%±3%]), relative to CONs. Representative photomicrographs of ChAT+IR cells in Ch1/Ch2 of CON- and AIE-exposed basal forebrain samples from P220 subjects. (B) Quantification of ChAT immunoreactivity in the horizontal limb of the diagonal band/nucleus basalis magnocellularis (Ch3/Ch4) revealed that AIE reduced ChAT expression by 31% (±4%) at P56 that persisted to P220 (19%±3%), relative to CONs. Representative photomicrographs of ChAT+IR cells in Ch3/Ch4 of CON- and AIE-exposed basal forebrain samples from P220 subjects. Data are presented as mean ± SEM. * indicates $p<0.05$ and ** indicates $p<0.01$, relative to CON rats.

basal forebrain cholinergic system, our finding that cholinergic cell protein expression is significantly diminished in the human alcoholic basal forebrain might underlie some of the cognitive dysfunction that characterizes alcoholism.

The AIE-associated reduction in ChAT expression throughout Ch1–Ch4 of late adolescent rats (P56) that persisted into adulthood (P220) replicates similar findings in young adult rats and mice exposed to AIE [2,19]. The cholinergic system of the basal forebrain is an important neuromodulator of memory and attention due to its innervation of the hippocampus and cortex [7,36]. It undergoes significant refinement during adolescent maturation [2], which increases its vulnerability to the neurotoxic effects of ethanol [37] and these reductions likely contribute to the neurocognitive deficits associated with adolescent binge ethanol exposure. For instance, our laboratory found deficits in reversal learning, which refers to the ability to alter a previously learned behavioral response with a new response when task demands change (i.e., a loss of behavioral flexibility), in young adult rats and mice following AIE exposure [2,27]. Reversal learning deficits are associated with prefrontal cortex dysfunction, and have also been observed in rats following 192 IgG-saporin lesions of cholinergic cells in the basal forebrain [38]. These deficits might be due to diminished cholinergic innervation of prefrontal cortex structures critical for this form of learning. In addition to involvement of the basal forebrain cholinergic system in cognition, it also plays a significant role in olfactory processes, given the projections from the horizontal limb of the diagonal band (Ch3) to the olfactory bulbs [7]. Olfactory deficits are reported in human alcoholics [39], and loss of cholinergic inputs to this region could also contribute to these deficits [40]. While adolescent binge ethanol exposure has been shown to alter glutamatergic and dopaminergic neuronal functioning [41], previous work from our laboratory found that parvalbumin+IR GABAergic interneurons of the basal forebrain are unaffected in an animal model of AIE [2], suggesting that cholinergic neurons of the basal forebrain are particularly vulnerable to the neurotoxic effects of ethanol. Thus, AIE-induced reductions of ChAT+IR in the basal forebrain may contribute to

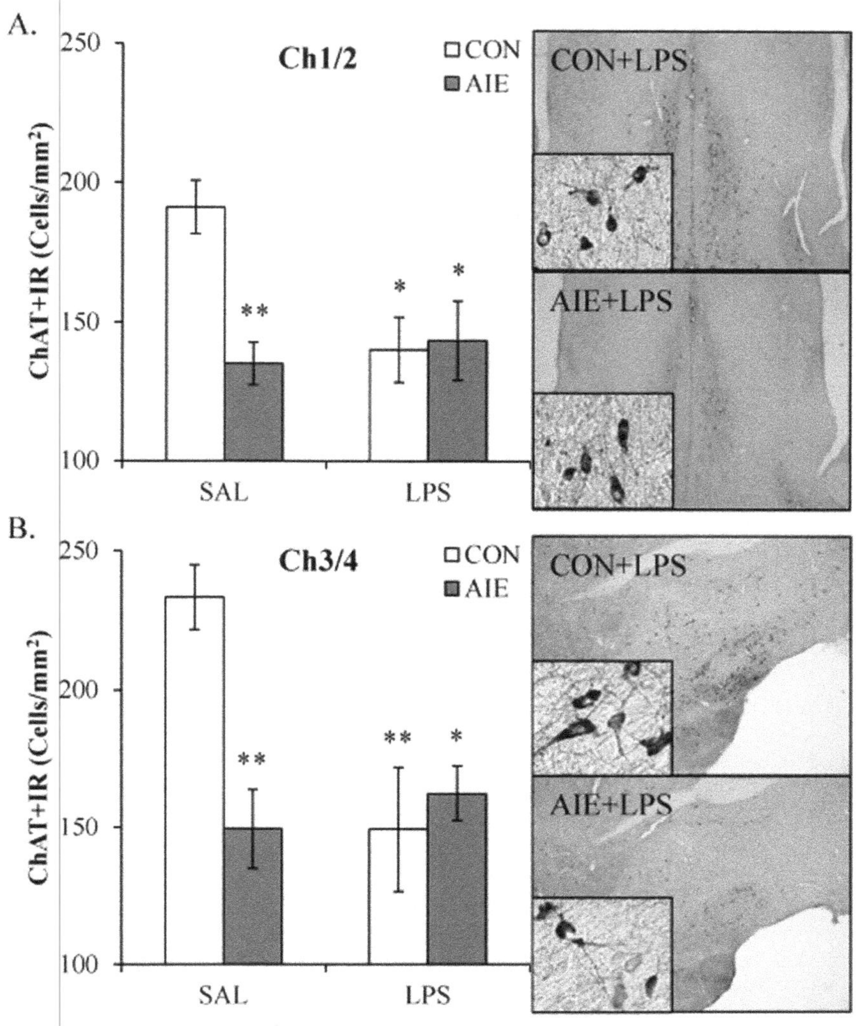

Figure 7. Exposure to lipopolysaccharide (LPS) mimics the choline acetyltransferase (ChAT) reductions associated with adolescent intermittent ethanol (AIE) exposure. (A) Profile counts in the medial septum/vertical limb of the diagonal band (Ch1/Ch2) of young adult rats (P80) revealed a significant reduction of ChAT+IR cells in AIE- (29%±6%), CON+LPS- (27%±6%), and AIE+LPS-exposed (25%±6%) rats, relative to CONs. Representative photomicrographs of ChAT+IR cells in Ch1/Ch2 of CON+LPS- and AIE+LPS-exposed rats. (B) Profile counts in the horizontal limb of the diagonal band/nucleus basalis magnocellularis (Ch3/Ch4) of young adult rats (P80) revealed a significant reduction of ChAT+IR cells in AIE- (36%±7%), CON+LPS- (36%±7%), and AIE+LPS-exposed (30%±7%) rats, relative to CONs. Representative photomicrographs of ChAT+IR cells in Ch3/Ch4 of CON+LPS- and AIE+LPS-exposed rats. Although LPS did not potentiate AIE-induced decreases of ChAT expression, it did result in a similar reduction in CON animals. Data are presented as mean ± SEM. * indicates $p<0.05$ and ** indicates $p<0.01$, relative to CON rats.

persistent behavioral flexibility deficits and olfaction in adults and adult alcoholics following adolescent binge drinking.

Brainstem cholinergic neurons, which are distributed throughout Ch5 and Ch6, provide ACh input to the reticular formation, and are involved in the regulation of sleep and wakefulness. Webster and colleagues [42] found that lesions of cholinergic cells within the brainstem disrupted REM sleep. Further, reduction of ChAT expression observed in the pedunculopontine nucleus (Ch5) of a rat model of myocardial infarction was accompanied by diminished REM sleep [43]. Sleep disturbances are associated with a variety of psychopathologies, including alcoholism [44]. In humans, alcohol dependence is associated with sleep disruption both during active drinking as well as abstinence [45]. Our findings of reduced ChAT expression in the pedunculopontine nucleus (Ch5) and laterodorsal tegmental nucleus (Ch6) of young adult rats (P80) after AIE might contribute to lasting sleep disturbances in adults. Indeed, although there are no direct studies on the effects of adolescent ethanol exposure on cholinergic function and sleep, adolescent rats exposed to ethanol vapor from P24 to P60 were found to exhibit diminished slow-wave sleep in adulthood [46].

We also observed reductions of ChAT+IR in the medial habenula (Ch7) and interpeduncular nuclei as well as the striatum. Reductions of ChAT in these regions may increase the risk for development of alcoholism and other drug dependence. The medial habenula-interpeduncular pathway is critically involved in inhibitory control and aversive conditioning [10]. Employing selective ablation techniques to lesion the medial habenula, Kobayashi and colleagues [10] found increased nocturnal hyperactivity as well as increased impulsivity and compulsivity on the 5-choice serial reaction time test. This was accompanied by a 60% reduction of ACh concentration in the interpeduncular nucleus in these mice. Although the present study is the first study to describe AIE-induced reductions of ChAT in the medial

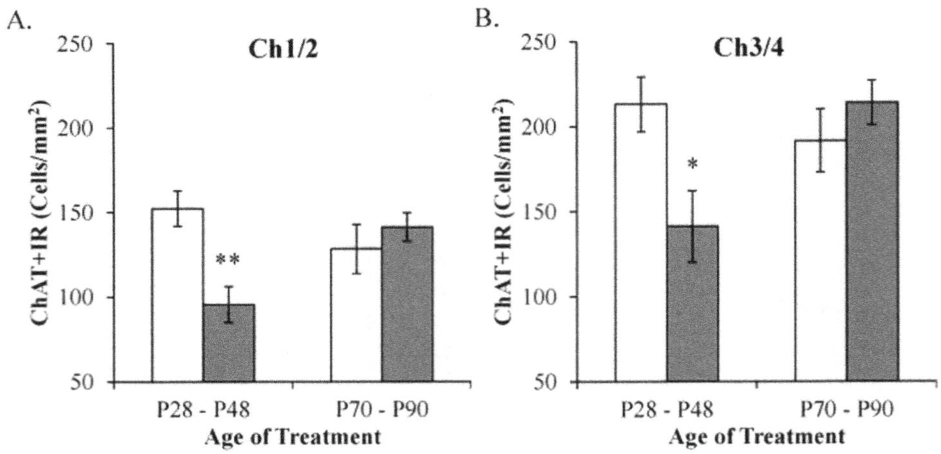

Figure 8. Binge ethanol exposure during adolescence, but not adulthood, decreases choline acetyltransferase (ChAT) expression in the young adult basal forebrain. (A) Immunohistochemical assessment of ChAT+IR in the medial septum/vertical limb of the diagonal band (Ch1/Ch2) revealed a significant 37% (±6%) reduction in subjects that received binge ethanol during adolescence (P28–P48), but not in adulthood (P70–P90). (B) Profile counts of ChAT+IR in the horizontal limb of the diagonal band/nucleus basalis magnocellularis (Ch3/Ch4) revealed a significant 34% (±10%) reduction in subjects that received binge ethanol during adolescence (P28–P48), but not in adulthood (P70–P90). Data are presented as mean ± SEM. * indicates $p<0.05$, relative to CON rats.

habenula and interpeduncular nuclei of young adult rats (P80), nicotine dependence is associated with degeneration of this pathway. Specifically, both continuous and intermittent nicotine exposure increases silver staining, a marker of neurodegeneration, in the medial habenula (Ch7) and the fasciculus retroflexus, a descending fiber pathway that connects the habenula with the interpeduncular nucleus [47,48]. Interestingly, continuous nicotine exposure at doses that resulted in degeneration of this pathway also increased self-administration of ethanol in rats [49]. Throughout the dorsal and ventral striatum, cholinergic interneurons modulate dopamine release from nerve terminals originating in the substantia nigra and ventral tegmental area, respectively [50,51]. Both pharmacological depletion of ACh stores in in the striatum with vesamicol, an inhibitor of vesicular ACh transport, and pharmacological blockade of nicotinic ACh receptors, inhibit dopamine release in the striatum [51]. Choline acetyltransferase is essential for the biosynthesis of acetylcholine, and diminished ChAT expression in the striatum might lead to a disruption of the balance between ACh and dopamine. Dysregulation of the neuromodulatory interaction between these two neurotransmitter systems might contribute to compulsive drug taking and addiction. Taken together, disruption of the cholinergic systems of the medial habenula-interpeduncular pathway and striatum might contribute to the development of alcohol dependence through alterations of dopamine-mediated reward responses, diminished inhibitory control, and increased compulsivity. Further research is needed to further elucidate cholinergic interactions with dopaminergic innervation of the striatum as it relates to the development of alcohol dependence.

While the precise mechanism underlying AIE-induced reductions of ChAT expression throughout the brain remain to be fully elucidated, it does appear that the innate immune system might be involved. We previously found persistently upregulated innate immune gene expression in the frontal cortex of young adult rats (P80) exposed to AIE [22,27]. In the present study, administration of LPS, a prototypical TLR4 agonist, decreased ChAT expression in CON rats to a similar degree to that observed in AIE-exposed animals. Surprisingly, we did not observe a potentiation of ChAT+

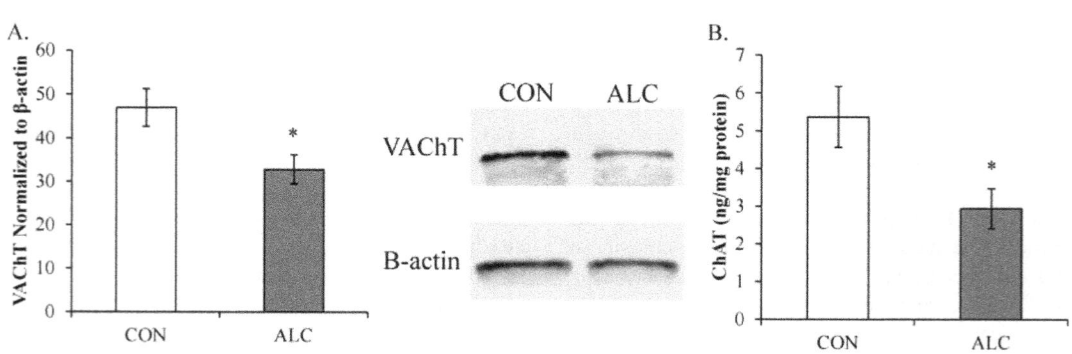

Figure 9. Vesicular acetylcholine transporter (VAChT) and choline acetyltransferase (ChAT) expression is reduced in the human post-mortem alcoholic basal forebrain. (A) Western blot assessment of VAChT protein expression revealed a significant 30% (±7%) reduction in the alcoholic basal forebrain, relative to moderate drinking controls. Representative lanes from Western blot analysis of VAChT. CON is moderate drinking controls and ALC is alcoholic subjects. Western blot analyses were run in triplicate and the mean was reported. (B) ELISA revealed a significant 51% (±11%) reduction of ChAT in the basal forebrain of human alcoholics, relative to moderate drinking controls. Data are presented as mean ± SEM. * indicates $p<0.05$, relative to CONs.

IR cell loss in the LPS-treated AIE subjects. This is might be due to the vulnerability of a distinct population of basal forebrain cholinergic cells [52,53] that were diminished during AIE treatment. A consequence of TLR4 activation is induction of oxidative stress due to the production of proinflammatory oxidases [54]. Oxidative stress has been shown to decrease ChAT expression. In basal forebrain cell culture, LPS (10 μg/mL, 2 days) resulted in a pronounced, selective decrease in ChAT-positive neurons, which might be due to nitric oxide (NO) production as microglia produce NO in response to LPS, and the NOS inhibitor NAME blocked the reduction in ChAT expression [55]. In *in vitro* differentiated cholinergic cells models, administration of sodium nitroprusside and aluminum, both of which increase generation of free radicals, reduced ChAT activity. Pyruvate dehydrogenase, an enzyme that converts pyruvate to acetyl-CoA, was also reduced in cultured cholinergic cells following administration of sodium nitroprusside and aluminum [56]. Thus, generation of NO and free radicals might contribute to the reduction of ChAT-immunopositive cells following AIE exposure. Although we find evidence of diminished cholinergic marker expression in the basal forebrain, it is unknown whether ethanol causes cholinergic cell death or down regulation of cholinergic markers. Further research is needed to elucidate this mechanism.

The effects of alcohol on the developing adolescent brain are different from those observed in adulthood. Adolescents are less sensitive to the sedative effects of alcohol [57], but are more vulnerable to alcohol-induced neurotoxicity [37]. In the present study, we found that binge ethanol exposure during adolescence, but not adulthood, led to long-term reductions of ChAT+IR cells in the basal forebrain. Similarly, our laboratory found persistently reduced hippocampal neurogenesis following adolescent, but not adult, binge ethanol exposure [30,31]. In contrast to the adolescent findings of persistent ChAT loss, chronic ethanol exposure in adulthood transiently reduces cholinergic cell populations in the basal forebrain. In a chronic ethanol exposure model in which rats received 20% ethanol as their sole source of fluid for 12 weeks, expression of acetylcholinesterase (AChE), an enzyme that hydrolyzes ACh into choline and acetyl-CoA, was reduced throughout the basal forebrain immediately following the conclusion of ethanol exposure. In a follow-up study, Arendt and colleagues [58] found progressive reductions of ACh content, release, and synthesis as well as decreased ChAT and AChE activity, and choline reuptake. Interestingly, 4 weeks of abstinence lead to recovery of cholinergic deficits, except in those subjects exposed to 28 weeks of 20% ethanol as their sole source of fluid. Thus, these data support the heightened vulnerability of the developing cholinergic system to the neurotoxic effects of ethanol.

In conclusion, ChAT expression is persistently diminished throughout the adult rat brain following adolescent, but not adult, binge ethanol exposure. Although a mechanism underlying this reduction remains to be fully elucidates, the endotoxin (LPS) data supports the hypothesis that AIE-induced innate immune gene induction contributes to the reduction in ChAT expression. These novel findings suggest that some of the behavioral deficits observed in humans and in animal models of adolescent binge drinking might be the result of a global cholinergic dysfunction. These novel findings reveal that early life insults can have long-lasting effects on the maturing cholinergic system of the CNS and might contribute to some of the behavioral deficits observed in humans and in animal models of adolescent binge drinking.

Acknowledgments

The authors thank Diana Lotito for help with preparation of the manuscript.

Author Contributions

Conceived and designed the experiments: RPV MB WL LPS FTC. Performed the experiments: RPV MB WL LPS FTC. Analyzed the data: RPV MB WL LPS FTC. Contributed reagents/materials/analysis tools: RPV MB WL LPS FTC. Wrote the paper: RPV MB WL LPS FTC.

References

1. Spear LP (2011) Rewards, aversions and affect in adolescence: emerging convergences across laboratory animal and human data. Developmental cognitive neuroscience 1: 392–400.
2. Coleman LG Jr, He J, Lee J, Styner M, Crews FT (2011) Adolescent binge drinking alters adult brain neurotransmitter gene expression, behavior, brain regional volumes, and neurochemistry in mice. Alcoholism, clinical and experimental research 35: 671–688.
3. Spear LP (2000) The adolescent brain and age-related behavioral manifestations. Neuroscience and biobehavioral reviews 24: 417–463.
4. Smith HR, Pang KC (2005) Orexin-saporin lesions of the medial septum impair spatial memory. Neuroscience 132: 261–271.
5. Power AE, McGaugh JL (2002) Cholinergic activation of the basolateral amygdala regulates unlearned freezing behavior in rats. Behavioural brain research 134: 307–315.
6. Knox D, Berntson GG (2006) Effect of nucleus basalis magnocellularis cholinergic lesions on fear-like and anxiety-like behavior. Behavioral neuroscience 120: 307–312.
7. Mesulam MM, Mufson EJ, Wainer BH, Levey AI (1983) Central cholinergic pathways in the rat: an overview based on an alternative nomenclature (Ch1–Ch6). Neuroscience 10: 1185–1201.
8. Benarroch EE (2013) Pedunculopontine nucleus: functional organization and clinical implications. Neurology 80: 1148–1155.
9. Herkenham M, Nauta WJ (1979) Efferent connections of the habenular nuclei in the rat. The Journal of comparative neurology 187: 19–47.
10. Kobayashi Y, Sano Y, Vannoni E, Goto H, Suzuki H, et al. (2013) Genetic dissection of medial habenula-interpeduncular nucleus pathway function in mice. Frontiers in behavioral neuroscience 7: 17.
11. Stamatakis AM, Stuber GD (2012) Activation of lateral habenula inputs to the ventral midbrain promotes behavioral avoidance. Nature neuroscience 15: 1105–1107.
12. Usunoff KG, Schmitt O, Itzev DE, Rolfs A, Wree A (2007) Efferent connections of the parabigeminal nucleus to the amygdala and the superior colliculus in the rat: a double-labeling fluorescent retrograde tracing study. Brain research 1133: 87–91.
13. Oda Y, Nakanishi I (2000) The distribution of cholinergic neurons in the human central nervous system. Histology and histopathology 15: 825–834.
14. Windle M, Spear LP, Fuligni AJ, Angold A, Brown JD, et al. (2008) Transitions into underage and problem drinking: developmental processes and mechanisms between 10 and 15 years of age. Pediatrics 121 Suppl 4: S273–289.
15. Johnston L, O'Malley P, Bachman J, Schulenberg JE (2009) Monitoring the future: National survey results on drug use, 1975–2008. Vol. 1: Secondary school students, 2008. Bethesda: National Institute on Drug Abuse.
16. Sher KJ, Gotham HJ (1999) Pathological alcohol involvement: a developmental disorder of young adulthood. Development and psychopathology 11: 933–956.
17. Crews FT, Boettiger CA (2009) Impulsivity, frontal lobes and risk for addiction. Pharmacology, biochemistry, and behavior 93: 237–247.
18. Slotkin TA, Ryde IT, Mackillop EA, Bodwell BE, Seidler FJ (2008) Adolescent nicotine administration changes the responses to nicotine given subsequently in adulthood: adenylyl cyclase cell signaling in brain regions during nicotine administration and withdrawal, and lasting effects. Brain research bulletin 76: 522–530.
19. Ehlers CL, Criado JR, Wills DN, Liu W, Crews FT (2011) Periadolescent ethanol exposure reduces adult forebrain ChAT+IR neurons: correlation with behavioral pathology. Neuroscience 199: 333–345.
20. Broadwater M, Spear LP (2013) Consequences of ethanol exposure on cued and contextual fear conditioning and extinction differ depending on timing of exposure during adolescence or adulthood. Behavioural brain research 256: 10–19.
21. Paxinos G, Watson C (1998) The Rat Brain in Stereotaxic Coordinates.
22. Vetreno RP, Qin L, Crews FT (2013) Increased receptor for advanced glycation end product expression in the human alcoholic prefrontal cortex is linked to adolescent drinking. Neurobiology of disease 59: 52–62.
23. Beynon SB, Walker FR (2012) Microglial activation in the injured and healthy brain: what are we really talking about? Practical and theoretical issues

associated with the measurement of changes in microglial morphology. Neuroscience 225: 162–171.

24. Dedova I, Harding A, Sheedy D, Garrick T, Sundqvist N, et al. (2009) The importance of brain banks for molecular neuropathological research: The New South wales tissue resource centre experience. International journal of molecular sciences 10: 366–384.
25. Levey AI, Armstrong DM, Atweh SF, Terry RD, Wainer BH (1983) Monoclonal antibodies to choline acetyltransferase: production, specificity, and immunohistochemistry. The Journal of neuroscience: the official journal of the Society for Neuroscience 3: 1–9.
26. Arvidsson U, Riedl M, Elde R, Meister B (1997) Vesicular acetylcholine transporter (VAChT) protein: a novel and unique marker for cholinergic neurons in the central and peripheral nervous systems. The Journal of comparative neurology 378: 454–467.
27. Vetreno RP, Crews FT (2012) Adolescent binge drinking increases expression of the danger signal receptor agonist HMGB1 and Toll-like receptors in the adult prefrontal cortex. Neuroscience 226: 475–488.
28. Qin L, Wu X, Block ML, Liu Y, Breese GR, et al. (2007) Systemic LPS causes chronic neuroinflammation and progressive neurodegeneration. Glia 55: 453–462.
29. Crews FT, Braun CJ, Hoplight B, Switzer RC 3rd, Knapp DJ (2000) Binge ethanol consumption causes differential brain damage in young adolescent rats compared with adult rats. Alcoholism, clinical and experimental research 24: 1712–1723.
30. Crews FT, Mdzinarishvili A, Kim D, He J, Nixon K (2006) Neurogenesis in adolescent brain is potently inhibited by ethanol. Neuroscience 137: 437–445.
31. Nixon K, Crews FT (2002) Binge ethanol exposure decreases neurogenesis in adult rat hippocampus. Journal of neurochemistry 83: 1087–1093.
32. Grant BF, Dawson DA (1998) Age of onset of drug use and its association with DSM-IV drug abuse and dependence: results from the National Longitudinal Alcohol Epidemiologic Survey. Journal of substance abuse 10: 163–173.
33. Hingson R, Heeren T, Zakocs R (2001) Age of drinking onset and involvement in physical fights after drinking. Pediatrics 108: 872–877.
34. Sullivan EV, Pfefferbaum A (2005) Neurocircuitry in alcoholism: a substrate of disruption and repair. Psychopharmacology 180: 583–594.
35. De Rosa E, Desmond JE, Anderson AK, Pfefferbaum A, Sullivan EV (2004) The Human Basal Forebrain Integrates the Old and the New. Neuron 41: 825–837.
36. Baxter MG, Chiba AA (1999) Cognitive functions of the basal forebrain. Current opinion in neurobiology 9: 178–183.
37. Crews F, He J, Hodge C (2007) Adolescent cortical development: a critical period of vulnerability for addiction. Pharmacology, biochemistry, and behavior 86: 189–199.
38. Cabrera SM, Chavez CM, Corley SR, Kitto MR, Butt AE (2006) Selective lesions of the nucleus basalis magnocellularis impair cognitive flexibility. Behavioral neuroscience 120: 298–306.
39. Rupp CI, Kurz M, Kemmler G, Mair D, Hausmann A, et al. (2003) Reduced olfactory sensitivity, discrimination, and identification in patients with alcohol dependence. Alcoholism, clinical and experimental research 27: 432–439.
40. Ma M, Luo M (2012) Optogenetic activation of basal forebrain cholinergic neurons modulates neuronal excitability and sensory responses in the main olfactory bulb. The Journal of neuroscience: the official journal of the Society for Neuroscience 32: 10105–10116.
41. Guerri C, Pascual M (2010) Mechanisms involved in the neurotoxic, cognitive, and neurobehavioral effects of alcohol consumption during adolescence. Alcohol 44: 15–26.
42. Webster HH, Jones BE (1988) Neurotoxic lesions of the dorsolateral pontomesencephalic tegmentum-cholinergic cell area in the cat. II. Effects upon sleep-waking states. Brain research 458: 285–302.
43. Bah TM, Laplante F, Wann BP, Sullivan R, Rousseau G, et al. (2010) Paradoxical sleep insomnia and decreased cholinergic neurons after myocardial infarction in rats. Sleep 33: 1703–1710.
44. Jones BE (1991) Paradoxical sleep and its chemical/structural substrates in the brain. Neuroscience 40: 637–656.
45. Roehrs T, Roth T (2001) Sleep, sleepiness, sleep disorders and alcohol use and abuse. Sleep medicine reviews 5: 287–297.
46. Criado JR, Wills DN, Walker BM, Ehlers CL (2008) Effects of adolescent ethanol exposure on sleep in adult rats. Alcohol 42: 631–639.
47. Carlson J, Armstrong B, Switzer RC 3rd, Ellison G (2000) Selective neurotoxic effects of nicotine on axons in fasciculus retroflexus further support evidence that this a weak link in brain across multiple drugs of abuse. Neuropharmacology 39: 2792–2798.
48. Carlson J, Noguchi K, Ellison G (2001) Nicotine produces selective degeneration in the medial habenula and fasciculus retroflexus. Brain research 906: 127–134.
49. Potthoff AD, Ellison G, Nelson L (1983) Ethanol intake increases during continuous administration of amphetamine and nicotine, but not several other drugs. Pharmacology, biochemistry, and behavior 18: 489–493.
50. Cachope R, Mateo Y, Mathur BN, Irving J, Wang HL, et al. (2012) Selective activation of cholinergic interneurons enhances accumbal phasic dopamine release: setting the tone for reward processing. Cell reports 2: 33–41.
51. Zhou FM, Liang Y, Dani JA (2001) Endogenous nicotinic cholinergic activity regulates dopamine release in the striatum. Nature neuroscience 4: 1224–1229.
52. Guo KH, Zhu JH, Yao ZB, Gu HY, Zou JT, et al. (2010) Chemical identification of nestin-immunoreactive neurons in the rat basal forebrain: a re-examination. Neurochemistry international 56: 694–702.
53. Unal CT, Golowasch JP, Zaborszky L (2012) Adult mouse basal forebrain harbors two distinct cholinergic populations defined by their electrophysiology. Frontiers in behavioral neuroscience 6: 21.
54. Park HS, Jung HY, Park EY, Kim J, Lee WJ, et al. (2004) Cutting edge: direct interaction of TLR4 with NAD(P)H oxidase 4 isozyme is essential for lipopolysaccharide-induced production of reactive oxygen species and activation of NF-kappa B. Journal of immunology 173: 3589–3593.
55. McMillian M, Kong LY, Sawin SM, Wilson B, Das K, et al. (1995) Selective killing of cholinergic neurons by microglial activation in basal forebrain mixed neuronal/glial cultures. Biochemical and biophysical research communications 215: 572–577.
56. Szutowicz A, Bielarczyk H, Gul S, Ronowska A, Pawelczyk T, et al. (2006) Phenotype-dependent susceptibility of cholinergic neuroblastoma cells to neurotoxic inputs. Metabolic brain disease 21: 149–161.
57. Silveri MM, Spear LP (1998) Decreased sensitivity to the hypnotic effects of ethanol early in ontogeny. Alcoholism, clinical and experimental research 22: 670–676.
58. Arendt T, Allen Y, Marchbanks RM, Schugens MM, Sinden J, et al. (1989) Cholinergic system and memory in the rat: effects of chronic ethanol, embryonic basal forebrain brain transplants and excitotoxic lesions of cholinergic basal forebrain projection system. Neuroscience 33: 435–462.

16

Larger Mid-Dorsolateral Prefrontal Gray Matter Volume in Young Binge Drinkers Revealed by Voxel-Based Morphometry

Sonia Doallo*, Fernando Cadaveira, Montserrat Corral, Nayara Mota, Eduardo López-Caneda, Socorro Rodríguez Holguín

Department of Clinical Psychology and Psychobiology, University of Santiago de Compostela, Santiago de Compostela, Spain

Abstract

Binge drinking or heavy episodic drinking is a high prevalent pattern of alcohol consumption among young people in several countries. Despite increasing evidence that binge drinking is associated with impairments in executive aspects of working memory (i.e. self-ordered working memory), processes known to depend on the mid-dorsolateral prefrontal cortex (Brodmann areas 46 and 9), less is known about the impact of binge drinking on prefrontal gray matter integrity. Here, we investigated the effects of binge drinking on gray matter volume of mid- dorsolateral prefrontal cortex in youths. We used voxel-based morphometry on the structural magnetic resonance images of subjects reporting a persistent (at least three years) binge drinking pattern of alcohol use ($n=11$; age 22.43 ± 1.03) and control subjects ($n=21$; age 22.18 ± 1.08) to measure differences in gray matter volume between both groups. In a region of interest analysis of the mid-dorsolateral prefrontal cortex, after co-varying for age and gender, we observed significantly larger gray matter volume in the left mid-dorsolateral prefrontal cortex (Brodmann areas 46 and 9) in binge drinkers in comparison with control subjects. Furthermore, there was a significant positive correlation between left mid-dorsolateral prefrontal cortex volume and Self-Ordered Pointing Test (SOPT) total errors score in binge drinkers. The left mid-dorsolateral prefrontal cortex volume also correlated with the quantity and speed of alcohol intake. These findings indicate that a repeated exposure to alcohol −that does not meet criteria for alcohol dependence− throughout post-adolescent years and young adulthood is linked with structural anomalies in mid-dorsolateral prefrontal regions critically involved in executive aspects of working memory.

Editor: Francisco J. Esteban, University of Jaén, Spain

Funding: This study was supported by a grant from the Consellería de Industria e Innovación, Xunta de Galicia (INCITE08PXIB211015PR) and by two grants from the Ministerio de Ciencia e Innovación of Spain (EDU2008-03400; PSI2011-22575). SD was supported by a postdoctoral contract from the Isidro Parga Pondal program (Xunta de Galicia, Spain). The funders had no role in study design, data collection and analysis, decision to publish, or preparation of the manuscript.

Competing Interests: The authors have declared that no competing interests exist.

* E-mail: sonia.doallo@usc.es

Introduction

Binge drinking (BD), or heavy episodic drinking, is characterized by repeated episodes of heavy alcohol consumption (leading to intoxication) followed by abstinence, and is now acknowledged as being the most common type of alcohol misuse among young people in several countries [1]. Despite the increased prevalence of this pattern of alcohol consumption during adolescence and early adulthood, the extent to which BD may affect brain integrity and cortical maturation has only been investigated recently. Of particular importance is how this pattern of repeated alcohol exposure affects the prefrontal cortex, one of the last brain regions to develop and that undergoes substantial developmental changes during this age span.

Studies of gray matter (GM) maturation show a loss in cortical GM density over time [2]–[3], which has been attributed to synaptic pruning and myelination, cellular changes known to occur throughout adolescence in humans [4]. Magnetic resonance imaging (MRI) studies have reported that, in the frontal lobe, the GM maturation ultimately involves the dorsolateral prefrontal cortex (DLPFC), which shows an increase in GM density reduction during the post-adolescent years [2]–[3]. In close parallel, significant improvements in high-order executive functions are observed at this stage of development [5].

Animal studies indicate that adolescence is a period of particular vulnerability to alcohol-induced neurotoxic effects. Intermittent administration of ethanol during adolescence induces prefrontal cortex damage [6]–[7].

In humans, alcohol-induced executive dysfunction and anomalous prefrontal functioning have been reported in adolescents and young people with Alcohol Use Disorder (AUD, defined as DSM-IV alcohol dependence or abuse), e.g. [8]–[11]. Regarding those studies in adolescents and young people reporting a BD pattern of alcohol consumption, alcohol-related functional abnormalities have been reported both in electrophysiological and hemodynamic correlates of cognitive function [12]–[18], including prefrontal-cortex dependent executive functioning [19]–[27]; for reviews see [1], [28]–[30]. At a neuropsychological level, binge drinkers show a variety of deficits on tasks assessing frontal executive function, such as attention and planning, cognitive flexibility, working memory, decision-making, word fluency, task switching and inhibitory control tasks [31]–[36]; for reviews see [1], [28]). Consistently, and importantly for the present study, in a recent work from our group [37], we found that adolescent binge drinkers performed worse than non-BD adolescents in tasks that depend on the integrity of the DLPFC. Specifically, BD resulted in poorer performance on tasks involving executive aspects of working memory (i.e. monitoring of information in working memory, such as self-generated responses) that have been consistently associated with activity in the mid-DLPFC (which comprises Brodmann's areas [BA] 46 and 9) [38]–[41]. These findings were in agreement with previous research by Scaife and Duka [34] also showing an impaired (gender-specific) performance in a spatial self-ordered task. Remarkably, we found these difficulties in self-ordered working memory to persist after maintenance of a binge-pattern of alcohol use over a 2-year period [42]. These results are also in line with other longitudinal studies showing a relationship between BD and altered executive functioning. For instance, prolonged BD has been associated with diminished decision-making [33]; furthermore, pre-existing altered activation in frontal regions has been observed in future alcohol-using adolescents during response inhibition [43] (see also [44]) and visual working memory [45].

Despite this increasing evidence for functional prefrontal impairments associated with BD, as well as for altered microstructural white matter integrity as measured by diffusion tensor imaging (DTI) [46]–[47], less is known about the impact of heavy episodic drinking on adolescents' prefrontal GM integrity. MRI studies in adolescents with AUD with [48] and without [49] comorbid psychiatric disorders have revealed smaller prefrontal total volume and prefrontal white matter volume in AUD adolescents compared to non-AUD adolescents. However, whether the observed abnormalities in total prefrontal volume among AUD adolescents were primarily due to white or gray matter pathology could not be established in these studies. Only very recently, one MRI study has provided evidence of differences (gender-specific) in cortical thickness in left frontal regions related to binge drinking in a non-clinical adolescent sample. Thicker frontal cortices were linked to poorer neuropsychological performance and were interpreted to represent altered pruning [50].

In this study, we used MRI and voxel-based morphometry (VBM) employing a region-of-interest (ROI) approach, to examine, based on our previous work, the effects of a persistent (at least three years) binge-pattern of alcohol use on GM volume of DLPFC (specifically, mid-DLPFC) in youths. We hypothesized that young binge drinkers would show structural abnormalities in mid-DLPFC compared with sociodemographically similar control subjects. Based on the scarce and inconclusive structural MRI literature available examining the effects of heavy alcohol use or abuse on GM integrity, we based our specific hypothesis about the direction of this effect in the work from Squeglia et al. [50]; i.e. we expected these alterations to be reflected as larger prefrontal volumes in binge drinkers relative to controls.

Materials and Methods

Participants

The neuroimaging assessment of participants was performed during their fourth academic year of attendance at the University of Santiago de Compostela, within the framework of a longitudinal study examining the neurocognitive consequences of BD on the young university population, and in which they had been assessed in their first [37] and third [42] academic year. Participants were contacted again and invited to participate in a MRI study. The 36 participants who agreed to participate were questioned about their current drinking pattern. Subjects were classified as binge drinkers (BD) if they reported drinking (i) six or more standard alcoholic drinks (10 g of alcohol according to the Spanish Health Authority's reference) on the same occasion at least once per week, or (ii) six or more standard alcoholic drinks on the same occasion at least once a month and, during these episodes, drank at a speed of consumption of at least three drinks per hour. They were classified as controls (CG) if they reported drinking six standard alcoholic drinks on the same occasion less than once per month and at a maximum speed of consumption of two drinks per hour. Participants had thus maintained these patterns (BD/control) of alcohol consumption for at least three years, according to our previous assessments. For sample consistency, four BD participants from the longitudinal study who did not report a current binge-drinking pattern of alcohol consumption were excluded from the analysis.

Sociodemographic and substance use data were collected through a questionnaire that included the Alcohol Use Disorders Identification Test (AUDIT)[51] and questions about consumption of other psychoactive substances (specific type of substance used, frequency of consumption, etc). The AUDIT has been validated to assess alcohol-related problems or disorders [51], and specifically in university students, for a review see [52]. The Galician validated version of the AUDIT [53] was used. Personal and family history of alcoholism and medical or psychopathological disorders information was collected through a semi-structured interview that comprised: a translated and adapted version of the Semi-Structured Assessment for the Genetics of Alcoholism (SSAGA), Individual Assessment Module (IAM) and Family History Assessment Module (FHAM), designed by the Collaborative Study on the Genetics of Alcoholism (COGA)[54]; and the Symptom Checklist-90-Revised (SCL-90-R)[55], which is a questionnaire for self-report of a range of current psychological symptoms and distress and measures nine primary symptom dimensions (interpersonal sensitivity, depression, anxiety, hostility, phobic anxiety, paranoid ideation and psychoticism).

The exclusion criteria were as follow: a score above 90 in the Global Severity Index (GSI) of the SCL-90-R(GSI is the average rating given to all 90 items and provides a measure of overall psychological distress) or in at least two of the symptomatic dimensions; personal history of neurological disorders; regular (i.e. on a weekly basis) consumption of cannabis or other drugs (legal or illegal) with psychoactive effects (whether prescribed or not); alcohol abuse/dependence according to the DSM-III-R criteria; personal and/or family history of major mental disorder and history of alcoholism in first-degree relatives; and MRI contraindications. Finally, 32 participants (mean age = 22.34, SD = 1.04, range 20–24) were selected for neuroimaging assessment: 11 binge drinkers (7 males, 4 females) and 21 non-binge drinkers (10 males, 11 females). All subjects gave written informed consent after the procedure had been carefully explained and received 30 € for their participation.

Ethics Statement

All participants were volunteers recruited from the University of Santiago de Compostela, and gave written consent to participate in this study for monetary compensation. The research was carried out in accordance with the ethical principles for research involving human subjects outlined in the Declaration of Helsinki, European Council Agreements and regulations on bioethics of Spain. The protocol was approved by the Bioethics Committee of the University of Santiago de Compostela.

MRI Data Acquisition

Subjects were scanned with a Siemens 1.5 Tesla scanner (Siemens, Erlangen, Germany). High-resolution T1-weighted transversal images covering the whole brain were acquired with a magnetization-prepared rapid gradient echo (MP-RAGE) sequence: 192 slices with section thickness of 1.0 mm; flip angle $=8°$; echo time $=4.38$ ms; repetition time $=2040$ ms; field of view $=192$ mm. A neuroradiologist evaluated all scans for gross structural abnormalities. No participants were excluded.

Image Processing

Structural images were processed with the voxel-based morphometry toolbox (VBM8) (http://dbm.neuro.uni-jena.de/vbm8/) implemented in Statistical Parametric Mapping (SPM8) (Wellcome Department of Imaging Neuroscience, London, UK) running on MATLAB 7.9.0 (R2009b; The Mathworks, Inc., Natick, MA, USA). VBM is a whole-brain, unbiased, semi-automated technique for characterizing regional cerebral differences in structural magnetic resonance images [56]. Segmentation of individual brains into gray matter, white matter, and cerebrospinal fluid was based on VBM8 using the default estimation options (i.e. very light bias regularization, 60 mm cut-off for estimating the Gaussian smoothness of bias in image intensity; ICBM [International Consortium for Brain Mapping] European template for initial affine transformation). Spatial normalization into the Montreal Neurological Institute (MNI) standard space was done by the high-dimensional DARTEL (Diffeomorphic Anatomical Registration Through Exponentiated Lie Algebra) approach implemented in VBM8. To this end, default options such as SANLM (spatial adaptive non local means) de-noising, light clean-up of partitions, and weighting of Hidden Markov-Random Fields by a factor of .15 were used. Subsequently, gray matter segments were modulated only by the nonlinear components to locally preserve actual GM values (so-called modulated volumes). Finally, the modulated volumes were smoothed with a 6-mm full-width-at-half-maximum (FWHM) Gaussian kernel. Normalized, modulated, smoothed images were submitted to group-level analyses.

Statistical Analysis

To assess differences in regional gray matter volume between groups, two-sample t-tests analyses (CG >BD, CG <BD) were performed in SPM8. Age and gender were entered as covariates in all analyses. Because we had a strong a priori hypothesis targeting the mid-DLPFC, a region-of-interest (ROI) approach was used. These analyses were carried out using the Wake Forest University (WFU) Pickatlas toolbox (Version 2.5)[57] implemented in SPM8, with the left and right mid-DLPFC ROIs being anatomically defined as BA46 and BA9 in the Talairach Daemon [TD] Brodmann area atlas [58]. Although our primary focus was the mid-DLPFC because we had a strong hypothesis about a specific alteration of this region in BD, in order to additionally test whether there is a specific deficit among BD in the DLPFC or whether potential BD-related GM alterations could extend to other frontal regions (which are the brain regions more vulnerable to the neurotoxic effects of alcohol), further ROI analysis were performed on the following frontal areas: ventrolateral prefrontal cortex (BA44, BA45, BA47), orbitofrontal cortex (BA11, BA10), anterior cingulate cortex (BA24, BA32, BA33) and dorsolateral premotor cortex (BA6, BA8). To control for multiple statistical testing within our ROIs, a family-wise error (FWE) at $P<0.05$ was applied. For completeness of reporting, an exploratory whole-brain analysis was also carried out with a statistical threshold of $P<0.001$ (uncorrected for multiple comparisons) and minimum cluster size of 100 voxels.

We also examined the relationship between mid-dorsolateral prefrontal GM volumes and both neuropsychological executive performance and alcohol consumption variables. The neuropsychological data used for this study were collected as part of a study in which we reported poorer performance in young binge drinkers compared with control subjects in neuropsychological tests of executive functions that depend on DLPFC integrity [42]. Our main objective was to examine the relationship between mid-DLPFC volumes and the test in which significant differences in performance were found between BD and CG over the 2-year follow-up period (as reported in 37 and 42); namely, the Self-Ordered Pointing Test (SOPT)[59]. In the SOPT —abstract design version, 108 sheets are shown to the subject, each of which shows a series of abstract designs. This task is composed of four blocks with three trials each, in which the number of stimuli per sheet increases block by block (6, 8, 10 and 12). The stimuli are repeated on every sheet of each trial but the position changes at random from sheet to sheet. The task is to point to one design on each sheet, without repeating previously indicated designs. For each participant, the number of perseverative errors (errors that occurred as a result of pointing to the same item that was chosen on the immediately preceding sheet) and the total number of errors (the sum of perseverative and non-perseverative errors) are recorded. The SOPT assesses planning and self-monitoring aspects of working memory. In addition, in order to test whether there is a specific link between mid-DLPFC volume and performance on the SOPT or whether a relationship could be observed with other tests assessing executive functioning in our longitudinal study, further correlation analyses were performed between volumetric data and the scores in the Digit Span backward and the Spatial Location backward subtests of WAIS-III [60] that assess working memory, as well as in the Zoo Map and Key Search subtests of the Behavioral Assessment of Dysexecutive Syndrome (BADS)[61] that assess planning (details of these tests have been previously described, [37], [42]). Performance data on the neuropsychological tests were available for all the 32 subjects included in the present study (the average time elapsed between accomplishment of the neuropsychological assessment and acquisition of T1 images was from 0.7 to 2.4 years [1.8 years on average, SD = 0.63]). Participants were asked to abstain from consuming drugs and alcohol within 24 h prior to neuropsychological assessment. Table 1 contains descriptive demographic and neuropsychological data for the two groups. Differences between groups in frequency, quantity and intensity of alcohol consumption are also reported.

For the correlation analysis, the mid-DLPFC GM volumetric data were extracted from the coordinates of cluster maxima revealed by the ROI analyses using the MarsBar toolbox (v0.43) (http://marsbar.sourceforge.net/) for further analysis in PASW Statistics 18.0. Correlations between mid-dorsolateral prefrontal volumes and neuropsychological measures (scores on the tests) for the BD group were calculated by Pearson correlations. For BD and CG, GM mid-dorsolateral prefrontal volumes were also correlated with alcohol consumption variables measuring Speed of consumption (number of drinks consumed within one hour of a binge episode); Frequency (number of times consuming alcohol in a standard week); and Quantity (total grams of alcohol in a standard week; total grams of alcohol in a binge drinking day; estimated grams of alcohol within 2 hours of a binge drinking episode) as well as with the variable age of onset of alcohol use.

Results

Group Differences in Mid-Dorsolateral Prefrontal GM Volumes

BD > Control Subjects. The region-of-interest analysis revealed that the BD group had a greater GM volume of the

Table 1. Demographic, Neuropsychological and Drinking data (mean ± standard deviation) for Binge Drinking (BD) and Control samples.

	Control	BD
N (males/females)	21 (10/11)	11 (7/4)
Age (range)	22.43 (1.03)	22.18 (1.08)
White ethnicity (%)	100	100
Tobacco smokers	0	4a
Occasional use of cannabis	0	3b
SOPT total errors	7.29±4.29	9.45±4.85
Digits backward	5.24±1.38	5.64±1.36
Spatial location backward	5.86±1.2	6.45±0.82
Zoo Map, raw score	12.29±3.23	12.27±4.67
Key Search, raw score	11.62±3.49	12.55±2.50
Speed of consumption: drinks per hour*	0.62±0.57	2.23±0.88
Number of times consuming alcohol in the last week*	0.93±1.03	2.18±1.10
Grams of alcohol in a standard week*	29.90±35.46	225.91±57.22
Grams of alcohol in a BD day*	2.86±13.09	100.45±20.94
Grams of alcohol (estimated) within 2 hours of a BD episode*	1.43±6.55	67.73±26.21
Age of onset of alcohol use*	15.81±0.98	14.81±1.4

a<10 cigarettes per day (3 males, 1 female).
b<10 per month (one male BD participant consumed 10 cannabis cigarettes per month; one male and one female BD participants consumed one cannabis cigarette per month or less).
*t<0.05 significant group differences.

left mid-DLPFC (BA46 and BA9) compared to the CG (MNI coordinates, −44, 42, 18; $t=5.10$; $k=11$; $P=0.012$ FWE-corrected at the voxel-level; $P=0.017$ FWE-corrected at the cluster-level)(Figure 1). No suprathreshold clusters were present for right mid-DLPFC ROI using the same thresholding criteria. The exploratory whole-brain analysis confirmed a significantly greater volume in a cluster in the left mid-DLPFC (MNI coordinates, −44, 42, 18; $t=5.10$; $k=115$; $P<0.001$ uncorrected)(Figure 1 and Table S1). At the exploratory whole-brain threshold, the BD group showed a greater GM volume in a number of brain regions, including occipital, limbic and frontal areas, compared to the control subjects (see Table S1 for details).

Control subjects > BD. Neither the ROI analysis, nor the whole brain analysis revealed any significant regions of increased GM in control subjects compared with binge drinkers.

Additional ROI analysis of frontal regions

Additional ROI analysis of other anatomically defined frontal regions showed that in comparison to the CG, the BD group had greater GM volumes of the bilateral anterior cingulate cortex (ACC)(left: MNI coordinates, −2, 36, 24; $t=4.87$; $k=8$; $P=0.014$ FWE-corrected at the voxel-level, $P=0.023$ FWE-corrected at the cluster-level; right: 15, 2, 43; $t=5.88$; $k=12$; $P=0.001$ FWE-

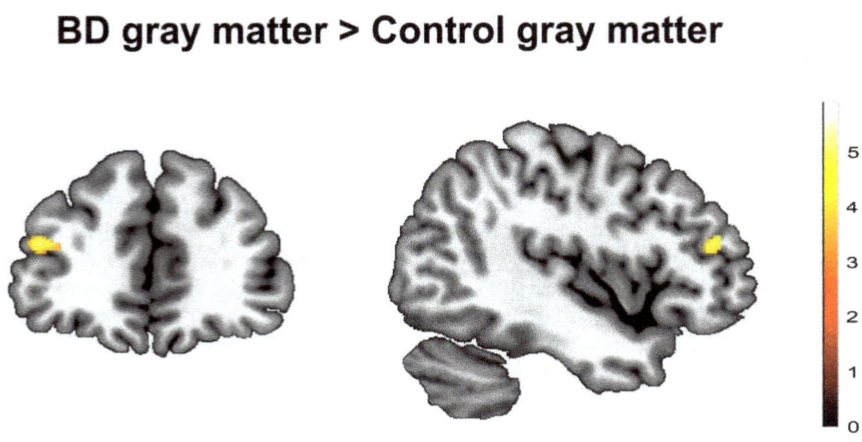

Figure 1. Group differences in gray matter volume. Color map showing larger gray matter volume in left mid-DLPFC (BA46 and BA9) in the binge drinking (BD) group compared with control subjects, after co-varying for age and gender (significant $P<0.05$ FWE-corrected at the voxel-level and at the cluster-level within regions of interest, and $P<0.001$ uncorrected on whole-brain analysis with minimum cluster size of 100 voxels). Color bar represents t-values.

corrected at the voxel-level, $P=0.018$ FWE-corrected at the cluster-level); no significant differences were found in the ventrolateral prefrontal cortex, orbitofrontal cortex or dorsolateral premotor cortex. There were no significant regions of increased GM in CG relative to BD group.

Correlation between Mid-Dorsolateral Prefrontal GM Volume and Executive Neuropsychological Performance

The correlation analyses for the BD subjects indicated that the left mid-DLPFC (BA46 and BA9) volume was positively correlated with SOPT total errors score ($r=0.558$, $P=0.037$). The same analysis for the control group was no significant ($r=0.092$, $P=0.346$). There were no significant correlations between the left mid-DLPFC volume and the other neuropsychological tests assessing executive functioning, neither in the BD group (Zoo Map, direct score: $r=-0.226$, $P=0.252$; Key Search, direct score: $r=-0.434$, $P=0.091$; Digit Span backward: $r=-0.316$, $P=0.172$; Spatial Location backward: $r=-0.414$, $P=0.103$) nor in the CG (Zoo Map, direct score: $r=-0.125$, $P=0.295$; Key Search, direct score: $r=-0.169$, $P=0.232$; Digit Span backward: $r=0.291$, $P=0.100$; Spatial Location backward: $r=0.082$, $P=0.361$).

Correlation between Mid-Dorsolateral Prefrontal GM Volume and Pattern of Alcohol Consumption

Significant positive correlations between the left mid-DLPFC volume and variables measuring Speed (number of drinks consumed within one hour of a binge episode, $r=0.323$, $P=0.036$) and Quantity of consumption (total grams of alcohol in a standard week, $r=0.418$, $P=0.009$; total grams of alcohol in a binge drinking day, $r=0.472$, $P=0.003$; estimated grams of alcohol within 2 hours of a binge drinking episode, $r=0.450$, $P=0.005$) were observed across groups. A significant negative correlation was also found with the variable age of onset of alcohol use ($r=-0.486$, $P=0.005$). There was no correlation between left mid-DLPFC volume and the variable measuring frequency of alcohol use (i.e. number of times consuming alcohol in a standard week; $r=0.118$, $P=0.261$).

BD without regular consumption of cannabis

To be sure that the difference in cannabis consumption between groups was not confounding the results, we re-analyzed the data excluding one male BD participant who reported a consumption of cannabis that could be considered as more regular (i.e. 10 cannabis cigarrettes per month).

The results confirmed the larger volume of the left mid-DLPFC [BA46 and BA9) in the BD group relative to the CG (−45, 42, 18; $t=5.32$, $k=17$, $P=0.008$ FWE-corrected at the voxel-level, $P=0.012$ FWE-corrected at the cluster-level) and the significant positive correlations between left mid-DLPFC volume and (i) SOPT total errors score ($r=0.692$, $P=0.013$) and (ii) consumption variables measuring Speed of consumption (number of drinks consumed within one hour of a binge episode, $r=0.322$, $P=0.039$) and Quantity of consumption (total grams of alcohol in a standard week, $r=0.441$, $P=0.007$; total grams of alcohol in a binge drinking day, $r=0.477$, $P=0.003$; estimated grams of alcohol within 2 hours of a binge drinking episode, $r=0.453$, $P=0.005$); again, no correlations were observed with frequency of consumption. The significant negative correlation of left mid-DLPFC volume with age of onset of alcohol use was also corroborated ($r=-0.492$, $P=0.005$).

The additional ROI analysis of other anatomically defined frontal regions showed again greater GM volumes of the bilateral ACC in BD relative to CG (left: MNI coordinates, −2, 36, 24; $t=4.61$; $k=3$; $P=0.027$ FWE-corrected at the voxel-level, $P=0.033$ FWE-corrected at the cluster-level; right: 15, 3, 43; $t=6.40$; $k=20$; $P=0.0005$ FWE-corrected at the voxel-level, $P=0.012$ FWE-corrected at the cluster-level).

The correlation analysis between the left mid-DLPFC volume and the other neuropsychological tests assessing executive functioning did not show either any significant effect for the BD group.

Discussion

The major finding of the present study is that young university students reporting a binge drinking pattern of alcohol consumption, with a history of at least three years of binge drinking (and who started alcohol consumption during adolescence), had a significantly larger GM volume of left mid-DLPFC (BA46 and BA9) than age-matched non-binge drinkers students. Furthermore, our results indicate that these cortical volume differences in GM were positively associated with poorer performance in neurocognitive measures of executive functioning (i.e. monitoring of information in working memory) that are known to depend on the integrity of the mid-DLPFC, as well as with the quantity and intensity of alcohol intake.

Our results are in line with a recent study indicating that repeated binge drinking during adolescence is associated with differences in left frontal cortical thickness [50], and proposing a relationship between thicker frontal cortices and less neurodevelopment. MRI studies have revealed a robust increase in local GM density loss in the dorsal frontal regions that control executive functioning between adolescence and adulthood [2], being one of the last brain regions to develop fully [3]. These post-adolescent changes in GM density have been attributed to both regressive (i.e. synaptic pruning) and progressive (i.e. myelination) cellular changes known to occur simultaneously in the brain during childhood, adolescence and young adulthood, and considered indices of neural maturation and enhanced neural processing efficiency [2]–[4]. Although care should be taken in interpreting our present results (it is possible that the differences in brain structure were premorbid to BD and predisposed subjects to heavy episodic alcohol use), the larger GM mid-DLPFC volume associated with BD might reflect the deleterious effects of heavy episodic alcohol exposure on typical development of prefrontal cortex, a region particularly sensitive to alcohol neurotoxicity [62]. Support for this hypothesis comes from the following several findings. Firstly, the positive relationship between the left mid-DLPFC volume and quantity and speed of alcohol intake, variables that actually define a risky binge drinking behavior (i.e. the high quantity and the speed at which alcohol is consumed during a single session). Secondly, the negative relationship between the left mid-DLPFC volume and age of onset of alcohol use, suggesting that as earlier the onset of consumption during adolescence the larger the volume in comparison to non-binge drinkers youths. Thirdly, other frontal anatomically defined regions of interest showed a similar pattern of volume alterations, namely the bilateral ACC. The ACC has been proposed to form part of a cognitive-control network (together with the lateral prefrontal and parietal cortices) subserving regulatory control over impulsive and risky behavior [63] and has been included in neural models of addiction, e.g. [64]–[65]. Structural GM abnormalities involving the ACC have been reported in drug abuser populations, such as cocaine-dependent subjects [66]; interestingly, work by Cheetham et al. [67] indicates that pre-existing individual differences in structural morphology (i.e. smaller volumes) of the left dorsal and rostral paralimbic ACC in adolescents (age 12) predicted problematic alcohol use four years later (age 16).

Finally, to highlight that a similar interpretation has been proposed very recently in a VBM study [68] examining subcortical GM differences (in ventral striatum, hippocampus and amygdala) related to BD in college-aged young adults, which found larger bilateral ventral striatum volumes in binge drinkers compared to controls. Based on evidence indicating that striatal volumes decline in GM between adolescence and young adulthood, the authors interpreted the enlarged volumes in terms of relative neuroanatomical inmaturity in this population.

Despite these convergent observations from the present and previous studies, further longitudinal VBM studies examining the effects of a binge pattern of alcohol use from adolescence to young adulthood are warranted to confirm this hypothesis.

The finding that the increase in volume in left mid-DLPFC was positively associated with poorer performance in the SOPT may also provide support for this hypothesis. The SOPT assesses executive aspects of working memory, specifically the ability of monitoring a sequence of responses in working memory. Importantly, lesion studies in non-human primates [40], [69] and functional neuroimaging studies [38], [41] have shown that successful performance of this task is associated with activity in the mid-DLPFC (BA46 and BA9). Based on this well-established association, hypothesis-driven correlation analysis between GM volume in mid-DLPFC and the performance on the SOPT was conducted. In agreement with this evidence, our results indicate that the larger mid-DLPFC volume of binge drinkers, which could be considered as an index of less neural processing efficiency in this region, was linked to less efficient executive functioning as measured by the SOPT. However, to interpret the present results, the following limitation should be acknowledged: all participants of this cross-sectional neuroimaging study came from a longitudinal study by our group examining the neurocognitive consequences of BD on the young university population, in which students had been assessed during a follow-up period of 2-years [37], [42], and which revealed that maintenance of a binge-drinking pattern was associated with poorer performance in the SOPT at both assessment times. Given that the neuropsychological data used in this study was taken from the assessment closer in time to MRI data acquisition (i.e. second evaluation time, see [42]), the time interval between scan and neuropsychological data collection could span from 0.7 to 2.4 years. Acknowledging the limitation of comparing structural and cognitive measures collected with such time lapse between them, we focused our main analysis on the one test in which performance has been consistently associated to mid-DLPFC (BA46 and BA9) functioning and in which performance impairments have been repeatedly found at different follow-ups in our sample (thus suggesting the high sensitivity of the SOPT to BD-related alterations). In line with the expected specific link between mid-DLPFC volume and SOPT performance, no significant correlations were found between volume of this brain region and performance in others tests assessing executive function in our sample. Nevertheless, because neural maturation is still expected to continue over that time period, caution should be taken when interpreting these results.

Taken together, the present neuroimaging findings extend our previous neuropsychological work by revealing that a repeated exposure to alcohol throughout post-adolescent years and young adulthood is linked with structural anomalies in mid-dorsolateral prefrontal regions critically involved in executive aspects of working memory (i.e. monitoring of information within working memory)[70]. Our results are also consistent with recent studies [36] showing that heavy social drinking adversely affects performance on random letter generation tasks, which engage working memory and executive processes (i.e. holding information 'on line', suppression of habitual response patterns, internally driven response generation and monitoring of responses) and which has been shown to be linked to the left dorsolateral prefrontal cortex [71].

Several limitations of this study warrant consideration. First, recruitment of subjects was limited to students who participated in a five-year longitudinal follow-up study and, within the binge-drinking group, to those who maintained this pattern of alcohol use over time. The selection criteria resulted in a small, unequal, sample size, thus rendering our analysis susceptible to a type-II error and low statistical power to detect differences between the groups (although effects were indeed observed). Additionally, the unequal number of males and females within and between groups precluded us from exploring the influence of gender, which has been shown to moderate the relationship between structural abnormalities and alcohol consumption (e.g. [49], [50]). Future studies with larger, even sample sizes will be necessary to confirm the present results. A second limitation already mentioned is that the cross-sectional nature of this study makes it difficult to draw conclusions about causal relationships between larger mid-DLPFC gray matter volumes and BD. Longitudinal studies are necessary to examine if larger mid-DLPFC volume represents a vulnerability to, or a consequence of, heavy episodic drinking during adolescence.

Despite these limitations, we were still able to demonstrate reliable structural differences between a BD group and control subjects in the mid-DLPFC (BA46 and BA9), a brain region critically involved in high-level executive control. Our work has thus significant implications for understanding the potential deleterious consequences of a binge pattern of alcohol consumption – that does not meet criteria for alcohol dependence – on the neurodevelopment of prefrontal regions during the post-adolescent years.

Acknowledgments

We thank to the personnel of the Imaging Diagnosis Service of the Hospital "Nuestra Señora de la Esperanza" in Santiago de Compostela for technical assistance in MRI data acquisition. We thank Dr Bo-Cheng Kuo for advice in the analysis.

Author Contributions

Conceived and designed the experiments: SD FC MC SRH. Performed the experiments: SD MC SRH NM ELC. Analyzed the data: SD. Contributed reagents/materials/analysis tools: FC SRH. Wrote the paper: SD. Assisted with data analysis: MC SRH. Assisted with interpretation of findings: SD FC MC ELC SRH. Provided critical revision of the manuscript for important intellectual content: SD FC MC NM ELC SRH.

References

1. Hermens DF, Lagopoulos J, Tobias-Webb J, De Regt T, Dore G, et al. (2013) Pathways to alcohol-induced brain impairment in young people: A review. Cortex 49: 3–17.
2. Sowell ER, Thompson PM, Tessner KD, Toga AW (2001) Mapping continued brain growth and gray matter density reduction in dorsal frontal cortex: Inverse relationships during postadolescent brain maturation. J Neurosci 21: 8819–8829.
3. Gogtay N, Giedd JN, Lusk L, Hayashi KM, Greenstein D, et al. (2004) Dynamic mapping of human cortical development during childhood through early adulthood. Proc Natl Acad Sci USA 101: 8174–8179.
4. Sowell ER, Thompson PM, Toga AW (2004) Mapping changes in the human cortex throughout the span of life. Neuroscientist 10: 372–392.
5. Yurgelun-Todd D (2007) Emotional and cognitive changes during adolescence. Curr Opin Neurobiol 17: 251–257.
6. Crews FT, Braun CJ, Hoplight B, Switzer RC 3rd, Knapp DJ (2000) Binge ethanol consumption causes differential brain damage in young adolescent rats compared with adult rats. Alcohol Clin Exp Res 24: 1712–1723.
7. Pascual M, Blanco AM, Cauli O, Miñarro J, Guerri C (2007) Intermittent ethanol exposure induces inflammatory brain damage and causes long-term behavioural alterations in adolescent rats. Eur J Neurosci 25: 541–550.
8. Tapert SF, Brown SA (1999) Neuropsychological correlates of adolescent substance abuse: Four-year outcomes. J Int Neuropsychol Soc 5: 481–493.
9. Tapert SF, Broen GG, Kindermann SS, Cheung EH, Frank LR, et al. (2001) fMRI measurements of brain dysfunction in alcohol-dependent young women. Alcohol Clin Exp Res 25: 236–245.
10. Tapert SF, Schweinsburg AD, Barlett VC, Brown SA, Frank LR, et al. (2004) Blood oxygen level dependent response and spatial working memory in adolescents with alcohol use disorders. Alcohol Clin Exp Res 28: 1577–1586.
11. Caldwell LC, Schweinsburg AD, Nagel BJ, Barlett VC, Brown SA, et al. (2005) Gender and adolescent alcohol use disorders on BOLD (blood oxygen level dependent) response to spatial working memory. Alcohol Alcohol 40: 194–200.
12. Ehlers CL, Phillips E, Finnerman G, Gilder D, Lau P, et al. (2007) P3 components and adolescent binge drinking in Southwest California Indians. Neurotoxicol Teratol 29: 153–163.
13. Maurage P, Pesenti M, Philippot P, Joassin F, Campanella S (2009) Latent deleterious effects of binge drinking over a short period of time revealed only by electrophysiological measures. J Psychiatry Neurosci 34: 111–118.
14. Maurage P, Joassin F, Speth A, Modave J, Philippot P, et al. (2012) Cerebral effects of binge drinking: respective influences of global alcohol intake and consumption pattern. Clin Neurophysiol 123: 892–901.
15. Maurage P, Bestelmeyer PE, Rouger J, Charest I, Belin P (2013) Binge drinking influences the cerebral processing of vocal affective bursts in young adults. Neuroimage Clin 3: 218–225.
16. Crego A, Cadaveira F, Parada M, Corral M, Caamaño-Isorna F, et al. (2012) Increased amplitude of P3 event-related potential in young binge drinkers. Alcohol 46: 415–425.
17. Petit G, Kornreich C, Maurage P, Noël X, Letesson C, et al. (2012) Early attentional modulation by alcohol-related cues in young binge drinkers: an event-related potentials study. Clin Neurophysiol 123: 925–936.
18. Petit G, Kornreich C, Verbanck P, Campanella S (2013) Gender differences in reactivity to alcohol cues in binge drinkers: a preliminary assessment of event-related potentials. Psychiatry Res 209: 494–503.
19. Crego A, Rodríguez Holguín S, Parada M, Mota N, Corral M, et al. (2009) Binge drinking affects attentional and visual working memory processing in young university students. Alcohol Clin Exp Res 33: 1870–1879.
20. Crego A, Rodríguez Holguín S, Parada M, Mota N, Corral M, et al. (2010) Reduced anterior prefrontal cortex activation in young binge drinkers during a visual working memory task. Drug Alcohol Depend 109: 45–56.
21. Schweinsburg AD, McQueeny T, Nagel BJ, Eyler LT, Tapert SF (2010) A preliminary study of functional magnetic resonance imaging response during verbal encoding among adolescent binge drinkers. Alcohol 44: 111–117.
22. Schweinsburg AD, Schweinsburg BC, Nagel BJ, Eyler LT, Tapert SF (2011) Neural correlates of verbal learning in adolescent alcohol and marijuana users. Addiction 106: 564–573.
23. Squeglia LM, Schweinsburg AD, Pulido C, Tapert SF (2011) Adolescent binge drinking linked to abnormal spatial working memory brain activation: differential gender effects. Alcohol Clin Exp Res 35: 1831–1841.
24. López-Caneda E, Cadaveira F, Crego A, Gómez-Suárez A, Corral M, et al. (2012) Hyperactivation of right inferior frontal cortex in young binge drinkers during response inhibition: a follow-up study. Addiction 107: 1796–1808.
25. López-Caneda E, Cadaveira F, Crego A, Doallo S, Corral M, et al. (2013) Effects of a persistent binge drinking pattern of alcohol consumption in young people: a follow-up study using event-related potentials. Alcohol Alcohol 48: 464–471.
26. Campanella S, Peigneux P, Petit G, Lallemand F, Saeremans M, et al. (2013) Increased cortical activity in binge drinkers during working memory task: a preliminary assessment through a functional magnetic resonance imaging study. PLoS One 8: e62260.
27. Xiao L, Bechara A, Gong Q, Huang X, Li X, et al. (2013) Abnormal affective decision making revealed in adolescent binge drinkers using a functional magnetic resonance imaging study. Psychol Addict Behav 27: 443–454.
28. Jacobus J, Tapert SA (2013) Neurotoxic effects of alcohol in adolescence. Annu Rev Clin Psychol 9: 703–721.
29. Maurage P, Petit G, Campanella S (2013). Pathways to alcohol-induced brain impairment in young people: a review by Hermens, et al., 2013. Cortex 49: 1155–1159.
30. Petit G, Maurage P, Kornreich C, Verbanck P, Campanella S (2013) Binge drinking in adolescents: a review of neurophysiological and neuroimaging research. Alcohol Alcohol 49: 198–206.
31. Hartley DE, Elsabagh S, File SE (2004) Binge drinking and sex: effects on mood and cognitive function in healthy young volunteers. Pharmacol Biochem Behav 78: 611–619.
32. Townsend JM, Duka T (2005) Binge drinking, cognitive performance and mood in a population of young social drinkers. Alcohol Clin Exp Res 29: 317–325.
33. Goudriaan AE, Grekin ER, Sher KJ (2007) Decision making and binge drinking: a longitudinal study. Alcohol Clin Exp Res 31: 928–938.
34. Scaife JC, Duka T (2009) Behavioural measures of frontal lobe function in a population of young social drinkers with binge drinking pattern. Pharmacol Biochem Behav 93: 354–362.
35. Sanhueza C, García-Moreno LM, Exposito J (2011) Weekend alcoholism in youth and neurocognitive aging. Psicothema 23: 209–214.
36. Montgomery C, Fisk JE, Murphy PN, Ryland I, Hilton J (2012) The effects of heavy social drinking on executive function: a systematic review and meta-analytic study of existing literature and new empirical findings. Hum Psychopharmacol Clin Exp 27: 187–199.
37. Parada M, Corral M, Mota N, Crego A, Rodríguez Holguín S, et al. (2012) Executive functioning and alcohol binge drinking in university students. Addict Behav 37: 167–172.
38. Petrides M, Alivisatos B, Evans AC, Meyer E (1993) Dissociation of human mid-dorsolateral from posterior dorsolateral frontal cortex in memory processing. Proc Natl Acad Sci USA 90: 873–877.
39. Petrides M, Alivisatos B, Meyer E, Evans AC (1993) Functional activation of the human frontal cortex during the performance of verbal working memory tasks. Proc Natl Acad Sci USA 90: 878–882.
40. Petrides M (1995) Impairments on nonspatial self-ordered and externally ordered working memory tasks after lesions of the mid-dorsal part of the lateral frontal cortex in the monkey. J Neurosci 15: 359–375.
41. Curtis CE, Zald DH, Pardo JV (2000) Organization of working memory within the human prefrontal cortex: a PET study of self-ordered object working memory. Neuropsychologia 38: 1503–1510.
42. Mota N, Parada M, Crego A, Doallo S, Caamaño-Isorna F, et al. (2013) Binge drinking trajectory and neuropsychological functioning among university students: a longitudinal study. Drug Alcohol Depend 133: 108–114.
43. Norman AL, Pulido C, Squeglia LM, Spadoni AD, Paulus MP, et al. (2011) Neural activation during inhibition predicts initiation of substance use in adolescence. Drug Alcohol Depend 119: 216–223.
44. Wetherill RR, Squeglia LM, Yang TT, Tapert SF (2013) A longitudinal examination of adolescent response inhibition: neural differences before and after the initiation of heavy drinking. Psychopharmacology 230: 663–671.
45. Squeglia LM, Pulido C, Wetherill RR, Jacobus J, Brown GG, et al. (2012) Brain response to working memory over three years of adolescence: influence of initiating heavy drinking. J Stud Alcohol Drugs 73: 749–760.
46. Jacobus J, McQueeny T, Bava S, Schweinsburg BC, Frank LR, et al. (2009) White matter integrity in adolescents with histories of marijuana use and binge drinking. Neurotoxicol Teratol 31: 349–355.
47. McQueeny T, Schweinsburg BC, Schweinsburg AD, Jacobus J, Bava S, et al. (2009) Altered white matter integrity in adolescent binge drinkers. Alcohol Clin Exp Res 33: 1278–1285.
48. De Bellis MD, Narasimhan A, Thatcher DL, Keshavan MS, Soloff P, et al. (2005) Prefrontal cortex, thalamus, and cerebellar volumes in adolescents and young adults with adolescent-onset alcohol use disorders and comorbid mental disorders. Alcohol Clin Exp Res 29: 1590–1600.
49. Medina KL, McQueeny T, Nagel BJ, Hanson KL, Schweinsburg AD, et al. (2008) Prefrontal cortex volumes in adolescents with alcohol use disorders: unique gender effects. Alcohol Clin Exp Res 32: 386–394.
50. Squeglia LM, Sorg SF, Schweinsburg AD, Wetherill RR, Pulido C, et al. (2012) Binge drinking differentially affects adolescent male and female brain morphometry. Psychopharmacology (Berl) 220: 529–539.
51. Babor TF, Higgins-Biddle JC, Saunders JB, Monteiro MG (2001) AUDIT. The Alcohol Use Disorders Identification Test. Guidelines for use in primary health care (2nd ed.). Geneva: World Health Organization.
52. Reinet DF, Allen JP (2007) The alcohol use disorders identification test: an update of research findings. Alcohol Clin Exp Res 31: 185–199.
53. Varela J, Braña T, Real E, Rial A (2005) Validación empírica do AUDIT (Cuestionario de Identificación dos Trastornos debido ó consumo de alcohol) na poboación xeral galega [Validation of AUDIT for Galician population].Santiago de Compostela, Spain: Consellería de Sanidade-Sergas (Xunta de Galicia).
54. Hesselbrock M, Easton C, Bucholz KK, Schuckit M, Hesselbrock VM (1999) A validity study of the SSAGA - A comparison with the SCAN. Addiction 94: 1361–1370.

55. Degoratis LR (1983) SCL-90-R. Administration, scoring and procedures manual II for the revised version of the SCL-90-R. John Hopkins University Press: Baltimore.
56. Good CD, Johnsrude IS, Ashburner J, Henson RNA, Friston KJ, et al. (2001) A voxel-based morphometric study of ageing in 465 normal adult human brains. Neuroimage 14: 21–36.
57. Maldjian JA, Laurienti PJ, Kraft RA, Burdette JH (2003) An automated method for neuroanatomic and cytoarchitectonic atlas-based interrogation of fMRI data sets. Neuroimage 19: 1233–1239.
58. Lancaster JL, Woldorff MG, Parsons LM, Liotti M, Freitas CS, et al. (2000) Automated Talairach atlas labels for functional brain mapping. Hum Brain Mapp 10: 120–131.
59. Petrides M, Milner B (1982) Deficits on subject-ordered tasks after frontal- and temporal-lobe lesions in man. Neuropsychologia 20: 249–262.
60. Wechsler D (1999) Escala de Inteligencia de Wechsler para adultos: III. Adaptación española (Wechsler Intelligence Scale for adults: III. Spanish adaptation). TEA Ediciones: Madrid.
61. Wilson BA, Evans JJ, Alderman N, Burgess PW, Emslec H, et al. (1996) Behavioral Assessment of the Dysexecutive Syndrome. Thames Valley Company. Bury St Edmunds: England.
62. Oscar-Berman M, Marinkovic K (2007) Alcohol: effects on neurobehavioral functions and the brain. Neuropsychol Rev 17: 239–257.
63. Steinberg L (2007) Risk taking in adolescence. New perspectives from brain and behavioural science. Curr Dir Psychol Sci 22: 45–50.
64. Goldstein RZ, Volkow ND (2002) Drug addiction and its underlying neurobiological basis: neuroimaging evidence for the involvement of the frontal cortex. Am J Psyhiatry 159: 1642–1652.
65. Koob GF (2006) The neurobiology of addiction: a neuroadaptational view relevant for diagnosis. Addiction 101: 23–30.
66. Franklin TR, Acton PD, Maldjian JA, Gray JD, Croft JR, et al. (2002) Decreased gray matter concentration in the insular, orbitofrontal, cingulate, and temporal cortices of cocaine patients. Biol Psychiatry 51: 134–142.
67. Cheetham A, Allen NB, Whittle S, Simmons J, Yücel M, et al. (2014) Volumetric differences in the anterior cingulate cortex prospectively predict alcohol-related problems in adolescence. Psychopharmacology DOI 10.10007/s00213-014-3483-8.
68. Howell NA, Worbe Y, Lange I, Tait R, Irvine M, et al. (2013) Increased ventral striatal volume in college-aged binge drinkers. PLoS One 8(9): e74164.
69. Petrides M (1991) Functional specialization within the dorsolateral frontal cortex for serial order memory. Proc Biol Sci 246: 299–306.
70. Petrides M (2005) Lateral prefrontal cortex: architectonic and functional organization. Philos Trans R Soc Lond B Biol Sci 360: 781–795.
71. Jahanshahi M, Dirnberger G (1999) The left dorsolateral prefrontal cortex and random generation of responses: studies with transcranial magnetic stimulation. Neuropsychologia 37: 181–190.

Dopamine Release Dynamics Change during Adolescence and after Voluntary Alcohol Intake

Sara Palm*, Ingrid Nylander

Neuropharmacology, Addiction & Behaviour, Department of Pharmaceutical Biosciences, Uppsala University, Uppsala, Sweden

Abstract

Adolescence is associated with high impulsivity and risk taking, making adolescent individuals more inclined to use drugs. Early drug use is correlated to increased risk for substance use disorders later in life but the neurobiological basis is unclear. The brain undergoes extensive development during adolescence and disturbances at this time are hypothesized to contribute to increased vulnerability. The transition from controlled to compulsive drug use and addiction involve long-lasting changes in neural networks including a shift from the nucleus accumbens, mediating acute reinforcing effects, to recruitment of the dorsal striatum and habit formation. This study aimed to test the hypothesis of increased dopamine release after a pharmacological challenge in adolescent rats. Potassium-evoked dopamine release and uptake was investigated using chronoamperometric dopamine recordings in combination with a challenge by amphetamine in early and late adolescent rats and in adult rats. In addition, the consequences of voluntary alcohol intake during adolescence on these effects were investigated. The data show a gradual increase of evoked dopamine release with age, supporting previous studies suggesting that the pool of releasable dopamine increases with age. In contrast, a gradual decrease in evoked release with age was seen in response to amphetamine, supporting a proportionally larger storage pool of dopamine in younger animals. Dopamine measures after voluntary alcohol intake resulted in lower release amplitudes in response to potassium-chloride, indicating that alcohol affects the releasable pool of dopamine and this may have implications for vulnerability to addiction and other psychiatric diagnoses involving dopamine in the dorsal striatum.

Editor: Ryan K. Bachtell, University of Colorado, United States of America

Funding: Financial support from the Alcohol Research Council of the Swedish Alcohol Retailing Monopoly, ERAB: the European Foundation for Alcohol Research (EA 11 30) and the Swedish Research Council (K2012-61X-22090-01-3; IN) is gratefully acknowledged. The funders had no role in study design, data collection and analysis, decision to publish, or preparation of the manuscript.

Competing Interests: The authors have declared that no competing interests exist.

* E-mail: Sara.Palm@farmbio.uu.se

Introduction

Adolescence is associated with high impulsivity and risk-taking behavior, making adolescent individuals more inclined to use drugs [1]. Nicotine, alcohol or cannabis are likely tested before psychostimulants or opiates [2,3] and early drug use is correlated to increased substance use disorders (SUD) later in life [4–6]. The neurobiology underlying this increased risk of SUD is unclear, but adolescence is a time of extensive brain development and disturbances of normal brain development by drugs of abuse is hypothesized to contribute to the increased vulnerability after adolescent drug use [7].

Drugs of abuse commonly act on the reward system and increase extracellular levels of dopamine in the nucleus accumbens acutely after intake [8]. However, the transition from initial drug use to compulsive use and addiction involve long-lasting changes in many of the neural networks [9] and one of them is hypothesized to involve a shift from the nucleus accumbens, mediating acute reinforcing effects, to recruitment of the dorsal striatum and habit formation [10]. The dopaminergic activity in the dorsal striatum could therefore also be a factor in the vulnerability of adolescent individuals.

Animal models are of great importance to our understanding of these mechanisms and the age window identified as adolescence in rodents is between postnatal day (PND) 28 and 50 [11]. Previous studies have shown that adolescent rats have a reduced basal rate of dopamine release, a reduced pool of readily releasable dopamine, but also a larger storage pool of dopamine compared to adults [12]. It has also been suggested that despite the reduced dopamine release under basal conditions, the adolescent individuals may be able to release more dopamine if stimulated by pharmacological challenges [13]. The first of objective of this study was therefore to test the hypothesis of increased dopamine release after a pharmacological challenge in adolescent animals. Dopamine release and uptake was investigated using chronoamperometric dopamine recordings in combination with a challenge by amphetamine in early and late adolescent, as well as adult, outbred Wistar rats.

The second objective of this study was to investigate the effect of environmental influence by voluntary alcohol intake during adolescence. The rationale behind this was that previous studies show that environmental factors during the adolescent period, such as intraperitoneally administered alcohol, increase basal extracellular levels of dopamine [14] while voluntary alcohol intake in alcohol-preferring P rats increase dopamine uptake, without affecting basal extracellular levels [15]. Discrepancies between these studies can be explained by a number of factors, such as route of administration, dose, rat strain and exact time period, but in both cases, adolescent alcohol intake affects the dopamine dynamics and this is well worth investigating further.

Materials and Methods

Ethics Statement

All animal experiments were performed under a protocol approved by the Uppsala Animal Ethical Committee and followed the guidelines of the Swedish Legislation on Animal Experimentation (Animal Welfare Act SFS1998:56) and the European Communities Council Directive (86/609/EEC).

Animals

Pregnant Wistar rats (RccHan: WI, Harlan Laboratories B.V., Horst, The Netherlands) arrived at the animal facility at gestation day 16. The animals arrived in batches over several weeks in order to accommodate the timing of the chronoamperometric recordings. The dams were single housed in macrolon cages (59 cm×38 cm×20 cm) with pellet food (Type R36; Lantmännen, Kimstad, Sweden) and tap water *ad libitum.* The cages contained wood-chip bedding and paper sheets (40×60 cm; Cellstoff, Papyrus) and were changed once a week by animal care personnel. The animal room was kept at constant temperature (22±1°C) and humidity (50±10%) on a regular 12 h light/dark cycle with lights on at 06:00 am. All rooms had a masking background noise to minimize unexpected sounds that could disturb the animals.

An overview of the experimental outline can be found in Figure 1. The litters that were born on the same day (postnatal day (PND) 0) were cross-fostered to include 6 males and 4 females in order to control for maternal shipping stress, maternal behavior and genetics. The pups were weaned on PND 22 and housed 3 per cage until PND 28 (±1 day) or PND 42 (±1 day) when chronoamperometric recordings were made. Only male pups were further used in this study. A group of thirty male rats were given voluntary binge-like access to 20% ethanol in a two-bottle free-choice paradigm from PND28 to PND65. The animals were given 24 hours access to ethanol for three consecutive days per week, i.e. Tuesday through Thursday for six weeks, a total of 18 sessions. For measures of ethanol intake, the bottles were weighed before and after each session and grams pure ethanol per kilogram body weight were calculated. Bottle positions were changed between sessions to avoid position preference. The ethanol-drinking animals were individually housed from PND 28 until PND 70. The animals with the highest cumulative ethanol intake (g/kg) were selected and electrochemical recordings were then made at PND 70 (±2 days). Age-matched water-drinking controls were also housed individually during the same period.

Chronoamperometric Recordings of Dopamine *In vivo*

Materials. Inactin, Nafion 5% solution, dopamine hydrochloride, L-ascorbic acid, potassium chloride, sodium chloride, sodium phosphate, calcium chloride and d-amphetamine sulfate

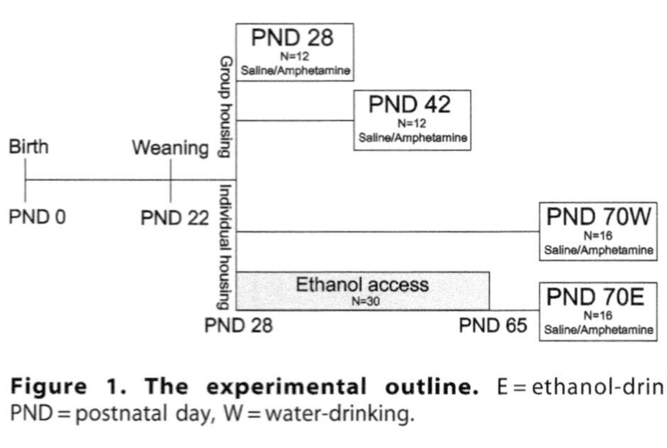

Figure 1. The experimental outline. E = ethanol-drinking, PND = postnatal day, W = water-drinking.

were obtained from Sigma-Aldrich, LLC (St Louis, MO, USA). Kerr sticky wax was obtained from DAB LAB AB (Upplands Väsby, Sweden). Carbon fibre microelectrodes (SF1A; 30 µm outer diameter×150 µm length) were purchased from Quanteon, LLC (Nicholasville, KY, USA), the reference electrode silver wire (200 µm, Teflon-insulated) was purchased from A-M Systems Inc. (Carlborg, WA, USA) and glass capillaries (0.58 mm inner diameter) for the micropipettes were purchased from World Precision Instruments Ltd (Stevenage, UK).

Surgery. Dopamine recordings were made at PND 28 (±1 day), PND 42 (±1 day) or PND 70 (±2 days). Surgery was performed immediately prior to the electrochemical recordings. A water-circulating heating pad (Gaymar Industries, Inc., Orchard Park, New York) was used to maintain body temperature. The animals were anesthetized with Inactin 125 mg/kg intraperitoneally (i.p.) and placed in a stereotaxic frame (Stoelting Co., Wood Dale, IL, USA). A hole in the skull was drilled overlying the recording site for the electrode, and another hole was drilled remote from the recording site for the placement of the Ag/AgCl reference electrode.

High-speed chronoamperometric recordings of dopamine release and uptake. High-speed chronoamperometric measurements (1 Hz sampling rate, 200 ms total) were performed using the FAST16-mkII recording system (Fast Analytical Sensing Technology, Quanteon, LLC, Nicholasville, KY, USA) according to a previously described procedure [16]. Carbon fibre microelectrodes (SF1A) were coated with three coats of Nafion with 5 min heating at 200°C before the first coating and after each coating [17]. The electrodes were then calibrated *in vitro* in 0.05 M phosphate buffered saline to determine selectivity, limit of detection (LOD) and slope before use *in vivo* [16]. The microelectrodes showed linear responses to serial additions of dopamine (2–6 µM), with an average correlation coefficient (R2) of 0.999±0.0003. The average selectivity for all electrodes used in this study was 14482±3005 µM for dopamine over ascorbic acid. The average LOD was 0.026±0.004 µM dopamine, and the average slope was −1.00±0.03 nA/µM dopamine. The average reduction/oxidation ratio measured during the reference peak responses of dopamine was 0.67±0.02, which is indicative of the detection of predominantly dopamine [17]. A silver wire was plated and used as the *in vivo* Ag/AgCl reference electrode [18].

In vivo experimental protocol. A micropipette (10–15 µm inner diameter) was filled with isotonic potassium chloride solution (120 mM KCl, 29 mM NaCl, 2.5 mM $CaCl_2 \cdot 2H_2O$) (pH 7.2–7.4) using a pipette-filling needle (28G, World Precision Instruments, Aston, UK). The micropipette was affixed approximately 150–200 µm from the carbon fibre tip using sticky wax. The electrode was stereotactically placed in the dorsal striatum, AP: +1.0 mm, L: +3.0 mm from bregma, the incisor bar was adjusted according to age and weight [19,20]. The electrode was initially placed dorsal (−3.0 mm) to the recording site, using a micromanipulator (Narishige International Ltd, London, UK) to lower it, and allowed to reach a stable baseline for about 45–60 min before being lowered to a depth of −4.0 mm from bregma. The electrode was then allowed another 5–10 min to stabilize at the recording site before the effect of a single injection of potassium chloride on dopamine release was determined. The potassium solution was locally applied using pressure ejection controlled by a PicoSpritzer III (Parker Hannifin Corporation, Pine Brook, NJ, USA) and the pressure (10–20 psi) and time (0.5–1.0 s) was adjusted to deliver 100 nl of the potassium solution, measured by a surgical microscope fitted with an eyepiece reticule [21].

Potassium evoked release was used in combination with subcutaneous injections of amphetamine or saline. Three reference peaks similar in amplitude were produced, 10 min apart. Five min after the last reference peak, rats were given either 2 mg/kg amphetamine or the equivalent amount of saline (1 ml/kg) and after another 5 min release was again evoked every 10 min, producing peaks at 5, 15, 25, 35, 45, 55 and 65 min after the systemic injection, see Figure 2A for a representative trace. The dose of amphetamine was chosen based on behavioral effects in locomotion and self-administration studies [22–24].

Verification of electrode placement and exclusions. The electrodes were cut off and left in place after the finished experiment and the brains were frozen. The placement was verified by sectioning of the frozen brains. From the 12 animals at PND28, 1 was excluded due to wrongful placement, and 2 because of recording errors. For the 12 animals at PND 42, 1 animal was excluded due to wrongful placement. For the 16 animals at PND 70, 3 were excluded due to recording errors. For the 16 ethanol-drinking animals at PND 70, 2 were excluded due to recording errors. Recording errors include pipette clogging and electrical disturbances such as power cuts and disturbances of the general power supply to the recording unit.

Data analysis. The maximal amplitude of the evoked peaks and the time for the peak to decline to 80% of its amplitude (T80) were calculated using the FAST Analysis software version 4.4 (Quanteon, LLC, Nicholasville, KY, USA), see Figure 2B for a representative trace. The three reference peaks were averaged and the percentage of these peaks were calculated for the peaks following injection. For statistical analysis, repeated measures analysis of variance (ANOVA) was used to compare chronoamperometric data over time between ages or drinking groups and

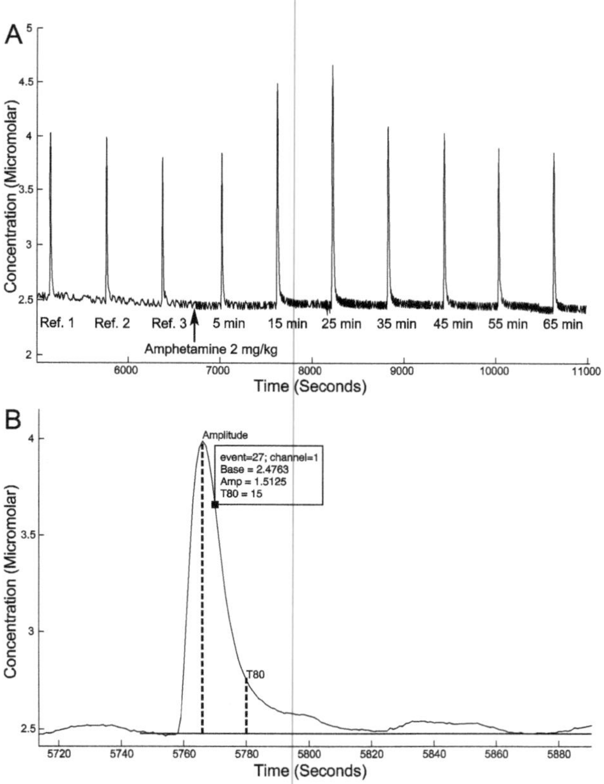

Figure 2. Representative traces. A) A representative trace of the oxidation current for a rat at postnatal day 28 receiving amphetamine and B) a close-up of the second reference peak for the same animal showing how amplitude and T80 were calculated. Amp = amplitude, Base = baseline, Ref = reference.

treatment (saline or amphetamine), followed by Fisher's least significant difference (LSD) post-hoc test. For ethanol intake data, which was not normally distributed, Friedman ANOVA was used. Statistical analyses were performed using Statistica 10 (StatSoft Inc., Tulsa, OK, USA). Differences were considered statistically significant at $p<0.05$.

Results

Age-dependent Effects

Differences in reference amplitudes between the age groups are shown in Figure 3. A repeated measures ANOVA comparing age and time, showed a main effect of age [$F(2,22) = 5.81$; $p = 0.009$], but no effect of time [$F(2,44) = 1.43$; $p = 0.25$] or any interaction effect between time and age [$F(4,44) = 1.70$; $p = 0.17$].

No effects of age [$F(2,24) = 1.02$; $p = 0.38$], time [$F(2,48) = 0.94$; $p = 0.40$] or time and age [$F(4,48) = 0.22$; $p = 0.93$] were found for the reference T80 values. The mean $\pm$ standard error of the mean (SEM) reference T80 values were 17.3 ± 1.3 for the PND 28, 19.5 ± 0.9 for the PND 42 and 20.5 ± 1.0 for the PND70.

Differences between the age groups in amplitude response to amphetamine are shown in Figure 4A–C. Amphetamine treatment resulted in main effects of age [$F(2,26) = 3.95$; $p = 0.03$], treatment [$F(1,26) = 10.77$; $p = 0.003$] and time [$F(6,156) = 3.32$; $p = 0.004$], and interaction effects between time and age [$F(12,156) = 2.23$; $p = 0.01$], time and treatment [$F(6,156) = 4.20$; $p<0.001$], but no interaction between age and treatment [$F(2,26) = 2.37$; $p = 0.11$] or time, age and treatment [$F(12,156) = 0.77$; $p = 0.68$].

The T80 response to amphetamine is shown in Figure 4D–E. There was no main effect of age [$F(2,25) = 1.87$; $p = 0.17$], but there were effects of treatment [$F(1,25) = 26.52$; $p<0.001$], time [$F(6,150) = 7.70$; $p<0.001$] and an interaction effect of time and treatment [$F(6,150) = 12.29$; $p<0.001$]. There was no interaction between age and treatment [$F(2,25) = 1.29$; $p = 0.29$], time and age [$F(12,150) = 0.66$; $p = 0.78$] and a trend towards an interaction between time, age and treatment [$F(12,150) = 1.60$; $p = 0.098$].

Voluntary Adolescent Alcohol Intake

Ethanol intake data for the 14 rats that were used in the chronoamperometric recordings are shown in Table 1. A Friedman ANOVA showed no significant differences in intake over time, although there was a trend [$\chi^2 = 9.80$; $p = 0.08$] towards differences driven by the intake during the second week (PND 35–37), which was slightly higher than the following weeks. A Friedman ANOVA of the preference showed an increase over time [$\chi^2 = 19.7$; $p = 0.001$], mainly as a result from increases over the first three weeks, see Table 1.

Differences in reference amplitudes between the ethanol- and water-drinking groups are shown in Figure 5. A repeated measures ANOVA comparing drinking group and time, showed a main effect of drinking group [$F(1,17) = 16.22$; $p<0.001$], but no effect of time [$F(2,34) = 1.76$; $p = 0.19$] or any interaction effect between time and drinking group [$F(4,44) = 1.32$; $p = 0.28$].

No effects of drinking group [$F(1,18) = 0.04$; $p = 0.85$], time [$F(2,36) = 1.96$; $p = 0.16$] or time and drinking group [$F(2,36) = 0.22$; $p = 0.81$] were found for the reference T80 values. The mean $\pm$ SEM reference T80 values were 20.5 ± 1.0 for the water-drinking rats, and 19.1 ± 1.3 for the ethanol-drinking rats.

The response to amphetamine in the ethanol- and water-drinking groups is shown in Figure 6. For the amplitudes, as shown in Figure 6A, there was a trend to an effect of treatment [$F(1,19) = 3.01$; $p = 0.099$] and there was a main effect of time [$F(6,114) = 2.30$; $p = 0.04$], but no effect of drinking group

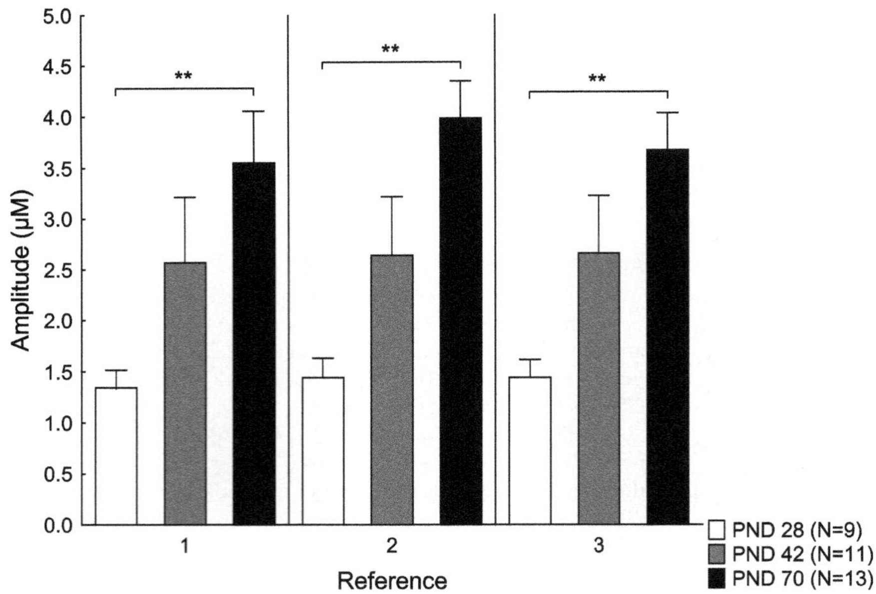

Figure 3. Reference peak amplitudes in different ages. Amplitudes (μM) (mean ± SEM) of the three reference peaks before treatment with either amphetamine or saline in the three age groups; postnatal day (PND) 28, 42 and 70. **p<0.01.

[F(1,19) = 0.39; p = 0.54] or any interaction effects between treatment and drinking group [F(1,19) = 0.83; p = 0.37] or time and treatment [F(6,114) = 1.13; p = 0.35], time and drinking group [F(6,114) = 0.44; p = 0.85] or time, treatment and drinking group [F(6,114) = 0.27; p = 0.95].

For the T80 values, Figure 6B, there was a main effect of treatment [F(1,19) = 17.35; p<0.001] and time [F(6,114) = 2.42; p = 0.03], and an interaction effect between time and treatment [F(6,114) = 10.28; p<0.001]. There was no effect of drinking group [F(1,19) = 0.33; p = 0.57], or any interaction effect between treatment and drinking group [F(1,19) = 0.76; p = 0.40], time and drinking group [F(6,114) = 1.66; p = 0.14], or time, treatment and drinking group [F(6,114) = 1.75; p = 0.12].

Discussion

Age-dependent effects on dopamine release and uptake was investigated under basal conditions and in response to amphetamine in early and late adolescent, as well as adult, rats. The impact of alcohol drinking during adolescence was also examined and is, to our knowledge, the first study investigating release and uptake in voluntary drinking adolescent rats with a chronoamperometric technique.

Age-dependent Effects

The age-dependent differences in reference amplitudes are in agreement with a previous study using voltammetry in combination with electrical stimulation, which showed that adult rats released more dopamine upon stimulation than young rats [12]. The time-point for adolescence used by Stamford (1989) was approximately PND 30, but since then studies have shown that around PND 40–45 there are peaks in basal extracellular levels of dopamine [25–27] and dopamine receptor D_2 density [28], while tyrosine hydroxylase levels are lower than both early adolescence and adulthood [29]. The current study therefore included two time-points during adolescence, PND 28 and PND 42, equivalent to early and late adolescence [11]. Amplitudes in late adolescent animals were intermediate to amplitudes in early adolescence and adulthood, indicating that development from adolescence into adulthood involved a gradual increase in the release capacity of dopamine in response to potassium chloride in the dorsal striatum. This is consistent with reports of increased extracellular levels of dopamine in the nucleus accumbens in adulthood compared to adolescence [30,31]. As previously mentioned, some studies also show peak levels at PND 45 [25–27] and they can be reconciled with the current study through reports of increased firing rates around the same PND [32,33]. The current study did not measure basal extracellular levels and it is possible that an increased firing rate results in increased basal levels without any peak in potassium-induced release. Furthermore, one of the studies showing potassium-induced extracellular levels in the nucleus accumbens to peak around PND 42 [25] contrasts to data from the dorsal striatum, from Stamford (1989) and the current study, which indicate regional differences.

The uptake measure, T80, did not reveal any differences between the ages in the current study, whereas Stamford (1989) found that the rate of uptake was higher in adult rats. This can be due to methodological differences in the measure of uptake; T80 includes both the linear and the curvilinear part of the curve, whereas Stamford used the linear part of the curve [34]. The concentrations reached in this study are only a tenth of the concentrations in the previous study and V_{max} should therefore not be reached. Using the linear part of the peak curve to calculate uptake rate under these conditions will only produce uptake rates dependent on amplitudes [35]. T80 was chosen because it also takes into account the curvilinear part of the curve, where dopamine concentrations are lower and is more sensitive to dopamine uptake blockers [35,36]. Naturally, T80 is also dependent on the amplitude, but as can be seen in this study, differences in amplitude do not automatically result in differences in T80, suggesting that the ratio of uptake to release is shifted towards uptake in the younger animals. Supporting the current findings is a study that used quantitative microdialysis and found no differences in the extraction fraction, an indirect measure of uptake rate, in the nucleus accumbens of rats at PND 35, 45 and 60 [26].

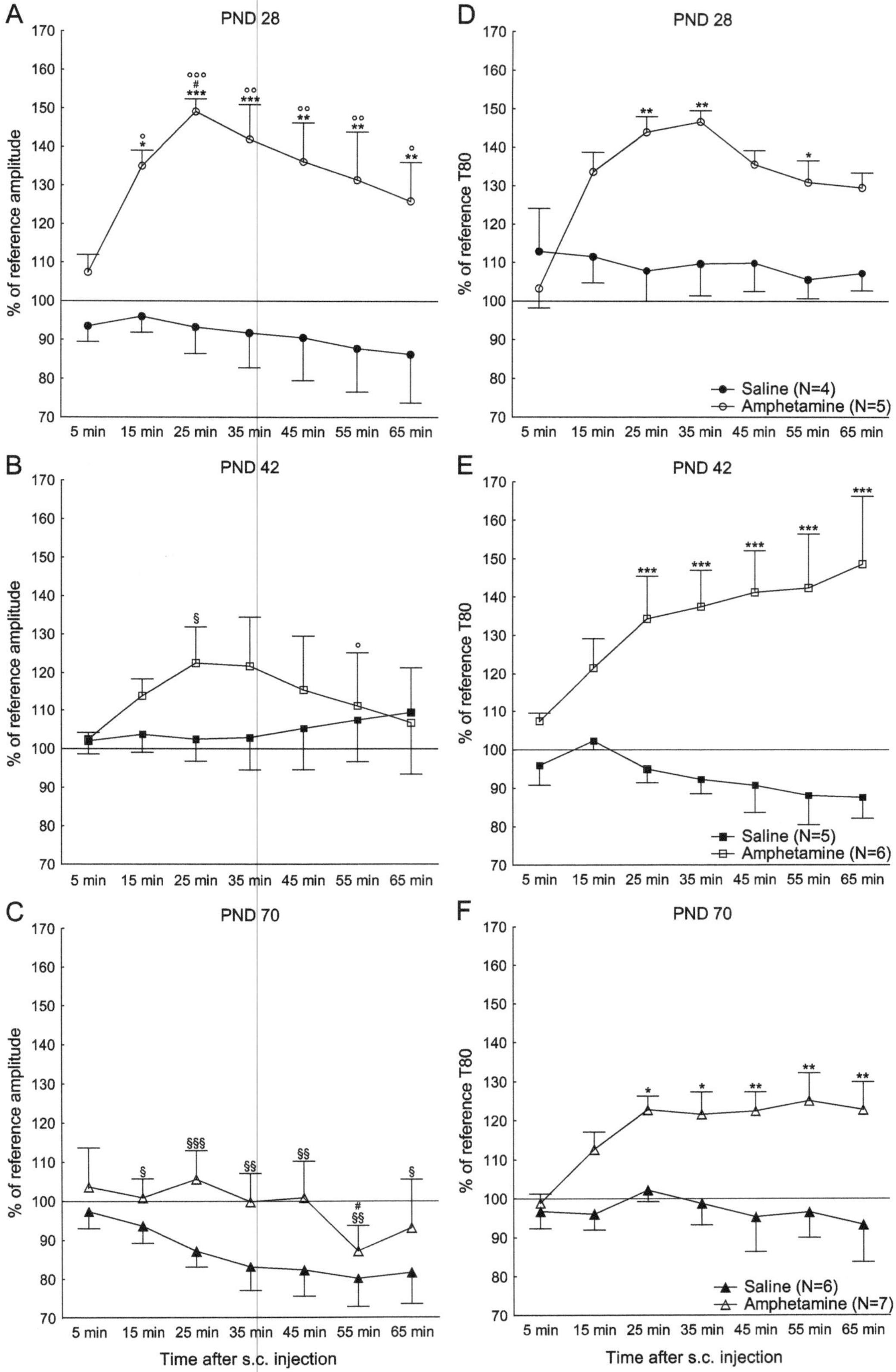

Figure 4. Amplitudes and T80 responses over time in different ages. Responses over time after subcutaneous (s.c.) injections of saline or amphetamine, as percent of reference values (mean ± SEM), for the amplitudes at A) postnatal day (PND) 28, B) PND 42 and C) PND 70, and for the T80 values at D) PND 28, E) PND 42 and F) PND 70. *$p<0.05$, **$p<0.01$, ***$p<0.001$ compared to saline controls, $^{\#}p<0.05$ compared to the equivalent time-point at PND 42, $^{\circ}p<0.05$, $^{\circ\circ}p<0.01$, $^{\circ\circ\circ}p<0.001$ compared to the equivalent time-point at PND 70, $^{\S}p<0.05$, $^{\S\S}p<0.01$, $^{\S\S\S}p<0.001$ compared to the equivalent time-point at PND 28.

Table 1. The median, minimum and maximum alcohol intake (g/kg/24 h) and preference (%) for the six weeks of alcohol access and the median, minimum and maximum cumulative intake (g) after the 18 sessions.

Week	Median intake	Min	Max	Median preference	Min	Max
1	3.5	3.1	7.5	11.9	9.6	19.1
2	4.1	2.6	8.9	15.2*	8.9	31.0
3	3.6	2.2	6.5	16.9*	9.5	35.3
4	3.5	1.8	7.0	17.5	9.3	35.5
5	3.3	1.9	6.0	19.4	9.8	36.9
6	3.6	1.7	5.6	22.9	10.4	34.5
Cumulative	12.5	9.0	22.0			

*p<0.05 compared to the previous week.

The greater potassium-evoked release in adulthood could be due to a larger releasable pool of dopamine [12] and a number of factors could be involved, such as age-dependent differences in dopamine synthesis by tyrosine hydroxylase [29,37], vesicular monoamine transporter-2 (VMAT-2)-containing vesicles [38], and kinetics of the VMAT-2 [39], as well as D2 receptor pruning [28] and function [40]. These factors could also help explain the increased amplitudes seen after amphetamine in early adolescent animals. Again, the current data are consistent with data showing a larger increase in dopamine release in young compared to adult animals in response to nomifensine [12] indicating that early adolescent rats have a proportionally larger storage pool, which can be released upon stimulation by psychoactive substances. This is further supported by data showing a larger increase in stimulated extracellular dopamine after amphetamine in adolescent animals [22]. However, there are microdialysis studies showing lower extracellular levels of dopamine after amphetamine in adolescents compared to adults [30,37], which again underline that a possibility of increase in stimulated release does not necessarily mean an increase in extracellular levels and that different techniques can add complementing information.

No age-dependent effects on T80 after amphetamine was found, which indicates that amphetamine exerts similar effects on dopamine uptake in all ages. This is again supported by the results from Stamford (1989), showing no differences in the degree of uptake blockade after nomifensine between age groups. There are also studies suggesting that age-related differences in dopamine transporter structure and function are related to the cocaine-binding site on the transporter, but not the amphetamine-binding site [22] which could indicate that age-dependent effects of amphetamine on uptake do not exist. However, there was a trend towards an interaction between time, age and treatment, suggesting that they responded differently over time to amphetamine depending on age. Further studies investigating the uptake by applying exogenous dopamine could also help separate amplitude-dependent uptake from transporter function [41–43]. Studies in awake rats would also be of importance, as the current study was done in anesthetized animals. The anesthesia used was the barbiturate thiobutabarbital (Inactin), a positive allosteric

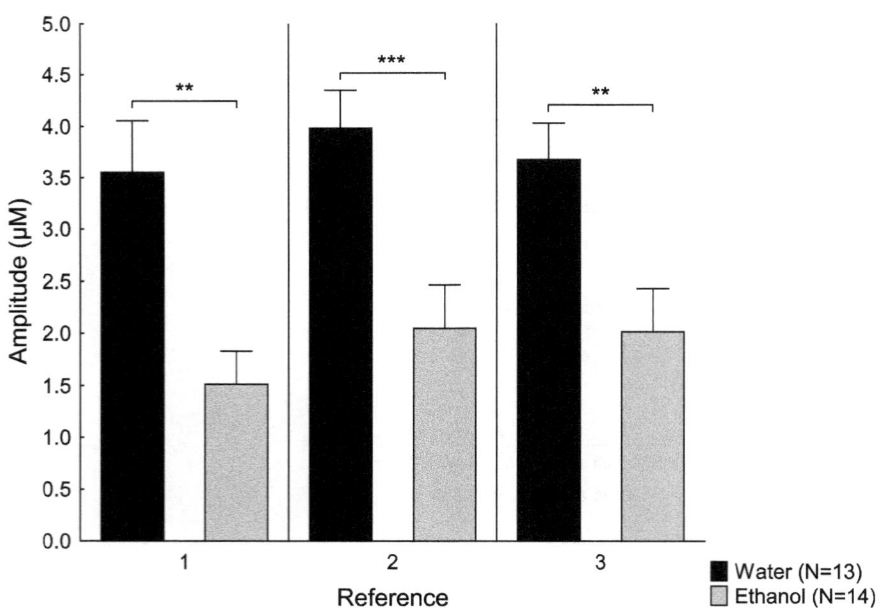

Figure 5. Reference peak amplitudes in water- or ethanol-drinking animals. Amplitudes (μM) (mean ± SEM) of the three reference peaks before treatment with either amphetamine or saline in the water- and ethanol-drinking groups. **p<0.01, ***p<0.001.

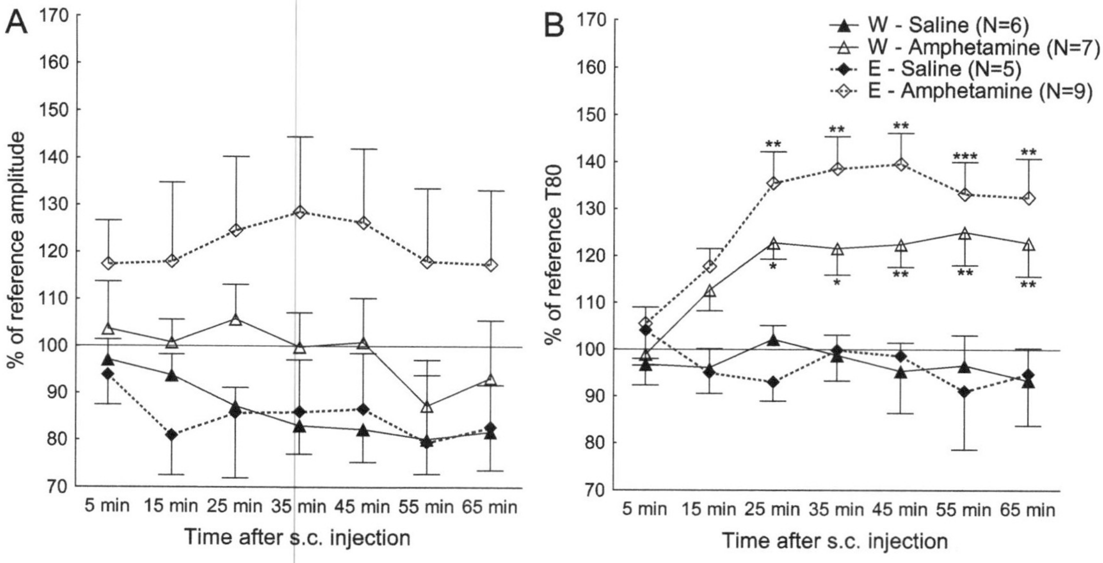

Figure 6. Amplitudes and T80 responses over time in water- or ethanol-drinking animals. Responses over time after subcutaneous (s.c.) injections of saline or amphetamine, as percent of reference values (mean ± SEM), for the A) amplitudes and B) T80 values in the water (W)- or ethanol (E)-drinking groups. *$p<0.05$, **$p<0.01$, ***$p<0.001$ compared to saline controls.

modulator of gamma-aminobutyric acid (GABA) A receptors, which produces a prolonged and stable anesthesia in rats [44]. GABA may exert different effects depending on age and alcohol-drinking history [45] and therefore, the anesthesia could interact with age or treatment and produce confounding effects. However, pentobarbital, another barbiturate, has been shown to have little effect on dopamine levels in the striatum [46]. Furthermore, in the current study, release was induced using potassium chloride and did not rely on spontaneous events, which should decrease the importance of GABAergic tone on release. As for the dopamine uptake there are reports that barbiturates may affect dopamine uptake specifically [47], but whether there could also be an interaction with age or treatment is unclear.

Voluntary Adolescent Alcohol Intake

Voluntary adolescent alcohol intake for six weeks resulted in lower reference amplitudes compared to water-drinking controls. The amplitudes were similar to those seen in early adolescent rats. Since the effects were seen in amplitudes and not uptake time, it is conceivable that alcohol affects factors controlling the releasable pool of dopamine rather than the dopamine transporter and there are data supporting unaffected uptake after adolescent alcohol [14]. There are also microdialysis data showing increased extracellular levels of dopamine after adolescent exposure to intraperitoneal injections of alcohol [14,27,48], and this is somewhat contradictory to the current findings of decreased releasable dopamine. As mentioned earlier, increased firing rates may be a way of reconciling the microdialysis data with the current data, but there are no studies to support this. Furthermore, there are studies showing that the mode of alcohol exposure, i.e. voluntary or forced, may have different effects on the neurobiology [49].

When treated with amphetamine, there were no significant differences between the alcohol- and water-drinking groups in amplitudes or T80. However, there was a trend towards an effect on amplitudes, due to the increase displayed by the alcohol-drinking group. There is also more variation in the response to amphetamine in the alcohol-drinking group, which could be due to a variation in alcohol intake, although this variation is not correlated to the response (data not shown). This also points to a limitation with this study, namely that blood alcohol levels were not measured. The study was based on undisturbed access for 24 h and for blood alcohol levels to be measured the access would have had to be limited and the stress involved in blood sampling would have risked to disturb the intake patterns of the animals. Thus, correlations between response and individual blood alcohol levels cannot be ruled out. However, the intake data presented in this study is similar to other studies, showing neurobiological effects of alcohol, using Wistar rats in similar ages or intake paradigms[50–52]. This suggests that not only individuals prone to high intake, but also modest drinkers from a cross-section of a general population, risk changes in neurobiology after voluntary adolescent alcohol intake.

No differences in uptake time after amphetamine suggests that adolescent alcohol has no effect on dopamine transporter function in response to amphetamine, but would also benefit from investigation by application of exogenous dopamine [41–43].

Furthermore, two interesting observations were made. Firstly, the reference amplitudes after alcohol intake are similar to those seen in animals at the beginning of the alcohol intake period, i.e. PND 28. Secondly, the size of the increase in amplitudes after amphetamine in the alcohol-drinking animals is similar to the late adolescent rats, i.e. PND 42. Whether these findings relate to altered development of the releasable pool and the storage pool of dopamine in the neurons remains to be elucidated. The current study did not include a group of adult alcohol-drinking rats so conclusions about the possibility of age-specific effects cannot be drawn. However, indications of age-specific effects can be found in the discrepancies between studies of adolescent alcohol-exposed rats that show unaffected dopamine uptake [14] and studies of adult alcohol-exposed rats and monkeys that show increased uptake, but no effects on evoked dopamine overflow [53,54]. For future studies, it would therefore be of great interest to investigate alcohol exposure and the mechanisms behind its effect in different ages. Further investigations into factors such as tyrosine hydroxylase, dopamine receptor density and function, and vesicular monoamine transporter could help shed some light on possible age-specific alcohol effects on the releasable pool and the storage pool of dopamine. To our knowledge, these factors have not been investigated after adolescent alcohol.

Conclusion

The data show a gradual increase of evoked dopamine overflow with age, supporting previous studies suggesting that the pool of releasable dopamine increases with age. In contrast, a gradual decrease in evoked overflow with age was seen in response to amphetamine, supporting a proportionally larger storage pool of dopamine in younger animals, making them potentially more sensitive to dopamine-releasing drugs. Adolescent alcohol intake resulted in overflow lower than in water-drinking controls., indicating that alcohol affects the releasable pool of dopamine and this may have implications for vulnerability to addiction and other psychiatric diagnoses involving the dopamine system in the dorsal striatum.

Acknowledgments

The authors wish to thank Ms. Marita Berg for technical assistance and Dr. Martin Lundblad for methodological discussions.

Author Contributions

Conceived and designed the experiments: SP IN. Performed the experiments: SP. Analyzed the data: SP IN. Wrote the paper: SP.

References

1. Arnett J (1992) Reckless Behavior in Adolescence - a Developmental Perspective. Developmental Review 12: 339–373.
2. Yamaguchi K, Kandel DB (1984) Patterns of drug use from adolescence to young adulthood: II. Sequences of progression. Am J Public Health 74: 668–672.
3. Degenhardt L, Chiu WT, Conway K, Dierker L, Glantz M, et al. (2009) Does the 'gateway' matter? Associations between the order of drug use initiation and the development of drug dependence in the National Comorbidity Study Replication. Psychol Med 39: 157–167.
4. Anthony JC, Petronis KR (1995) Early-onset drug use and risk of later drug problems. Drug Alcohol Depend 40: 9–15.
5. Grant BF, Dawson DA (1997) Age at onset of alcohol use and its association with DSM-IV alcohol abuse and dependence: results from the National Longitudinal Alcohol Epidemiologic Survey. J Subst Abuse 9: 103–110.
6. DeWit DJ, Adlaf EM, Offord DR, Ogborne AC (2000) Age at first alcohol use: a risk factor for the development of alcohol disorders. Am J Psychiatry 157: 745–750.
7. Crews F, He J, Hodge C (2007) Adolescent cortical development: a critical period of vulnerability for addiction. Pharmacol Biochem Behav 86: 189–199.
8. Di Chiara G, Imperato A (1988) Drugs abused by humans preferentially increase synaptic dopamine concentrations in the mesolimbic system of freely moving rats. Proc Natl Acad Sci U S A 85: 5274–5278.
9. Koob GF, Volkow ND (2010) Neurocircuitry of addiction. Neuropsychopharmacology 35: 217–238.
10. Everitt BJ, Robbins TW (2013) From the ventral to the dorsal striatum: Devolving views of their roles in drug addiction. Neurosci Biobehav Rev.
11. Spear LP (2000) The adolescent brain and age-related behavioral manifestations. Neurosci Biobehav Rev 24: 417–463.
12. Stamford JA (1989) Development and ageing of the rat nigrostriatal dopamine system studied with fast cyclic voltammetry. J Neurochem 52: 1582–1589.
13. Marco EM, Adriani W, Ruocco LA, Canese R, Sadile AG, et al. (2011) Neurobehavioral adaptations to methylphenidate: the issue of early adolescent exposure. Neurosci Biobehav Rev 35: 1722–1739.
14. Badanich KA, Maldonado AM, Kirstein CL (2007) Chronic ethanol exposure during adolescence increases basal dopamine in the nucleus accumbens septi during adulthood. Alcohol Clin Exp Res 31: 895–900.
15. Sahr AE, Thielen RJ, Lumeng L, Li TK, McBride WJ (2004) Long-lasting alterations of the mesolimbic dopamine system after periadolescent ethanol drinking by alcohol-preferring rats. Alcohol Clin Exp Res 28: 702–711.
16. Littrell OM, Pomerleau F, Huettl P, Surgener S, McGinty JF, et al. (2012) Enhanced dopamine transporter activity in middle-aged Gdnf heterozygous mice. Neurobiol Aging 33: 427 e421–414.
17. Gerhardt GA, Hoffman AF (2001) Effects of recording media composition on the responses of Nafion-coated carbon fiber microelectrodes measured using high-speed chronoamperometry. J Neurosci Methods 109: 13–21.
18. Lundblad M, af Bjerken S, Cenci MA, Pomerleau F, Gerhardt GA, et al. (2009) Chronic intermittent L-DOPA treatment induces changes in dopamine release. J Neurochem 108: 998–1008.
19. Paxinos G, Watson C (2007) The Rat Brain in Stereotaxic Coordinates. New York: Academic Press.
20. Sherwood NM, Timiras PS (1970) A stereotaxic atlas of the developing rat brain. Berkeley,: University of California Press. 209 p. (p. 214–203 illus.) p.
21. Friedemann MN, Gerhardt GA (1992) Regional effects of aging on dopaminergic function in the Fischer-344 rat. Neurobiol Aging 13: 325–332.
22. Walker QD, Morris SE, Arrant AE, Nagel JM, Parylak S, et al. (2010) Dopamine uptake inhibitors but not dopamine releasers induce greater increases in motor behavior and extracellular dopamine in adolescent rats than in adult male rats. J Pharmacol Exp Ther 335: 124–132.
23. Hooks MS, Jones GH, Neill DB, Justice JB Jr (1992) Individual differences in amphetamine sensitization: dose-dependent effects. Pharmacol Biochem Behav 41: 203–210.
24. Dellu F, Piazza PV, Mayo W, Le Moal M, Simon H (1996) Novelty-seeking in rats–biobehavioral characteristics and possible relationship with the sensation-seeking trait in man. Neuropsychobiology 34: 136–145.
25. Nakano M, Mizuno T (1996) Age-related changes in the metabolism of neurotransmitters in rat striatum: a microdialysis study. Mech Ageing Dev 86: 95–104.
26. Badanich KA, Adler KJ, Kirstein CL (2006) Adolescents differ from adults in cocaine conditioned place preference and cocaine-induced dopamine in the nucleus accumbens septi. Eur J Pharmacol 550: 95–106.
27. Philpot RM, Wecker L, Kirstein CL (2009) Repeated ethanol exposure during adolescence alters the developmental trajectory of dopaminergic output from the nucleus accumbens septi. Int J Dev Neurosci 27: 805–815.
28. Teicher MH, Andersen SL, Hostetter JC Jr (1995) Evidence for dopamine receptor pruning between adolescence and adulthood in striatum but not nucleus accumbens. Brain Res Dev Brain Res 89: 167–172.
29. Mathews IZ, Waters P, McCormick CM (2009) Changes in hyporesponsiveness to acute amphetamine and age differences in tyrosine hydroxylase immunoreactivity in the brain over adolescence in male and female rats. Dev Psychobiol 51: 417–428.
30. Laviola G, Pascucci T, Pieretti S (2001) Striatal dopamine sensitization to D-amphetamine in periadolescent but not in adult rats. Pharmacol Biochem Behav 68: 115–124.
31. Gazzara RA, Andersen SL (1994) The ontogeny of apomorphine-induced alterations of neostriatal dopamine release: effects on potassium-evoked release. Neurochem Res 19: 339–345.
32. McCutcheon JE, Marinelli M (2009) Age matters. Eur J Neurosci 29: 997–1014.
33. Wong WC, Ford KA, Pagels NE, McCutcheon JE, Marinelli M (2013) Adolescents are more vulnerable to cocaine addiction: behavioral and electrophysiological evidence. J Neurosci 33: 4913–4922.
34. Stamford JA, Kruk ZL, Millar J, Wightman RM (1984) Striatal dopamine uptake in the rat: in vivo analysis by fast cyclic voltammetry. Neurosci Lett 51: 133–138.
35. Wightman RM, Zimmerman JB (1990) Control of dopamine extracellular concentration in rat striatum by impulse flow and uptake. Brain Res Brain Res Rev 15: 135–144.
36. Zahniser NR, Dickinson SD, Gerhardt GA (1998) High-speed chronoamperometric electrochemical measurements of dopamine clearance. Methods Enzymol 296: 708–719.
37. Matthews M, Bondi C, Torres G, Moghaddam B (2013) Reduced presynaptic dopamine activity in adolescent dorsal striatum. Neuropsychopharmacology 38: 1344–1351.
38. Truong JG, Wilkins DG, Baudys J, Crouch DJ, Johnson-Davis KL, et al. (2005) Age-dependent methamphetamine-induced alterations in vesicular monoamine transporter-2 function: implications for neurotoxicity. J Pharmacol Exp Ther 314: 1087–1092.
39. Volz TJ, Farnsworth SJ, Rowley SD, Hanson GR, Fleckenstein AE (2009) Age-dependent differences in dopamine transporter and vesicular monoamine transporter-2 function and their implications for methamphetamine neurotoxicity. Synapse 63: 147–151.
40. Benoit-Marand M, O'Donnell P (2008) D2 dopamine modulation of corticoaccumbens synaptic responses changes during adolescence. Eur J Neurosci 27: 1364–1372.
41. Cass WA, Gerhardt GA (1995) In vivo assessment of dopamine uptake in rat medial prefrontal cortex: comparison with dorsal striatum and nucleus accumbens. J Neurochem 65: 201–207.
42. Cass WA, Zahniser NR, Flach KA, Gerhardt GA (1993) Clearance of exogenous dopamine in rat dorsal striatum and nucleus accumbens: role of metabolism and effects of locally applied uptake inhibitors. J Neurochem 61: 2269–2278.
43. Miller EM, Pomerleau F, Huettl P, Russell VA, Gerhardt GA, et al. (2012) The spontaneously hypertensive and Wistar Kyoto rat models of ADHD exhibit sub-regional differences in dopamine release and uptake in the striatum and nucleus accumbens. Neuropharmacology 63: 1327–1334.

44. Fish RE (2008) Anesthesia and Analgesia in Laboratory Animals. San Diego: Academic Press.
45. Silveri MM (2014) Contributions of GABA to alcohol responsivity during adolescence: Insights from preclinical and clinical studies. Pharmacol Ther.
46. Semba K, Adachi N, Arai T (2005) Facilitation of serotonergic activity and amnesia in rats caused by intravenous anesthetics. Anesthesiology 102: 616–623.
47. Keita H, Lecharny JB, Henzel D, Desmonts JM, Mantz J (1996) Is inhibition of dopamine uptake relevant to the hypnotic action of i.v. anaesthetics? Br J Anaesth 77: 254–256.
48. Pascual M, Boix J, Felipo V, Guerri C (2009) Repeated alcohol administration during adolescence causes changes in the mesolimbic dopaminergic and glutamatergic systems and promotes alcohol intake in the adult rat. J Neurochem 108: 920–931.
49. Spanagel R (2003) Alcohol addiction research: from animal models to clinics. Best Pract Res Clin Gastroenterol 17: 507–518.
50. Adermark L, Jonsson S, Ericson M, Soderpalm B (2011) Intermittent ethanol consumption depresses endocannabinoid-signaling in the dorsolateral striatum of rat. Neuropharmacology 61: 1160–1165.
51. García-Burgos D, González F, Manrique T, Gallo M (2009) Patterns of ethanol intake in preadolescent, adolescent, and adult Wistar rats under acquisition, maintenance and relapse-like conditions. Alcoholism: Clinical and Experimental Research 33: 722–728.
52. Steensland P, Fredriksson I, Holst S, Feltmann K, Franck J, et al. (2012) The monoamine stabilizer (-)-OSU6162 attenuates voluntary ethanol intake and ethanol-induced dopamine output in nucleus accumbens. Biol Psychiatry 72: 823–831.
53. Budygin EA, John CE, Mateo Y, Daunais JB, Friedman DP, et al. (2003) Chronic ethanol exposure alters presynaptic dopamine function in the striatum of monkeys: a preliminary study. Synapse 50: 266–268.
54. Budygin EA, Oleson EB, Mathews TA, Lack AK, Diaz MR, et al. (2007) Effects of chronic alcohol exposure on dopamine uptake in rat nucleus accumbens and caudate putamen. Psychopharmacology (Berl) 193: 495–501.

18

Effectiveness of Guided and Unguided Low-Intensity Internet Interventions for Adult Alcohol Misuse

Heleen Riper[1,2]*, Matthijs Blankers[3,4,5], Hana Hadiwijaya[1,11], John Cunningham[6,7], Stella Clarke[8], Reinout Wiers[9], David Ebert[2,10], Pim Cuijpers[1,2]

1 Department of Clinical Psychology and EMGO Institute, VU University Amsterdam, Amsterdam, Netherlands, **2** Division Health Trainings online, EU innovation Incubator, Leuphana University, Lüneburg, Germany, **3** Arkin Mental Health Care, Amsterdam, the Netherlands, **4** Trimbos Institute, Netherlands Institute of Mental Health and Addiction, Utrecht, The Netherlands, **5** Amsterdam Institute for Addiction Research, Department of Psychiatry, Academic Medical Centre, University of Amsterdam, the Netherlands, **6** Centre for Mental Health Research, the Australian National University, Canberra, Australia, **7** Centre for Addiction and Mental Health, Toronto, Canada, **8** NHS Fife, Edinburgh, Scotland, United Kingdom, **9** Addiction, Development and Psychopathology (ADAPT) lab, Department of Psychology, University of Amsterdam, Amsterdam, The Netherlands, **10** Division for Clinical Psychology and Psychotherapy, Department for Psychology, Philipp's University Marburg, Marburg, Germany, **11** TS Social and Behavioral Sciences, Department of Developmental Psychology, Tilburg University, Tilburg, the Netherlands

Abstract

Background: Alcohol misuse ranks within the top ten health conditions with the highest global burden of disease. Low-intensity, Internet interventions for curbing adult alcohol misuse have been shown effective. Few meta-analyses have been carried out, however, and they have involved small numbers of studies, lacked indicators of drinking within low risk guidelines, and examined the effectiveness of *unguided* self-help only. We therefore conducted a more thorough meta-analysis that included both *guided* and *unguided* interventions.

Methods: Systematic literature searches were performed up to September 2013. Primary outcome was the mean level of alcohol consumption and drinking within low risk guidelines for alcohol consumption at post-treatment.

Findings: We selected 16 randomised controlled trials (with 23 comparisons and 5,612 participants) for inclusion. Results, showed a small but significant overall effect size in favour of Internet interventions ($g = 0.20$, 95% CI: 0.13–0.27, $p < .001$). Participants in Internet interventions drunk on average 22 grams of ethanol less than controls and were significantly more likely to be adhering to low-risk drinking guidelines at post-treatment (RD 0.13, 95% CI: 0.09–0.17, $p < .001$). Subgroup analyses revealed no significant differences in potential moderators for the outcome of alcohol consumption, although there was a near-significant difference between comparisons with waitlist control and those with assessment-only or alcohol information control conditions ($p = .056$).

Conclusions: Internet interventions are effective in reducing adult alcohol consumption and inducing alcohol users to adhere to guidelines for low-risk drinking. This effect is small but from a public health point of view this may warrant large scale implementation at low cost of Internet interventions for adult alcohol misuse. Moderator analyses with sufficient power are, however, needed in order to assess the robustness of these overall results and to assess whether these interventions may impact on subgroups with different levels of success.

Editor: Robert Stewart, Institute of Psychiatry, United Kingdom

Funding: The authors have no support or funding to report.

Competing Interests: The authors have declared that no competing interests exist.

* Email: h.riper@vu.nl

Introduction

The *Global Burden of Disease Study 2010* from the World Health Organization has documented a growing health burden from Alcohol Use Disorders (AUDs) over the past two decades among adults in both developed and developing societies [1,2]. The health burden increases further if the whole spectrum of alcohol misuse [3] is taken into account, whereby people consume alcohol in excess of the low-risk drinking guidelines but do not meet AUD criteria [1,4,5]. They include people who engage in *hazardous alcohol use* – and who may thereby develop physical, psychological and social problems in the short term and alcohol dependency and serious or fatal illness later on – or *harmful alcohol use*, meaning that they are already experiencing such problems [4]. This mounting health burden is due not just to population growth or ageing, but also to an absolute increase in alcohol consumption by adults [1,6]. It affects both traditional groups of drinkers and newer groups such as women [7] and the elderly [8]. The risks of problem drinking multiply with every increment in alcohol consumption or every heavier drinking pattern [9,10]. Estimates reveal that eight out of ten adults who drink too much alcohol lack professional help; if they do receive it, that is often at a very late stage in their drinking career [11]. Studies also show that whilst a high number of people who misuse alcohol do desire help, they prefer it outside conventional health care settings [12]. Public health strategies to curb alcohol misuse therefore have considerable room for improvement. One particular enhancement could lie in an expanded availability of brief, low-intensity Internet interventions for use both in and beyond the primary care sector [13,14].

Conventional (that is, non-Internet) Screening and Brief Interventions (SBIs) have been evaluated mostly in their delivery to non–alcohol-dependent, non–treatment-seeking adults whose alcohol misuse was identified in opportunistic health screening in primary care. Numerous meta-analyses and systematic reviews have convincingly shown the clinical effectiveness of SBIs in reducing alcohol consumption in comparison to non-intervention controls. The results of all these studies have recently been synthesised in studies by Jonas and colleagues [15,16], and these in turn by Moyer in her 2013 update to the United States Preventive Services Task Force's earlier recommendation statement on screening and brief interventions in primary care for alcohol misuse [3]. Overall, the results show significant effect sizes in the small to moderate range for low-intensity interventions in comparison to control conditions in terms of average decreases in alcohol consumption [3,15,16]. Cost-effectiveness studies, albeit limited in number, also report promising results [17–19]. Effectiveness studies on the reduction of alcohol consumption through SBIs provided in other settings such as general hospitals, emergency departments or work environments have been inconclusive [20–23].

Providing Internet self-help interventions both in primary care and directly to people in the community appears a promising strategy to overcome the gap between the high number of people that misuse alcohol and the low number that actually receive or seek help in primary care [24]. Studies on web-based self-help interventions for adult problem drinking show that (1) the interventions are mostly of an unguided nature and are delivered as stand-alone procedures directly to participants in the community, and to a far lesser extent via primary care, clinical or employment settings [25,26]; (2) they largely reach first-time help seekers (with rates varying from 80% to 90% [27,28]); (3) people who misuse alcohol take up these services on a much wider scale than the available brief, low-intensity face-to-face interventions in primary care settings [24,29]; and (4) people differ in whether they desire additional help from professionals [28]. Studies have also shown such unguided interventions to be effective in reducing adult alcohol misuse as compared to no-intervention control conditions. A 2011 meta-analysis by Riper and colleagues [26] found a small but significant effect size of $g = 0.39$ (95% CI: 0.23–0.56) for unguided self-help interventions via the Internet. Numbers needed to treat (NNT = 5) were comparable to those for face-to-face brief interventions in primary care settings [30]. Small effect sizes also emerged in meta-analyses on various health promotion interventions, including alcohol use [31,32]. Few cost-effectiveness studies are available, but they indicate potential economic gain from Internet-based interventions for adult alcohol misuse [33].

The number of eligible randomised controlled trials on web-based interventions for alcohol misuse was rather limited in these systematic reviews and meta-analyses. The Riper meta-analysis [26], for example, identified only 7 eligible randomised controlled trials. This sharply contrasts with meta-analyses assessing the clinical and cost-effectiveness of Internet interventions for depression or anxiety. For example, Richards and Richardson [34] were able to include 19 RCTs on depression in their 2012 meta-analysis. For these disorders, overall evidence is accumulating that guided interventions generally lead to a greater reduction of depressive or anxiety symptoms than unguided interventions [34,35] and that guided Internet interventions are as effective as face to face interventions [36].

Recently, the numbers of published randomised controlled trials on Internet-based interventions for alcohol misuse has increased, including some that evaluate therapist-led self-help interventions [37,38]. We therefore decided to conduct this meta-analysis. We investigated the overall effectiveness of alcohol interventions in comparison to no-intervention controls and, if possible in terms of alcohol consumption reduction, drinking within the guidelines for low risk drinking and actual amounts reduced. We then examined whether certain study characteristics, such as the guided or unguided design of interventions, affected the primary outcome measure of alcohol consumption. To the best of our knowledge, this is the first meta-analysis that includes both guided and unguided Internet interventions to address problematic alcohol consumption among adults.

Methods

Identification of Studies

We conducted literature searches up to September 2013 in the following bibliographic databases: MEDLINE, PsycINFO, Science Citation Index Expanded, Social Sciences Citation Index, Arts and Humanities Citation Index, CINAHL, PUBMED and EMBASE, using key words and text words. Words indicating online interventions (Internet, Web, online, computer, mobile) were combined with terms indicative of type of treatment (self-help, brief intervention, treatment, unguided, guided, supported, low-intensity) and problematic alcohol use (alcohol abuse, alcohol misuse, problem drinking, hazardous, harmful, dependence, abstinence). We also re-examined exclusion lists of papers retrieved for our previous meta-analysis [26] to see if any would meet the inclusion criteria for the current study. No language restrictions were applied.

Our initial selection was based on titles and abstracts. If these yielded insufficient information to assess the eligibility criteria, full-text articles were retrieved and assessed in terms of our inclusion criteria. All papers included or excluded at all stages were assessed by two independent raters (authors HR and HH) (see figure 1). The same raters assessed the effect sizes and moderator variables in the included studies. Any disagreement was resolved by discussion. A protocol does not exist for this meta-analysis; steps undertaken are described in this method section.

Eligibility Criteria

Randomised controlled trials were included that (1) compared a web-based intervention with a control group (in an assessment-only, waitlisted or alcohol information brochure control condition); (2) included a low-intensity self-help intervention that the participant could perform on a computer or mobile phone, with or without guidance from a professional; (3) assessed alcohol drinking behaviour in terms of quantity consumed as a primary outcome measure; (4) studied adults aged 18 or older; (5) included alcohol drinkers who exceeded local guidelines for low-risk drinking (if lower-risk participants were also included, we retained only the results of those with alcohol misuse).

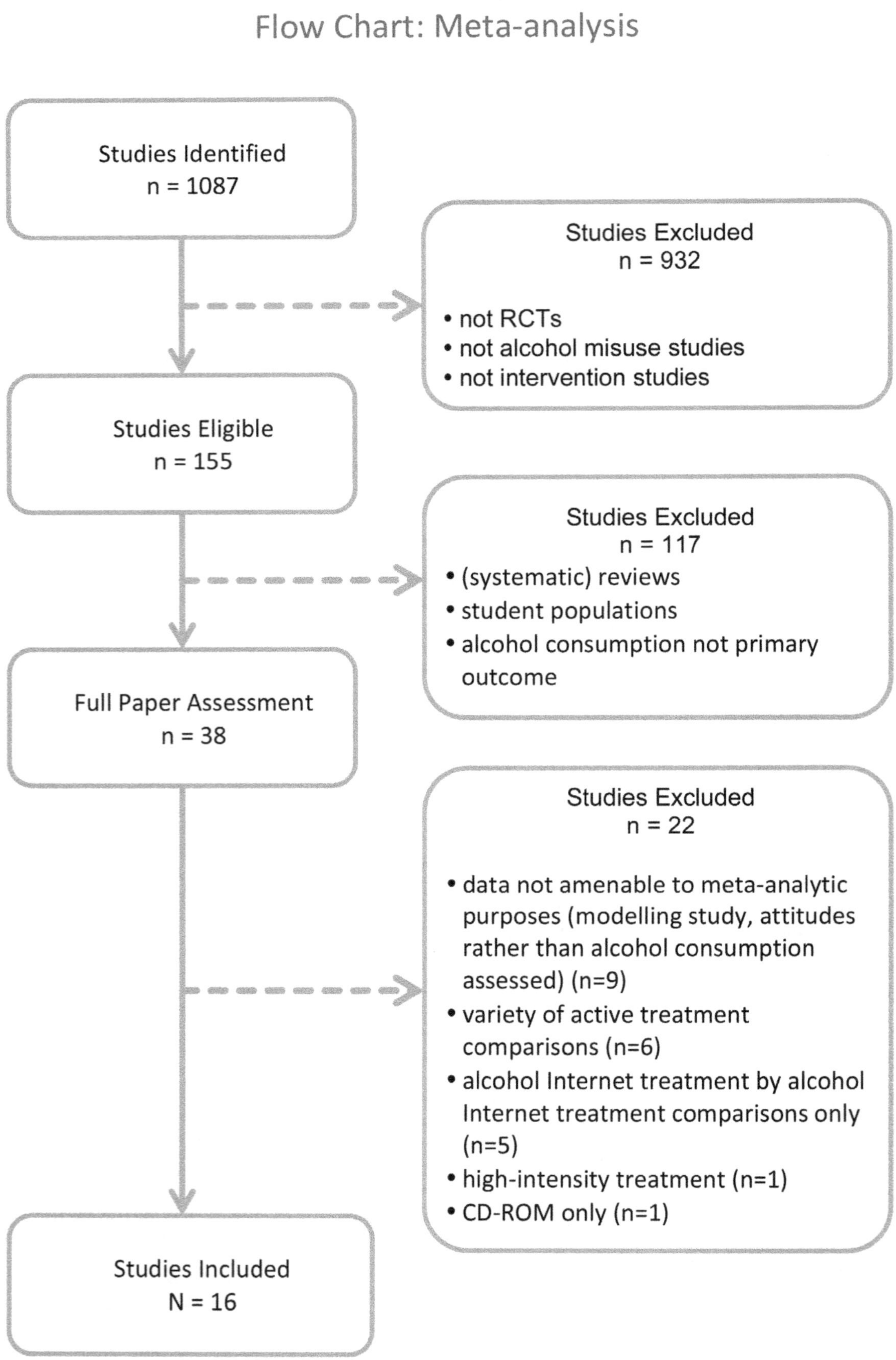

Figure 1. Study inclusion meta-analysis: flow chart.

Risk-of-bias Assessment and Data Extraction

We assessed the validity of the included studies on the basis of four criteria from the risk-of-bias assessment tool developed by the Cochrane Collaboration [39]. It verifies study attributes in randomised controlled trials that are potential sources of bias, including (1) adequacy of allocation sequence generation, (2) concealment of the allocation to the different conditions, (3) blinding of assessors and outcomes and (4) handling of incomplete outcome data using intention-to-treat analyses (this was rated as positive if intention-to-treat analyses were performed, thus retaining all randomised participants in the analyses; see table 1). Authors HH and MB assessed risk of bias as Yes, No or Unclear using the Cochrane Collaboration tool (see 2.3).

Study Characteristics

Characteristics of the analysed studies are described in table 1. We coded (1) year of study and country of origin; (2) participant characteristics: alcohol consumption level at baseline, recruitment setting, target group; (3) intervention characteristics: therapeutic principles, mode and setting of delivery, guided or unguided self-help format, number of sessions; and (4) other study characteristics: type of control condition, number of participants in each comparative condition, primary outcome measure (how consumed quantities of alcohol were assessed), intention-to-treat (ITT) versus completers-only (CO) analyses, post-treatment assessments in months, dropout rate and risk of bias. The brief self-help alcohol interventions we identified were based on one or more of the following principles: behavioural self-control [40], motivational interviewing [41], transtheoretical model of change [42], cognitive-behavioural therapy (CBT, [43]), and personalised normative feedback (PNF [44]).

Meta-analyses

We first calculated a mean alcohol consumption effect size for each comparison between an alcohol intervention and a control group. Effect sizes were calculated by subtracting the average post-test score of the alcohol self-help group from the average score of the comparison group and dividing the result by the pooled standard deviations of the two groups. This effect size is known as Cohen's *d*. As the effect size *d* is subject to small-sample bias, it can be adjusted by using a scaling factor, which is multiplied by *d* to arrive at Hedges's bias-corrected effect size *g*, so that $g = d\,(1-[3/4(n_1+n_0]-9)$. An effect size of 0.50 indicates that the mean of the experimental group is half a standard deviation larger than the mean of the control group. Effect sizes of approximately 0.80 can be considered large, 0.5 as moderate, and 0.2 small [45]. Participant adherence to low-risk alcohol guidelines (by either abstaining or not exceeding recommended limits) was assessed in terms of percentages (yes/no).

If means and standard deviations were not reported, we contacted the study authors to obtain these and/or we used the procedures of the Comprehensive Meta-Analysis software (CMA, version 2.2.021) to calculate the effect size using continuous or dichotomous outcomes. In the event these were not available either, we used other statistics (such a *t*- or *p*-value). Where possible, data from intention-to-treat analyses were used; completers-only data were used if the former were unavailable. If more than one alcohol consumption outcome measure was reported in a single study, we averaged the effect sizes from those measures to produce a single summary effect size for use in the meta-analysis, statistically adjusting those calculations to account for variance introduced by the multiple measures [46].

We calculated the mean effect sizes using a random effects model. This assumes that the included studies were drawn from 'populations' of studies that systematically differed from one another (heterogeneity). As a test of homogeneity of effect sizes, we calculated the I^2 statistic, an indicator of heterogeneity in percentages. A value of 0% indicates no observed heterogeneity, and larger values show increasing heterogeneity, with 25% as low, 50% as moderate and 75% as high [47]. As the I^2 statistic is known to be imprecise [48], we calculated the 95% confidence interval using the non-central chi-squared-based approach within the heterogi module in Stata [49]. We also estimated numbers needed to treat (NNTs) [50].

Subgroup analyses. In consideration of the literature, ten subgroups analyses were carried out using the mixed effects model, whereby studies within subgroups are pooled with the random effects model (see table 2). Tests for significant differences between subgroups are then performed with the fixed effects model. For continuous variables, we used bivariate meta-regression analyses to test whether there was a significant relationship between each variable and the alcohol effect size, as indicated by a *Z*-value and an associated *p*-value.

Power Calculations

We calculated both beforehand and afterwards how many studies would be needed to ensure sufficient statistical power to identify relevant effects as we expected a small to moderate effect size [26,51]. The power calculations were carried out according to the procedures described by Borenstein and colleagues [46]. Beforehand we hoped to find enough studies to enable identification of a small effect size of $d = 0.40$ based on the random effects model. The power calculations indicated that this would require at least ten studies with a mean sample size of 70 participants per condition. That conservatively assumes a medium level of between-study variance (τ^2), a statistical power of .80 and a significance level of $\alpha < .05$.

Publication Bias

To detect possible publication bias, we visually examined the funnel plots of the primary outcome measures for symmetry. We conducted Egger's linear regression test of the intercept to quantify the bias captured by the funnel plot and test whether it was significant [52]. Duval and Tweedie trim-and-fill procedure was performed to further verify whether the pooled effect size estimate was unbiased [53]. These procedures were all performed with CMA.

Results

Selection and Inclusion of Studies

A flowchart depicting our study selection procedure is shown in figure 1. In reporting the results we followed the guidelines of the PRISMA statement (see Checklist S1) [54].

Characteristics of Included Studies

Table 1 summarises the selected characteristics of the 16 studies (containing 23 comparisons) included in the meta-analysis. The studies assessed a total of 5,612 participants (3,268 in experimental and 2,344 in control conditions) and thus provided sufficient statistical power to detect a small effect size (see section 2.6).

In five studies, sample inclusion was based on self-reported alcohol consumption, using cut-off points indicative of alcohol use exceeding low-risk guidelines, with differing levels for men and women. Five other studies applied the Alcohol Use Identification Test (AUDIT [55]) or the Fast Alcohol Screening Test (FAST [56]). Two studies applied both AUDIT and alcohol consumption cut-off points; one selected on the basis of GGT (gamma-glutamyl

Table 1. Study characteristics of 16 randomised controlled trials of Internet-based interventions for adult alcohol misuse.

<table>
<tr><th>Author, year, country</th><th>Recruitment</th><th>Target group, inclusion criteria</th><th>Delivery mode | setting</th><th>Type of support | intervention(s) | dosage</th><th>Comparison (intervention vs control)</th><th>N[a]/N[b]</th><th>Outcome measure</th><th>ITT or CO</th><th>Post-treat-ment assessment</th><th>DO</th><th>Risk of bias[1–4]</th><th>Baseline: M (SD) drinks[k] per week | and/or AUDIT score</th></tr>
<tr><td>Araki, 2006, Japan</td><td>Workplace</td><td>Males, GGT ≥60 IU/l</td><td>E-mail | workplace</td><td>Guided |HE | 2 sessions</td><td>Guided vs AO</td><td>12/12</td><td>Drinks per day</td><td>CO</td><td>2 months</td><td>3%</td><td>1) Unclear* 2) No 3) Unclear* 4) No</td><td>Drinks: 18.6 (12.2) | AUDIT: -</td></tr>
<tr><td>Bischof, 2008, Germany</td><td>General practice</td><td>GP patients age 18–64, alcohol dependence or abuse, or >20/30 g of alcohol per day for females/males in past 4 weeks, or >60/80 g for females/males on >1 occasion in the past 4 weeks</td><td>E-mail, phone | home</td><td>Guided |BCC, MI, TTM | 4 sessions (FC) or max. 3 sessions (SC)</td><td>1) Guided SC[c] vs AB/H; 2) Guided FC[d] vs AB/H</td><td>1) 131/139^; 2) 138/139^</td><td>Grams of alcohol per day</td><td>ITT</td><td>12 months</td><td>8%</td><td>1) Yes 2) No 3) Yes 4) Yes</td><td>Drinks: 31.9 (35.2) | AUDIT: -</td></tr>
<tr><td>Blankers, 2011, Netherlands</td><td>Community</td><td>Males/females, AUDIT ≥8 and ≥14 units/week</td><td>Internet | home</td><td>Guided and unguided |CBT, MI | 7 sessions guided, 6 modules unguided</td><td>1) Guided vs WL; 2) Unguided vs WL</td><td>1) 68/69^; 2) 68/69^</td><td>Drinks in past week</td><td>ITT</td><td>3 months; 6 months</td><td>30%</td><td>1) Yes 2) No 3) Yes 4) Yes</td><td>Drinks: 44.7 (26.4) | AUDIT: 19.5 (5.1)</td></tr>
<tr><td>Boon & Huiberts, 2006, Netherlands</td><td>Community</td><td>Males/females, ≥21/14 units/week; or ≥6/4 units on ≥1 day/week</td><td>Internet | research setting</td><td>Unguided |PNF | single-session</td><td>Unguided vs AB</td><td>102/89</td><td>Drinks per week</td><td>CO</td><td>9 months</td><td>32%</td><td>1) Yes 2) No 3) Yes 4) No</td><td>Drinks: - | AUDIT: -</td></tr>
<tr><td>Boon, 2011, Netherlands</td><td>Community</td><td>Males, ≥21 units/week or ≥6 units ≥1 day per week</td><td>Internet | research setting</td><td>Unguided |PNF | single-session</td><td>Unguided vs AB</td><td>230/220</td><td>Drinks per week</td><td>ITT</td><td>1 month; 6 months</td><td>8%</td><td>1) Yes 2) Yes 3) Yes 4) Yes</td><td>Drinks: 31.3 (16.8) | AUDIT: -</td></tr>
<tr><td>Brendryen, 2013, Norway</td><td>Community</td><td>FAST ≥3</td><td>Internet | home</td><td>Unguided | PNF, CBT | multiple sessions</td><td>Unguided vs AB</td><td>125/119</td><td>Drinks per week</td><td>ITT</td><td>2 months; 6 months*</td><td>37%</td><td>1) Yes 2) Yes 3) Yes 4) Yes</td><td>Drinks: 23.5 (16.1) | AUDIT: -</td></tr>
<tr><td>Cunningham, 2009, Canada</td><td>Community</td><td>Males/females, AUDIT ≥11</td><td>Internet | home</td><td>Unguided |PNF | single-session</td><td>Unguided vs AB</td><td>35/37</td><td>Drinks per week</td><td>ITT</td><td>3 months; 6 months</td><td>8%</td><td>1) Yes 2) No 3) Yes 4) Yes</td><td>Drinks: 22.5 (12.6) | AUDIT-C: 8.9-</td></tr>
<tr><td>Delrahim-Howlett, 2011, USA</td><td>Women's and infant services</td><td>Females, ≥3 units on ≥1 day/month</td><td>Internet | health care</td><td>Unguided |PNF | single-session</td><td>Unguided vs AB double-blind</td><td>68/67</td><td>Drinks per occasion</td><td>CO</td><td>1 month; 2 months</td><td>10%</td><td>1) Yes 2) Yes 3) Yes 4) No</td><td>Drinks: 8.2 (7.5) | AUDIT: -</td></tr>
<tr><td>Doumas & Hannah, 2008, USA</td><td>Workplace</td><td>Males/females[&], ≥1 occasions with ≥5/4 units/past 2 weeks</td><td>Internet | workplace</td><td>Guided and unguided |PNF, MI | single-session</td><td>1) Guided vs AO 2) Unguided vs AO</td><td>1)12/16; 2) 8/7 [l]</td><td>Drinks per week</td><td>CO</td><td>1 month</td><td>37%</td><td>1) Yes 2) No 3) Yes 4) No</td><td>Drinks: 3.89 (2.44) | AUDIT: -</td></tr>
<tr><td>Hansen, 2012, Denmark</td><td>Community</td><td>Males/females, ≥21/14 units/week</td><td>Internet | home</td><td>Unguided |PNF | single-session</td><td>1) Unguided advice vs AO 2) Unguided PF[f] vs AO</td><td>1) 476/454; 2) 450/454</td><td>Drinks per week</td><td>ITT</td><td>6 months; 12 months</td><td>37%</td><td>1) Yes 2) No 3) Yes 4) Yes</td><td>Drinks: 32.8 (13.5) | AUDIT: -</td></tr>
<tr><td>Hester, 2005, USA</td><td>Community</td><td>Males/females, AUDIT ≥8</td><td>CD-ROM | health care</td><td>Unguided |PNF, BSC, MI |single-session extended</td><td>Unguided vs WL</td><td>35/26</td><td>Drinks per day</td><td>CO</td><td>4 weeks</td><td>0%</td><td>1) Yes 2) No 3) Yes 4) No</td><td>Drinks: 47.6 (42.9) | AUDIT: 19.7 (-)</td></tr>
<tr><td>Pemberton[m], 2011, USA</td><td>Military</td><td>Males/females[&],/all interested (we assessed high-risk group only)</td><td>Internet | home</td><td>Unguided |HBM, MI, SCM | 3 modules</td><td>1) Unguided combined vs AO; 2) Unguided MI[h] vs AO</td><td>1) 144/72; 2) 95/73 [l]</td><td>Drinks per occasion</td><td>ITT</td><td>1 month</td><td></td><td>1) No 2) NA* 3) Yes 4) Yes</td><td>Drinks: - | AUDIT: -</td></tr>
</table>

Table 1. Cont.

Author, year, country	Recruitment	Target group, inclusion criteria	Delivery mode | setting	Type of support | intervention(s) | dosage	Comparison (intervention vs control)	N[a]/N[b]	Outcome measure	ITT or CO	Post-treat-ment assessment	DO	Risk of bias[1–4]	Baseline: M (SD) drinks[k] per week | and/or AUDIT score
Riper, 2007, Netherlands	Community	Males/females, >21/14 units/week; or ≥6/4 units ≥1 day for past 3 months	Internet | home	Unguided |BSC, CBT, MI |6 weeks	Unguided vs AB	130/131	Drinks per week	ITT	6 months	42%	1) Yes 2) No 3) Yes 4) Yes	Drinks: 43.6 (21.7) | AUDIT: -
Schulz, 2013, Netherlands	Community/ online access panel	AUDIT; (1) >1 drink (females) or >2 drinks (males) per day, (2) drinking more than 5 days per week; (3) >7 AUDIT	Internet | home	PNF | 3 sessions	1) Alternating vs AO 2) Summative vs AO	1) 132/135^; 2) 181/135^	Mean drinks per week	ITT	6 months		1) Yes 2) Yes 3) Yes 4) Yes	Drinks: 12.9 (11.2) | AUDIT: -
Suffoletto, 2012, USA	Emergency department	Males/females, AUDIT-C ≥4/3	SMS | home	Unguided |PNF | 12 weeks	1) Unguided[i] vs AO; 2) Unguided[j] vs AO	1) 14/13^; 2) 12/13^	Drinks per drinking day	CO	3 months	13%	1) Yes 2) Yes 3) Yes 4) No	Drinks: - | AUDIT: -
Wallace, 2011, UK	Alcohol website	Males/females, AUDIT-C ≥5	Internet | home	Unguided |CBT | 3 modules	Unguided vs CW	582/695	Drinks in past week	ITT	3 months	45%	1) Yes 2) Yes 3) Yes 4) Yes	36.8 (25.0) | AUDIT: 18.8 (7.3)

Notes: [1–4]: Risk of bias: 1): adequate sequence generation; 2): report of conditions by an independent party; 3): blinding of outcome assessor or using self-report outcomes only; 4): intention to treat analyses; *: in regression analysis coded as NO; ^ control group reported twice; &: at risk group drinkers only; [a]intervention group size; control group size; [c]full-care intervention; ?stepped-care intervention; [e]brief personalised feedback intervention; [f]brief personalised advice intervention; [g]Alcohol Savvy intervention; [h]Drinker's Check-Up intervention; [i]text message feedback intervention; [j]text message assessment intervention; [k]1 'drink' contains 10 grams of ethanol; [l]only a subsample included; [m]not all participants randomly allocated; AB alcohol brochure control; AB/H alcohol/health brochure control; AO assessment-only control; AUDIT: Alcohol Use Disorders Identification Test; AUDI-C [brief AUDIT, composite] measure that consists of respondents' scores on frequency of drinking, drinks per drinking day and frequency of five or more drinks on one occasion; BSC behavioural self-control training; CBT cognitive-behavioural therapy; CO completers-only analysis; CW comparator website control; DO Study dropout; FAST Fast Alcohol Screening Test; GGT gamma-glutamyl transpeptidase test; HB Health booklet control; HBM Health Belief model; HE health education; ITT intention-to-treat analysis; MI motivational interviewing; PFGS personalised feedback with goal setting; PNF personalised normative feedback; SCM stages of change model; TTM transtheoretical model of change.

Table 2. Effects of low-intensity Internet alcohol treatment on alcohol consumption in comparison with no-intervention controls, and subgroup analyses of associations between effect sizes and study characteristics (Hedges's *g*).

Experimental/Control	subgroup	n comparisons	*g*	95% CI	I^{2b}	95% CI	p^{d}	NNT[e]
All studies[a]		23	0.20	0.13–0.27***	27	0~56		8.93
One effect size per study (lowest excluded)		16	0.23	0.15–0.32***	34	0~64		7.69
One effect size per study (highest excluded)		16	0.20	0.10–0.29***	39*	0~66		8.93
Lowest effect size removed		22	0.20	0.13–0.27***	24	0~55		8.93
Highest effect size removed		22	0.19	0.12–0.25***	20	0~53		9.43
Subgroup analyses (N = 23)								
Type of control	Assessment-only	11	0.15	0.06–0.24***	0	0~60	**.056**	11.90
	Waitlist	3	0.48	0.22–0.73***	0	0~90		3.76
	Alcohol brochure	9	0.20	0.08–0.31***	48	0~76		8.93
Blinding of participants	Yes	8	0.16	0.04–0.28**	30	0~69	.393	11.11
	No	15	0.23	0.14–0.32***	23	0~58		7.69
Analyses	ITT	13	0.22	0.13–0.31***	30	0~64	.600	8.06
	CO	10	0.18	0.05–0.30**	19	0~60		9.80
Recruitment	Community	11	0.21	0.11–0.31***	52*	4~76	.962	8.47
	Primary care/clinic	7	0.21	0.04–0.39**	24	0~66		8.47
	Work	5	0.24	0.05–0.412**	0	0~71		7.46
Population for inclusion	At-risk drinking cut-off	12	0.19	0.09–0.28***	40	0~70	.530	9.43
	AUDIT (10)/(FAST (1)	11	0.24	0.12–0.35***	1	0~61		7.46
Focus of treatment	PNF	9	0.16	0.07–0.24***	0	0~65	.236	11.11
	Combined	14	0.24	0.13–0.35***	42*	0~69		7.46
Professional guidance	Yes	5	0.23	0.05–0.41**	10	0~81	.730	7.69
	No	18	0.20	0.12–0.28***	33	43~87		8.93
Number of sessions	Single	8	0.16	0.08–0.25***	0	0~68	.399	11.11
	More than one	15	0.22	0.12–0.33***	42*	0~68		8.06
Gender	Male only	4	0.26	0.12–0.40***	0	0~85	.484	8.06
	Male and female	19	0.20	0.11–0.28***	35	0~63		8.93

Notes: **bold** – near significance; [a]-1 according to the random effects model; [a]-2: according to the mixed effects model [b]The P-values in this column indicatewhether the Q-statistic is significant (I2-statistics do not include a test of significance).; [c]The P-values in this column indicate whether the difference between the effect sizes in the subgroups is significant.; *P≤0.05; **P<0.01; ***P≤0.001; AUDIT: Alcohol Use Disorders Identification Test; CBT cognitive-behavioural therapy; CI = confidence interval; CO completers-only analysis; DSM = Diagnostic Statistical Manual of Mental Disorders; FAST: Fast Alcohol Screening Test; ITT intention-to-treat analysis; MI motivational interviewing; n comp = number of comparisons; NNT = number needed to treat; PNF personalised normative feedback.

transpeptidase) testing. Two of the sixteen studies [57,58] included anyone interested in participating; for these studies, we confined our analysis to subgroups belonging to the at-risk drinking population.

Seven studies applied a single-focus therapeutic strategy, which in six cases was personalised normative feedback (PNF) and in one case a generic health education approach. The other nine studies used combined treatment approaches consisting of motivational interviewing (MI), personalised normative feedback (PNF), cognitive-behavioural therapy (CBT) and/or behavioural self-control and change principles. The control groups represented assessment-only ($n = 6$), waitlisted ($n = 3$) or alcohol information brochure conditions ($n = 7$). The outcome assessments to indicate alcohol consumption were expressed in terms of mean standard drinks per drinking day, total numbers of standard drinks in the previous week, mean standard drinks per drinking occasion or amounts of alcohol in grams.

The risk of bias varied among the studies (table 1), with 14 studies reporting adequate sequence generation, 6 reporting allocation to conditions by an independent party, 15 reporting blinding of outcome assessors or using self-report outcomes only, and 10 using intention-to-treat analyses. Dropout rates varied from 0% to 42%.

Meta-analysis

The effect of low-intensity Internet-based alcohol interventions to reduce alcohol consumption in comparison to controls was small but significant at post-test ($g = 0.20$, random effects model, 95% CI: 0.13–0.27, $p < .001$, NNT = 8.93). Results are shown in figure 2 (from high to low study effect sizes) and table 2. Heterogeneity was low but with a moderate confidence interval ($I^2 = 27$, 95% CI: 0–56). A post-hoc power calculation showed that our set of studies had sufficient statistical power (0.99) on the basis of the random effects model (with a low level of between-study variance, $\tau^2 = .001$, and a significance level of $\alpha < .05$).

Seven studies [37,57–62] compared more than one group receiving differing types of Internet-based brief treatment with a single control group, so that our analysis included multiple comparisons from these studies. The fact that the comparisons were not independent of one another could have artificially reduced the heterogeneity of the analysed studies, thereby affecting the pooled effect size. To test this, we carried out sensitivity analyses that included only one effect size per study. As table 2 shows, removal of the comparisons with the highest effect sizes had almost no influence on the pooled effect size nor did removing the comparisons with the lowest effect sizes. Removal of the one guided intervention comparison with the highest effect size (in Blankers [37]) did not influence the observed effect size either, nor did removal of that with the lowest effect size [62].

Mean Alcohol Consumption Reduction and Drinking within Low Risk Guidelines

On average, the intervention participants were drinking 2,2 alcohol consumptions (22 grams of ethanol) less per week at post-treatment than controls ($n = 14$; 95% CI: 0.87–3.46, $p = .001$, $I^2 = 0$, $p < .001$; mean difference). Post-test differences [37,61,63–65]) revealed that intervention participants were significantly more likely than controls to have reduced their alcohol consumption to within the low-risk guidelines as compared to controls ($n = 6$; RD 0.13, 95% CI: 0.09–0.17, $p < .001$, $I^2 = 0$, non-significant).

Subgroup Analyses

Subgroup analyses revealed no significant differences between study characteristics and effect sizes for alcohol consumption (see table 2). The differences between types of control conditions bordered on significance ($p = .056$). We found a higher effect size for decreased alcohol consumption for studies applying a waitlist control condition ($g = 0.48$) than those applying an alcohol brochure condition ($g = 0.20$) or an assessment-only condition ($g = 0.15$).

Follow-up Assessments

No significant differences in effect remained at follow-up (6 to 12 months after baseline) between the six unguided interventions (8 comparisons) and control groups ($g = 0.06$, 95% CI: −0.14–0.25, $p = .567$, random effects model) for which such follow-up assessments were available. No follow-up assessments were available for the guided interventions.

Low Intensity Internet Alcohol Interventions versus Controls

Study name	Comparison	Outcome	Statistics for each study: Hedges's g	Standard error	Variance	Lower limit	Upper limit	Z-Value	p-Value
Blankers 2011a	Guided vs C-WL	Drinks/lastweek	0.588	0.211	0.044	0.176	1.001	2.795	0.005
Riper 2008	Unguided vs C-B	Drinks/week	0.522	0.126	0.016	0.275	0.769	4.143	0.000
Hester 2005	Unguided vs C- WL	Drinks/day	0.511	0.260	0.067	0.002	1.020	1.966	0.049
Suffoletto 2012a	Unguided advice + feedback vs C-AO	Drinks/drinkday	0.395	0.449	0.201	-0.484	1.274	0.881	0.378
Blankers 2011b	Unguided vs C-WL	Drinks/lastweek	0.346	0.210	0.044	-0.066	0.757	1.647	0.100
Schultz 2013b	Unguided vs AO	drinks/week	0.337	0.163	0.027	0.018	0.657	2.070	0.038
Araki 2006	Guided vs C-AO	Drinks/day	0.336	0.232	0.054	-0.119	0.791	1.448	0.148
Doumas 2008a	Guided vs C-AO	Drinks/weekend	0.312	0.457	0.209	-0.584	1.208	0.683	0.495
Boon 2011	Unguided vs C-B	Drinks/week	0.281	0.109	0.012	0.067	0.495	2.578	0.010
Pemberton 2011a	DCUunguided SL/SC v C-AO	Combined	0.279	0.144	0.021	-0.005	0.562	1.929	0.054
Cunningham 2009	Unguided vs C-B	Drinks/week	0.277	0.234	0.055	-0.182	0.737	1.182	0.237
Boon 2006	Unguided vs C-B	Drinks/week	0.261	0.145	0.021	-0.023	0.545	1.800	0.072
Schulz 2013a	Unguided vs AO	Drinks/week	0.260	0.168	0.028	-0.069	0.589	1.548	0.122
Delrahim 2011a	Unguided PF vs AB	Combined	0.200	0.172	0.029	-0.136	0.537	1.167	0.243
Pemberton 2011b	SAunguided MI v C-AO	Combined	0.148	0.155	0.024	-0.156	0.452	0.956	0.339
Hansen 2012b	Unguided PF vs C-AO	Drinks/week	0.137	0.081	0.007	-0.021	0.295	1.696	0.090
Brendryen2013	Unguided vs C-B	Drinks/week	0.136	0.128	0.016	-0.114	0.387	1.066	0.286
Bischof 2007a	Guided full care vs C-B	Combined	0.126	0.148	0.022	-0.163	0.415	0.853	0.394
Bischof 2007b	Guided stepped vs C-B	Combined	0.097	0.146	0.021	-0.190	0.383	0.660	0.509
Doumas 2008b	Unguided vs-AO	Drinks/week	0.092	0.487	0.238	-0.863	1.048	0.189	0.850
Hansen 2012a	Unguided advice vs C-AO	Drinks/week	0.040	0.081	0.007	-0.119	0.200	0.496	0.620
Wallace 2011	Unguided vs C-PL	Drinks/lastweek	0.036	0.056	0.003	-0.074	0.146	0.641	0.521
Suffoletto 2012b	Unguideds-a only vs C-AO	Drinks/drinkday	-0.654	0.488	0.239	-1.611	0.304	-1.338	0.181
		Overall Effect Size	0.203	0.037	0.001	0.131	0.275	5.508	0.000

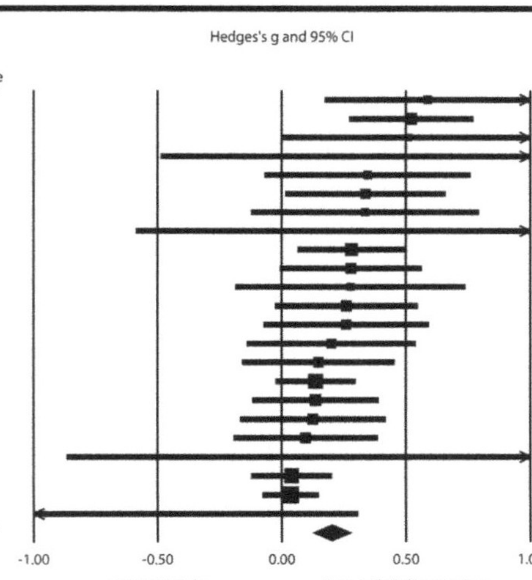

Figure 2. Results of meta-analysis: forest plot.

Regression Analyses

Meta-regression analyses with Hedges's g as the dependent variable uncovered no significant associations between effect size and either the number of alcohol intervention sessions ($\beta = -0.0001$, 95% CI: -0.004–0.003, $p = .938$) or the risk of bias ($\beta = 0.068$, 95% CI: -0.15–0.01, $p = .089$) in the studies assessed.

Publication Bias

There was evidence of publication bias in terms of Duval and Tweedie's trim-and-fill method. After adjustment for missing studies, the effect size for decreased alcohol consumption diminished from $g = 0.20$ to $g = 0.14$ (95% CI: 0.06–0.22; trimmed studies $n = 8$, random effects model). Egger's test indicated an asymmetric funnel plot ($p = .028$, two-tailed).

Discussion

This meta-analysis showed a small but significant overall effect size ($g = 0.20$) in favour of low-intensity Internet-based self-help interventions to curb alcohol misuse over control conditions. At post-treatment, intervention participants were consuming an average of 22 grams of alcohol less per week than controls. The reduction appears lower than those found in analyses of face-to-face brief interventions in primary care. The latter include a Cochrane Collaboration systematic review of 29 primary care trials [30], which reported a significantly reduced weekly consumption of 38 grams at one-year follow-up (see also the study by Jonas and colleagues [15]). In our study, Internet intervention participants were 13% more likely than controls to stay within the guidelines after treatment ($n = 6$). This is in line with the study of Jonas and colleagues [15] who showed that those receiving primary care alcohol interventions were 11% more likely to do so when compared with controls.

The overall effect size in this meta-analysis is lower than, the effect size found in our previous study that focused solely on *unguided* e-interventions (7 studies, $g = 0.39$) [26]. Some explanations for this may lie in the three-times-higher number of comparisons involved in the current analysis and the fact that studies with null findings were now included [60,66]. The current overall effect also compares with meta-analyses of face-to-face primary care samples [3,30,67,68] and of non-clinical samples performing postal self-help interventions based on bibliotherapy [69–71]. These studies all showed significant small to moderate effect sizes for curbing alcohol misuse. We found no significant differences between experimental and control conditions for those studies that assessed follow-up outcomes up to twelve months. Such a decay of intervention effects is not uncommon; larger effect sizes are generally found at the earliest follow-ups [15,68]. Some studies of brief interventions for problem drinking have nonetheless reported positive influences on alcohol reduction up to four years later [67] and on mortality [72].

Subgroup Analyses

Results of the subgroup analyses did not reveal any significant differences between experimental and control conditions. All these results need to be interpreted with caution, as the number of studies included in the subgroup analyses was low. This means that there where either no real differences between these conditions or that real difference may have gone undetected. The variation in types of control predictors was of borderline significance ($p = .056$) in terms of effect. A moderate effect size was found for studies using waitlist control conditions, while those with assessment-only or alcohol brochure control showed small ones. Other studies have similarly reported higher effect sizes for intervention studies that used waitlisted groups as comparators [73]. One explanation could be that waitlisted participants tend to delay behavioural change because they anticipate professional help in the near future; that could cause overestimation of the intervention effect.

We did not find a significantly greater effect size for guided ($g = 0.23$) than for unguided ($g = 0.20$) alcohol interventions, even though such significant differences in benefit have been overwhelmingly established for web-based treatment of depression and anxiety [34,74]. Our lack of significant effect might be due to the fact that many participants in web-based alcohol interventions are first-time help seekers; they may hence derive health gains from their first formal attempt at behavioural change, whether unguided or guided. Alternatively, a real difference may have gone undetected as a consequence of the low number of guided interventions in our analysis (5 comparisons. Only the Blankers and colleagues [37], and the Doumas and Hannah [57] studies provided direct comparisons between guided and unguided interventions. Both showed a small, but non significant, difference in effect in terms of alcohol consumption reduction in favour of guided interventions. These non-significant results are probably due to lack of power in both studies as well.

In contrast with our previous analysis from 2011 [26], we now found no significant differences in alcohol reduction between single-session interventions and more extended ones. Although the literature is somewhat inconclusive [75], it provides some confirmation for our current findings [30,68,76].

Web-based interventions may offer considerable promise for reducing alcohol misuse by women. We found no difference in alcohol consumption outcomes between all-male and mixed-gender samples, whereas several studies on face-to-face alcohol interventions in primary care had reported that men were more likely to benefit than women [30,67]. In the case of Internet-based interventions for alcohol misuse, however, female uptake appears equally as high as male uptake [28,77] and have been seen to have similar impacts on female and on male drinking, or possibly even greater influence on females, as suggested by Riper and colleagues (2008, [78]).

No difference in effect sizes emerged between studies that used cut-off points in alcohol consumption as study inclusion criteria and those that applied stricter measurements such as AUDIT [55]. AUDIT scores among the latter were high (averaging around 20, indicating a potentially high risk of alcohol dependence amongst participants. Internet interventions might thus well be effective for a broad spectrum of people who misuse alcohol. Just as in many trials of brief alcohol interventions and routine practice studies [18,79], the studies in our analysis did not conduct diagnostic interviews to assess for alcohol dependence. This lack of actual diagnoses also hampers any attempt to use the available data to test the common view that self-help interventions are particularly suited to people with less serious alcohol problems, but less appropriate for those with alcohol dependence [3,80].

Several limitations underlie our meta-analysis that may have affected our overall results. First, as indicated the number of studies included in the subgroup analyses was low. The resulting insufficient statistical power may call into question our outcomes whereby no significant difference between a number of conditions could be observed. Second, some included studies had substantial dropout rates (above 30%; see table 1). High study (and treatment) dropout rates are a common phenomenon in both online and offline self-help interventions for alcohol misuse and in Internet interventions in general [81,82]. Third, the impact of online self-help in reducing alcohol consumption may have been underestimated here because control group drinking was also assessed; such assessment alone possibly motivates controls to reduce their consumption [83,84]. Last but not least, we were not able to evaluate possible negative side-effects of Internet-based interventions for problem drinking, as the studies lack reports on such effects.

Clinical Implications

The results of this study support the use of guided and unguided Internet-based self-help interventions for curbing alcohol misuse in various settings (primary health care, work environments and the community). Although the overall effect size for these interventions was small, the public health impact could be substantial if large numbers of people who misuse alcohol were to take part in these interventions. Decreasing alcohol consumption as well as abstinence and adherence to low-risk guidelines are health benefits in their own right and potential predictors of longer-term maintenance of decreased alcohol consumption [85]. A modelling study by Smit and colleagues [86] has suggested that if online interventions were to partially replace conventional face-to-face brief alcohol interventions, that could sustain comparable levels of population health at lower costs.

Future Research

Future studies should try to assess which type (s) of alcohol misuse populations could benefit most from brief online alcohol interventions. More studies with longer-term follow-up periods (over 12 months) are needed, too, to assess the maintenance of intervention effects over time in terms of reduced consumption and other health outcomes. Studies focusing on the effects of guided self-help interventions in curbing alcohol misuse, in direct comparison with unguided interventions, could shed light on whether the former produce better outcomes and, if so, at what costs. It is also important to investigate whether combining low-intensity Internet interventions with brief face-to-face interventions (blending of channels) would increase the effectiveness of interventions to curb alcohol misuse.

Conclusion

Internet interventions are capable of reaching out effectively to the large group of people who engage in alcohol misuse. From a public health perspective, this justifies an upscaling of such interventions in routine practice as well as in a wide range of community settings.

Author Contributions

Conceived and designed the experiments: HR HH PC. Performed the experiments: HR HH MB. Analyzed the data: HR HH MB PC. Contributed reagents/materials/analysis tools: HR PC. Contributed to the writing of the manuscript: HR MB HH JC SC DE RW PC.

References

1. Whiteford HA, Degenhardt L, Rehm J, Baxter AJ, Ferrari AJ, et al. (2013) Global burden of disease attributable to mental and substance use disorders: findings from the Global Burden of Disease Study 2010. Lancet 382: 1575–1586.
2. Tang YL, Xiang XJ, Wang XY, Cubells JF, Babor TF, et al. (2013) Alcohol and alcohol-related harm in China: policy changes needed. Bull World Health Organ 91: 270–276.
3. Moyer VA (2013) Screening and behavioral counseling interventions in primary care to reduce alcohol misuse: U.S. preventive services task force recommendation statement. Ann Intern Med 159: 210–218.
4. Saunders JB, Lee NK (2000) Hazardous alcohol use: its delineation as a subthreshold disorder, and approaches to its diagnosis and management. Compr Psychiatry 41: 95–103.
5. WHO (2000) International guide for monitoring alcohol consumption and related harm. Geneva.: World Health Organization.
6. Degenhardt L, Whiteford HA, Ferrari AJ, Baxter AJ, Charlson FJ, et al. (2013) Global burden of disease attributable to illicit drug use and dependence: findings from the Global Burden of Disease Study 2010. Lancet 382: 1564–1574.
7. Grucza RA, Bucholz KK, Rice JP, Bierut LJ (2008) Secular trends in the lifetime prevalence of alcohol dependence in the United States: a re-evaluation. Alcohol Clin Exp Res 32: 763–770.
8. Watson HE (1999) Minimal interventions for problem drinkers: a review of the literature. J Adv Nurs 30: 513–519.
9. Parry CD, Patra J, Rehm J (2011) Alcohol consumption and non-communicable diseases: epidemiology and policy implications. Addiction 106: 1718–1724.
10. Rehm J, Mathers C, Popova S, Thavorncharoensap M, Teerawattananon Y, et al. (2009) Global burden of disease and injury and economic cost attributable to alcohol use and alcohol-use disorders. Lancet 373: 2223–2233.
11. Cunningham JA, Breslin FC (2004) Only one in three people with alcohol abuse or dependence ever seek treatment. Addict Behav 29: 221–223.
12. Koski-Janne A, Cunningham J (2001) Interest in different forms of self-help in a general population sample of drinkers. Addict Behav 26: 91–99.
13. Nilsen P, McCambridge J, Karlsson N, Bendtsen P (2011) Brief interventions in routine health care: a population-based study of conversations about alcohol in Sweden. Addiction 106: 1748–1756.
14. Wilson GB, Heather N, Kaner EF (2011) New developments in brief interventions to treat problem drinking in nonspecialty health care settings. Curr Psychiatry Rep 13: 422–429.
15. Jonas DE, Garbutt JC, Amick HR, Brown JM, Brownley KA, et al. (2012) Behavioral counseling after screening for alcohol misuse in primary care: a systematic review and meta-analysis for the U.S. Preventive Services Task Force. Ann Intern Med 157: 645–654.
16. Jonas DE, Garbutt JC, Brown JM, Amick HR, Brownley KA, et al. (2012) Screening, Behavioral Counseling, and Referral in Primary Care To Reduce Alcohol Misuse. Rockville (MD): Agency for Healthcare Research and Quality (US). Report No.: 12-EHC055-EF.
17. Latimer N, Guillaume L (2009) Prevention and early identification of alcohol use disorders in adults and young people: screening and brief interventions: cost effectiveness review. Sheffield: ScHARR Public Health Collaborating Centre.
18. Purshouse RC, Brennan A, Rafia R, Latimer NR, Archer RJ, et al. (2013) Modelling the cost-effectiveness of alcohol screening and brief interventions in primary care in England. Alcohol Alcohol 48: 180–188.
19. Tariq L, van den Berg M, Hoogenveen RT, van Baal PH (2009) Cost-effectiveness of an opportunistic screening programme and brief intervention for excessive alcohol use in primary care. PLoS One 4: e5696.
20. Mdege ND, Fayter D, Watson JM, Stirk L, Sowden A, et al. (2013) Interventions for reducing alcohol consumption among general hospital inpatient heavy alcohol users: a systematic review. Drug Alcohol Depend 131: 1–22.
21. Watson JM, Fayter D, Mdege N, Stirk L, Sowden AJ, et al. (2013) Interventions for alcohol and drug problems in outpatient settings: a systematic review. Drug Alcohol Rev 32: 356–367.
22. Pedersen B, Oppedal K, Egund L, Tonnesen H (2011) Will emergency and surgical patients participate in and complete alcohol interventions? A systematic review. BMC Surg 11: 26.
23. Osilla KC, Van Busum K, Schnyer C, Larkin JW, Eibner C, et al. (2012) Systematic review of the impact of worksite wellness programs. Am J Manag Care 18: e68–e81.
24. Hester RK, Lenberg KL, Campbell W, Delaney HD (2013) Overcoming Addictions, a Web-based application, and SMART Recovery, an online and in-person mutual help group for problem drinkers, part 1: three-month outcomes of a randomized controlled trial. J Med Internet Res 15: e134.
25. White A, Kavanagh D, Stallman H, Klein B, Kay-Lambkin F, et al. (2010) Online alcohol interventions: a systematic review. J Med Internet Res 12: e62.
26. Riper H, Spek V, Boon B, Conijn B, Kramer J, et al. (2011) Effectiveness of E-self-help interventions for curbing adult problem drinking: a meta-analysis. J Med Internet Res 13: e42.
27. Cunningham JA, Wild TC, Cordingley J, Van Mierlo T, Humphreys K (2009) A randomized controlled trial of an internet-based intervention for alcohol abusers. Addiction 104: 2023–2032.
28. Riper H, Kramer J, Conijn B, Smit F, Schippers G, et al. (2009) Translating effective web-based self-help for problem drinking into the real world. Alcohol Clin Exp Res 33: 1401–1408.
29. Vernon ML (2010) A review of computer-based alcohol problem services designed for the general public. J Subst Abuse Treat 38: 203–211.
30. Kaner EF, Beyer F, Dickinson HO, Pienaar E, Campbell F, et al. (2007) Effectiveness of brief alcohol interventions in primary care populations. Cochrane Database Syst Rev CD004148.

31. Rooke S, Thorsteinsson E, Karpin A, Copeland J, Allsop D (2010) Computer-delivered interventions for alcohol and tobacco use: a meta-analysis. Addiction 105: 1381–1390.
32. Portnoy DB, Scott-Sheldon LA, Johnson BT, Carey MP (2008) Computer-delivered interventions for health promotion and behavioral risk reduction: a meta-analysis of 75 randomized controlled trials, 1988–2007. Prev Med 47: 3–16.
33. Blankers M, Nabitz U, Smit F, Koeter MW, Schippers GM (2012) Economic evaluation of internet-based interventions for harmful alcohol use alongside a pragmatic randomized controlled trial. J Med Internet Res 14: e134.
34. Richards D, Richardson T (2012) Computer-based psychological treatments for depression: a systematic review and meta-analysis. Clin Psychol Rev 32: 329–342.
35. Cuijpers P, Marks IM, van Straten A, Cavanagh K, Gega L, et al. (2009) Computer-aided psychotherapy for anxiety disorders: a meta-analytic review. Cogn Behav Ther 38: 66–82.
36. Cuijpers P, Donker T, van Straten A, Li J, Andersson G (2010) Is guided self-help as effective as face-to-face psychotherapy for depression and anxiety disorders? A systematic review and meta-analysis of comparative outcome studies. Psychol Med 1–15.
37. Blankers M, Koeter MW, Schippers GM (2011) Internet therapy versus internet self-help versus no treatment for problematic alcohol use: A randomized controlled trial. J Consult Clin Psychol 79: 330–341.
38. Postel MG, de Haan HA, ter Huurne ED, Becker ES, de Jong CA (2010) Effectiveness of a web-based intervention for problem drinkers and reasons for dropout: randomized controlled trial. J Med Internet Res 12: e68.
39. Higgins JPT, Green S (2008 February) Higgins JPT, Green S (editors). Cochrane Handbook for Systematic Reviews of Interventions Version 5.0.0. The Cochrane Collaboration. Available.
40. Hester RK (1995) Behavioral self-control training. In: Hester RK, Miller WR, editors. Handbook of Alcoholism Treatment Approaches: Effective Alternatives. Needham Heights, MA: Allyn and Bacon. 148–159.
41. Miller WR, Rollnick S (2002) Motivational Interviewing: Preparing people to change addictive behavior. New York: Guilford Press.
42. Prochaska JO, Velicer WF (1997) The transtheoretical model of health behavior change. Am J Health Promot 12: 38–48.
43. Kalden R, Caroll K, Donovan D, Cooney N, Monti P, et al. (1992) Cognitive behavioral Coping Skills Therapy Manual: A Clinical Research Guide for Therapists Treating Individuals With Alcohol Abuse and Dependence. In: Mattson MEM, editors. NIAAA Project MATCH Monograph Series. Rockville, Md: National Institute on Alcoholism and Alcohol Abuse.
44. Chan KK, Neighbors C, Gilson M, Larimer ME, Alan MG (2007) Epidemiological trends in drinking by age and gender: providing normative feedback to adults. Addict Behav 32: 967–976.
45. Cohen J (1997) Statistical power analyses for the behavioral sciences (revised ed.). New York: Academic Press.
46. Borenstein M, Hedges L, Higgins JPT, Rothstein HR (2009) Introduction to meta-analysis. Chichester, UK: Wiley.
47. Higgins JP, Thompson SG, Deeks JJ, Altman DG (2003) Measuring inconsistency in meta-analyses. BMJ 327: 557–560.
48. Ioannidis JP, Patsopoulos NA, Evangelou E (2007) Uncertainty in heterogeneity estimates in meta-analyses. BMJ 335: 914–916.
49. Orsini N, Bottai M, Higgins JP, Buchan I (2006) Heterogi: Stata module to quantify heterogeneity in a meta-analysis. [Computer Software].
50. Kraemer HC, Kupfer DJ (2006) Size of treatment effects and their importance to clinical research and practice. Biol Psychiatry 59: 990–996.
51. Riper H, van Straten A, Keuken M, Smit F, Schippers G, et al. (2009) Curbing problem drinking with personalized-feedback interventions: a meta-analysis. Am J Prev Med 36: 247–255.
52. Egger M, Davey SG, Schneider M, Minder C (1997) Bias in meta-analysis detected by a simple, graphical test. BMJ 315: 629–634.
53. Duval S, Tweedie R (2000) Trim and fill: A simple funnel-plot-based method of testing and adjusting for publication bias in meta-analysis. Biometrics 56: 455–463.
54. Moher D, Liberati A, Tetzlaff J, Altman DG (2010) Preferred reporting items for systematic reviews and meta-analyses: the PRISMA statement. Int J Surg 8: 336–341.
55. Saunders JB, Aasland OG, Babor TF, Defuentes-Merillas L, Grant M (1993) Development of the Alcohol Use Disorders Identification Test (AUDIT): WHO Collaborative Project on Early Detection of Persons with Harmful Alcohol Consumption II. Addiction 88: 791–804.
56. Hodgson R, Alwyn T, John B, Thom B, Smith A (2002) The FAST Alcohol Screening Test. Alcohol Alcohol 37: 61–66.
57. Doumas DM, Hannah E (2008) Preventing high-risk drinking in youth in the workplace: a web-based normative feedback program. J Subst Abuse Treat 34: 263–271.
58. Pemberton MR, Williams J, Herman-Stahl M, Calvin SL, Bradshaw MR, et al. (2011) Evaluation of two web-based alcohol interventions in the U.S. military. J Stud Alcohol Drugs 72: 480–489.
59. Bischof G, Grothues JM, Reinhardt S, Meyer C, John U, et al. (2008) Evaluation of a telephone-based stepped care intervention for alcohol-related disorders: a randomized controlled trial. Drug Alcohol Depend 93: 244–251.
60. Hansen AB, Becker U, Nielsen AS, Gronbaek M, Tolstrup JS, et al. (2012) Internet-based brief personalized feedback intervention in a non-treatment-seeking population of adult heavy drinkers: a randomized controlled trial. J Med Internet Res 14: e98.
61. Schulz DN, Candel MJ, Kremers SP, Reinwand DA, Jander A, et al. (2013) Effects of a web-based tailored intervention to reduce alcohol consumption in adults: randomized controlled trial. J Med Internet Res 15: e206.
62. Suffoletto B, Callaway C, Kristan J, Kraemer K, Clark DB (2012) Text-message-based drinking assessments and brief interventions for young adults discharged from the emergency department. Alcohol Clin Exp Res 36: 552–560.
63. Boon B, Risselada A, Huiberts A, Riper H, Smit F (2011) Curbing alcohol use in male adults through computer generated personalized advice: randomized controlled trial. J Med Internet Res.13(2): e43.
64. Boon B, Huibers A (2006) Preventie problematisch alcoholgebruik. In: Meijer SA, Smit F, Schoemaker CG, Cuijpers P, editors. Gezond verstand. Evidence-based preventie van psychische stoornissen [Common sense. Evidence-based prevention of mental disorders]. VTV Themarapport (RIVM-rapportnummer: 270061003. Bilthoven: RIVM.
65. Riper H, Kramer J, Smit F, Conijn B, Schippers G, et al. (2008) Web-based self-help for problem drinkers: a pragmatic randomized trial. Addiction 103: 218–227.
66. Wallace P, Murray E, McCambridge J, Khadjesari Z, White IR, et al. (2011) On-line randomized controlled trial of an internet based psychologically enhanced intervention for people with hazardous alcohol consumption. PLoS One 6: e14740.
67. O'Donnell A, Anderson P, Newbury-Birch D, Schulte B, Schmidt C, et al. (2014) The impact of brief alcohol interventions in primary healthcare: a systematic review of reviews. Alcohol Alcohol 49: 66–78.
68. Moyer A, Finney JW, Swearingen CE, Vergun P (2002) Brief interventions for alcohol problems: a meta-analytic review of controlled investigations in treatment-seeking and non-treatment-seeking populations. Addiction 97: 279–292.
69. Apodaca TR, Miller WR (2003) A meta-analysis of the effectiveness of bibliotherapy for alcohol problems. J Clin Psychol 59: 289–304.
70. Vasilaki EI, Hosier SG, Cox WM (2006) The efficacy of motivational interviewing as a brief intervention for excessive drinking: a meta-analytic review. Alcohol Alcohol 41: 328–335.
71. Burke BL, Arkowitz H, Menchola M (2003) The efficacy of motivational interviewing: a meta-analysis of controlled clinical trials. J Consult Clin Psychol 71: 843–861.
72. Cuijpers P, Riper H, Lemmers L (2004) The effects on mortality of brief interventions for problem drinking: a meta-analysis. Addiction 99: 839–845.
73. Cunningham JA, Kypri K, McCambridge J (2013) Exploratory randomized controlled trial evaluating the impact of a waiting list control design. BMC Med Res Methodol 13: 150.
74. Donker T, van SA, Riper H, Marks I, Andersson G, et al. (2009) Implementation of Internet-based preventive interventions for depression and anxiety: role of support? The design of a randomized controlled trial. Trials 10: 59.
75. Moyer VA (2013) Screening and behavioral counseling interventions in primary care to reduce alcohol misuse: U.S. preventive services task force recommendation statement. Ann Intern Med 159: 210–218.
76. Kaner E, Bland M, Cassidy P, Coulton S, Dale V, et al. (2013) Effectiveness of screening and brief alcohol intervention in primary care (SIPS trial): pragmatic cluster randomised controlled trial. BMJ 346: e8501.
77. Cunningham JA, Khadjesari Z, Bewick BM, Riper H (2010) Internet-based interventions for problem drinkers: From efficacy trials to implementation. Drug Alcohol Rev 29: 617–622.
78. Riper H, Kramer J, Keuken M, Smit F, Schippers G, et al. (2008) Predicting successful treatment outcome of web-based self-help for problem drinkers: secondary analysis from a randomized controlled trial. J Med Internet Res 10: e46.
79. Robinson SM, Sobell LC, Sobell MB, Arcidiacono S, Tzall D (2014) Alcohol and drug treatment outcome studies: new methodological review (2005–2010) and comparison with past reviews. Addict Behav 39: 39–47.
80. Saitz R (2010) Alcohol screening and brief intervention in primary care: Absence of evidence for efficacy in people with dependence or very heavy drinking. Drug Alcohol Rev 29: 631–640.
81. Eysenbach G (2005) The law of attrition. J Med Internet Res 7: e11.
82. Postel MG, de Haan HA, ter Huurne ED, van der Palen J, Becker ES, et al. (2011) Attrition in web-based treatment for problem drinkers. J Med Internet Res 13: e117.
83. McCambridge J, Kypri K, McElduff P (2013) Regression to the mean and alcohol consumption: A cohort study exploring implications for the interpretation of change in control groups in brief intervention trials. Drug Alcohol Depend.
84. McCambridge J, Kypri K, McElduff P (2014) Regression to the mean and alcohol consumption: a cohort study exploring implications for the interpretation of change in control groups in brief intervention trials. Drug Alcohol Depend 135: 156–159.
85. Roerecke M, Gual A, Rehm J (2013) Reduction of alcohol consumption and subsequent mortality in alcohol use disorders: systematic review and meta-analyses. J Clin Psychiatry 74: e1181–e1189.
86. Smit F, Lokkerbol J, Riper H, Majo MC, Boon B, et al. (2011) Modeling the cost-effectiveness of health care systems for alcohol use disorders: how implementation of eHealth interventions improves cost-effectiveness. J Med Internet Res 13: e56.

19

Neuroinflammation and Neurodegeneration in Adult Rat Brain from Binge Ethanol Exposure: Abrogation by Docosahexaenoic Acid

Nuzhath Tajuddin[1], Kwan-Hoon Moon[1], S. Alex Marshall[2], Kimberly Nixon[2], Edward J. Neafsey[1], Hee-Yong Kim[3], Michael A. Collins[1]*

1 Department of Molecular Pharmacology & Therapeutics, Loyola University Chicago, Stritch School of Medicine, Maywood, Illinois, United States of America, 2 Department of Pharmaceutical Sciences, University of Kentucky, Lexington, Kentucky, United States of America, 3 Laboratory of Molecular Signaling, NIAAA, National Institutes of Health, Bethesda, Maryland, United States of America

Abstract

Evidence that brain edema and aquaporin-4 (AQP4) water channels have roles in experimental binge ethanol-induced neurodegeneration has stimulated interest in swelling/edema-linked neuroinflammatory pathways leading to oxidative stress. We report here that neurotoxic binge ethanol exposure produces comparable significant effects *in vivo* and *in vitro* on adult rat brain levels of AQP4 as well as neuroinflammation-linked enzymes: key phospholipase A2 (PLA2) family members and poly (ADP-ribose) polymerase-1 (PARP-1). In adult male rats, repetitive ethanol intoxication (3 gavages/d for 4 d, ~9 g/kg/d, achieving blood ethanol levels ~375 mg/dl; "Majchrowicz" model) significantly increased AQP4, Ca^{+2}-dependent PLA2 GIVA (cPLA2), phospho-cPLA2 GIVA (p-cPLA2), secretory PLA2 GIIA (sPLA2) and PARP-1 in regions incurring extensive neurodegeneration in this model—hippocampus, entorhinal cortex, and olfactory bulb—but not in two regions typically lacking neurodamage, frontal cortex and cerebellum. Also, ethanol reduced hippocampal Ca^{+2}-independent PLA2 GVIA (iPLA2) levels and increased brain "oxidative stress footprints" (4-hydroxynonenal-adducted proteins). For *in vitro* studies, organotypic cultures of rat hippocampal-entorhinocortical slices of adult age (~60 d) were ethanol-binged (100 mM or ~450 mg/dl) for 4 d, which augments AQP4 and causes neurodegeneration (Collins et al. 2013). Reproducing the *in vivo* results, cPLA2, p-cPLA2, sPLA2 and PARP-1 were significantly elevated while iPLA2 was decreased. Furthermore, supplementation with docosahexaenoic acid (DHA; 22:6n-3), known to quell AQP4 and neurodegeneration in ethanol-treated slices, blocked PARP-1 and PLA2 changes while counteracting endogenous DHA reduction and increases in oxidative stress footprints (3-nitrotyrosinated proteins). Notably, the PARP-1 inhibitor PJ-34 suppressed binge ethanol-dependent neurodegeneration, indicating PARP upstream involvement. The results with corresponding models support involvement of AQP4- and PLA2-associated neuroinflammatory pro-oxidative pathways in the neurodamage, with potential regulation by PARP-1 as well. Furthermore, DHA emerges as an effective inhibitor of these binge ethanol-dependent neuroinflammatory pathways as well as associated neurodegeneration in adult-age brain.

Editor: Vinod K. Yaragudri, Nathan Kline Institute for Psychiatric Research and New York School of Medicine, United States of America

Funding: Supported by NIH U01 AA018279 (MAC), R01 AA0016959 (KN), and T32 DA016176 (SAM). The funders had no role in study design, data collection and analysis, decision to publish, or preparation of the manuscript.

Competing Interests: The authors have declared that no competing interests exist.

* Email: mcollin@luc.edu

Introduction

Alcohol (ethanol) use disorders constitute a major worldwide cause of health impairment and productivity loss [1,2]. Amidst a range of organ damage outcomes, chronic ethanol abuse—and particularly binge-type alcoholism [3,4]—causes neuropathological sequelae leading to brain dysfunction and dementia [5]. A repetitive binge intoxication adult rat model developed by Majchrowicz nearly 40 years ago to study alcoholic withdrawal seizures [6] was later shown to have surprisingly regionalized neurodegeneration in the temporal (particularly entorhinal) cortex (EC) and the hippocampus (HC) (mainly dentate gyrus granule cells), as well as olfactory bulb neurons [7,8]. Results indicating the involvement of oxidative stress but not excitotoxicity [9] in this *in vivo* model of acquired neurodegeneration point to neuroinflammatory (glial-neuronal) pro-oxidative mechanisms; however, the detailed pathways remain uncertain. The Majchrowicz adult rat intoxication model or a variant has been used by a number of laboratories to examine underlying mechanisms. Apoptosis as a chief neurodegenerative pathway was ruled out by the absence of TUNEL staining [10]. Evidence that diuretics such as furosemide and acetazolamide prevent ethanol-induced elevations in rat brain water content while reducing or blocking neurodegeneration indicated that brain edema was important [11,12]. Cellular edema, a major and often intractable clinical problem that exacerbates neuropathology in brain ischemia and trauma, thus might elicit neuroinflammatory processes in binge ethanol abuse. A further contributor to the neurodamage in this binge model may well be stress-elevated circulating glucocorticoid (corticosterone), as recently reported [13]. (However, it is worth noting a paradox in that glucocorticoids have well-known edema-resolving effects, particularly under cerebral acidotic conditions [14]).

Neuroinflammation—brain pro-oxidative processes dependent on glia acting on neurons—has assumed a more general focus in alcohol neuropathology studies. While there is considerable interest in the role of microglial activation, it is unclear in the above binged rat model whether microglia contribute directly to neurodegeneration [15,16]. Astroglia could have key roles, since they are enriched in membrane aquaporin-4 (AQP4) water channels that mediate glial edema during brain insults [17]. Furthermore, such brain astroglial swelling due to binge ethanol could promote phospholipid-instigated neuroinflammation—e.g., increased phospholipase A2 (PLA2) activities, which release excessive quantities of arachidonic acid (ARA, 20:4n-6) from membrane phospholipids [18,19]. ARA can be a major source of reactive oxygen species (ROS) via autoxidation and its metabolism to eicosanoid products. Specific families of PLA2 known to mobilize ARA during brain insults and neuroinflammatory stresses were the focus of our studies here. Calcium (Ca^{+2})-dependent (cytosolic) PLA2 (cPLA2), which has received the most attention [20]—and particularly the cPLA2 GIVA isoform—was examined. Small secreted PLA2 (sPLA2) enzymes have gained interest in neuroinflammatory models [21], among which sPLA2 GIIA received our focus. In contrast, Ca^{+2}-independent PLA2 (iPLA2) isoforms may have brain homeostatic roles; we were principally interested in iPLA2 GVIA, because of its importance in the turnover of endogenous docosahexaenoic acid (DHA, 22:6n-3) [22]. Moreover, we were guided by our results from brain regions of adult rats given moderate rather than high ethanol doses in a "binge-pattern" [23], which showed reduced iPLA2 GVIA and significantly elevated expression levels of cPLA2 GIVA, sPLA2 GIIA, and AQP4, as well as poly (ADP-ribose) polymerase-1 (PARP-1). PARP-1 is a key nuclear DNA repair enzyme, but when hyperactivated, it can promote a form of regulated necrosis (termed parthanatos) by oxidative stress routes involving glial activation [24,25].

The above neuroinflammation-related enzymes were examined in the Majchrowicz *in vivo* intoxication model, in parallel with a somewhat unique *in vitro* model, binge ethanol-treated adult-age rat organotypic hippocampal-entorhinal cortical (HEC) slices in culture. Organotypic brain slice cultures (typically hippocampal and only occasionally HEC) have often been used in neurodegeneration studies [26,27], but invariably at adolescent or developing brain ages. It seemed reasonable that data with adult-age HEC slice preparations would more reliably correlate with results from intact adult brain. For example, the adult-age rat HEC slices incur neurodamage and AQP4 elevations when subjected to binging that closely approximates the *in vivo* model (four successive [overnight] exposures to 100 mM ethanol—a concentration not unusual in the blood of severe alcoholics [28,29] that is frequently used in neurodegeneration studies—whereas developing HEC slice cultures require ~6 exposure days) [30]. At least with entorhinal cortex, the above suggestion that adult brain neurons are more susceptible than developing neurons to binge ethanol-induced neurodegeneration corresponds well with binge ethanol results *in vivo* [31]. Since edema is linked at times to reactive oxygen/nitrogen species, we also assessed the extent of oxidative stress in the ethanol-binged slices using "oxidative footprints"—levels of 4-hydroxynonenal (4HNE)-adducted and/or 3-nitrotyrosinated (3NT-) proteins. In part, the latter assays were motivated by indications in other disease conditions involving brain oxidative stress, e.g., hepatic encephalopathy, that protein tyrosine nitration is associated with brain edema [32].

An important facet of this study is the investigation of the neuroprotective effects of DHA against ethanol-dependent brain damage [30,33]. Endogenous rat brain levels of this essential n-3 unsaturated fatty acid are equal to those of n-6 ARA, but in contrast to the latter, DHA is often anti-oxidative and anti-inflammatory rather than pro-inflammatory [34–36]. Depletion of brain DHA, principally within membrane phosphatidylserine, could underlie aberrant neuroapoptosis in fetal alcoholism models [37,38], and dietary DHA can counter the brain oxidative damage and neurobehavioral deficits of ethanol exposure in utero [39–41]. We find with the ethanol-binged adult-age HEC slice cultures that endogenous DHA is indeed reduced, and that supplemented DHA normalizes those levels, reduces oxidative stress, and exerts global suppression of the above neuroinflammatory proteins. One of these, PARP-1, may be a crucial regulatory enzyme in a pro-inflammatory phospholipid-dependent cascade.

Materials and Methods

Materials

Antibodies. AQP4 (sc-20812), cPLA2 IVA (sc-454), ser 505 p-cPLA2 IVA (sc-34391), and glyceraldehyde phosphate dehydrogenase (GAPDH, sc-166545) were from Santa Cruz Biotechnology, Santa Cruz CA; iPLA2 VIβ (07-169) was from Upstate Biotech, Lake Placid NY; sPLA2 IIA (181055100) was from BioVendor, Candler NC; PARP-1 (9542s) was from Cell Signaling, Danvers MA; Anti-3NT-protein (AB7048) was from Abcam Co., Cambridge MA; and anti-4HNE-adducted protein (AB5605) was from Millipore Corp., Temecula CA. Secondary antibodies were from Jackson ImmunoResearch, West Grove PA, and luminol reagent for immunoblot detection was from Pierce Chemicals, Rockford IL. DHA was from Cayman Chemicals, Ann Arbor MI, PJ34 was from Enzo Life Sciences, Farmingdale NY, and other chemicals/reagents were from Sigma Chemicals, St. Louis MO.

Animal experiments

These studies were carried out in accordance with the recommendations in the Guide for the Care and Use of Laboratory Animals of the National Institutes of Health. The *in vivo* protocol was approved by the Institutional Animal Care and Use Committee of the University of Kentucky, and all efforts were made to minimize suffering during treatments and sacrifice. The *in vitro* protocol was approved by the Institutional Animal Care and Use Committee of Loyola University Medical Center, and all efforts were made to minimize suffering during anesthesia and sacrifice.

Binge ethanol intoxication in vivo

Adult male SD rats (275–300 g) were subjected to the 4-day binge intoxication protocol modified from Majchrowicz that has a well-documented neurodegeneration profile [8,42,43]. The model mimics the high blood ethanol levels of binge pattern alcoholics [3]. Rats were provided nutritionally complete liquid diets containing either ethanol (25%w/v) or isocaloric dextrose in vanilla Ensure Plus (Abbott Laboratories, Columbus OH) every 8 hr via intragastric gavage (range: 8.3–9.7 g/kg/d). Rats in the ethanol group received an initial loading dose of 5 g/kg, with subsequent doses adjusted based on a behavioral intoxication scale detailed in earlier reports [44,45]. Control rats were given volumes of diet equal to the average volumes given the ethanol-treated rats. Water was freely available but not chow. Serum ethanol levels, which averaged ~375 mg/dl (~82 mM), were ascertained in blood samples taken 90 min after the 6th ethanol dose using an

AM1 Alcohol Analyzer (Analox, London UK) calibrated against a 300 mg/dl external standard. Rats were sacrificed by decapitation on the morning of the 5th day, 8–10 hr after the last ethanol or control gavage treatment. Intact brains were quickly removed, divided in half and quick-frozen in liquid nitrogen. At appropriate times, brains were thawed on ice and respective brain regions were taken for protein extraction as described under Immunoblotting.

Adult-age HEC slice cultures

Male Sprague-Dawley rats (Harlan, Indianapolis IN), 40±2 days old, were anesthetized with isoflurane and thoroughly perfused *via* the intracardiac route with ~150 ml of ice-cold lactate-Ringer's solution. When translucent, rat brains were placed in ice-cold Gey's buffer solution; the hippocampal-entorhinal cortical complex was removed and slices (250–300 μ) were prepared using a McIlwain tissue chopper. Slices were carefully placed on Millipore 0.4 μ membrane inserts (2–3 slices/insert), which were placed in 6-well plates, with each well containing 1.2 ml of MEM media with 25% heat-inactivated horse serum (HS). Slices were incubated at 32°C and 5% CO2 for the first 48 hr, and media was then changed to 20% heat-inactivated HS, and slices were transferred to a 37°C incubator (5% CO2). Cultures were then maintained 17–19 days, with the media changed every 2–3 days. Slices were monitored visually and those appearing unusually dark or broken were discarded.

Binge ethanol and DHA treatment of HEC slice cultures

At a brain age of 60±3 days, slices in experimental groups were treated overnight for ~16 h with 100 mM ethanol in MEM/20% HS for 4 successive nights, media without ethanol for ~8 h during daylight hours for 3 d and then ~4 h on the 4th day, to permit slice assays. Control slices were subjected to similar changes throughout the 4 d period with HS-containing MEM media without ethanol. Half of experimental and control slices were treated with DHA (25–50 μM) or PJ34 (10 μM) beginning 4 h prior to the start of ethanol treatment and throughout both overnight ethanol/media and daytime media exposures. The DHA concentrations used, reported to sustain neuronal viability in primary brain cultures [46], border physiological values for n-3 fatty acids [47]. Slices then were treated as described below with propidium iodide (PI), a fluorescent dye selectively accumulated by dying and dead neurons in organotypic brain slices [48,49], or pooled for immunoblot analyses.

PI staining for assessment of neurodegeneration in HEC slices

Media were removed from the wells and slices were incubated for 20–30 min with 1.2 ml fresh serum-free media containing 10 μM PI. After removal of PI-containing media, slices were washed twice with serum-free media, followed by addition of complete media with 20% HS for 1 hr before observing fluorescence results of PI labeling.

Immunoblotting with rat brain tissues

For HNE- and 3NT-proteins in brain regions of binge ethanol-treated and control rats and in pooled HEC slices, isolated brain regions or slices (rinsed with phosphate-buffered saline (PBS) and pooled—6-9 slices) were lysed in an isotonic buffer (50 mM Tris, 1 mM EDTA, protease and phosphatase inhibitor cocktail, pH 7.4), and then centrifuged for 10 min @ 13,000 rpm. For the neuroinflammation-associated proteins (cPLA2, p-cPLA2, sPLA2, iPLA2, AQP4, PARP-1), isolated brain regions or slices as above were sonicated 15–20 sec in a different lysis buffer (0.1% SDS, 1% sodium deoxycholate, 1% triton X-100, 150 mM NaCl, and 25 mM Tris HCl, pH 7.6) containing protease and phosphatase inhibitor cocktail. After centrifugation as above, protein concentrations were acquired with a bicinchoninic acid (BCA)–based method (Pierce Biotech, Rockford, IL); Aliquots (10 μg protein) of supernatants were then separated by 12% SDS-PAGE, transferred to PVDF-immobilon membranes, and subjected to immunoblot analysis by using appropriate protein antibodies. The intensities of immunoblots were normalized to GAPDH immunoblots, obtained on the same gels following stripping and reprobing, after scanning images with LABwork 4.5 image acquisition and analysis software (UltraViolet Products, Upland CA).

Unsaturated fatty acid assay

Lipids were extracted in the presence of internal standard (IS), tricosanoic acid (23:0), following established procedures in the Kim laboratory [50]. Aliquots were transmethylated by reaction with BF_3-methanol (14%, w/v) at 100°C for 2 h under nitrogen, and the methyl esters were then extracted with hexane and analyzed by gas chromatography-flame ionization detection. Individual fatty acids were identified by comparing retention times with known fatty acid standards (GLC-411 from Nu-Chek Prep., Elysian MN, USA). After comparing peak areas to IS in the conventional way, the contents of individual fatty acids were expressed as percent of total identified fatty acids [50].

Statistical analyses

Unless indicated otherwise, results were reproduced with 6–15 brain slices per group in each experiment. Quantitation of PI fluorescence with 1.99 NIH Image J software was as previously described in detail [33]. For the protein extracts of both *in vivo* brain regions and HEC slices, immunoblot levels were determined relative to levels of GAPDH as housekeeping protein, and expressed as percent of control (mean ± sem). Results were analyzed for statistically significant differences ($p<0.05$ or $p<0.01$) by Tukey's t-test and one-way analysis of variance (ANOVA) with completely randomized design.

Results

In vivo study

Figure 1 confirms the presence of substantial oxidative stress, i.e., 4HNE-adducted proteins that arise from peroxidation of endogenous/released AA and adduction of the peroxidative aldehyde product, 4HNE, with protein sidechains [51], in two susceptible brain regions *in vivo* (Majchrowicz rat model) after 4 days of repetitive ethanol gavages and morning sacrifice on day 5. It is very likely that the large immunoblots in the range of 50–55 KDa for both regions and also ~70+ KDa in EC constitute not just single proteins but an appreciable number of 4HNE-adducted proteins, based on 2-dimensional gel studies with such adducts [52]. When all discernible 4HNE-immunoblots are combined in the quantitation, significant elevations in levels of 4HNE-adducted oxidative footprints in HC and EC are observed, consistent the reported effectiveness of antioxidants in reducing neurodegeneration in this in vivo model [53].

Figures 2 and 3 are representative immunoblots of the neuroinflammation-associated proteins—cPLA2, p-cPLA2, sPLA2, iPLA2, AQP4 and PARP-1—and their *in vivo* levels, normalized to GAPDH, in five brain regions of adult male rats after neurotoxic binge ethanol or control treatments. Figure 2A shows that levels of cPLA2 and its phosphorylated/activated form, p-cPLA2, were significantly increased 40–140% above controls in the three regions that sustain appreciable neurodegeneration in

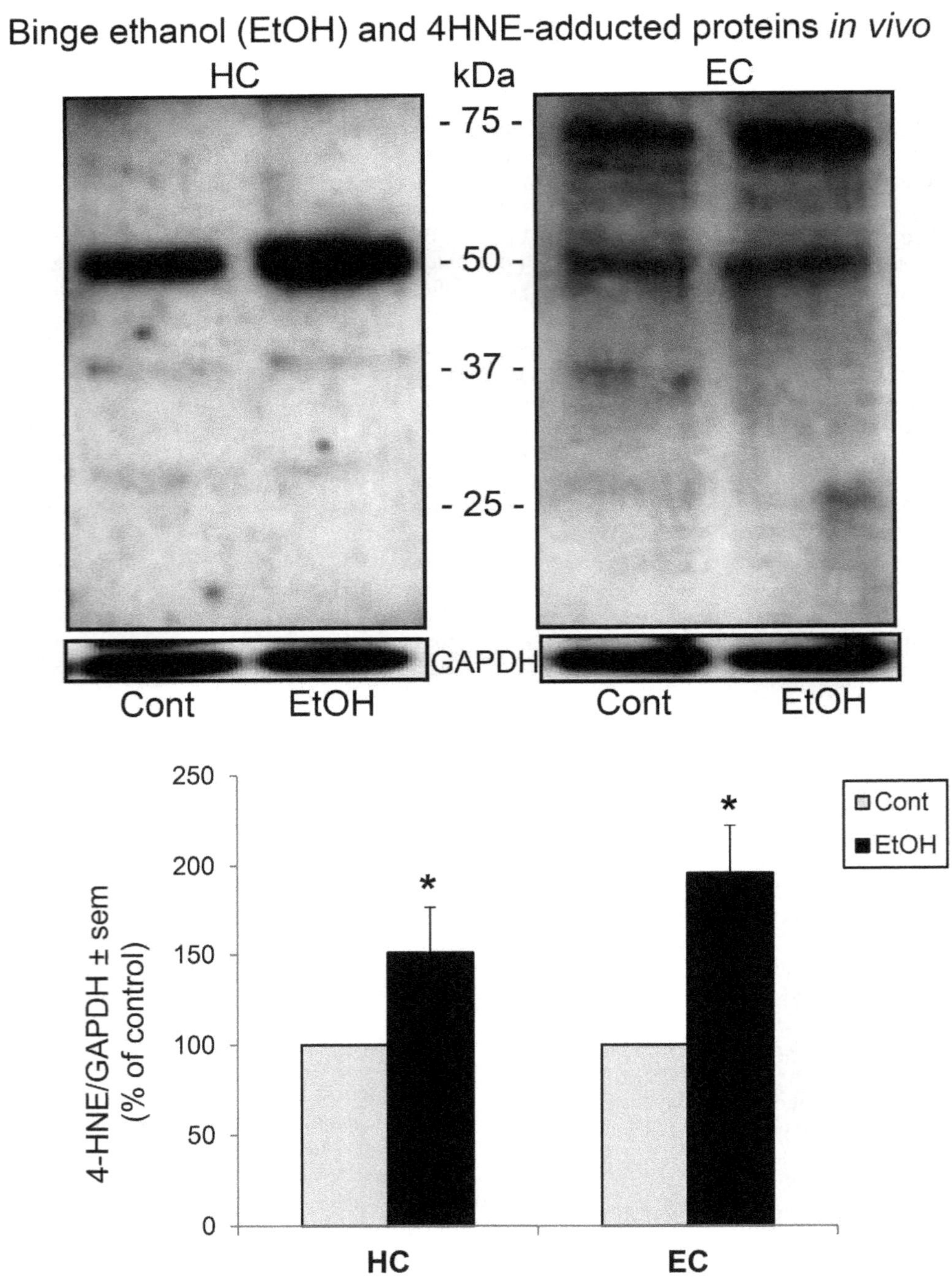

Figure 1. Effects of binge ethanol exposure on oxidative stress (4HNE-) protein footprint levels *in vivo*. Significant increases over respective controls (Cont) in levels of oxidative stress footprint, 4-hydroxynonenal (4HNE)-adducted proteins, in hippocampus (HC) and entorhinal cortex (EC) following neurotoxic binge ethanol treatment of adult male rats for 4 days (Majchrowicz model). Top: representative immunoblots of 4HNE-adducted proteins in HC and EC. Bottom: quantitation of immunoblots of 4HNE-adducted proteins in HC and EC. *$p<0.01$ vs. control (Cont); n = 4–7 rats per group.

the model—HC, EC and OB [8]. In contrast, cPLA2 and p-cPLA2 levels did not differ from control values in the CB and FC, two regions typically having little or no neurodamage. In Fig. 2B, the regional changes in sPLA2 mirrored cPLA2—significant elevations ranging from 75% to 240% above control levels in the three vulnerable regions of HC, EC and OB, but no significant changes in CB or FC. Figure 2C shows that iPLA2 was affected differently by binge ethanol treatment, being significantly reduced 35% below control values in the HC. It was not appreciably changed from control values in the other brain regions.

Figure 3 shows that *in vivo* responses to neurotoxic ethanol binging for AQP4 and PARP-1 mirrored those of cPLA2, p-cPLA2 and sPLA2. As with the cPLA2 and sPLA2 families, ethanol binges significantly increased AQP4 levels 65–110% above controls in the HC, EC and OB, whereas levels of the water channel did not differ from controls in the CB and FC. As shown in Figure 3B, PARP-1 also corresponded with the AQP4,

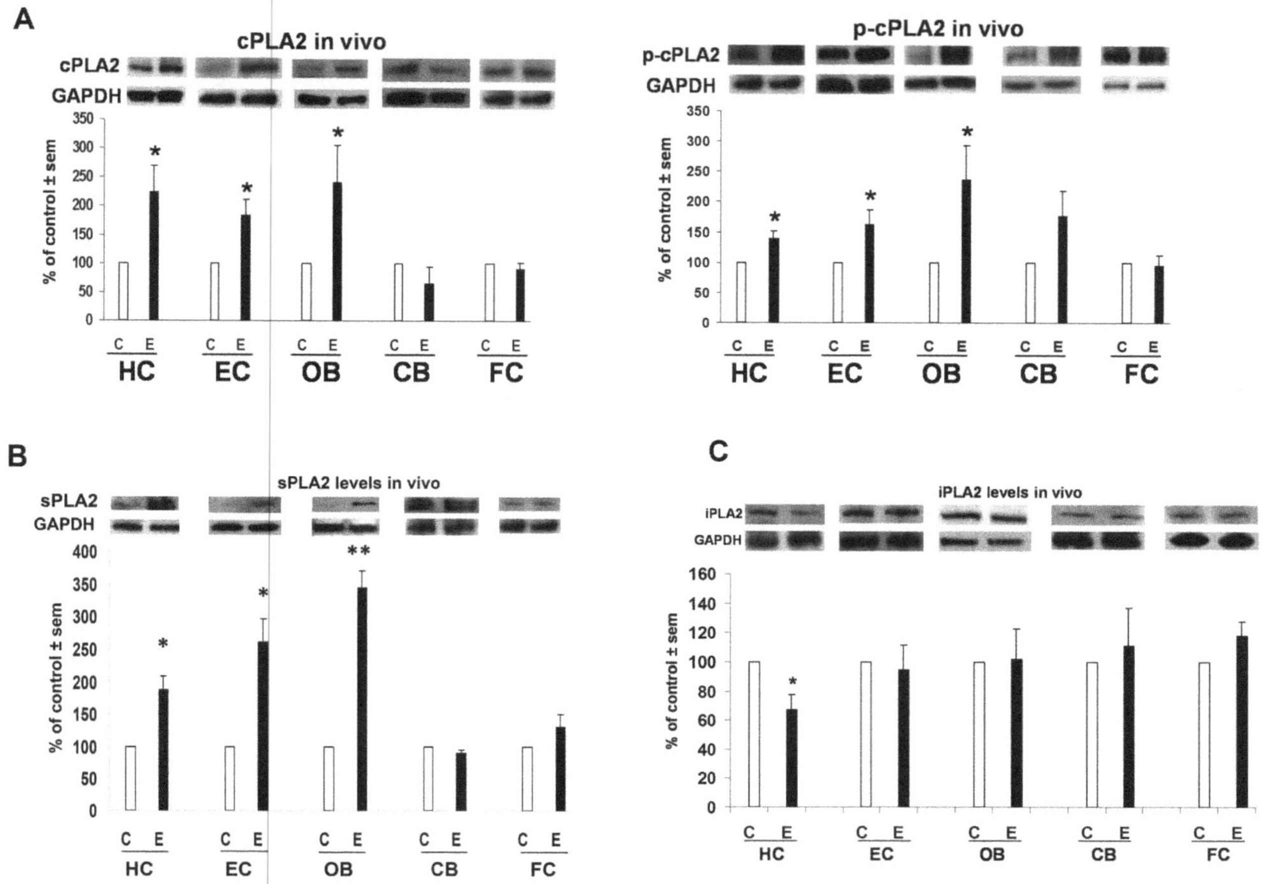

Figure 2. Selective effects of binge ethanol exposure on brain PLA2 levels *in vivo*. Significant alterations compared to respective controls (C) in protein expression (immunoblots) of PLA2 enzymes in brain regions selectively incurring neurodamage due to binge ethanol (E) treatment in adult male rats for 4 days (Majchrowicz model). Fig. 2A: Significantly increased levels of cPLA2 (top) and p-cPLA2 (bottom) in the hippocampus (HC), entorhinal cortex (EC) and olfactory bulb (OB), but not in cerebellum (CB) and frontal cortex (FC). Fig. 2B: Significantly increased sPLA2 levels in the HC, EC and OB, but not in CB and FC. Fig. 2C. Significantly decreased levels of iPLA2 in the HC. *$p<0.05$ vs. C. **$p<0.01$ vs. C. n = 4–7 rats/group.

cPLA2, p-cPLA2 and sPLA2 results. Quantitation of PARP-1 immunoblots revealed significant elevations of 125–150% above controls in the neurovulnerable regions of HC, EC and OB, but there were no changes in its levels in CB and FC.

In vitro studies

Figure 4, Figure 5 and Figure 6 demonstrate the effects in the rat adult-age HEC slice cultures of binge ethanol exposure on key neurotoxic outcomes, the above neuroinflammation-associated enzymes, and specific unsaturated fatty acid levels, and moreover, the effects of DHA supplementation on these measures. Figure 4A (top) shows representative images of HEC slices from control, DHA (25 μM), ethanol and ethanol+DHA groups at the 3 day treatment timepoint showing intensified PI labeling of degenerating neurons due to binge ethanol, and the relative absence of PI-stained neurons in the ethanol+DHA co-treated slice. The bottom graph shows that DHA concentrations of 25 and 50 μM potently inhibit binge ethanol-induced PI labeling (degenerating neurons), and to approximately the same extent. In Figure 4B, the quantitation of the time course of PI-stained neurons over 4 days of binge ethanol treatment demonstrates that degenerating neuron levels rose significantly above control levels on day 2, and continued to moderately increase for the two remaining days. The co-presence of DHA effectively prevented the increased neurodegeneration in HEC slices on each of those three ethanol exposure days. Although not used in these DHA experiments, adrenic acid, an analogous 22-carbon n-6 fatty acid and a negative control which was previously added to HEC slice cultures in place of DHA, had no effect on binge ethanol-dependent neurodegeneration [33].

In Figure 4C the results show that binge ethanol treatment of the HEC slice cultures for 4 days significantly augmented oxidative stress as indicated by elevations above basal levels in 3NT-proteins derived from reactions of peroxynitrite (product of the free radicals, superoxide and nitric oxide) with proteins. As with the Figure 1 oxidative protein footprints, the large immunoblots contain a number of proteins with nitrotyrosine sidechains that react to antibody, and quantitation encompassed all observable immunoblots. Consistent with its effects on neurodegeneration, co-exposure of ethanol-binged slices with DHA (25 μM) largely abolished elevations in this oxidative footprint. Parenthetically, we found that HNE-adducted proteins as in the *in vivo* brain samples could not be reliably determined in the slices because of interference from aldehydic adducts derived from supplemented DHA.

Figure 5 displays the immunoblot levels of five of the six neuroinflammation-related proteins (i.e., in Figures 2 and 3) in adult-age HEC slice cultures that were binge-exposed for 4 days to ethanol (100 mM) or control media, with and without DHA supplementation. AQP4 augmentation by binge ethanol in these

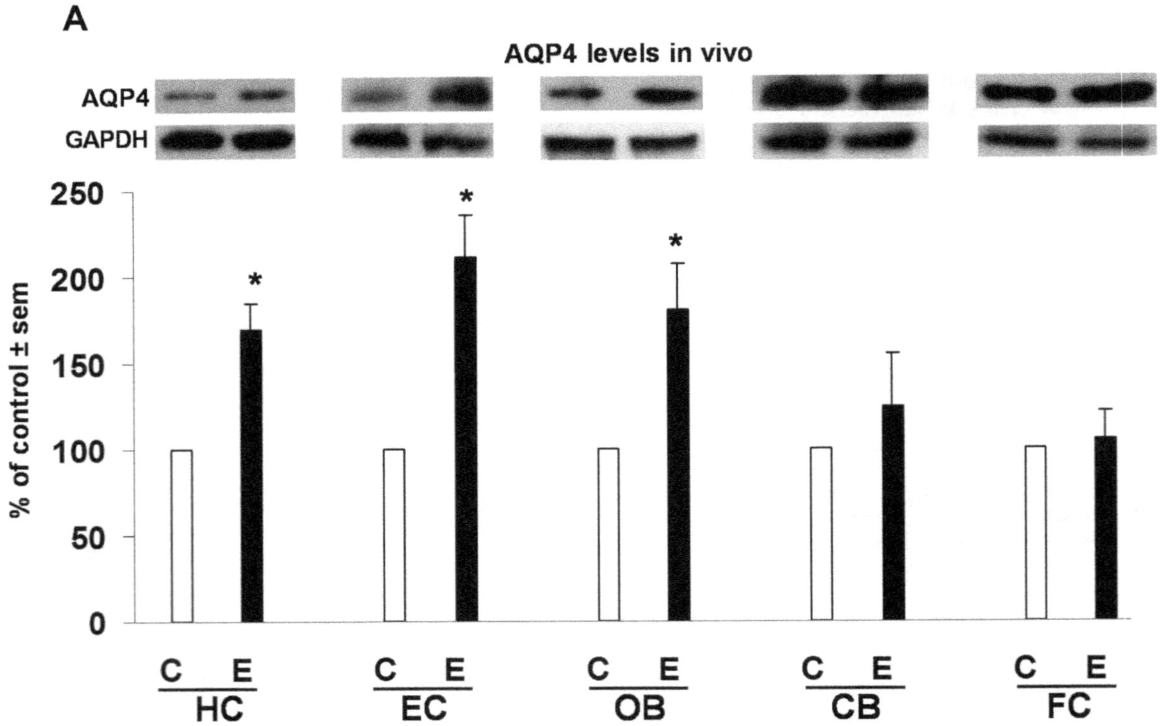

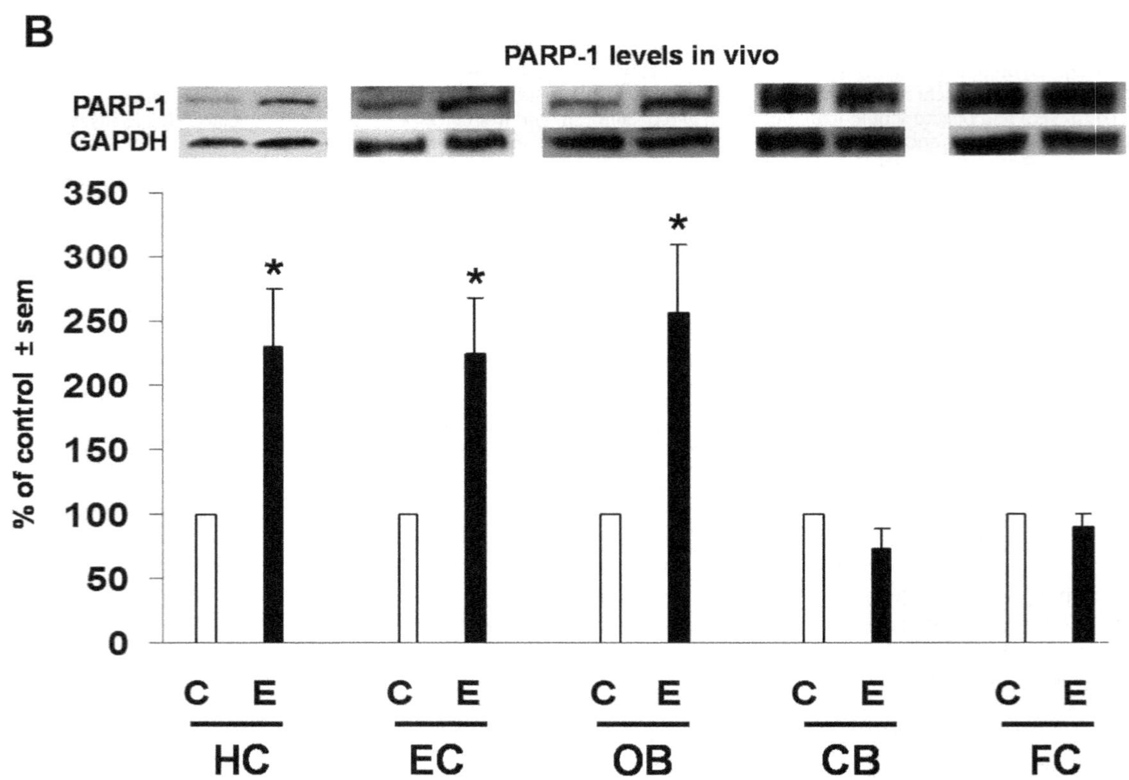

Figure 3. Selective effects of binge ethanol exposure on brain AQP4 and PARP-1 levels *in vivo*. Significant elevations over respective controls (C) in levels of AQP4 and PARP-1 in those brain regions selectively incurring neurodamage due to binge ethanol (E) treatment in adult male rats for 4 days (Majchrowicz model). Fig. 3A: Significantly increased AQP4 levels in the HC, EC and OB, but not in CB and FC. Fig. 3B: Significantly increased PARP-1 levels in the HC, EC and OB, but not in CB and FC. *$p < 0.05$ vs. C. n = 4–7 rats/group.

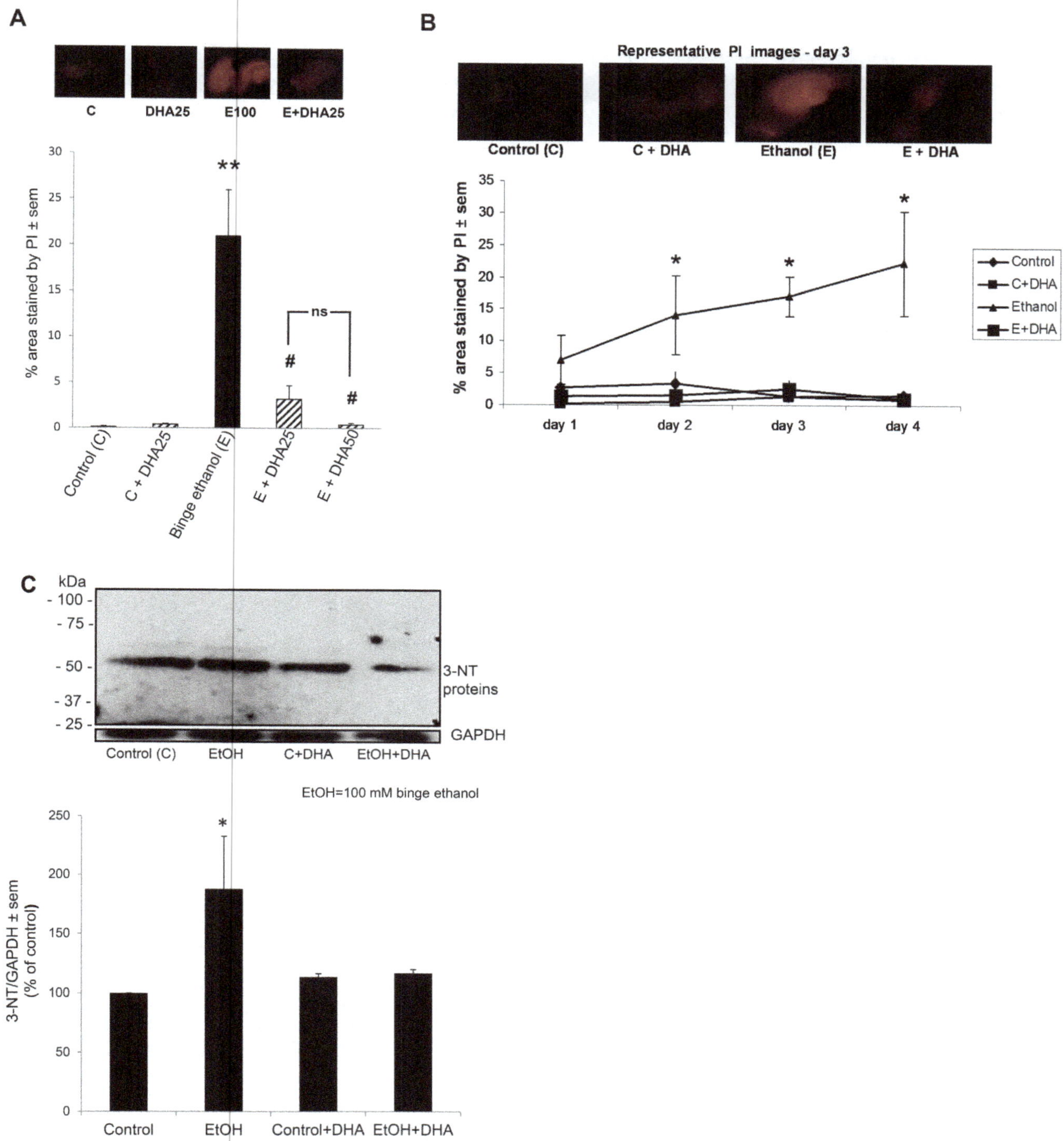

Figure 4. Effects of binge ethanol treatment and DHA supplementation on neurodegeneration and oxidative (3NT-) protein footprints in adult-age HEC slice cultures. Binge ethanol treatment of adult-age rat HEC slice cultures for 4 days as described in Methods significantly increases degenerating neurons (PI staining) and the levels of oxidative stress footprints (3NT-proteins), and supplementation of cultures with DHA prevents the increases. Fig. 4A: (top) Representative PI-stained images showing increased neurodegeneration after 3 days of binge ethanol treatment (100 mM), with DHA supplementation (25 μM) suppressing PI staining (neurodegeneration). (Bottom) Quantitation of PI labeling shows significant neurodegeneration due to 4 days of binge ethanol exposure (E), and neuroprotection against E by DHA at 25 and 50 μM. **$p<0.01$ vs. C. #$p<0.05$ vs. E. Fig. 4B. Quantitation of PI labeling reveals significantly increased neurodegeneration over control due to binge E as early as 2 days of binge ethanol treatment, with prevention of the neurodegeneration throughout the 4 days of treatment by DHA supplementation. *$p<0.05$ vs. control (C) or E+DHA. Fig. 4C (Top) Representative immunoblots of 3NT-proteins in HEC slice cultures following binge ethanol exposure (100 mM) for 4 days. (Bottom) Quantitation of immunoblots showing that binge ethanol exposure causes increased 3NT-proteins in the HEC slice cultures, and DHA supplementation (25 μM) prevents the increases. *$p<0.05$ vs. Control.

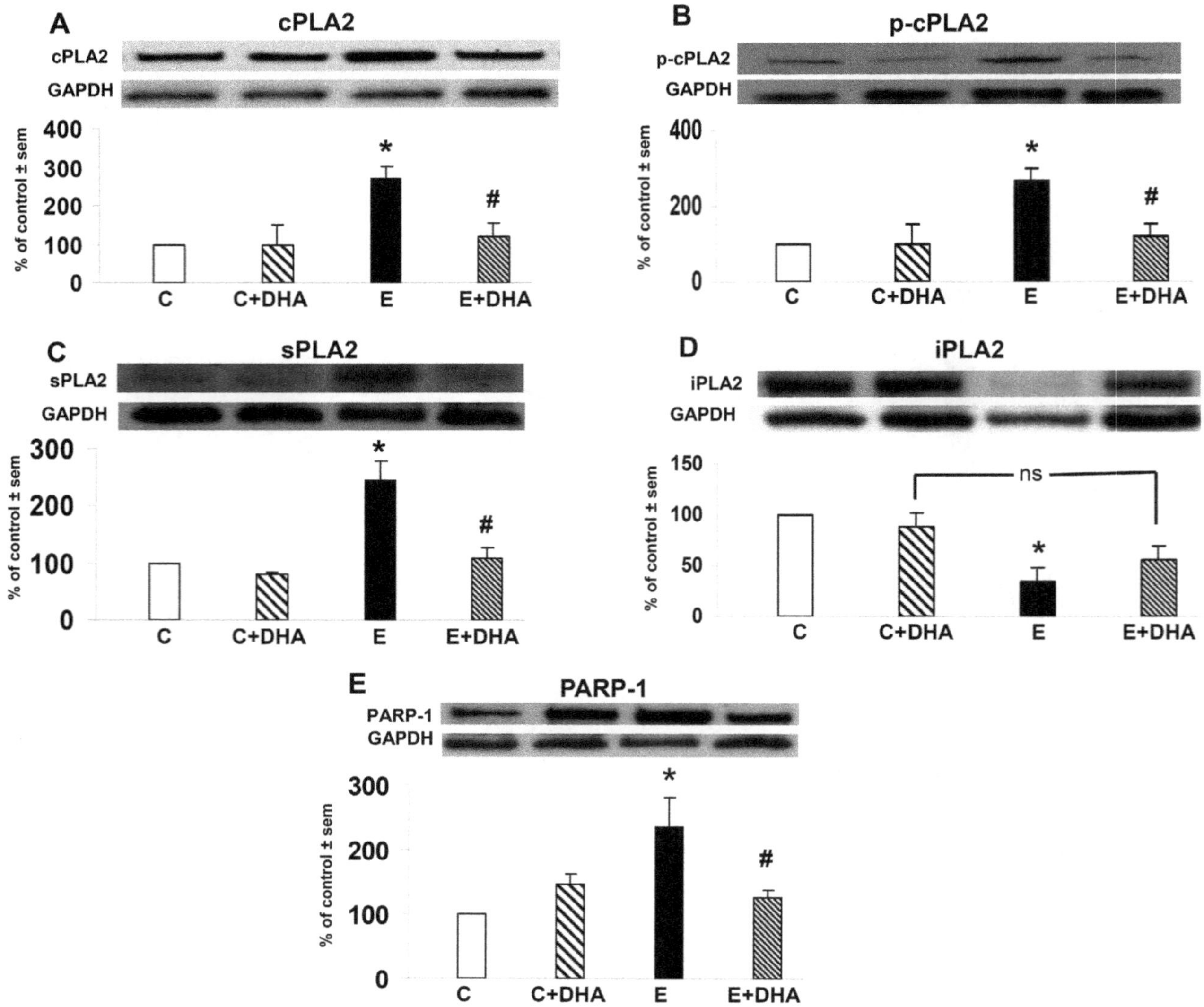

Figure 5. Effects of binge ethanol treatment and DHA supplementation on PLA2 and PARP-1 levels in adult-age HEC slice cultures. Significant neuroinflammatory enzyme alterations compared to control (C) caused by 4 days of binge ethanol (E) treatment (100 mM) of adult-age rat HEC slice cultures, and prevention of the alterations by supplementation of cultures with DHA (25 μM). Fig. 5A: Increased levels of cPLA2 GIVA over control levels due to binge E and inhibition of the increase by DHA supplementation (E+ DHA). *$p<0.05$ vs. C; #$p<0.05$ vs. E. Fig. 5B: Increased levels of p-cPLA2 GIVA over control levels due to binge E and inhibition of the increase by DHA supplementation (E+DHA). *$p<0.05$ vs. C; #$p<0.05$ vs. E. Fig. 5C: Increased levels of sPLA2 GIIA over control levels due to binge E and inhibition of the increase by DHA supplementation (E+DHA). *$p<0.05$ vs. C; #$p<0.05$ vs. E. Fig. 5D: Reduced levels of iPLA2 GVIA with respect to control levels due to binge E and partial blockade of the reduction by DHA supplementation (E+DHA). *$p<0.05$ vs. C. Fig. 5E: Increased levels of PARP-1 over control levels due to binge E and inhibition of the increase by DHA supplementation (E+DHA). *$p<0.05$ vs. C; #$p<0.05$ vs. E.

adult-age slice cultures and suppression by added DHA were previously communicated [30]. Here it is evident that neurotoxic binge ethanol treatment caused significant elevations (160–240% above controls) in levels of cPLA2 (Figure 5A) and p-cPLA2 (Figure 5B), the latter confirming cPLA2 activation. Whereas added DHA alone had no effects relative to controls, its supplementation throughout ethanol treatment prevented increases in both proteins. Similarly, in Figure 5C, HEC slice sPLA2 levels were potentiated ~150% above controls by the binge ethanol exposure; as with cPLA2, added DHA only did not change sPLA2, but supplementation abolished ethanol-induced sPLA2 elevations. With iPLA2 (Figure 5D), consistent with *in vivo* HC results in Fig. 2C, its levels in the HEC slices were significantly reduced ~65% by binge ethanol. DHA alone had no effect on iPLA2 levels, but its supplementation with binge ethanol countered the reduction in iPLA2, thus normalizing its levels. In Figure 5E, also coinciding with *in vivo* findings, PARP-1 levels were significantly enhanced ~130% over control values by the binge ethanol exposure. DHA alone did not alter PARP-1 levels, but consistent with DHA's PLA2 and AQP4 suppression and its prevention of neurodegeneration (Figure 4), co-treatment with the n-3 fatty acid nullified binge ethanol's potentiation of PARP-1 levels.

Figure 6 shows quantitative results of assays of selected endogenous long-chain unsaturated fatty acids in lipid extracts of the binge ethanol-exposed adult rat HEC slices, with and without DHA supplementation. Expressed as percent of total fatty acids, endogenous brain content of DHA (22:6n−3) was significantly

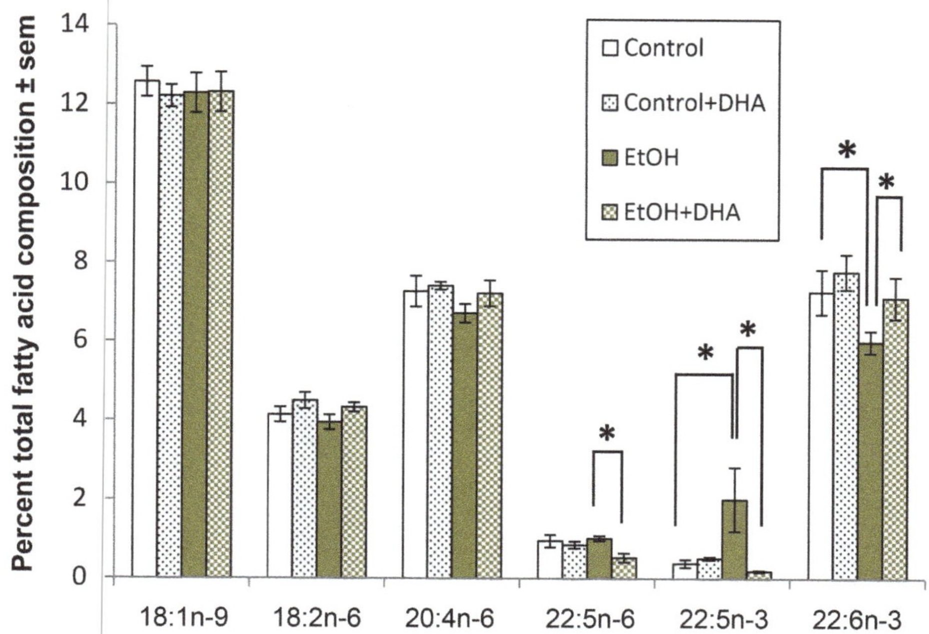

Figure 6. Effect of binge ethanol treatment and DHA supplementation on contents of DHA and selected unsaturated fatty acids in adult-age HEC slice cultures. Binge ethanol treatment (EtOH, 100 mM) of adult-age rat HEC slice cultures for 4 days as described in Methods significantly decreases the slice content of endogenous DHA (22:6n−3); supplementation of ethanol-binged cultures throughout with 25 μM DHA normalizes the DHA content. Binge ethanol treatment also increased the endogenous content of 22:5n−3, and DHA supplementation reduced the levels of this potential DHA precursor, as well as reduced the endogenous levels of ARA (22:4n−6). All other unsaturated fatty acids (not shown) were not significantly changed by binge ethanol treatment and DHA supplementation. $^*p<0.05$ (n = 3/group, Tukey's t-test).

depleted by ethanol exposure, and supplementation with DHA (25 μM) prevented the depletion—results agreeing with earlier *in vivo* findings in the Kim laboratory. Concomitantly, binge ethanol treatment significantly increased a likely DHA precursor, 22:5n−3, with DHA supplementation promoting a normalization of this fatty acid's contents.

Interested in the possibility that PARP-1, known to be activated by oxidative stress and DNA strand breaks, could have direct upstream actions on ethanol-induced neurodegeneration in the adult-age organotypic HEC slices, we used the relatively specific PARP-1 inhibitor PJ-34 [54] at 10 μM for the initial assessment. In Figure 7 (upper) are representative images of HEC slices showing increased PI staining (neurodegeneration) after 4 days of binge exposure to ethanol (100 mM) without PJ-34, and apparent suppression of fluorescence by PJ-34 co-administration. Quantitation in Figure 7 (lower) of fluorescence verified significant neurotoxicity in ethanol-binged slices, and while PI staining with PARP-1 inhibitor PJ-34 alone was not different from controls, its co-presence exerted significant neuroprotection against the ethanol-induced neurotoxicity.

Discussion

We demonstrate with age-complementary *in vivo* and *in vitro* adult rat brain models that major neuroinflammation-associated pro-oxidative pathways encompassing AQP4, key PLA2 families, and PARP-1 are significantly altered in binge ethanol-dependent neurodegeneration. Specifically, neurotoxic ethanol binging promotes significant elevations in cPLA2, p-cPLA2, and sPLA2 and decrements in iPLA2 in both models. The *in vivo* results with the well-documented "Majchrowicz" binge model [6] were distinguished by the fact that, along with AQP4 and PARP-1, the above PLA2 elevations occurred in three brain regions that typically sustain neurodegeneration, but not in two regions having few if any degenerating neurons. In adult-age rat organotypic HEC slice cultures the ethanol-induced changes in these neuroinflammation-linked proteins agreed well with the *in vivo* findings, and furthermore, were in accord with recent binge ethanol results *in vivo* [45] in that the neurodegeneration becomes manifested within a few days of exposure. Whether the above proteins constitute a relatively unified cohesive pathway or are components of interacting, even redundant, signaling routes for induced oxidative neurodamage is yet to be established; however, the results (Figure 7) with a PARP-1 inhibitor provide preliminary evidence implicating a PARP-1-contingent neurotoxic process. The results further indicate that supplementation with an essential n-3 fatty acid, DHA—previously reported to halt ethanol-engendered neurodegeneration in binge-treated brain slices—additionally suppresses alterations in the neuroinflammatory proteins and oxidative stress footprints.

Among the proteins examined, AQP4 is of particular interest, as research principally with ischemic or traumatic brain damage models, but also with water intoxication and certain brain infections, demonstrates that increased activity or levels of the astroglial water channel regulates cytotoxic (cellular) brain edema [17,55]. Astroglial overexpression of AQP4 in mice accelerates ischemia-induced brain edema [56], and AQP4 knockdown in traumatized astroglial cultures reduces cell swelling [57]. AQP4 may have a prominent neuroinflammatory role in brain insults, since experiments with AQP4 knockout mice confirm the protein's requirement for full induction of brain proinflammatory cytokines (notably tumor necrosis factor alpha) during endotoxin treatment or experimental allergic encephalomyelitis [58]. Thus AQP4 acts as a brain neuroinflammatory channel during particular stresses or insults.

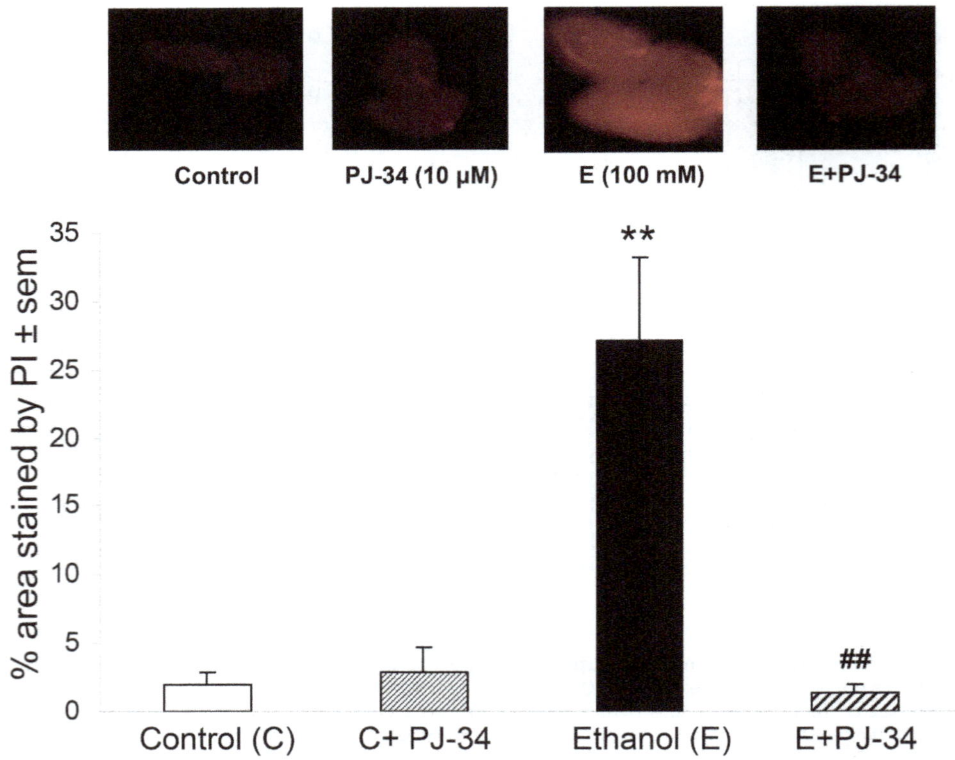

Figure 7. Effect of PARP-1 inhibitor PJ-34 on ethanol-induced neurodegeneration in adult-age HEC slice cultures. Neurodegeneration (PI staining) due to 4 days of binge ethanol treatment (100 mM) of rat adult-age organotypic HEC slice cultures is suppressed by co-treatment with PARP-1 inhibitor, PJ-34 (10 μM). (Top) Images of representative PI-stained slices from C, PJ-34, E and E+PJ-34 slice cultures indicate increased neurodegeneration (E) that is reduced in E+PJ-34. (Bottom) Quantitation of PI staining demonstrates increased neurodegeneration due to binge ethanol (E) that is significantly suppressed by PJ-34 (E + PJ-34). **$p<0.01$ vs. C. ##$p<0.01$ vs. E.

After finding moderate brain edema in a once-daily adaptation of the Majchrowicz ethanol gavage model, we determined that edema's deterrence with furosemide in that model and in ethanol-binged HEC slice cultures was neuroprotective [11]—as it was with the diuretic, acetazolamide [12], which fortuitously is an AQP4 inhibitor. Astroglial cells in culture swell due to ethanol exposure and withdrawal, but previous evidence of blockade by diuretics has been conflicting [59,60]. However, acceleration of trauma-related cerebral edema by ethanol has been linked to increased AQP4 upregulation and activity, with acetazolamide, presumably through inhibition of AQP4, exerting protection [61]. Herein, binge ethanol-induced AQP4 elevations in brain regions that sustain neurodegeneration, but not in regions known to lack neurodamage, indicate that the water channel could be an important factor in the regioselective neurodegeneration. Furthermore, increased AQP4 in the binge-treated adult-age HEC slice cultures, as well as being in accord with *in vivo* results, is in harmony with our findings in developing HEC slice cultures [12]. How AQP4 levels are altered by ethanol binges requires study, but several stimuli known to potentiate brain or astroglial AQP4 levels/activity are reported by others to be increased by ethanol in various exposure protocols. For example, ROS [62], lactic acid [[63], proinflammatory cytokines [64], and glutamate [65] have been shown to increase the water channel. Depending on the model, ethanol and/or ethanol withdrawal can promote or potentiate brain levels of all of these factors [9,66,67].

PLA2 isoforms, and chiefly those of Ca^{+2}-dependent cPLA2 and sPLA2 families, are rate-controlling for normal or excessive release of ARA. This essential n-6 fatty acid is precursor for neuroinflammatory eicosanoids as well as ROS generation *via* subsequent action of cyclooxygenases and/or autooxidation. Interestingly, a feed-forward mechanism could also operate, since ARA-derived eicosanoids (leukotrienes) can increase AQP4 and promote edema [68]. Of the two PLA2 families, cPLA2 (~85 kDa) and its hyperactivation have been most frequently linked to AA-derived neuroinflammation and neurodegeneration [20,69]. Furthermore, PLA2 isoforms are prone to be increased and/or activated by brain cell swelling and deformation [18], and cPLA2 can act as a mechanosensitive transducer to cellular osmotic stress and membrane stretching [70,71]. Also, phosphorylation by mitogen-activated protein kinase (MAPK) family members, a catalytic step producing activated p-cPLA2, is similarly modulated by osmotic or stretch-induced stress [72,73], which is entirely compatible with the mechanisms in these binge ethanol models.

The smaller sPLA2 family members (13–20 KDa), either independently or complicit with cPLA2, could be involved in brain neuroinflammatory mechanisms [74]. Notably, inhibition of sPLA2 has been found to reduce neuroinflammation and ischemic injury in adult rats [75]. Brain sPLA2 IIA elevations have been documented in rat stroke models [76], during Alzheimer's disease [77], and now in the acquired brain damage caused by binge ethanol in organotypic brain slice cultures. However, other sPLA2 family members such as sPLA2 V and most recently sPLA2 III, expressed intraneuronally in synaptic regions [78], also could be important in ethanol's mechanism and should be investigated. It has been known for some time that chronic ethanol in vivo increases brain PLA2 activity in general [79], so at this juncture it is plausible to consider that the elevated cPLA2 and sPLA2 activities are components of downstream neuroinflammatory activation and ROS increases during binge ethanol exposure.

Furthermore, the observed reduction in iPLA2 GVI levels due to ethanol is in harmony with neuroinflammatory outcomes that indicate a reciprocal relationship between iPLA2 and cPLA2/sPLA2 [80,81]. This could relate to iPLA2 possibly serving as a mitochondrial housekeeping and protective enzyme [22]. Studies have associated iPLA2 with suppression of lipid peroxidation [82], and such an anti-oxidant function could be explained by the enzyme's activity in sustaining endogenous DHA turnover in brain membrane phospholipids [83]. Reduced DHA turnover related to iPLA2 depletion in binge ethanol-exposed brain could portend diminished endogenous neuroprotection associated with this n-3 fatty acid (discussed in more detail below).

Binge ethanol's significant potentiation of multi-faceted PARP-1 selectively *in vivo* as well as in HEC slices, in concert with a PARP-1 inhibitor's suppression of neurodegeneration (and also our previous report with a relatively moderate binge rat model for robust PARP-1 augmentation [23]), support a role in ethanol neurotoxicity for this previously underappreciated player. Nuclear PARP-1 responds to oxidative stress and DNA strand breaks to synthesize polyADP-ribose (PAR) chains that then recruit DNA repair protein assemblies. However, PARP-1 hyperactivation can deplete essential cellular NAD+ levels and ATP, as well as trigger PAR-directed mitochondrial non-apoptotic death, which is termed parthanatos [24]. Parthanatos is a probable neuronal death pathway in a transgenic Parkinsonian mouse model [84] and in endotoxin-induced neuroinflammation [85]. To our knowledge, PARP-1-dependent neuronal demise has not been linked convincingly to ethanol, nor has the enzyme been experimentally associated with brain AQP4- or PLA2-dependent neuroinflammatory pathways. However, a functional link between PARP-1 activity and binge ethanol neuropathology as indicated by PJ-34 inhibitor results (Figure 6) is consistent with elevated brain oxidative stress in chronic ethanol-treated rodents [9], oxidative DNA damage in brain of alcoholics [86], and—in regard to parthanatos—the absence of neuronal apoptosis (i.e., predominance of necrosis) in the Majchrowicz binge ethanol model [10]. Future experiments with the binge models should employ RNA interference and other inhibitors together with PAR measurements in order to more firmly establish PARP-1's role in binge ethanol-induced neurodegenerative signaling.

The prominent actions of supplemented DHA in the adult HEC slices may provide insights into neuroinflammatory protein mechanisms in the binge ethanol models. Growing evidence indicates that DHA administration during other neurodamaging conditions or diseases can promote prosurvival and/or neuroprotection [87,88]. The data herein show that DHA supplementation of binge ethanol-treated HEC slice cultures inhibits elevations in the selected PLA2 families, PARP-1, and as reported, AQP4 water channels [30], concomitant with inhibiting neurodegeneration. To be noted is that DHA's suppression of these neuroinflammatory pathways *in vitro* is highly consistent with protective findings previously reported with the Majchrowicz binge intoxication model—(1), with furosemide, a diuretic having anti-oxidative and potentially anti-inflammatory effects [89]; (2) with cannabidiol, an anti-inflammatory compound that also exerts neuroprotection [89]; and (3) with metabotropic glutamate receptor stimulation, which selectively elevates transforming growth factor-β (suppressed by the binging) and inhibits entorhinal cortex neurodegeneration [90].

We consider that two overall neuroprotective mechanisms for DHA in the experimental literature could be functioning. The first advances that enriched esterification in the 2-position of phospholipids with DHA, and in particular, inner neuronal membrane phosphatidylserine, sustains neuronal survival against insults. In part such phosphatidylserine enrichment with DHA favors translocation and activation of PKB/Akt, a key pro-survival kinase that antagonizes oxidative signaling [91,92]. Indeed, as Figure 6 demonstrates, gas chromatography assays of the HEC slice cultures reveal relatively selective reductions in endogenous DHA levels from binge ethanol treatment, with restoration by supplemented DHA.

A second mechanism relates to unesterified or "free" DHA and its metabolic products. Considerable attention has focused on DHA's dihydroxylation initiated by 15-lipoxygenase-1 to generate 10R,17S-dihydroxydocosa-4Z,7Z,11E,13E,15Z,19Z-hexaenoic acid or neuroprotectin-1 (NPD1); other oxidized isomers, inclusively termed resolvins, also may be produced *via* this or a related enzyme [93,94]. NPD1, formed primarily in brain astroglia from DHA, is a highly potent cytoprotectant and antioxidant against retinal and brain ischemic insults, and can suppress brain neuroinflammation [95]. Another potentially neuroprotective product of nonesterified DHA that has received recent attention is amidated docosahexaenoylethanolamide (synaptamide) [96], which is structurally analogous to the arachidonic acid-derived cannabinoid, arachidonoylethanolamide (anandamide). Synaptamide has been shown to promote neurite growth and preserve synaptic function [97], and it is tenable that it, like the hydroxylated DHA derivatives, NPD1 and other resolvins, might wield antioxidant-related neurosurvival effects.

Integrating our findings within a mechanistic scheme, the speculation is that the first ethanol binges trigger limited but still effectual increases in ROS primarily during withdrawals (or its nadirs in vivo), somewhat akin to ischemia-reperfusion. Possible ROS sources include NADPH oxidase stimulation, ethanol metabolism (cytochrome P450, catalase, peroxidases), and/or mitochondrial membrane damage/leakage. Such early ROS generation could be sufficient to boost AQP4 expression via unspecified oxidative transcription factors, while also initiating nuclear DNA fragmentation and thus enhancing upregulation of PARP-1. Repetitive binges would greatly augment these events, leading to astroglial swelling-related activation/expression of cPLA2 and sPLA2, which evoke excessive AA mobilization, loss of endogenous DHA turnover due to decreased iPLA2, and greater increases in neuron-damaging ROS levels, concomitant with PAR-mediated glial activation [54] and associated parthanatos.

Supplemented DHA, exerting anti-oxidant actions through routes outlined above, could overcome immediate ROS generation triggered by the first several ethanol binges and basically inhibit the cascade of downstream ROS-augmenting cascades that depend upon PARP-1, AQP4, and PLA2. Relevant to this scheme is that DHA co-treatment in a DNA alkylating agent-treated hippocampal cell line blocks PARP-1 activity (PAR formation) while preventing oxidative stress and neuronal death [98]. In view of PET neuroimaging results indicating DHA metabolic deficits in brains of chronic alcoholics [99], our DHA findings *in vitro* reinforce an implication from that report that n-3 fatty acid supplementation during withdrawal therapy could be beneficial for cognitive support and even neuroprotection. Indeed, enrichment of neuronal cell phospholipids and particularly phosphatidylserine with supplemental DHA has been known for some time to effect neuroprotection against a range of insults [100].

Author Contributions

Conceived and designed the experiments: MAC EJN NT KHM KN SAM. Performed the experiments: NT KHM. Analyzed the data: MAC NT

HYK EJN KN. Contributed reagents/materials/analysis tools: NT KHM HYK KN EJN. Wrote the paper: MAC EJN KN HYK.

References

1. Rehm J, Mathers C, Popova S, Thavorncharoensap M, Teerawattananon Y, et al. (2009) Global burden of disease and injury and economic cost attributable to alcohol use and alcohol-use disorders. Lancet 373: 2223–33.
2. Shield KD, Gmel G, Kehoe-Chan T, Dawson DA, Grant BF, et al. (2013) Mortality and potential years of life lost attributable to alcohol consumption by race and sex in the united states in 2005. PLoS ONE [Electronic Resource] 8: e51923.
3. Hunt WA (1993) Are binge drinkers more at risk of developing brain damage? Alcohol 10: 559–61.
4. Virta JJ, Järvenpää T, Heikkilä K, Perola M, Koskenvuo M, et al. (2010) Midlife alcohol consumption and later risk of cognitive impairment: A twin follow-up study. Journal of Alzheimer's Disease 22: 939–948.
5. Ridley NJ, Draper B, Withall A (2013) Alcohol-related dementia: An update of the evidence. Alzheimer's research & therapy 5: 1–8.
6. Majchrowicz E (1975) Induction of physical dependence upon ethanol and the associated behavioral changes in rats. Psychopharmacologia 43: 245–54.
7. Switzer RC, Majchrowicz E, Weight F (1982) Ethanol-induced argyrophilia in entorhinal cortex of rat. Anatomical Record 202: 186A.
8. Collins MA, Corso TD, Neafsey EJ (1996) Neuronal degeneration in rat cerebrocortical and olfactory regions during subchronic "binge" intoxication with ethanol: Possible explanation for olfactory deficits in alcoholics. Alcoholism: Clinical & Experimental Research 20: 284–92.
9. Collins MA, Neafsey EJ (2012) Ethanol and adult CNS neurodamage: Oxidative stress, but possibly not excitotoxicity. Frontiers in Bioscience 4: 1358–67.
10. Obernier JA, Bouldin TW, Crews FT (2002) Binge ethanol exposure in adult rats causes necrotic cell death. Alcoholism: Clinical & Experimental Research 26: 547–57.
11. Collins MA, Zou JY, Neafsey EJ (1998) Brain damage due to episodic alcohol exposure in vivo and in vitro: Furosemide neuroprotection implicates edema-based mechanism. Faseb J 12: 221–30.
12. Sripathirathan K, Brown J, Neafsey EJ, Collins MA (2009) Linking binge alcohol-induced neurodamage to brain edema and potential aquaporin-4 upregulation: Evidence in rat organotypic brain slice cultures and in vivo. Journal of Neurotrauma 26: 261–73.
13. Cippitelli A, Damadzic R, Hamelink C, Brunnquell M, Thorsell A, et al. (2014) Binge-like ethanol consumption increases corticosterone levels and neurodegneration whereas occupancy of type II glucocorticoid receptors with mifepristone is neuroprotective. Addict Biol 19: 27–36.
14. Tran ND, Kim S, Vincent HK, Rodriguez A, Hinton DR, et al. (2010) Aquaporin-1-mediated cerebral edema following traumatic brain injury: Effects of acidosis and corticosteroid administration. J Neurosurg 112: 1095–1104.
15. Zhao YN, Wang F, Fan YX, Ping GF, Yang JY, et al. (2013) Activated microglia are implicated in cognitive deficits, neuronal death, and successful recovery following intermittent ethanol exposure. Behav Brain Res 236: 270–282.
16. Marshall SA, McClain JA, Kelso ML, Hopkins DM, Pauly JR, et al. (2013) Microglial activation is not equivalent to neuroinflammation in alcohol-induced neurodegeneration: The importance of microglia phenotype. Neurobiol Dis 54: 239–251.
17. Saadoun S, Papadopoulos MC (2010) Aquaporin-4 in brain and spinal cord oedema. Neuroscience 168: 1036–46.
18. Lambert IH, Pedersen SF, Poulsen KA (2006) Activation of PLA2 isoforms by cell swelling and ischaemia/hypoxia. Acta Physiol (Oxf) 187: 75–85.
19. Basavappa S, Pedersen SF, Jorgensen NK, Ellory JC, Hoffmann EK (1998) Swelling-induced arachidonic acid release via the 85-kDa cPLA2 in human neuroblastoma cells. J Neurophysiol 79: 1441–9.
20. Sun GY, He Y, Chuang DY, Lee JC, Gu Z, et al. (2012) Integrating cytosolic phospholipase A2 with oxidative/nitrosative signaling pathways in neurons: A novel therapeutic strategy for AD. Molecular Neurobiology 46: 85–95.
21. Ong WY, Farooqui T, Farooqui AA (2010) Involvement of cytosolic phospholipase A(2), calcium independent phospholipase A(2) and plasmalogen selective phospholipase A(2) in neurodegenerative and neuropsychiatric conditions. Current Medicinal Chemistry 17: 2746–63.
22. Green JT, Orr SK, Bazinet RP (2008) The emerging role of group VI calcium-independent phospholipase A2 in releasing docosahexaenoic acid from brain phospholipids. Journal of Lipid Research 49: 939–44.
23. Tajuddin N, Przybycien-Szymanska MM, Pak TR, Neafsey EJ, Collins MA (2013) Effect of repetitive daily ethanol intoxication on adult rat brain: Significant changes in phospholipase A2 enzyme levels in association with increased PARP-1 indicate neuroinflammatory pathway activation. Alcohol 47: 39–45.
24. David KK, Andrabi SA, Dawson TM, Dawson VL (2009) Parthanatos, a messenger of death. Frontiers in Bioscience 14: 1116–28.
25. Galluzzi L, Kepp O, Krautwald S, Kroemer G, Linkermann A (2014) Molecular mechanisms of regulated necrosis.
26. Barron S, Mulholland PJ, Littleton JM, Prendergast MA (2008) Age and gender differences in response to neonatal ethanol withdrawal and polyamine challenge in organotypic hippocampal cultures. Alcoholism: Clinical & Experimental Research 32: 929–36.
27. Zou JY, Crews FT (2005) TNF alpha potentiates glutamate neurotoxicity by inhibiting glutamate uptake in organotypic brain slice cultures: Neuroprotection by NF kappa B inhibition. Brain Res 1034: 11–24.
28. Adachi J, Mizoi Y, Fukunaga T, Ogawa Y, Ueno Y, et al. (1991) Degrees of alcohol intoxication in 117 hospitalized cases. Journal of Studies on Alcohol 52: 448–53.
29. Jones AW (1999) The drunkest drinking driver in sweden: Blood alcohol concentration 0.545% w/v. Journal of Studies on Alcohol 60: 400–6.
30. Collins MA, Moon KH, Tajuddin N, Neafsey EJ, Kim HY (2013) Docosahexaenoic acid (DHA) prevents binge ethanol-dependent aquaporin-4 elevations while inhibiting neurodegeneration: Experiments in rat adult-age entorhino-hippocampal slice cultures. Neurotoxicity research 23: 105–110.
31. Crews FT, Braun CJ, Hoplight B, Switzer RC,3rd, Knapp DJ (2000) Binge ethanol consumption causes differential brain damage in young adolescent rats compared with adult rats. Alcoholism: Clinical & Experimental Research 24: 1712–23.
32. Haussinger D, Gorg B, Reinehr R, Schliess F (2005) Protein tyrosine nitration in hyperammonemia and hepatic encephalopathy. Metab Brain Dis 20: 285–294.
33. Brown J, 3rd, Achille N, Neafsey EJ, Collins MA (2009) Binge ethanol-induced neurodegeneration in rat organotypic brain slice cultures: Effects of PLA2 inhibitor mepacrine and docosahexaenoic acid (DHA). Neurochemical Research 34: 260–7.
34. Bazan NG, Molina MF, Gordon WC (2011) Docosahexaenoic acid signalolipidomics in nutrition: Significance in aging, neuroinflammation, macular degeneration, alzheimer's, and other neurodegenerative diseases. Annual Review of Nutrition 31: 321–51.
35. Farooqui AA, Horrocks LA, Farooqui T (2007) Modulation of inflammation in brain: A matter of fat. Journal of Neurochemistry 101: 577–99.
36. Orr SK, Trepanier MO, Bazinet RP (2013) N-3 polyunsaturated fatty acids in animal models with neuroinflammation. Prostaglandins Leukotrienes & Essential Fatty Acids 88: 97–103.
37. Wen Z, Kim HY (2007) Inhibition of phosphatidylserine biosynthesis in developing rat brain by maternal exposure to ethanol. J Neurosci Res 85: 1568–1578.
38. Akbar M, Baick J, Calderon F, Wen Z, Kim HY (2006) Ethanol promotes neuronal apoptosis by inhibiting phosphatidylserine accumulation. Journal of Neuroscience Research 83: 432–40.
39. Furuya H, Aikawa H, Yoshida T, Okazaki I (2000) The use of docosahexaenoic acid supplementation to ameliorate the hyperactivity of rat pups induced by in utero ethanol exposure. Environmental Health & Preventive Medicine 5: 103–110.
40. Patten AR, Sickmann HM, Dyer RA, Innis SM, Christie BR (2013) Omega-3 fatty acids can reverse the long-term deficits in hippocampal synaptic plasticity caused by prenatal ethanol exposure. Neurosci Lett 551: 7–11.
41. Patten AR, Brocardo PS, Christie BR (2013) Omega-3 supplementation can restore glutathione levels and prevent oxidative damage caused by prenatal ethanol exposure. J Nutr Biochem 24: 760–769.
42. Corso TD, Mostafa HM, Collins MA, Neafsey EJ (1998) Brain neuronal degeneration caused by episodic alcohol intoxication in rats: Effects of nimodipine, 6,7-dinitro-quinoxaline-2,3-dione, and MK-801. Alcohol Clin Exp Res 22: 217–24.
43. Marshall SA, McClain JA, Kelso ML, Hopkins DM, Pauly JR, et al. (2013) Microglial activation is not equivalent to neuroinflammation in alcohol-induced neurodegeneration: The importance of microglia phenotype. Neurobiol Dis.
44. Zou JY, Martinez DB, Neafsey EJ, Collins MA (1996) Binge ethanol-induced brain damage in rats: Effect of inhibitors of nitric oxide synthase. Alcoholism: Clinical & Experimental Research 20: 1406–11.
45. Hayes DM, Deeny MA, Shaner CA, Nixon K (2013) Determining the threshold for alcohol-induced brain damage: New evidence with gliosis markers. Alcoholism: Clinical & Experimental Research 37: 425–434.
46. Cao D, Li M, Xue R, Zheng W, Liu Z, et al. (2005) Chronic administration of ethyl docosahexaenoate decreases mortality and cerebral edema in ischemic gerbils. Life Sciences 78: 74–81.
47. Langelier B, Alessandri JM, Perruchot MH, Guesnet P, Lavialle M (2005) Changes of the transcriptional and fatty acid profiles in response to n-3 fatty acids in SH-SY5Y neuroblastoma cells. Lipids 40: 719–728.
48. Noraberg J, Poulsen FR, Blaabjerg M, Kristensen BW, Bonde C, et al. (2005) Organotypic hippocampal slice cultures for studies of brain damage, neuroprotection and neurorepair. Current Drug Targets - Cns & Neurological Disorders 4: 435–52.
49. Berry JN, Sharrett-Field LJ, Butler TR, Prendergast MA (2012) Temporal dependence of cysteine protease activation following excitotoxic hippocampal injury. Neuroscience 222: 147–158.
50. Wen Z, Kim HY (2004) Alterations in hippocampal phospholipid profile by prenatal exposure to ethanol. Journal of Neurochemistry 89: 1368–77.
51. Riahi Y, Cohen G, Shamni O, Sasson S (2010) Signaling and cytotoxic functions of 4-hydroxyalkenals. American Journal of Physiology - Endocrinology & Metabolism 299: E879–86.

52. Moon KH, Hood BL, Kim BJ, Hardwick JP, Conrads TP, et al. (2006) Inactivation of oxidized and S-nitrosylated mitochondrial proteins in alcoholic fatty liver of rats. Hepatology 44: 1218–30.
53. Crews F, Nixon K, Kim D, Joseph J, Shukitt-Hale B, et al. (2006) BHT blocks NF-kappaB activation and ethanol-induced brain damage. Alcoholism: Clinical & Experimental Research 30: 1938–49.
54. Kauppinen TM, Suh SW, Berman AE, Hamby AM, Swanson RA (2009) Inhibition of poly(ADP-ribose) polymerase suppresses inflammation and promotes recovery after ischemic injury. Journal of Cerebral Blood Flow & Metabolism 29: 820–829.
55. Fukuda AM, Badaut J (2012) Aquaporin 4: A player in cerebral edema and neuroinflammation. Journal of neuroinflammation 9: 279.
56. Yang B, Zador Z, Verkman AS (2008) Glial cell aquaporin-4 overexpression in transgenic mice accelerates cytotoxic brain swelling. Journal of Biological Chemistry 283: 15280–6.
57. Rao KV, Reddy PV, Curtis KM, Norenberg MD (2011) Aquaporin-4 expression in cultured astrocytes after fluid percussion injury. Journal of Neurotrauma 28: 371–81.
58. Li L, Zhang H, Varrin-Doyer M, Zamvil SS, Verkman AS (2011) Proinflammatory role of aquaporin-4 in autoimmune neuroinflammation. FASEB Journal 25: 1556–66.
59. Aschner M, Allen JW, Mutkus LA, Cao C (2001) Ethanol-induced swelling in neonatal rat primary astrocyte cultures. Brain Res 900: 219–226.
60. Adermark L, Clarke RB, Olsson T, Hansson E, Soderpalm B, et al. (2011) Implications for glycine receptors and astrocytes in ethanol-induced elevation of dopamine levels in the nucleus accumbens. Addict Biol 16: 43–54.
61. Katada R, Nishitani Y, Honmou O, Mizuo K, Okazaki S, et al. (2012) Expression of aquaporin-4 augments cytotoxic brain edema after traumatic brain injury during acute ethanol exposure. Am J Pathol 180: 17–23.
62. Esposito G, Imitola J, Lu J, De Filippis D, Scuderi C, et al. (2008) Genomic and functional profiling of human down syndrome neural progenitors implicates S100B and aquaporin 4 in cell injury. Human Molecular Genetics 17: 440–57.
63. Morishima T, Aoyama M, Iida Y, Yamamoto N, Hirate H, et al. (2008) Lactic acid increases aquaporin 4 expression on the cell membrane of cultured rat astrocytes. Neuroscience Research 61: 18–26.
64. Ito H, Yamamoto N, Arima H, Hirate H, Morishima T, et al. (2006) Interleukin-1beta induces the expression of aquaporin-4 through a nuclear factor-kappaB pathway in rat astrocytes. Journal of Neurochemistry 99: 107–18.
65. Gunnarson E, Zelenina M, Axehult G, Song Y, Bondar A, et al. (2008) Identification of a molecular target for glutamate regulation of astrocyte water permeability. GLIA 56: 587–96.
66. Oyama LM, Couto RC, Couto GE, Damaso AR, Oller do Nascimento CM (2000) Ethanol intake during lactation. II. effects on pups' liver and brain metabolism. Alcohol 21: 201–6.
67. Blanco AM, Guerri C (2007) Ethanol intake enhances inflammatory mediators in brain: Role of glial cells and TLR4/IL-1RI receptors. Frontiers in Bioscience 12: 2616–30.
68. Wang ML, Huang XJ, Fang SH, Yuan YM, Zhang WP, et al. (2006) Leukotriene D4 induces brain edema and enhances CysLT2 receptor-mediated aquaporin 4 expression. Biochemical & Biophysical Research Communications 350: 399–404.
69. Ghosh M, Tucker DE, Burchett SA, Leslie CC (2006) Properties of the group IV phospholipase A2 family. Prog Lipid Res 45: 487–510.
70. Lehtonen JY, Kinnunen PK (1995) Phospholipase A2 as a mechanosensor. Biophysical Journal 68: 1888–94.
71. Alexander LD, Alagarsamy S, Douglas JG (2004) Cyclic stretch-induced cPLA2 mediates ERK 1/2 signaling in rabbit proximal tubule cells. Kidney Int 65: 551–563.
72. Neary JT, Kang Y, Willoughby KA, Ellis EF (2003) Activation of extracellular signal-regulated kinase by stretch-induced injury in astrocytes involves extracellular ATP and P2 purinergic receptors. The Journal of neuroscience 23: 2348–2356.
73. Xu D, Wang L, Olson JE, Lu L (2001) Asymmetrical response of p38 kinase activation to volume changes in primary rat astrocytes. Exp Biol Med 226: 927–933.
74. Chen S, Yao L, Cunningham TJ (2012) Secreted phospholipase A2 involvement in neurodegeneration: Differential testing of prosurvival and anti-inflammatory effects of enzyme inhibition. PloS one 7: e39257.
75. Hoda MN, Singh I, Singh AK, Khan M (2009) Reduction of lipoxidative load by secretory phospholipase A2 inhibition protects against neurovascular injury following experimental stroke in rat. Journal of Neuroinflammation 6: 21.
76. Lin TN, Wang Q, Simonyi A, Chen JJ, Cheung WM, et al. (2004) Induction of secretory phospholipase A2 in reactive astrocytes in response to transient focal cerebral ischemia in the rat brain. J Neurochem 90: 637–645.
77. Moses GS, Jensen MD, Lue LF, Walker DG, Sun AY, et al. (2006) Secretory PLA2-IIA: A new inflammatory factor for alzheimer's disease. Journal of Neuroinflammation 3.
78. Yang H, Siddiqi NJ, Alhomida AS, Ong WY. (2013) Expression and localization of sPLA2-III in the rat CNS. Neurochem Res 38: 753–760.
79. Hudspith M, John GR, Nhamburo PT, Littleton JM (1985) Effect of ethanol in vitro and in vivo on Ca2+-activated metabolism of membrane phospholipids in rat synaptosomal and brain slice preparations. Alcohol 2: 133–8.
80. Rao JS, Kim HW, Kellom M, Greenstein D, Chen M, et al. (2011) Increased neuroinflammatory and arachidonic acid cascade markers, and reduced synaptic proteins, in brain of HIV-1 transgenic rats. Journal of Neuroinflammation 8: 101.
81. Sun GY, Shelat PB, Jensen MB, He Y, Sun AY, et al. (2010) Phospholipases A2 and inflammatory responses in the central nervous system. NeuroMolecular Medicine 12: 133–48.
82. Kinsey GR, Blum JL, Covington MD, Cummings BS, McHowat J, et al. (2008) Decreased iPLA2gamma expression induces lipid peroxidation and cell death and sensitizes cells to oxidant-induced apoptosis. Journal of Lipid Research 49: 1477–87.
83. Strokin M, Chechneva O, Reymann KG, Reiser G, Strokin M, et al. (2006) Neuroprotection of rat hippocampal slices exposed to oxygen-glucose deprivation by enrichment with docosahexaenoic acid and by inhibition of hydrolysis of docosahexaenoic acid-containing phospholipids by calcium independent phospholipase A2. Neuroscience 140: 547–53.
84. Lee Y, Karuppagounder SS, Shin JH, Lee YI, Ko HS, et al. (2013) Parthanatos mediates AIMP2-activated age-dependent dopaminergic neuronal loss. Nat Neurosci 16: 1392–1400.
85. Czapski GA, Adamczyk A, Strosznajder RP, Strosznajder JB (2013) Expression and activity of PARP family members in the hippocampus during systemic inflammation: Their role in the regulation of prooxidative genes. Neurochem Int 62: 664–673.
86. Gotz ME, Janetzky B, Pohli S, Gottschalk A, Gsell W, et al. (2001) Chronic alcohol consumption and cerebral indices of oxidative stress: Is there a link? Alcoholism: Clinical & Experimental Research 25: 717–25.
87. Eckert GP, Lipka U, Muller WE (2013) Omega-3 fatty acids in neurodegenerative diseases: Focus on mitochondria. Prostaglandins, Leukotrienes and Essential Fatty Acids 88: 105–114.
88. Mayurasakorn K, Williams JJ, Ten VS, Deckelbaum RJ (2011) Docosahexaenoic acid: Brain accretion and roles in neuroprotection after brain hypoxia and ischemia. Current Opinion in Clinical Nutrition & Metabolic Care 14: 158–167.
89. Hamelink C, Hampson A, Wink DA, Eiden LE, Eskay RL (2005) Comparison of cannabidiol, antioxidants, and diuretics in reversing binge ethanol-induced neurotoxicity. J Pharmacol Exp Ther 314: 780–8.
90. Cippitelli A, Damadzic R, Frankola K, Goldstein A, Thorsell A, et al. (2010) Alcohol-induced neurodegeneration, suppression of transforming growth factor-beta, and cognitive impairment in rats: Prevention by group II metabotropic glutamate receptor activation. Biological Psychiatry 67: 823–30.
91. Kim HY (2008) Biochemical and biological functions of docosahexaenoic acid in the nervous system: Modulation by ethanol. Chemistry & Physics of Lipids 153: 34–46.
92. Kim HY, Akbar M, Kim YS (2010) Phosphatidylserine-dependent neuroprotective signaling promoted by docosahexaenoic acid. Prostaglandins Leukotrienes & Essential Fatty Acids 82: 165–72.
93. Serhan CN, Arita M, Hong S, Gotlinger K (2004) Resolvins, docosatrienes, and neuroprotectins, novel omega-3-derived mediators, and their endogenous aspirin-triggered epimers. Lipids 39: 1125–32.
94. Orr SK, Palumbo S, Bosetti F, Mount HT, Kang JX, et al. (2013) Unesterified docosahexaenoic acid is protective in neuroinflammation. J Neurochem 127: 378–393.
95. Bazan NG (2013) The docosanoid neuroprotectin D1 induces homeostatic regulation of neuroinflammation and cell survival. Prostaglandins Leukotrienes & Essential Fatty Acids 88: 127–129.
96. Kim HY, Spector AA, Xiong ZM (2011) A synaptogenic amide N-docosahexaenoylethanolamide promotes hippocampal development. Prostaglandins Other Lipid Mediat 96: 114–120.
97. Rashid MA, Katakura M, Kharebava G, Kevala K, Kim H (2013) N-docosahexaenoylethanolamine is a potent neurogenic factor for neural stem cell differentiation. J Neurochem 125: 869–884.
98. Cieslik M, Pyszko J, Strosznajder JB (2013) Docosahexaenoic acid and tetracyclines as promising neuroprotective compounds with poly(ADP-ribose) polymerase inhibitory activities for oxidative/genotoxic stress treatment. Neurochem Int 62: 626–636.
99. Umhau JC, Zhou W, Thada S, Demar J, Hussein N, et al. (2013) Brain docosahexaenoic acid [DHA] incorporation and blood flow are increased in chronic alcoholics: A positron emission tomography study corrected for cerebral atrophy. PLoS ONE [Electronic Resource] 8: e75333.
100. Salem N Jr, Litman B, Kim HY, Gawrisch K (2001) Mechanisms of action of docosahexaenoic acid in the nervous system. Lipids 36: 945–959.

The Effectiveness of Alcohol Screening and Brief Intervention in Emergency Departments

Colin Drummond[1¶], Paolo Deluca[1*¶], Simon Coulton[2], Martin Bland[3], Paul Cassidy[4], Mike Crawford[5], Veronica Dale[3], Eilish Gilvarry[6,7], Christine Godfrey[3], Nick Heather[8], Ruth McGovern[6], Judy Myles[1], Dorothy Newbury-Birch[6], Adenekan Oyefeso[9,10], Steve Parrott[3], Robert Patton[1], Katherine Perryman[1], Tom Phillips[1,11], Jonathan Shepherd[12], Robin Touquet[13], Eileen Kaner[6]

1 Addictions Department, Institute of Psychiatry, King's College London, London, United Kingdom, **2** Centre for Health Service Studies, University of Kent, Canterbury, United Kingdom, **3** Department of Health Sciences, University of York, York, United Kingdom, **4** Teams Family Practice, Gateshead, United Kingdom, **5** Department of Psychological Medicine, Imperial College, London, United Kingdom, **6** Institute of Health and Society, Newcastle University, Newcastle, United Kingdom, **7** Northern Regional Drug and Alcohol Services, Newcastle, United Kingdom, **8** Faculty of Health and Life Sciences, Northumbria University, Newcastle, United Kingdom, **9** Division of Population Health Sciences and Education, St George's, University of London, London, United Kingdom, **10** Jeesal Cawston Park Hospital, Norfolk, United Kingdom, **11** Humber NHS Foundation Trust, Willerby, United Kingdom, **12** Violence Research Group, Cardiff University, Cardiff, United Kingdom, **13** Emergency Department, Kingston Hospital, Kingston upon Thames, London, United Kingdom

Abstract

Background: Alcohol misuse is common in people attending emergency departments (EDs) and there is some evidence of efficacy of alcohol screening and brief interventions (SBI). This study investigated the effectiveness of SBI approaches of different intensities delivered by ED staff in nine typical EDs in England: the SIPS ED trial.

Methods and Findings: Pragmatic multicentre cluster randomized controlled trial of SBI for hazardous and harmful drinkers presenting to ED. Nine EDs were randomized to three conditions: a patient information leaflet (PIL), 5 minutes of brief advice (BA), and referral to an alcohol health worker who provided 20 minutes of brief lifestyle counseling (BLC). The primary outcome measure was the Alcohol Use Disorders Identification Test (AUDIT) status at 6 months. Of 5899 patients aged 18 or more presenting to EDs, 3737 (63·3%) were eligible to participate and 1497 (40·1%) screened positive for hazardous or harmful drinking, of whom 1204 (80·4%) gave consent to participate in the trial. Follow up rates were 72% (n = 863) at six, and 67% (n = 810) at 12 months. There was no evidence of any differences between intervention conditions for AUDIT status or any other outcome measures at months 6 or 12 in an intention to treat analysis. At month 6, compared to the PIL group, the odds ratio of being AUDIT negative for brief advice was 1·103 (95% CI 0·328 to 3·715). The odds ratio comparing BLC to PIL was 1·247 (95% CI 0·315 to 4·939). A per protocol analysis confirmed these findings.

Conclusions: SBI is difficult to implement in typical EDs. The results do not support widespread implementation of alcohol SBI in ED beyond screening followed by simple clinical feedback and alcohol information, which is likely to be easier and less expensive to implement than more complex interventions.

Editor: Bernard Le Foll, Centre for Addiction and Mental Health, Canada

Funding: The study was funded by the UK Department of Health. The Department of Health, proposed the general study design, but the details of the methodology were determined by the study team. The sponsor had no role in data collection, data analysis, interpretation of the results or writing the report. The corresponding author had full access to the data and had final responsibility for the decision to submit for publication. The views expressed herein do not necessarily reflect those of the Department of Health or the National Health Service in England and Wales.

Competing Interests: All authors had financial support from the Department of Health in England (Alcohol Policy Unit) for the submitted work; no financial relationships with any organisations that might have an interest in the submitted work in the previous three years; no other relationships or activities that could appear to have influenced the submitted work. There are no further patents, products in development or marketed products to declare.

* Email: Paolo.Deluca@kcl.ac.uk

¶ These authors are joint first authors on this work.

Introduction

Alcohol makes a significant contribution to the global burden of disease, injury and economic cost [1]. Over 20 million people are treated in emergency departments (ED) in England each year of which 35% of attendances are alcohol related, rising to 40% of attendances at weekends and up to 70% at peak times [2,3]. Such presentations offer the opportunity for early identification and intervention to reduce hazardous and harmful drinking [4,5].

There is a substantial evidence base for the efficacy of opportunistic screening and brief interventions (SBI) to reduce hazardous and harmful drinking in primary health care [6]. The evidence in ED is currently inconclusive. We conducted a rapid systematic review of SBI trials in ED (S1 Text) excluding studies conducted in adolescents only, trauma centres, and ED studies only including injured patients, to allow comparability to the current study. We identified six randomized controlled trials and two systematic reviews [6–13]. All identified trials were single site studies, four of which were in university teaching hospitals and mostly delivered by specialist staff employed by the study team rather than ED staff. Four of the trials assessed efficacy rather than effectiveness. Only one trial had a significant effect of intervention on alcohol consumption at 12 months [12]. A further trial had a significant effect on consumption at 6 but not 12 months, and reduced re-attendances at 12 months [8]. One trial found that patients receiving no intervention fared significantly better than those randomized to motivational interviewing [9].

ED is a busy environment with high patient and junior doctor turnover making SBI challenging to implement: one UK trial was abandoned due to low uptake of screening and intervention, whilst in another trial, though successful, initial data collection by ED staff was of necessity limited [8,14]. So while alcohol SBI in ED shows some promise in single site trials, its effectiveness in the typical ED setting was unknown. Further the optimal intensity of SBI was unknown [6,15]. The current study (SIPS ED trial) is the first pragmatic multicentre RCT of SBI in typical EDs. It included a larger sample size than previous trials, and cluster randomization to reduce contamination between intervention conditions. It was commissioned by the UK Department of Health as a facet of the Alcohol Harm Reduction Strategy for England [16]. The wider SIPS research programme included two related cluster RCTs in primary health care and criminal justice agencies and a health economic evaluation which are reported separately [17–19].

Methods

Ethics statement

The study received ethical approval from the London Research Ethics Committee (reference number: 07/MRE02/06).

Trial design and participants

The trial methodology is described here in brief. The protocol for this trial and CONSORT checklist are available as Checklist S1 and Protocol S1. We conducted a pragmatic factorial cluster randomized trial of alcohol SBI in nine EDs across three English regions (North East, South East, London). Participating EDs were selected on the basis of having no current routine alcohol SBI programme, representing a broad cross section of EDs including rural, suburban, urban and metropolitan catchment areas with wide ethnic and sociocultural diversity, located in both teaching hospitals and typical district general hospitals.

Our aim was that all patients aged 18 years or older who attended the participating EDs and otherwise met the inclusion criteria would be screened by ED staff using one of three short validated alcohol screening tools: the modified Single Alcohol Screening Question (M-SASQ), FAST Alcohol Screening Test, or a modified version of Paddington Alcohol Test (SIPS-PAT) [19]. EDs were randomly assigned to one of the three screening approaches. Inclusion criteria were age $>= 18$ and screening positive on an alcohol screening test, being sufficiently alert and orientated to provide informed consent, living within the catchment area of the ED, and being able to speak read or write English sufficiently well to complete study questionnaires. Exclusion criteria were patients who were age <18, already seeking alcohol treatment, participating in another study of alcohol interventions, severe injury, or suffering from a serious mental health problem, or grossly intoxicated, or being of no fixed abode.

Procedures

Those patients screening positive on the relevant alcohol tool were invited by ED or research staff to provide informed written consent to participate in the trial. The aim was to have all eligibility, screening, consent and baseline data collection carried out by ED staff. Furthermore ED staff were trained to deliver the interventions according to the condition they were allocated to. However, due to a low level of ED staff participation, this was carried out by the research team in six of nine EDs. The baseline assessment included demographic data, an extended item version of the Alcohol Use Disorders Identification Test, and a modified Readiness Ruler [19]. Participants were sent a voucher with a value of £10 following completion of the baseline interview.

We compared three different alcohol interventions of different intensity and complexity, with three EDs randomized to each condition, creating nine clusters in total. Participants in the minimal intervention control group were provided with simple clinical feedback using a standard script that their test result indicated they were drinking above the government's "safe" drinking levels, and were given a Patient Information Leaflet (PIL): the Department of Health's "*Drinking and You: How Much is Too Much?*" leaflet, including information on local alcohol services where further help could be sought by the patient themselves [19].

The intermediate intervention was the provision of 5 minutes of brief advice (BA) about drinking using the SIPS brief advice tool (*Brief Advice About Alcohol Risk*) developed for the trial and was based on the *How much is too much?* intervention pack developed as part of the UK version of the WHO collaborative Drink-Less Brief Intervention programme by Northumbria and Newcastle Universities [19]. Following brief advice the PIL was delivered in the same manner as in the minimal intervention group.

The more intensive intervention was Brief Lifestyle Counseling (BLC) delivered by SIPS employed Alcohol Health Workers (AHW) with specialist training and experience in alcohol motivational interventions. This was a 20 min lifestyle counseling alcohol intervention based on the *How much is too much?* intervention pack originally developed by Northumbria and Newcastle Universities, informed by the work of Rollnick and colleagues [19–20]. The procedure was that ED staff would first deliver the BA and PIL as above and then refer the patient to the SIPS AHW with an appointment the following day or as soon as possible thereafter.

At the intake point participants were invited to give their preference of follow up method - either by telephone, email or postal questionnaire. The protocol allowed for changing from the preferred method of follow up to the other methods if this proved unsuccessful. Most opted for telephone follow up and many who preferred other methods were successfully followed up by telephone. Telephone follow up was conducted by researchers who were blind to the participants allocated intervention condition.

The primary outcome measure was the AUDIT status (score of <8 versus $>= 8$) on the extended item AUDIT questionnaire at 6 months post consent.

Secondary outcome measures were average number of drinks per day using the quantity-frequency questions of the extended AUDIT, alcohol related problems using the Alcohol Problems

Questionnaire (APQ), readiness to change using a modified Readiness Ruler, all of which were measured at 6 and 12 months, and patient satisfaction using a modified version of the Patient Satisfaction Questionnaire measured at 12 months only [19]. We have noted that there are some discrepancies in the definition of our primary outcome in previous published documents of our study: Primary outcome in trial registration: "Alcohol Use Disorders Identification Test (AUDIT) at baseline and 6 months".

Primary outcome in protocol paper: "the score on the AUDIT screen at 12 months post-consent".

Primary outcome in this manuscript: "the AUDIT status (score of <8 versus > = 8) on the extended item AUDIT questionnaire at 6 months post consent".

To clarify this issue the primary outcome as stated in the registration is the primary outcome tool and this is operationalised as AUDIT status (score of <8 versus > = 8) at 6 months, this is the same as in this manuscript. In the BMC protocol paper we use the term score on the AUDIT screen which in effect is an alternative term for the AUDIT status. We can see that an error has occurred in the BMC protocol paper as we have used a 12 month time-point for the primary outcome rather than 6, as stated in the registration and submitted paper and the outcome the original study was powered to assess. We will contact the relevant editor at BMC to have this amended.

Randomization and masking

Randomization was conducted using a secure remote randomization service. Nine allocations were generated for each of the possible factorial combinations of screening method (SIPS-PAT, FAST, M-SASQ) and intervention condition (PIL, BA, BLC). EDs and allocations were randomly sampled without replacement and paired to generate allocation groups.

Participants were informed that they would be taking part in a study comparing different types of alcohol intervention taking place in different EDs. However they were only informed of the intervention taking place in their ED. Staff in each ED were informed of the design of the study and provided with a basic description of the different interventions being compared in the trial. However local ED staff were only trained to administer the intervention appropriate to their randomized ED allocation. The research team and SIPS employed AHWs were aware of the study design and were trained in all intervention methods. Researchers conducting 6 and 12 month follow up were blinded to the participants' allocated treatment condition and efforts were made to prevent participants from inadvertently revealing the intervention they received.

Sample size and data analysis

Recent meta-analysis suggests that the difference between brief intervention and control in alcohol consumption is 13%; 5% reduction in the control group and 18% in the brief intervention group [21]. We employed an established formula in our sample size calculation [22] and in order to detect this difference at the 5% significance level with 80% power, for a two-sided test, requires 109 patients in each of the three groups, a total of 327. Assuming a loss to follow up of 25% inflates the sample required to 131 in each group, a total of 393 patients. The proposed study involves a cluster design and requires a statistical adjustment to account for any potential cluster effect. The literature and our previous experience of trials in primary care suggest that is appropriate. Assuming an intra-class correlation coefficient of 0·04, a cluster size of the order 44 patients, this inflates the sample size calculation by a factor of 2·7 requiring a total of 1179 patients, 393 in each group, with an expectation that at least 882 will be followed up at 6 months and 12 months.

The primary analysis was by intention to treat, whereby participants are analysed as members of their allocated group irrespective of the treatment received to provide a pragmatic estimate of effectiveness, using a weighted linear regression model. The data were summarised for each of the nine clusters, summing the total number of AUDIT positive and AUDIT negative patients. The average baseline AUDIT score for each cluster was also calculated. For each cluster the odds of being AUDIT negative (low alcohol risk) were computed. For the primary analysis, the log odds of being AUDIT negative at 6 months were used as the dependent variable. In order to adjust for baseline differences in clusters, baseline AUDIT score was included in the model in addition to intervention and screening method. The analysis was weighted for the number of patients in each cluster responding at month six. The results were transformed and then presented as odds ratios. We explored the impact of missing data on the primary outcome by conducting multiple imputations and assessing the impact of missing data using sensitivity analysis. Weighted analyses were conducted for all other binary measures. Continuous variables were analysed using the mean score from each cluster which was then used in a weighted linear regression model. A per protocol analysis was conducted for the primary outcome including only those who received their allocated intervention. For the analysis of readiness to change ruler, the four categories were collapsed to form two categories, effectively those who were thinking of changing or had actually changed drinking and those who had not. All analyses were performed in STATA version 10.

Results

Implementation, recruitment and follow up

Screening and interventions were carried out by ED staff in three of 9 EDs and of necessity, due to low ED staff participation, by SIPS employed staff in the remaining six: two of three in the PIL condition, one of three in the BA condition and all in the BLC condition.

Recruitment started in March 2008 and finished in April 2009, and 12 month follow up was completed in May 2010. The Consort statement for the study is shown in Figure 1. A total of 5899 potential participants were assessed for eligibility for the trial, of whom 3737 (63·3%) were eligible to participate. Reasons for ineligibility are shown in Table 1. The commonest reasons for ineligibility were not being alert and orientated (26·1%), unable to speak English (21·1%), and not providing verbal consent to be screened (16·1%). Of those eligible 1497 (40·1%) screened positive for alcohol misuse, of whom 1204 (80·4%) gave consent to participate in the trial, with similar numbers across intervention groups (PIL n = 406; BA n = 403; BLC n = 395).

All patients in EDs allocated to PIL condition received the intervention. In the BA condition all patients received the PIL and 97% received BA. In the BLC condition, all patients received PIL, 99% received BA, and 50% received BLC.

Overall the follow-up rate at 6 months was 72% (n = 863), and was higher for those in the BA group (75%) than those allocated to PIL (72%) and BLC (68%). At 12 months the follow up rate was 67% (n = 810), higher in the BA group (73%) than either the PIL group (65%) or the BLC group (64%). These differences in follow up rate were not statistically significant.

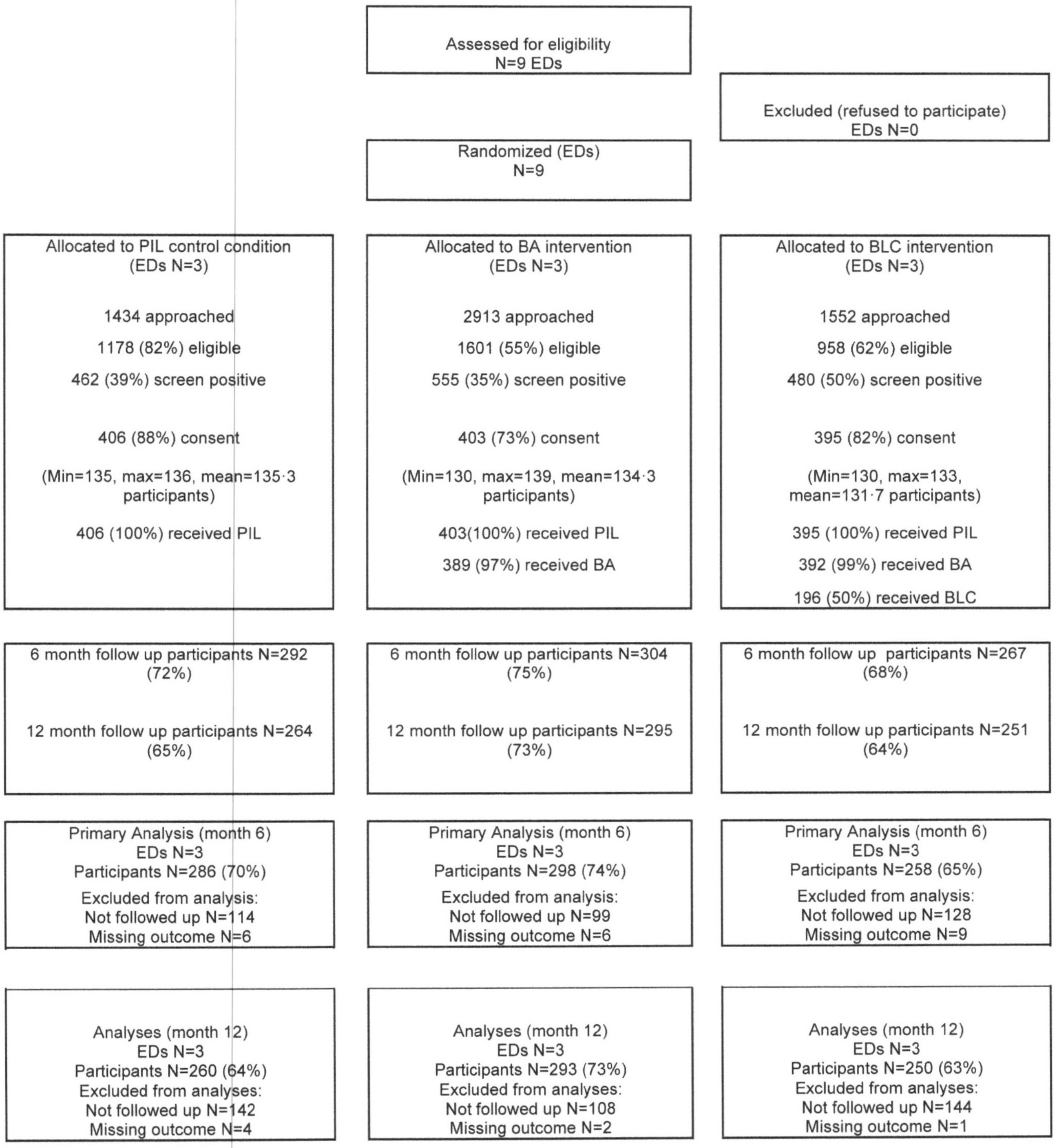

Figure 1. Consort Diagram.

Sample characteristics

The characteristics of the sample are shown in Table 2. Overall the mean age of those consenting to the study was 34·6 years and was similar across screening and intervention groups. The majority of the sample was male (65%). Overall 88% of the sample classified their ethnicity as white, with more white participants in the PIL group (93%) than either the BA or BLC groups (both 85%). The proportion of single people was 54%, with more in the BLC group (62%) than either the PIL (53%) or BA (48%) groups. Almost 65% of the sample continued with education after the age of 16 years. A smaller proportion of participants in the PIL group (59%) had continued in education than either the BA (66%) or BLC (69%) groups. Overall 39% of participants had a degree or equivalent. A higher proportion of those in the BLC group (48%) had a degree than either the BA (37%) or PIL (33%) groups. In excess of 45% of participants were current smokers.

Table 1. Reasons for ineligibility.

Reason	n	% of ineligible
Not alert and orientated	564	26·1
Does not speak English	457	21·1
Refused verbal consent to screen	349	16·1
Not resident within 20 miles of ED	260	12·0
Serious mental health problem	120	5·6
No fixed abode	113	5·2
Gross alcohol intoxication	106	4·9
Already seeking help for an alcohol problem	90	4·2
Severely injured	79	3·7
Already participating in a research project	24	1·1
Totals	**2162**	**100**

The mean AUDIT score at baseline was 12·4 (SD 6·9)(Table 3). The PIL group had a higher baseline AUDIT score 13·3 (SD 6·9) than either BA 12·2 (SD 7·0) or BLC 11·7 (SD 6·6). Overall 22·1% were AUDIT negative (PIL 14·9%, BA 24·5%, BLC 27·2%).

Clinical effectiveness

In the primary analysis, the proportion of AUDIT negative was 27·6% in PIL, 34·5% in BA and 39·5% BLC at 6 months (Table 4). The odds ratio comparing BA to PIL was 1·103 (95% CI 0·328 to 3·715) and comparing BLC to PIL was 0·690 (95% 0·315 to 4·939). These were not statistically significant differences. Multiple imputation of missing data found no significant differences so the outcome reported is based on observed values at 6 months. Differences in AUDIT status at 12 months also were not significantly different between intervention groups.

Similarly no significant differences were found between intervention conditions for average drinks per day, AUDIT score, APQ score or readiness to change, at 6 or 12 months. All results are presented in Tables 4 and 5.

A per protocol analysis based on interventions actually received by patients, and an analysis comparing both BA and BLC in a combined group to PIL also failed to find any significant differences between the intervention groups at 6 months (Tables 4 and 5).

Discussion

This study has important implications for alcohol screening and brief intervention (SBI) in ED. The original design of the study was for the SBI to be delivered by ED staff, apart from the BLC intervention. The latter required ED staff to refer patients to an alcohol health worker (AHW) for a subsequent consultation usually a few days after initial ED attendance, this being comparable to the St Mary's model [8]. However due to low participation of ED staff the study team had to deliver the SBI in six out of nine EDs. The implication is that, although there is some enthusiasm amongst ED staff to carry out alcohol interventions, it is likely to be difficult to implement SBI in the typical ED setting without significant external support from specialist alcohol staff.

The results showed that in a large pragmatic multicentre RCT, there was no significant difference in outcome between the three intervention conditions either in intention to treat or per protocol analyses on any of the outcome measures. These results are largely consistent with the systematic review, with the exception of two out of six single site efficacy studies conducted in university teaching hospitals which found significant effects of more intensive intervention [8–12]. This suggests that beyond the provision of simple clinical feedback and an alcohol information leaflet, more intensive interventions do not add significant clinical benefit.

Only 50% of patients referred for BLC intervention actually received it. Although this is a higher attendance rate than the previous UK ED trial (29·3%) and an Australian trial (10%), it suggests non-attendance at subsequent outpatient appointments following ED attendance may limit the effectiveness of BLC in typical practice [8,9]. Also previous research has shown that longer delay in receiving an appointment with an AHW results in greater attrition [23].

The strengths of this study include the fact that it is the first large pragmatic multicentre RCT of effectiveness of SBI in typical EDs, and rates of eligibility and consent were higher than in previous SBI studies, which adds weight to the generalisability of the research. Further we did not exclude patients with alcohol dependence as some previous studies have, since there is some evidence to suggest more dependent drinkers might benefit more from SBI in ED than hazardous drinkers [24,25]. Cluster randomization reduced the potential for contamination between interventions being delivered within a single clinical site with the potential for subversion of the protocol.

Weaknesses of the study include that we achieved a lower follow-up rate than planned (70% at 6 months and 67% at 12 months, compared to 75% planned) which will have reduced the statistical power, although these follow up rates are comparable with previous trials in ED. As this was a pragmatic effectiveness trial there was more limited measurement of the fidelity of the interventions in order to more closely represent typical practice. It is therefore possible that the lack of differences between intervention groups may have been due to unsuccessful implementation of the clinical protocols. Further, in six out of nine EDs the clinical protocols were implemented by study staff so the intervention being evaluated differed from the protocol. However as this was a pragmatic trial, the introduction of an AHW to deliver SBI reflects what is likely to have occurred with implementation in typical practice.

The study did not include a 'no intervention' group as a comparator with more intensive interventions. It is therefore not possible to conclude that the reductions in hazardous and harmful drinking in all three conditions can be attributed to the

Table 2. Demographic and baseline measures by intervention allocation.

		Minimal (N = 406)		Brief Advice (N = 403)		Brief Lifestyle Counseling (N = 395)		Total (N = 1204)	
		N	**Mean (SD)**	**N**	**Mean (SD)**	**N**	**Mean (SD)**	**N**	**Mean (SD)**
Age in years		402	34·1 (12·6)	402	35·2 (14·3)	394	34·5 (13·3)	1198	34·6 (13·4)
Average drinks per day		401	2·4 (2·1)	400	2·1 (2·0)	389	2·2 (2·1)	1190	2·3 (2·1)
		N	**%**	**N**	**%**	**N**	**%**	**N**	**%**
Gender	Male	272/404	67·3%	270/403	67·0%	242/395	61·3%	784/1202	65·2%
Ethnicity	White	372/401	92·8%	343/402	85·3%	334/395	84·6%	1049/1198	87·6%
Marital Status	Single	215/403	53·3%	192/402	47·8%	245/393	62·3%	652/1198	54·4%
Education after 16 years	Yes	240/404	59·4%	267/402	66·4%	273/395	69·1%	780/1201	64·9%
Possess degree or equivalent	Yes	130/398	32·7%	148/400	37·0%	182/382	47·6%	460/1180	39·0%
Smoke tobacco	Current smoker	198/404	49·0%	172/401	42·9%	172/395	43·5%	542/1200	45·2%
Readiness Ruler	Never think about drinking less	149/401	37·2%	141/397	35·5%	143/390	36·7%	433/1188	36·4%
	Sometimes think about drinking less	135/401	33·7%	145/397	36·5%	142/390	36·4%	422/1188	35·5%
	I have decided to drink less	41/401	10·2%	44/397	11·1%	43/390	11·0%	128/1188	10·8%
	Already trying to cut down	76/401	19·0%	67/397	16·9%	62/390	15·9%	205/1188	17·3%

Table 3. Baseline AUDIT score.

		Minimal		Brief Advice		Brief Lifestyle Counseling		Total		ICC
		N	**%**	**N**	**%**	**N**	**%**	**N**	**%**	
AUDIT Status	NEGATIVE (<8)	59	14·9%	96	24·5%	103	27·2%	258	22·1%	0·04 (0·02)
	POSITIVE (>=8)	336	85·1%	296	75·5%	276	72·8%	908	77·9%	
AUDIT Category	NEGATIVE (<8)	59	14·9%	96	24·5%	103	27·2%	258	22·1%	0·03 (0·02)
	HAZARDOUS (8–15)	228	57·7%	208	53·1%	199	52·5%	635	54·5%	
	HARMFUL (>=16)	108	27·3%	88	22·4%	77	20·3%	273	23·4%	
AUDIT score		**N**	**Mean (SD)**	**N**	**Mean (SD)**	**N**	**Mean (SD)**	**N**	**Mean (SD)**	
		395	13·3 (6·9)	392	12·2 (7·0)	379	11·7 (6.6)	1166	12·4 (6·9)	0·02 (0·01)

Table 4. Outcome measures at 6 and 12 months.

	Minimal Intervention	Brief Advice	Brief Lifestyle Counseling	Brief Advice/Minimal*		Brief Lifestyle Counseling/ Minimal*		ICC (se)
				OR	P-value	OR	P-value	
	N (%)	N (%)	N (%)	(95% CI)		(95% CI)		
Intention to treat analysis								
AUDIT Negative [a] - Month 6	79/286 (27·6)	103/298 (34·5)	102/258 (39·5)	1·1	0·81	1·2	0·65	0·02 (0·02)
				(0·3 to 3·7)		(0·3 to 4·9)		
AUDIT Negative [a] - Month 12	91/260 (35·0)	123/293 (42·0)	108/250 (43·2)	1·0	0·88	0·9	0·69	0·02 (0·01)
				(0·4 to 2·5)		(0·3 to 2·6)		
RCQ – Changed – Month 6[b]	121/287 (42·2)	105/297 (35·4)	94/261 (36·0)	0·8	0·23	0·8	0·36	0·01 (0·01)
				(0·5 to 1·3)		(0·5 to 1·4)		
RCQ – Changed – Month 12[b]	112/253 (44·3)	106/286 (37·1)	82/244 (33·6)	0·8	0·18	0.647	0·08	0·01 (0·01)
				(0·5 to 1·3)		(0·4 to 1·1)		

	N	N	N	Mean Difference	P-value	Mean Difference*	P-value	
	Mean (SE)	Mean (SE)	Mean (SE)	(95% CI)		(95% CI)		
AUDIT Score – Month 6 [a]	286	298	258	−0·4	0·72	−0·4	0·77	0·02 (0·02)
	11·2 (0·7)	10·8 (0·6)	10·8 (0·7)	(−3·5 to 2·7)		(−3·9 to 3·2)		
AUDIT Score – Month 12 [a]	260	293	250	−0·5	0·70	−0·5	0·71	0·02 (0·01)
	10·3 (0·9)	9·8 (0·7)	9·8 (0·8)	(−4·1 to 3·1)		(−4·7 to 3·6)		
APQ Score – Month 6[a]	286	298	258	0·2	0·75	0·4	0·47	0·01 (0·01)
	2.7 (0.3)	2.9 (0.3)	3.2 (0.3)	(−1·3 to 1·6)		(−1·2 to 2·1)		
APQ Score – Month 12[a]	263	295	251	−0·5	0·27	−0·1	0·89	0·01 (0·01)
	2.7 (0.3)	2.2 (0.2)	2.6 (0.2)	(−1·6 to 0·6)		(−1·3 to 1·2)		
ADD – Month 6[c,+]	291	300	264	0.0	0.95	−0.2	0.33	0.01 (0.01)
	2.4 (0.13)	2.1 (0.11)	2.0(0.12)	(−0.7 to 0.7)		(−0.8 to 0.4)		
ADD – Month 12[c,+]	263	294	251	0.1	0.78	−0.2	0.38	0.02 (0.02)
	2.2 (0.13)	1.9 (0.11)	1.8 (0.12)	(−0.6 to 0.7)		(−0.8 to 0.4)		

[a]adjusted for mean baseline AUDIT score and screening instrument.
[b]adjusted for baseline log odds of being in change group and screening instrument.
[c]adjusted for baseline ADD and screening instrument.
*estimates of differences are produced from weighted regression models.
[+]ADD – average drinks per day.

Table 5. Outcome measures at 6 and 12 months.

	Minimal Intervention N (%)	Brief Advice N (%)	Brief Lifestyle Counseling N (%)	Brief Advice/ Minimal*		Brief Lifestyle Counseling/ Minimal*		ICC (se)
	N	N	N	Mean Difference	P-value	Mean Difference*	P-value	
	Mean (SE)	Mean (SE)	Mean (SE)	(95% CI)		(95% CI)		
General Satisfaction – Month 12[d]	240	268	234	−0.06	0.31	−0.12	0.08	0.01 (0.01)
	4.01 (0.04)	3.95(0.04)	3.90 (0.04)	(−0.19 to 0.07)		(−0.26 to 0.02)		
Communication – Month 12[d]	241	269	231	−0.08	0.25	−0.04	0.52	0.01 (0.01)
	4.14 (0.04)	4.06 (0.04)	4.09 (0.04)	(−0.25 to 0.09)		(−0.22 to 0.13)		
Interpersonal manner – Month 12[d]	240	269	233	0.01	0.90	−0.02	0.81	0.01 (0.01)
	4.04 (0.04)	4.05 (0.03)	4.02 (0.04)	(−0.21 to 0.23)		(−0.25 to 0.21)		
Combined analysis	**Minimal N (%)**	**Combined Treatment N (%)**		**Combined/Minimal**				
				OR		**P-value**		
AUDIT Negative - Month 6[a]	79/286 (27·6)	205/556 (36·9)		1·1		0·69		0·02 (0·02)
				(0·5 to 2·8)				
Per protocol analysis								
AUDIT Negative - Month 6[a]	79/286 (27·6)	99/289 (34·3)	49/133 (36·8)	1·1	0·78	1·5	0·23	0·03 (0·02)
				(0·3 to 3·5)		(0·6 to 3·9)		

[a]adjusted for mean baseline AUDIT score and screening instrument.
[d]adjusted for screening instrument.
*estimates of differences are produced from weighted regression models.

interventions rather than 'assessment reactivity' or regression to the mean effects.[26] However three ED trials which have included patients who were only screened and followed up did not show differences in outcome with patients who were assessed and enrolled in the trial interventions [11,12,27].

Viewed in the context of our systematic review these findings add to a growing body of evidence that suggest ED is a less useful setting in which to implement alcohol SBI than in primary health care where the evidence is considerably stronger [6]. This might be related to several differences between the settings. Primary care staff are likely to have a more effective and ongoing therapeutic relationship with patients, which may provide a better context for SBI compared to the transient nature of ED attendance. Primary care has a more established role in providing preventive lifestyle interventions including diet and smoking, which may increase the legitimacy of alcohol SBI for both practitioners and patients. Patients often present to ED at a point of crisis which may be accompanied by distress and/or alcohol intoxication, and this might limit patients' receptiveness to alcohol or other lifestyle interventions [28,29].

It has been suggested that ED presents a 'teachable moment' when patients may be more amenable to an intervention making a connection between alcohol consumption and the presenting problem, increasing motivation to reduce drinking [23]. Alternatively it is possible that patients make this connection by virtue of the distress of their presenting condition and having to attend ED, without it being pointed out by clinical staff, which might obviate the need for, and limit the potential impact of SBI [28,29].

Nevertheless there is growing enthusiasm for implementation of SBI in ED in the UK and elsewhere [9,30,31]. A recent national survey of EDs in England conducted in 2011 reported that nearly half of EDs routinely ask patients about alcohol, 96% offer help or advice about alcohol, and 72% have access to an alcohol health worker or specialist nurse: significant increases on a 2006 survey [30]. Our results and the systematic review do not support widespread implementation of alcohol SBI in ED beyond the provision of screening followed by simple clinical feedback and alcohol information, which is likely to be easier and less expensive to implement than more complex interventions.

Acknowledgments

We would like to thank all the staff of the nine emergency departments for their support for the research. The participating hospitals were King's College Hospital (King's College Hospital NHS Foundation Trust), St Thomas's Hospital (Guy's and St Thomas's Hospital NHS Foundation Trust), North Middlesex Hospital (North Middlesex University Hospital NHS Trust) and Central Middlesex Hospital (North West London Hospitals NHS Trust), London, Royal Hampshire County Hospital (Hampshire Hospitals NHS Foundation Trust), Newcastle General Hospital (Newcastle upon Tyne Hospitals NHS Foundation Trust), Darlington Memorial Hospital (County Durham and Darlington NHS Foundation Trust), South Tyneside Hospital (South Tyneside NHS Foundation Trust), Hexham Hospital (Northumbria Healthcare NHS Foundation Trust). We also thank the Mental Health Research Network and the National Institute for Health Research Clinical Research Networks for their support.

Exclusive Licence

Ethical Approval

This study received multicentre ethical approval (07/MRE02/06) plus local agreement from all relevant local research ethics committees. Research governance approval was granted by all relevant primary care trusts. The research was done in accordance with the Helsinki declaration.

Author Contributions

Conceived and designed the experiments: CD, PD, SC, MB, PC, MC, VD, EG, CG, NH, RM, JM, DN, AO, SP, RP, KP, TP, JS, RT, and EK. Performed the experiments: PD, DNB, KP, AO, RM and RP. Analyzed the data: CG, SP, SC, VD and MB Contributed reagents/materials/analysis tools: CD, EK, NH and JS. Wrote the manuscript: CD, PD, SC, MB, PC, MC, VD, EG, CG, NH, RM, JM, DN, AO, SP, RP, KP, TP, JS, RT, and EK. Other (please specify): Expertise on clinical aspects of the research: RT JM PC Statistical input: SC VD MB.

References

1. Rehm J, Mathers C, Popova S, Thavorncharoensap M, Teerawattananon Y, et al. (2009) Global burden of disease and injury and economic cost attributable to alcohol use and alcohol-use disorders. Lancet 373: 2223–2233.
2. Waller S, Thom B, Harris S, Kelly M (1998) Perceptions of alcohol related attendances in accident and emergency departments in England: a national survey. Alcohol Alcohol 33(4): 354–361.
3. Drummond C, Phillips T, Coulton S, Barnaby B, Keating S, et al. (2005) National prevalence survey of alcohol-related attendances at accident and emergency departments in England. Alcohol Clin Exp Res 29(5): 36A (suppl)
4. French MT, Gumus G, Turner HL (2008) The role of alcohol use in emergency department episodes. Subst Use Misuse 43: 2074–2088.
5. Cunningham RM, Bernstein SL, Walton M, Broderick K, Vaca FE, et al. (2009) Alcohol, tobacco, and other drugs: future directions for screening and intervention in the emergency department. Acad Emerg Med 16:1078–1088.
6. Kaner EFS, Dickinson HO, Beyer F, Pienaar E, Schlesinger C, et al. (2009) The effectiveness of brief alcohol intervention in primary care settings: a systematic review. Drug Alc Rev 28: 301–323.
7. Bazargan-Hejazi S, Bing E, Bazargan M, Der-Martirosian C, Hardin E, et al. (2005) Evaluation of a brief intervention in an inner-city emergency department. Ann Emerg Med 46: 67–76.
8. Crawford MJ, Patton R, Touquet R, Drummond C, Byford S, et al. (2004) Screening and referral for brief intervention of alcohol misusing patient in and emergency department: a pragmatic randomized controlled trial. Lancet 364: 1334–1339.
9. Dent AW, Weiland TJ, Phillips GA, Lee NK (2008) Opportunistic screening and clinician-delivered brief intervention for high-risk alcohol use among emergency department attendees: a randomized controlled trial. Emerg Med Austral 20: 121–8.
10. D'Onofrio G, Pantalon MV, Degutis LC, Fiellin DA, Busch SH, et al. (2008) Brief intervention for hazardous and harmful drinkers in the emergency department. Ann Emerg Med 51:742–750.
11. Cherpitel CJ, Korcha RA, Moskalewicz J, Swiatkiewicz G, Ye Y, et al. (2010) Screening, brief intervention, and referral to treatment (SBIRT): 12 month outcomes of a randomised controlled trial in a Polish emergency department. Alc Clin Exp Res 34:1922–1928.
12. D'Onofrio G, Fiellin DA, Pantalon MV, Charwaski MC, Owens PH, et al. (2012) A brief intervention reduces hazardous and harmful drinking in emergency department patients. Ann Emerg Med 60:181–192.
13. D'Onofrio G, Degutis LC (2002) Preventive care in the emergency department: screening and brief intervention for alcohol problems in the emergency department: a systematic review. Acad Emerg Med 9: 627–638.

14. Peters J, Brooker C, McCabe C, Short N (1998) Problems encountered with opportunistic screening for alcohol-related problems in patients attending an accident and emergency department. *Addiction* 93: 589–594.
15. Drummond DC (1997) Alcohol interventions: do the best things come in small packages? Addiction 92: 375–379.
16. Prime Minister's Strategy Unit (2004) Alcohol Harm Reduction Strategy. London, Cabinet Office.
17. Kaner E, Bland M, Cassidy P, Coulton S, Dale V, et al. (2013) Pragmatic cluster randomized controlled trial of the effectiveness and cost-effectiveness of screening and brief alcohol intervention in primary care in England. Br Med J 346: e8501.
18. Newbury-Birch D, Bland M, Cassidy P, Coulton S, Deluca P, et al. (2009) Screening and brief interventions for hazardous and harmful alcohol use in probation services: a cluster randomized controlled trial protocol. BMC Public Health 18: 418.
19. Coulton S, Perryman K, Bland M, Cassidy P, Crawford M, et al. (2009) Screening and brief intervention for hazardous alcohol use in accident and emergency departments: a randomized controlled trial protocol. BMC Health Serv Res 9: 114.
20. Rollnick S, Mason P, Butler C (1999) Health Behaviour Change: A guide for practitioners. Edinburgh, Churchill Livingstone.
21. Moyer A, Finney JW, Swearingen CE, Vergun P (2002) Brief interventions for alcohol problems: a meta-analytic review of controlled investigations in treatment-seeking and non-treatment-seeking populations. Addiction 97: 279–292.
22. Wittes J (2002) Sample size calculations for randomized controlled trials. Epidemiol Rev 24 (1): 39–53.
23. Williams S, Brown A, Patton R, Crawford MJ, Touquet R (2005) The half-life of the 'teachable moment' for alcohol misusing patients in the emergency department. Drug Alc Dep 77: 205–208.
24. Blow FC, Ilgen MA, Walton MA, Czyz EK, McCammon R, et al. (2009) Severity of baseline alcohol use as a moderator of brief interventions in the emergency department. Alcohol Alcohol 44: 486–490.
25. Walton MA, Goldstein AL, Chermack ST, McCammon RJ, Cunningham RM, et al. (2008) Brief alcohol intervention in the emergency department: moderators of effectiveness. J Stud Alcohol Drugs 69: 550–560.
26. Bernstein JA, Bernstein E, Heeren TC (2010) Mechanisms of change in control group drinking in clinical trials of brief alcohol intervention: implications for bias toward the null. Drug Alc Rev 29: 498–507.
27. Daeppen J-B, Gaume J, Bady P, Yersin B, Clames J-M, et al. (2007) Brief alcohol intervention and alcohol assessment do not influence alcohol use in injured patients treated in the emergency department: a randomized controlled clinical trial. Addiction 102: 1224–1233.
28. Field CA, Baird J, Saitz R, Caetano R, Monti PM (2010) The mixed evidence for brief intervention in emergency departments, trauma centres, and inpatient hospital settings: what should we do? Alc Clin Exp Res 34: 2004–2010.
29. Trinks A, Festin K, Bendtsen P, Nilsen P (2013) What makes emergency department patients reduce their alcohol consumption? a computer based intervention study in Sweden. Int Emerg Nurs 21(1): 3–9.
30. Patton R, O'Hara P (2012) Alcohol: signs of improvement. The 2nd national emergency department survey of alcohol identification and intervention activity. Emerg Med J doi:10.1136/emermed-2012-201527
31. Cunningham RM, Harrison SR, McKay MP, Mello MJ, Sochor M, et al. (2010) National survey of emergency department alcohol screening and intervention practices. Ann Emerg Med 55: 556–562.

Chronic Ethanol Exposure during Adolescence in Rats Induces Motor Impairments and Cerebral Cortex Damage Associated with Oxidative Stress

Francisco Bruno Teixeira[1], Luana Nazaré da Silva Santana[1], Fernando Romualdo Bezerra[2], Sabrina De Carvalho[2], Enéas Andrade Fontes-Júnior[2,3], Rui Daniel Prediger[4], Maria Elena Crespo-López[3], Cristiane Socorro Ferraz Maia[2]*, Rafael Rodrigues Lima[1]

1 Laboratory of Functional and Structural Biology, Institute of Biological Sciences, Federal University of Pará, Belém-Pará, Brazil, **2** Laboratory Pharmacology of Inflammation and Behavior, Institute of Health Sciences, Federal University of Pará, Belém-Pará, Brazil, **3** Laboratory of Molecular Pharmacology, Institute of Biological Sciences, Federal University of Pará, Belém-Pará, Brazil, **4** Department of Pharmacology, Center of Biological Sciences, Federal University of Santa Catarina, Florianópolis, Santa Catarina, Brazil

Abstract

Binge drinking is common among adolescents, and this type of ethanol exposure may lead to long-term nervous system damage. In the current study, we evaluated motor performance and tissue alterations in the cerebral cortex of rats subjected to intermittent intoxication with ethanol from adolescence to adulthood. Adolescent male Wistar rats (35 days old) were treated with distilled water or ethanol (6.5 g/kg/day, 22.5% w/v) during 55 days by gavage to complete 90 days of age. The open field, inclined plane and the rotarod tests were used to assess the spontaneous locomotor activity and motor coordination performance in adult animals. Following completion of behavioral tests, half of animals were submitted to immunohistochemical evaluation of NeuN (marker of neuronal bodies), GFAP (a marker of astrocytes) and Iba1 (microglia marker) in the cerebral cortex while the other half of the animals were subjected to analysis of oxidative stress markers by biochemical assays. Chronic ethanol intoxication in rats from adolescence to adulthood induced significant motor deficits including impaired spontaneous locomotion, coordination and muscle strength. These behavioral impairments were accompanied by marked changes in all cellular populations evaluated as well as increased levels of nitrite and lipid peroxidation in the cerebral cortex. These findings indicate that continuous ethanol intoxication from adolescence to adulthood is able to provide neurobehavioral and neurodegenerative damage to cerebral cortex.

Editor: Viviana Trezza, Roma Tre University, Italy

Funding: Francisco Bruno Teixeira was supported by a Brazilian Government/Conselho Nacional de Desenvolvimento Científico e Tecnológico (CNPq) fellowship. Fernando Romualdo Bezerra was supported by a Brazilian Government/Coordenação de Aperfeiçoamento de Pessoal de Nível Superior (CAPES) fellowship. R.D.P. is supported by a research fellowship from CNPq. The authors would like to thank the PROPESP - UFPA for providing financial support (PAPQ). The funders had no role in study design, data collection and analysis, decision to publish, or preparation of the manuscript.

Competing Interests: The authors have declared that no competing interests exist.

* Email: crismaia@ufpa.br

Introduction

According to World Health Organization (WHO), the abusive consume of ethanol (EtOH) is responsible by over 2.5 million of premature deaths per year and almost 4% of all deaths worldwide are attributed to alcohol. Recent projections have indicated that EtOH consumption will continue to rise in coming decades, and that young adults are at highest increment in rising rates of consumption [1]. In this context, the last National Survey on Alcohol and Drug Use in Brazil [2] indicated that alcohol consumption is increasing, mainly among adolescents, becoming a serious health problem.

Some brain regions, such as the cerebral cortex, hippocampus and cerebellum, are highly vulnerable to chronic EtOH exposure and significant reduction in brain weight and volume has been found among alcoholics [3–5]. However, it must be stressed that brain damage severity is dependent of many variables including EtOH consumption profile (amount, frequency and duration) together with subject's variables (age, gender, etc) [6–11].

It is well documented that EtOH exposure during adolescence produces neurobehavioral alterations that differ from those seen in adults and that EtOH-induced structural modifications in specific brain regions including cerebral cortex and hippocampus may underlie these cognitive and affective impairments [12–14]. EtOH is more deleterious to brain during adolescence probably because during this period several CNS structures are under maturation, with changes from molecular components till brain weight [15]. Although the exact molecular mechanisms associated with EtOH-induced brain damage remain to be elucidated, previous studies have demonstrated the role of neuroinflammatory and oxidative stress processes [12,14,16,17].

Several studies have reported that chronic intoxication causes increased microglial activation and astrocytic hypertrophy, along with release of proinflammatory cytokines [18–22] and that those events may be associated with neurodegeneration induced ethanol [23].

Regarding oxidative stress, one of the main reactive nitrogen species is the nitric oxide (NO), produced by the enzyme nitric oxide synthase which is induced in pathological situations such as chronic EtOH intoxication [24].

Therefore, in the present study we investigated whether heavy chronic EtOH exposure during adolescence may induce motor impairments and histological damage in cerebral cortex of rats. We also addressed the putative involvement of neuroinflammatory and oxidative stress mechanisms in such effects of chronic EtOH exposure during adolescence.

Materials and Methods

Animals and experimental groups

A total of 20 adolescent male Wistar rats (35 days old), obtained from the Federal University of Pará (UFPA) were kept in collective cages (5 animals per cage). Animals were maintained in a climate-controlled room with a 12-h light/dark cycle (lights on 7:00 AM), and food and water *ad libitum*. All procedures were approved by the Ethics Committee on Experimental Animals of the Federal University of Pará (license number BIO- 007–09) and followed the guidelines suggested by the *NIH Guide for the Care and Use of Laboratory Animals*. Animals received orally (gavage) distilled water or EtOH (6.5 g/kg/day, 22.5% w/v) (n = 10 animals) once a day, for 55 days (i.e., until the 90th day of life), as previously described [14]. The current protocol of EtOH administration was based on previous studies from our group [14] showing that EtOH intoxication (6.5 g/kg/day) during the developing CNS may induce long-lasting neurobehavioral impairments and brain histochemical alterations in rats.

To investigate putative effects of EtOH intoxication on overall poor nutrition levels that may directly affect the motor performance and cortical damage, the animals' body weight was controlled during the entire period (55 days) of EtOH exposure (i.e., from the 35th day until the 90th day of life) at intervals of 7 days. The animals' survival rate in each group was assessed during the entire experimental protocol period and all animals survived the entire study. Moreover, all the behavioral and immunohistochemistry analyses were performed by an experienced experimenter who was unaware of the experimental group of the animals tested.

Behavioral assays

Twenty-four hours after the last EtOH or distilled water administration, animals were conducted to the room assay and acclimated by at least 1 h before the beginning of the behavioral tests, with attenuation of noise levels and low illumination (12 lux).

Open field. The spontaneous locomotor activity of the animals was evaluated in an open field arena during 5 min. The apparatus, made of wood covered with impermeable Formica, had a white floor of 100×100 cm (divided by black lines into 25 squares of 20×20 cm) and white walls, 40 cm high. Each rat was placed at the center of the open field and the numbers of squares crossed were registered.

Inclined plane. The animal's ability to maintain postural stability was evaluated with the inclined plane test. The rats were placed on the inclined plane which is raised in 5 degrees increments and can be used as an index of hind limb strength [14,25]. The maximum inclination at which the rat could maintain its position for 5 s was recorded as the final angle. Each rat was tested in five consecutive trials with an inter-trial interval of 60 s, and the average angle was calculated.

Rotarod. The rotarod apparatus (Insight Scientific Equipments, SP, Brazil) consists of a grooved metal roller (8 cm in diameter) and separated 9-cm wide compartments elevated 16 cm. As a part of the test procedure, animals were initially trained to maintain themselves on the rotating rod at 15 rotation per minute (RPM) for 3 min (habituation phase). After a period of 24 h, the animals were evaluated for their ability to remain on the rotating rod during 4 successive trials of 3 min at 15 RPM with an inter-trial interval of 60 s [14].

Histological evaluation

Perfusion and immunohistochemistry. Following behavioral assays, a set of animals (n = 5 animals per group) were deeply anesthetized with ketamine hydrochloride (90 mg/kg, i.p.) and xylazine hydrochloride (10 mg/kg, i.p.) and transcardially perfused with heparinized 0.9% saline solution followed by 4% paraformaldehyde in 0.2 M phosphate buffer. Surgical manipulation was performed only after both the corneal and the paw withdraw reflexes were abolished. Brains were removed from the skull and post-fixed for 12 h in the same fixative and cryoprotected in increasing concentrations gradients of sucrose-glycerol solutions over 7 days. The brain was then frozen in TissueTek, 20 μm coronal sections of cerebral cortex were cut using a cryostat (CarlZeissMicron, Germany). Sections were prepared on to gelatinized slides air dried for 24 h. They are stored in a freezer at −20°C for posterior analysis.

Sections of 20 μm were submitted to immunohistochemistry analysis as described previously [14,26]. Briefly, the slide-mounted sections were removed from the freezer, kept in an oven at 37°C for 30 min and rinsed in 0.1 M phosphate buffer saline (PBS) for 5 min. In order to improve labeling intensity, sections were treated with 0.2 M boric acid (pH 9.0) previously heated to 65°C for 25 min. The temperature was maintained constant over the treatment period. Sections were allowed to cool down for about 20 min and incubated under constant agitation in an 1% hydrogen peroxide solution in methanol for 20 min. Sections were then rinsed in 0.05% PBS/Tween (Sigma Company, USA) solution for 5 min for three times and incubated with 10% normal horse serum (NeuN) and goat serum (GFAP and Iba1) in PBS for 1 h. Without further rinsing, sections were then incubated overnight with the primary antibody in PBS, NeuN (1:500, Miliporere, USA), GFAP (1:1000, Sigma, USA) and Iba1 (1:1000, Dako, Denmark) rinsed in PBS/Tween solution for 5 min (3 times), and incubated with biotinylated horse anti-mouse (NeuN antibody) and goat anti-rabbit (GFAP and Iba1 antibodies) secondary antibodies (Vector Laboratories, USA) diluted at 1: 500 in PBS for 2 h. As a negative control, normal sera, rather the primary antibody, were used in some sections.

Sections were rinsed again for 5 min (three times) and incubated in the avidin-biotin-peroxidase complex (ABC Kit, Vector Laboratories, USA) for 2 h. Sections were rinsed four times (5 min each) and revealed with Diaminobenzidime (DAB) [14,26]. After the DAB reaction, sections were rinsed two times (5 min each) in 0.1 MPB, dehydrated, and coverslipped with Entellan (Merck, Germany).

Qualitative and quantitative analyses. All sections were initially surveyed by light microscopy. Illustrative images from all experimental groups were obtained with a digital camera (Moticam 2500, USA) attached to a microscope (Nikon, Eclipse 50i, USA). We used coronal sections containing cerebral cortex to count the numbers of neuron ($NeuN^+$ cells), microglia (Iba1+ cells) and astrocyte ($GFAP^+$ cells) using a 0.0665 mm^2 square graticule attached to the microscope eyepiece (objective 40x). We counted three fields per section and three sections per animal for control and EtOH groups (Fig. 1).

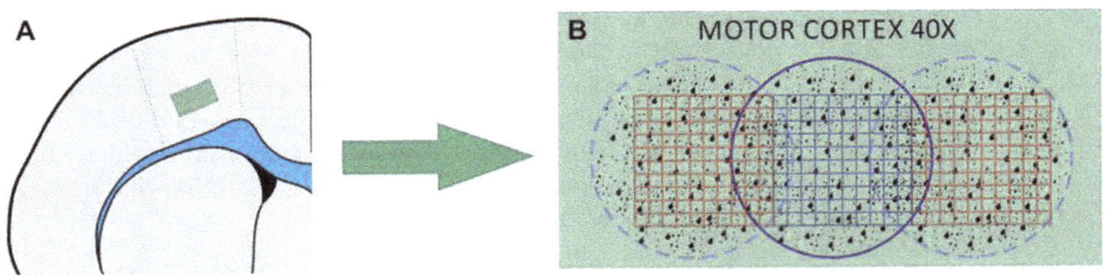

Figure 1. Schematic representation of the methodology utilized to count cells in the motor cortex area.

Biochemical analysis

After behavioural assays, a different set of animals from that used in histological studies (n = 5 animals per group) were sacrificed by cervical dislocation and brains were immediately removed and cooled on dry ice. Then, the entire cerebral cortex was separated from the rest of the encephalon and homogenized in ice-cold 20 mM Tris-HCl buffer (pH 7.4).

Nitrite assay. An aliquot of crude homogenate was centrifuged at 21,000 *g* for 20 min at 4°C, and supernatant was used to analyze nitrite levels as described elsewhere [27]. Briefly, samples were incubated at room temperature for 20 min with Griess reagent [0.1% N-(1-naphthyl) ethylenediaminedihydrochloride; 1% sulfanilamide in 5% phosphoric acid; 1:1]. The absorbance was measured at 550 nm and compared to that of standard solutions of sodium nitrite.

Lipid peroxidation (LPO) assay. Lipid peroxidation was evaluated by measuring malondialdehyde (MDA) and 4-hydroxyalkenals (4HDA) levels as previously showed [28]. Briefly, an aliquot of crude homogenate was centrifuged at 2,500 *g* for 30 min at 4°C, and supernatant was processed as described by the Bioxytech LPO-568 kit (Cayman Chemical). This kit takes advantage of a chromogenic reagent that reacts with MDA and 4HDA at 45°C, yielding a stable chromophore with maximal absorbance at the 586 nm wave length.

Protein content. Quantities of proteins in the supernatants (used for determination of lipid peroxidation and nitrite levels) were assayed as described elsewhere [29]. Thus, after corrected for protein concentration, results of lipid peroxidation and nitrite levels were expressed as percentages of control groups.

Statistical analyses

All values are expressed as means±S.E.M. (n = 10 animals per group for behavioral tests and n = 5 per group for immunohistochemistry and biochemical analyses). Statistical comparison of body weight gain between control and EtOH groups was performed using one-way analysis of variance (ANOVA) with repeated measures (days). Data from rotarod test were evaluated with one-way ANOVA (treatment) with repeated measures (trials). Following significant ANOVAs, multiple post-hoc comparisons were performed using the Tukey's test. The rest of data was compared using Student's t-test. The accepted level of significance was $P<0.05$. All tests were performed using the Statistica software package (StatSoft Inc., Tulsa, OK, USA).

Results

Effects of chronic EtOH exposure during adolescence on body weight gain in rats

As illustrated in Fig. 2, the body weight of the animals was evaluated during the entire period (55 days) of ethanol exposure (i.e., from the 35th day until the 90th day of life) at intervals of 7 days. One-way ANOVA with repeated measures revealed significant effects for the treatment factor ($F_{1,16} = 73.11$; $P< 0.0001$), for the repetition factor ($F_{8,128} = 84.67$; $P<0.0001$) and for the interaction factor between treatment and repetition ($F_{8,128} = 2.68$; $P<0.05$). Subsequent post-hoc comparisons using the Tukey's test revealed that ethanol induced a significant reduction in the body weight gain of rats specifically from the 63th to 77th days of life ($P<0.05$). However, the final body weight of control- and EtOH-treated rats after the period of 55 days of treatment did not differ statistically (Fig. 2).

Chronic EtOH exposure during adolescence disrupts the motor performance of rats

The results of locomotor activity evaluated in the open field arena (for 5 min) are summarized in Fig. 3A. Student's t-test indicated a significant reduction ($P<0.05$) in the total number of squares crossed by EtOH-treated rats in the open field test.

The effects of chronic ethanol administration during adolescence on the rats' ability to maintain postural stability evaluated in the inclined plane test are illustrated in Fig. 3B. Student's t-test comparisons indicated that EtOH administration induced a significant decrease in the mean angle score when compared to the control group ($P<0.05$).

The effects of chronic ethanol administration during adolescence on the motor coordination and balance of rats evaluated in the rotarod test are illustrated in Fig. 3C. One-way ANOVA with repeated measures revealed significant effects for the treatment [$F_{2,54} = 76.85$; $P<0.0001$] and the repetition factor [$F_{2,108} = 29.33$;

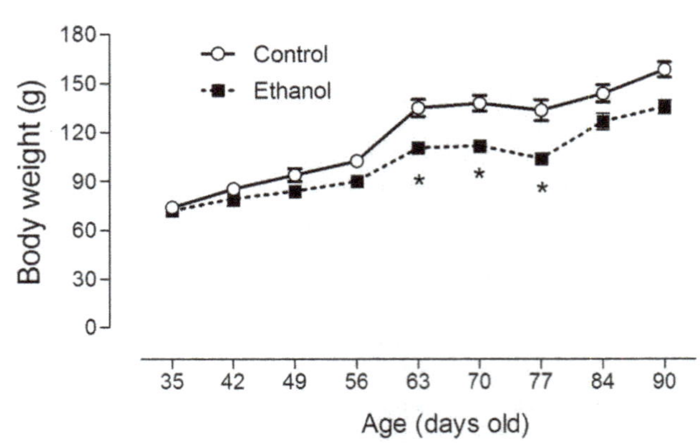

Figure 2. Effects of chronic ethanol (EtOH) administration (6.5 g/kg/day) during adolescence over a period of 55 days (i.e., from the 35th day until the 90th day of life) in the body weight gain of rats. The results are expressed as mean ± SEM of the body weight with interval of 7 days (n = 10 animals per group). *$P<0.05$ compared to control group (One-way ANOVA with repeated measures followed by Tukey's test).

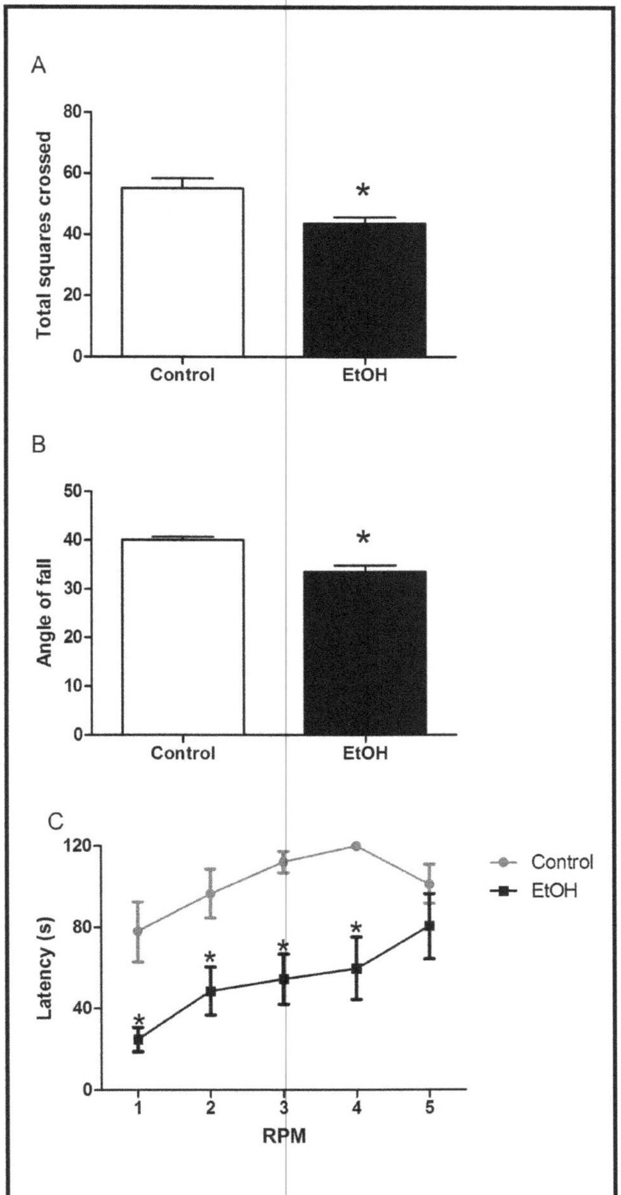

Figure 3. Effects of chronic ethanol (EtOH) administration (6.5 g/kg/day) during adolescence on the locomotor activity of male Wistar rats evaluated in the open field (OF), inclined plane and rotarod test. The results are expressed as mean ± SEM of the: (A) total squares crossed (OF test); (B) Angle of fall (inclined plane test); (C) Latency to fall during 5 sessions at 15 rotations per minute (rotarod test) (n = 10 animals per group). *P<0.05 compared to control group (t-Student test for A and B; One-way ANOVA with repeated measures followed by Tukey's test for C).

$P<0.0001$] and the interaction factor between treatment and repetition [$F_{4,108} = 4.59$; $P<0.01$] in the latency to fall of the rotarod. Post-hoc comparisons revealed that ethanol exposure during adolescence induced a significant decrease in the latencies to fall in the four test sessions of the rotarod (Fig. 3C).

Chronic EtOH exposure during adolescence induces neuronal loss and reduction in the number of microglial and astrocyte cells in the cerebral cortex of rats

The immunohistochemistry for neuronal cells (NeuN) identified that EtOH induced neuronal loss in the cerebral cortex of rats (Fig. 4 A–C).

After 55 days of ethanol exposure, it was observed a significant reduction in the number of GFAP+ cells revealed an expressive reduction in astrocyte cells in rats treated chronically with EtOH during adolescence (Fig. 4 D–F).

Moreover, a quantitative assessment of microglial measured by Iba-1+ cells labelled in the cerebral cortex revealed an expressive reduction of this cell (Fig. 4 G–I).

Chronic EtOH exposure during adolescence increases nitrite levels and lipid peroxidation in cerebral cortex of rats

Chronic exposure to ethanol during adolescence induced an increase in oxidative stress-related parameters in cerebral cortex of rats, as evidenced by a significant increase in both nitrite levels (an indirect marker of nitric oxide production) (Fig. 5A) and lipid peroxidation (Fig. 5B).

Discussion

The present study demonstrates, for the first time, that chronic EtOH intoxication during adolescence induces marked long-term motor disruption evaluated in different behavioral tasks (open field, inclined plane and rotarod) that were accompanied by cellular alterations in the cerebral cortex of rats. Additionally, biochemical assays revealed a main role for oxidative stress, and especially for nitrergic pathway in the present effects induced by chronic EtOH exposure during adolescence.

Epidemiological studies have been shown the increasing consume among adolescents in the world, that initiates around the 12 years old and increasing during overall adolescence, reaching about 45.5 % in young adults [30]. A recent survey about EtOH consume in Brazil has indicated similar data from that observed in other countries in which the consumption of alcohol is increasing among adolescents and in a heavy drinking profile [2].

Early evidence revealed that EtOH induces brain damage observed by brain atrophy that was more evident among alcoholics that have drunk heavily and during long-term periods [3–5]. Other studies also revealed marked impairments on motor and cognitive functions in both humans and laboratory animals following chronic ethanol exposure (for review see [31]). Indeed, it is well documented that adolescence is a period of vulnerability for drug abuse [32]. However, the long-term neurobehavioral consequences and molecular mechanisms remain poorly understood. It is well documented that the relationship between excessive alcohol consumption and neurotoxic levels among adolescents in a binge drinking episodes highlights to the fact that they are resistant to sedative effects and motor deficits induced by alcohol intake. On the other hand, adolescents have a profile of higher vulnerability to rewarding properties of alcohol when compared to adults [33].

Bell et al. [34] have investigated the acquisition of EtOH drinking behavior during adolescence in selectively bred alcohol-preferring rat model. The authors demonstrated that under 24-h of free-choice paradigm, adolescent alcohol-preferring rats intake 7.5 g/kg of alcohol per day till 10 mg/kg/day when offered multiple concentration of EtOH solution that can reflect the

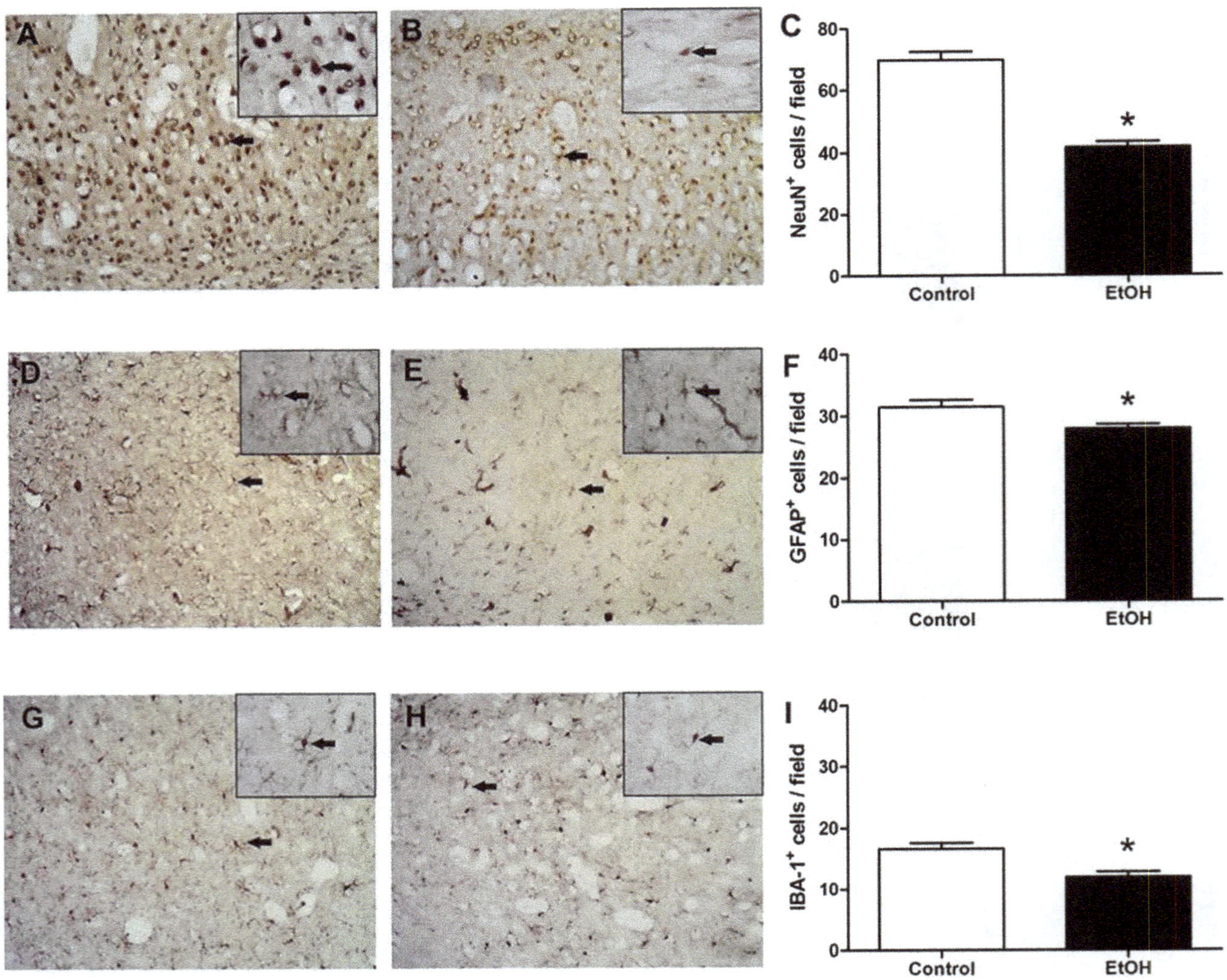

Figure 4. Effects of chronic ethanol (EtOH) administration (6.5 g/kg/day) during adolescence on the cell density of cortex motor. These results are expressed with photomicrographs and mean ± SEM. A (Control), B (EtOH), C: photomicrographs and graph expressing Neu-N label; D (Control), E (EtOH), F: photomicrographs and graph expressing GFAP label; G (Control), H (EtOH), I: photomicrographs and graph expressing Iba-1 label (n = 5 animals per group). *P<0.05 compared to control group (t-Student test). Scale = 200 µm. Inset, scale = 100 µm.

voluntary heavy consume during adolescence. Thus, in the present study we investigated whether heavy chronic ethanol exposure during adolescence induces long-term motor impairments and histological damage in cerebral cortex of rats.

Previous studies have shown that in the adolescence occurs structural and functional maturation of the brain. In this period, there are significant modifications in brain organization and cortical circuitry [35]. Alcohol inhibits brain maturation and neurogenesis, becoming adolescent brain more susceptible to the neurotoxic effects of alcohol abuse [36]. Motor coordination impairments following acute EtOH doses are more prominent in adult than adolescent rats. However, chronic alcohol exposure is more harmful during adolescence, mainly on motor function, that persists long-term after stopping alcohol administration [37,38].

The results of the present study showed that chronic EtOH exposure during adolescence affects locomotor activity of rats, as indicated by reduction in the number of squares crossed in the open field arena. Pascual et al. [39] demonstrated that adolescent rats exposed to EtOH (3.0 g/kg/day) for two consecutive days at 48-h intervals over 14 days display motor deficits related to cerebellar and neocortex damage by inflammatory mechanisms. We also observed that rats chronically exposure to EtOH during adolescence displayed a disruption in their ability to maintain postural stability and motor coordination on rotarod. These findings are in accordance with a recent study of our group [14] showing that chronic EtOH administration (6.5 g/kg/day during 55 days) during adolescence may potentiate the motor impairments and motor cortex damage induced by focal ischemia in female rats.

The motor cortex has long been viewed to play an important role in fine motor control and fractionation of movement [40,41], sensorimotor integration and higher-order cognitive-motor movements [42]. There are also other studies showing the role of motor cortex in the performance of behavioral tasks utilized in the current study [43] as well as showing that alterations on motor cortex can be associated with impaired spontaneous locomotion and incoordination in rodents following ethanol exposure [14,44].

Previous immunohistochemical studies demonstrated that alcohol exposure was related to neuronal loss in cortical regions [14,16,45], which is in agreement with our data showing reduction

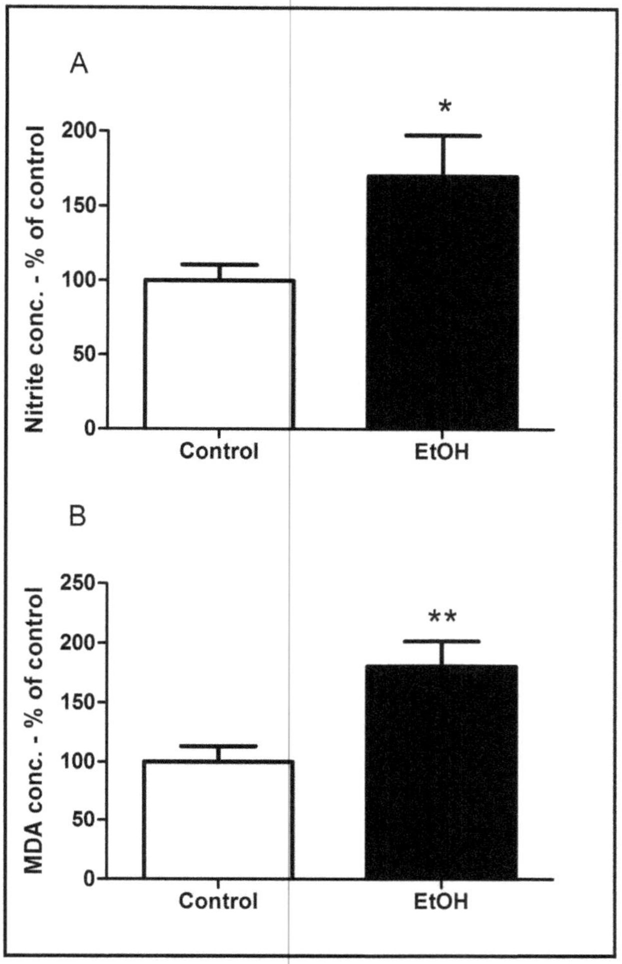

Figure 5. Effects of chronic ethanol (EtOH) administration (6.5 g/kg/day) during adolescence on the oxidative stress parameters of Wistar rats. The results are expressed as mean ± SEM of the: (A) Nitrite concentration per milligram of protein; (B) Malondialdehyde (MDA) concentration per miligrams of protein (n = 5 animals per group). *P<0.05 compared to control group (t-Student test).

in the anti-NeuN+ cells in the cerebral cortex. The mechanisms associated to ethanol-induced neuronal death in previous studies have been inferred as consequence of increase of oxidative stress and induction of pro-inflammatory mediators including cytokines, COX-2 and iNOS [12,14,16,23,24].

On the pathophysiology of ethanol intoxication, microglial activation seems to represent a pivotal step by releasing pro-inflammatory factors [22,46]. Moreover, during ethanol intoxication, there is an increase of nuclear factor kappa B (NF-kB) transcription [47] that plays a role in the signaling of immune and inflammatory responses [48], and a reduction of protein dependent of adenosine monophosphate cyclic (AMPc) family transcription [47] with neuroprotective functions against oxidative stress, excitotoxicity and apoptose [47,49,50].

Previous experimental [36,51] and *post-mortem* brain human studies [20] have shown that alcohol increases the expression of microglial markers after chronic alcohol exposure. Interestingly, and in accordance with previous findings from literature [10], we observed that chronic ethanol exposure during adolescence reduced microglial density in cerebral cortex of rats. Therefore, the current data suggests that ethanol exposure appears interfered with microglial proliferation.

It must be considered that microglial activation may also be related to neuroprotective events following stroke [52] and ethanol intoxication [53]. For instance, 3D two-photon microscopy analysis revealed that following oxygen-glucose deprivation (OGD) in hippocampal slices, microglia physically interacts with neurons protecting these cells from ischemic damage [54]. The same group showed that microglia provides protection following ischemia by phagocytosing [55]. In addition, genetic ablation of proliferating microglia exacerbates the ischemic damage, manifested by increases pro-inflammatory cytokines, apoptosis and infarct areas following middle cerebral artery occlusion (MCAO) in mice [52].

Following ethanol intoxication, microglia may serve both neuroprotective and detrimental actions [53]. While in the acute phase of ethanol intoxication microglia were shown to contribute to damage, they seem to be neuroprotective in the withdrawal phase [53]. Consequently, anti-inflammatory approaches must be devised to maximize the beneficial actions of neuroinflammation, while reducing their detrimental effects.

Moreover, our study demonstrated that alcohol reduced astrocyte population that was contradictory to other studies that inferred that alcohol increased astrocytes cells linked to increase production of reactive oxygen species (ROS) and calcium releasing in mitochondria of these cells [18,19,56]. In this sense, astrocytes protect against oxidative stress induced by alcohol perhaps by antioxidant factors production, such as glutathione peroxidase [57].

In addition to neuroinflammatory effects in binge alcohol-induced neuronal degeneration, oxidative stress has been largely associated to ethanol intoxication [58]. In cerebral cortex, chronic intake of alcohol alters cell membrane fluidity probably due to oxidative stress as indicated by increased nitrite and lipid peroxidation levels, enhanced presence of nitric oxide synthase and decreased superoxide dismutase [59]. However, all these effects were described for adult brains, and deleterious consequences for the developing brain with chronic intoxication from adolescence to adult age remains unknown.

Recently, damage by oxidative stress was showed in adolescent mice chronically exposed to alcohol for two weeks [60]. Interestingly, although this exposure caused a significant protein oxidative damage to hippocampus, no alterations were detected in prefrontal cortex [60]. By opposite, our data indicates that longer periods of exposure (55 days, from adolescence to adult age) lead to significantly raise both nitrite and lipid peroxidation levels in cerebral cortex of rats. These results are according to those described elsewhere in hippocampus and cerebral cortex of adult animals intoxicated with ethanol [61]. Therefore, we hypothesized that in adolescent rodents, a marked oxidative stress can be triggered initially in hippocampus, while longer periods of ethanol exposure are required to detect oxidative stress parameters in cerebral cortex. This constitutes a very interesting field that requires additional research.

Conclusions

Our results provide new evidence that heavy chronic ethanol intake during adolescence in male rats promotes long-term motor coordination deficits, as well as decreased spontaneous locomotion and balance. These behavioral changes were accompanied by a significant reduction in number of neurons and glia cells with increase in both nitrite levels (an indirect marker of nitric oxide production) and lipid peroxidation in the cerebral cortex. The exact mechanisms involved in reduction of glia cells remain unclear and more work is needed to understand how decrease in glia occurs in response to ethanol during adolescence.

Author Contributions

Conceived and designed the experiments: MEC CSFM RRL. Performed the experiments: FBT LNSS FRB SC EAF. Analyzed the data: RDP MEC CSFM RRL. Contributed reagents/materials/analysis tools: RDP EAF MEC CSFM RRL. Wrote the paper: FBT RDP MEC CSFM RRL.

References

1. World Health Organization (2011) Global status report on alcohol and health. Geneva, Switzerland, World Health Organization Press.
2. Instituto Nacional de Ciência e Tecnologia para Políticas Públicas do Álcool e Outras Drogas (2013) II Levantamento Nacional de Álcool e Drogas (LENAD). Available: http://inpad.org.br/wp-content/uploads/2013/04/LENAD_ALCOOL_Resultados-Preliminares.pdf. Accessed 25 July 2012.
3. Harper CG, Blumbergs PC (1982) Brain weights in alcoholics. J Neurol Neurosurg Psychiatry 45: 838–840.
4. Harding A, Halliday GM, Kril JJ (1996) Loss of vasopressin immunoreactive neurons in alcoholics is dose-related and time dependent. Neuroscience 72: 699–708.
5. Harper C (2009). The neuropatology of alcohol-related brain damage. Alcohol & Alcohol 44: 136–140.
6. Little PJ, Kuhn CM, Wilson WA, Swartzwelder HS (1996) Differential effects of ethanol in adolescent and adult rats. Alcohol Clini Exp Res 20: 1346–1351.
7. Maier SE, West JR (2001) Regional differences in cell loss associated with binge-like alcohol exposure during the first two trimesters equivalent in the rat. Alcohol 23: 49–57.
8. Varlinskaya EI, Spear LP (2004) Acute ethanol withdrawal (hangover) and social behavior in adolescent and adult male and female Sprague-Dawley rats. Alcohol Clin Exp Res 28: 40–50.
9. Doremus-Fitzwater TL, Spear LP (2007) Developmental differences in acute ethanol withdrawal in adolescent and adult rats. Alcohol Clin Exp Res 31: 1516–1527.
10. Koss WA, Sadowski RN, Sherril LK, Gulley JM, Juraska JM (2012) Effects of ethanol during adolescence on the number of neurons and glia in the medial prefrontal cortex and basolateral amygdale of adult male and female rats. Brain Res 1466: 24–32.
11. Schramm-Sapyta NL, Francis R, Macdonald A, Keistler C, O'Neill L, et al. (2014) Effect of sex on ethanol consumption and conditioned taste aversion in adolescent and adult rats. Psychopharmacology 231: 1831–1839.
12. Pascual M, Blanco AM, Cauli O, Minarro J, Guerri C (2007) Intermittent ethanol exposure induces inflammatory brain damage and causes long-term behavioural alterations in adolescent rats. Eur J Neurosci 25: 541–550.
13. Maia CS, Lucena GM, Correa PB, Serra RB, Matos RW, et al. (2009) Interference of ethanol and methylmercury in the developing central nervous system. Neurotoxicology 30: 23–30.
14. Oliveira GB, Fontes ED Jr, de Carvalho S, da Silva JB, Fernandes LM, et al. (2014) Mynocycline mitigates motor impairments and cortical neuronal loss induced by focal ischemia in rats chronically exposed to ethanol during adolescence. Brain Res Mar 15, doi: 10.1016/j.brainres.2014.03.005.
15. Toga AW, Thompson PM, Sowell ER (2006) Mapping brain maturation. Trends Neurosci 29: 148–59.
16. Valles SL, Blanco AM, Pascual M, Guerri C (2004) Chronic ethanol treatment enhances inflammatory mediators and cell death in the brain and in astrocytes. Brain Pathol 14: 365–371.
17. Blanco AM, Valles SL, Pascual M, Guerri C (2005) Involvement of TLR4/type I IL-1 receptor signaling in the induction of inflammatory mediators and cell death induced by ethanol in cultured astrocytes. J Immunol 175: 6893–6899.
18. Franke H (1995) Influence of chronic alcohol treatment on the GFAP-immunoreactivity in astrocytes of the hippocampus in rats. Acta Histochem 97: 263–271.
19. Franke H, Kittner H, Berger P, Wirkner K, Shramek J (1997) The reaction of astrocytes and neurons in the hippocampus of adult rats during chronic ethanol treatment and correlations to behavioral impairments. Alcohol 14: 445–454.
20. He J, Crews FT (2008) Increased MCP-1 and microglia in various regions of the human alcoholic brain. Exp Neurol 210: 349–358.
21. McClain JA, Hayes DM, Morris SA, Nixon K (2011) Adolescent binge alcohol exposure alters hippocampal progenitor cell proliferation in rats: effects on cell cycle kinetics. J Comp Neurol 519: 2697–2710.
22. Qin L, Crews FT (2012) NADPH oxidase and reactive oxygen species contribute to alcohol-induced microglial activation and neurodegeneration. J Neuroinflammation 9: 5.
23. Crews FT, Nixon K (2009) Mechanisms of neurodegeneration and regeneration in alcoholism. Alcohol Alcohol 44: 115–127.
24. Brocardo PS, Gil-Mohapel J, Christie BR (2011) The role of oxidative stress in fetal alcohol spectrum disorders. Brain Res Rev 67: 209–225.
25. Murphy MP, Rick JT, Milgram NW, Ivy GO (1995) A simple and rapid test of sensorimotor function in the aged rat. Neurobiol Learn Mem 64: 181–186.
26. Gomes-Leal W, Corkill DJ, Freire MA, Picanco-Diniz CW, Perry VH (2004) Astrocytosis, microglia activation, oligodendrocyte degeneration, and pyknosis following acute spinal cord injury. Exp Neurol 190: 456–467.
27. Green LC, Wagner DA, Glogowski J, Skipper PL, Wishnok JS, et al. (1982) Analysis of nitrate, nitrite, and [15N]nitrate in biological fluids. Anal Biochem 126: 131–138.
28. Esterbauer H, Cheeseman KH (1990) Determination of aldehydic lipid peroxidation products: malonaldehyde and 4-hydroxynonenal. Methods Enzymol 186: 407–421.
29. Lowry OH, Rosebrough NJ, Farr AL, Randall RJ (1951) Protein measurement with the Folin phenol reagent. J Biol Chem 193: 265–275.
30. Skala K, Walter H (2013). Adolescence and alcohol: a review of the literature. Neuropsychiatr. 27: 202–211.
31. López-Caneda E, Rodríguez Holguín S, Cadaveira F, Corral M, Doallo S (2014). Impact of Alcohol Use on Inhibitory Control (and Vice Versa) During Adolescence and Young Adulthood: A Review. Alcohol Alcohol 49: 173–181.
32. Toumbourou JW, Evans-Whipp TJ, Smith R, Hemphill SA, Herrenkohl TI, et al. (2014). Adolescent predictors and environmental correlates of young adult alcohol use problems. Addiction 109: 417–424.
33. Doremus F, Varlinskaya TL, Spear LP E (2010) Motivational systems in adolescence: possible implications for age differences in substance abuse and risk-taking behaviors. Brain Cogn 72: 114–123.
34. Bell RL, Rodd-Henricks ZA, Kuc KA, Lumeng L, Li TK, et al. (2003) Effects of concurrent access to a single concentration or multiple concentrations of ethanol on the intake of ethanol by male and female periadolescent alcohol-preferring (P) rats. Alcohol 29: 137–148.
35. Selemon LD (2013) A role for synaptic plasticity in the adolescent development of executive function. Transl Psychiatry 5;3:e238 DOI: 10.1038/tp.2013.7.
36. Crews FT, Mdzinarishvili A, Kim D, He J, Nixon K (2006) Neurogenesis in adolescent brain is potently inhibited by ethanol. Neuroscience 137: 437–445.
37. White A, Bae J, Truesdale M, Ahmad S, Wilson W, et al. (2002) Chronic intermittent alcohol exposure during adolescence prevents normal developmental changes in sensitivity to alcohol-induced motor impairments. Alcohol Clin Exp Res 26: 960–968.
38. White A, Truesdale M, Bae J, Ahmad S, Wilson W, et al. (2002) Differential effects of alcohol on motor coordination in adolescent and adult rats. Pharmacol Biochem Behav 73: 673–677.
39. Pascual M, Pla A, Miñarro J, Guerri C (2014) Neuroimmune Activation and Myelin Changes in Adolescent Rats Exposed to High-Dose Alcohol and Associated Cognitive Dysfunction: A Review with Reference to Human Adolescent Drinking. Alcohol Alcohol 49: 187–192.
40. Asanuma H (1973) Cerebral cortical control of movement. Physiologist 16: 143–166.
41. Evarts EV, Fromm C, Kroller J, Jennings VA (1983) Motor cortex control of finely graded forces. J Neurophysiol 49: 1199–1215.
42. Sanes JN, Donoghue JP (2000) Plasticity and primary motor cortex. Annu Rev Neurosci 23: 393–415.
43. Stigger F, Lovatel G, Marques M, Bertoldi K, Moysés F, et al. (2013) Inflammatory response and oxidative stress in developing rat brain and its consequences on motor behavior following maternal administration of LPS and perinatal anoxia. Int J Dev Neurosci. 31: 820–827.
44. Helfer JL, Calizo LH, Dong WK, Goodlett CR, Greenough WT, et al. (2009) Binge-like postnatal alcohol exposure triggers cortical gliogenesis in adolescent rats. J Comp Neurol 514: 259–271.
45. Obernier JA, Bouldin TW, Crews FT (2002) Binge ethanol exposure in adult rats causes necrotic cell death. Alcohol Clin Exp Res 26: 547–557.
46. Zhao YN, Wang F, Fan YX, Ping GF, Yang JY, et al. (2013) Activated microglia are implicated in cognitive deficits, neuronal death, and successful recovery following intermittent ethanol exposure. Behavi Brain Res 236: 270–282.
47. Zou JY and Crews FT (2005) TNF alpha potentiates glutamate neurotoxicity by inhibiting glutamate uptake in organotypic brain slice cultures: neuroprotection by nf kappa b inhibition. Brain Res 1034: 11–24.
48. O'Neill LA, Kaltschmidt C (1997) NF-kappa B: a crucial transcription factor for glial and neuronal cell function. Trends Neurosci 20: 252–258.
49. Lonze BE, Ginty DD (2002) Function and regulation of CREB family transcription factors in the nervous system. Neuron 35: 605–623.
50. Mantamadiotis T, Lemberger T, Bleckmann SC, Kern H, Kertz O, et al. (2002) Disruption of CREB function in brain leads to neurodegeneration. Nat Genet 31: 47–54.
51. Ward RJ, Colivicchi MA, Allen R, Schol F, Lallemand F, et al. (2009) Neuro-inflammation induced in the hippocampus of 'binge drinking' rats may be mediated by elevated extracellular glutamate content. J. Neurochem 111: 1119–1128.
52. Lalancette-Hebert M, Gowing G, Simard A, Weng YC, Kriz J (2007) Selective ablation of proliferating microglial cells exacerbates ischemic injury in the brain. J Neurosci 27: 2596–2605.

53. Zhao YN, Wang F, Fan YX, Ping GF, Yang JY, et al. (2012) Activated microglia are implicated in cognitive deficits, neuronal death, and successful recovery following intermittent ethanol exposure. Behav Brain Res 236: 270–282.
54. Neumann J, Gunzer M, Gutzeit HO, Ullrich O, Reymann KG, et al. (2006) Microglia provide neuroprotection after ischemia. FASEB J 20: 714–716.
55. Neumann J, Sauerzweig S, Rönicke R, Gunzer F, Dinkel K, et al. (2008) Microglia cells protect neurons by direct engulfment of invading neutrophil granulocytes: a new mechanism of CNS immune privilege. J Neurosci 28: 5965–5975.
56. González A, Pariente JA, Salido GM (2007) Ethanol stimulates ROS generation by mitochondria through Ca^{+2} mobilizations and increases GFAP content in rat hippocampal astrocytes. Brain Res 1178: 28–37.
57. Watts LT, Rathinam ML, Schenker S, Henderson GI (2005) Astrocytes protect neurons from ethanol-induced oxidative stress and apoptotic death. J Neurosci Res 80: 655–666.
58. Collins MA, Neafsey EJ (2012) Neuroinflammatory pathways in binge alcohol-induced neuronal degeneration: oxidative stress cascade involving aquaporin, brain edema, and phospholipase A2 activation. Neurotox Res 21: 70–78.
59. Reddy VD, Padmavathi P, Kavitha G, Saradamma B, Varadacharyulu N (2013) Alcohol-induced oxidative/nitrosative stress alters brain mitochondrial membrane properties. Mol Cell Biochem 375: 39–47.
60. Ros-Simó C, Moscoso-Castro M, Ruiz-Medina J, Ros J, Valverde O (2013) Memory impairment and hippocampus specific protein oxidation induced by ethanol intake and 3, 4-methylenedioxymethamphetamine (MDMA) in mice. J Neurochem 125: 736–746.
61. Tiwari V, Chopra K (2013) Protective effect of curcumin against chronic alcohol-induced cognitive deficits and neuroinflammation in the adult rat brain. Neuroscience 244: 147–158.

22

Prefrontal Response and Frontostriatal Functional Connectivity to Monetary Reward in Abstinent Alcohol-Dependent Young Adults

Erika E. Forbes[1,2,3]*, Eric E. Rodriguez[1], Samuel Musselman[1], Rajesh Narendran[1,4]

1 Department of Psychiatry, University of Pittsburgh School of Medicine, Pittsburgh, Pennsylvania, United States of America, 2 Department of Psychology, University of Pittsburgh, Pittsburgh, Pennsylvania, United States of America, 3 Department of Pediatrics, University of Pittsburgh School of Medicine, Pittsburgh, Pennsylvania, United States of America, 4 Department of Radiology, University of Pittsburgh School of Medicine, Pittsburgh, Pennsylvania, United States of America

Abstract

Although altered function in neural reward circuitry is widely proposed in models of addiction, more recent conceptual views have emphasized the role of disrupted response in prefrontal regions. Changes in regions such as the orbitofrontal cortex, medial prefrontal cortex, and dorsolateral prefrontal cortex are postulated to contribute to the compulsivity, impulsivity, and altered executive function that are central to addiction. In addition, few studies have examined function in these regions during young adulthood, when exposure is less chronic than in typical samples of alcohol-dependent adults. To address these issues, we examined neural response and functional connectivity during monetary reward in 24 adults with alcohol dependence and 24 psychiatrically healthy adults. Adults with alcohol dependence exhibited less response to the receipt of monetary reward in a set of prefrontal regions including the medial prefrontal cortex, lateral orbitofrontal cortex, and dorsolateral prefrontal cortex. Adults with alcohol dependence also exhibited greater negative correlation between function in each of these regions and that in the nucleus accumbens. Within the alcohol-dependent group, those with family history of alcohol dependence exhibited lower mPFC response, and those with more frequent drinking exhibited greater negative functional connectivity between the mPFC and the nucleus accumbens. These findings indicate that alcohol dependence is associated with less engagement of prefrontal cortical regions, suggesting weak or disrupted regulation of ventral striatal response. This pattern of prefrontal response and frontostriatal connectivity has consequences for the behavior patterns typical of addiction. Furthermore, brain-behavior findings indicate that the potential mechanisms of disruption in frontostriatal circuitry in alcohol dependence include family liability to alcohol use problems and more frequent use of alcohol. In all, these findings build on the extant literature on reward-circuit function in addiction and suggest mechanisms for disrupted function in alcohol dependence.

Editor: Ingmar H.A. Franken, Erasmus University Rotterdam, Netherlands

Funding: This study was funded by NIH R01 AA018330 (www.niaaa.nih.gov). The authors' work on this project was also supported by National Institutes of Health grants R01 DA026222 (Dr. Forbes, PI), R01 MH093605 (Dr. Forbes, PI), and R21DA 033612 (Dr. Forbes, PI). The funders had no role in study design, data collection and analysis, decision to publish, or preparation of the manuscript.

Competing Interests: Dr. Narendran's imaging group has done contractual research work at the University of Pittsburgh for GlaxoSmithKline Inc. and ONO Pharmaceutical Co., LTD.

* E-mail: forbese@upmc.edu

Introduction

Across conceptual models, disrupted function in neural reward circuitry is postulated to be a central mechanism of alcohol dependence and other forms of addiction [1,2,3]. Changes in reward circuitry with the development of addiction are thought to reflect a shift from reward-driven behavior during the initial stages of addiction to loss of reward function by later stages [4]. Recent models of addiction have focused on altered function in prefrontal regions that mediate behavioral processes such as compulsivity, impulsivity, and higher-order cognitive control [5,6]. Together, these constructs reflect difficulty in controlling behavior flexibly, as directed by future goals rather than short-term gains, and through inhibition of inappropriate or goal-inconsistent behaviors, respectively. Specifically, adaptations related to the development of addiction are posited to involve increased hypofrontality, which can be conceptualized as poor executive control over behavior, as well as poor modulation of responding in other reward regions. In terms of prefrontal function, these adaptations are likely to involve altered function in regions such as the orbitofrontal cortex (OFC), medial prefrontal cortex (mPFC), and dorsolateral prefrontal cortex (DLPFC), all of which contribute to function in reward circuitry but have differing roles. For example, although all of these regions process rewarding stimuli, the mPFC can have an excitatory influence on dopamine neurons [7] and seems to respond to contextual features of reward [8], while the OFC appears to specialize in inhibition of dopamine neurons [7]. Furthermore, subregions of the OFC differ: medial OFC appears specialized for responding to reward and lateral OFC for responding to punishment and to changing or suppressing previously rewarded behaviors [9,10]. In addition, Both imaging and basic science studies indicate that chronic drug or alcohol use leads to a disruption in the OFC regulation of ventral striatum (primarily, nucleus accumbens) DA transmission via glutamatergic projections (for a review, see [11]).

In addition, adaptations in dopamine-system function are postulated to disrupt the functional connectivity of these prefrontal regions with the ventral striatum (VS), especially the nucleus accumbens. For example, in a positron emission tomography study, Volkow and colleagues reported that controls—but not alcohol-dependent adults—exhibited an association between decreased glucose metabolism in the OFC and increased methylphenidate-induced dopamine release in the VS [12]. This finding suggests altered coupling between these two regions, with an association between lower response in the OFC and increased dopamine in the VS, which could indicate less effective regulation of VS responding by OFC. Furthermore, in detoxified alcohol-dependent adults, weaker OFC functional connectivity with the midbrain predicts the likelihood of relapse [13]. Similarly, this finding raises the possibility that poor or suboptimal connectivity between OFC and basic reward regions is a correlate or consequence of addiction. Given the role of the OFC in inhibitory control and self-regulation [14,15], these findings suggest that alcohol dependence involves reduced inhibition of ventral striatal response, which is relevant to compulsive use.

Non-drug rewards such as money or natural rewards can provide a valuable context for investigating hypofrontality in alcohol dependence. For two possible reasons, responding in frontostriatal circuitry is likely disrupted during the processing of non-drug rewards. First, lasting, generalized hypofrontality in people suffering from addiction could be evident in neural response to a variety of reward classes, including to non-drug rewards such as money or natural rewards such as food. Changes in the dopamine system influence response to both drug rewards (i.e., the drug itself, with its rewarding effects) and non-drug rewards [15], and it is likely that the neural adaptations that occur with addiction generalize to responding in the presence of other types of reward, including natural rewards and money. Thus, hypofrontality could reflect general disruption in reward circuitry, whether responding to drug or non-drug rewards. In the case of non-drug rewards, hypofrontality could have consequences for difficulty in guiding behavior to obtain these rewards as necessary for healthy functioning [11]. Second, another possibility is that hypofrontality is particularly evident in the context of response to non-drug or natural rewards in addiction, because reward circuitry adapts to focus on drug rewards at the expense of non-drug rewards. Consistent with this possibility, studies of alcohol dependence have revealed an opposite pattern of response to alcohol-related and non-alcohol-related stimuli in addiction. Specifically, it appears that in comparison with healthy adults, alcohol-dependent adults exhibit greater response in reward-related regions to alcohol-related reward [16,17,18,19], but *decreased* response to monetary (i.e., non-drug) reward [20,21]. Furthermore, response in the mPFC and VS to alcohol-related reward predict relapse among detoxified alcohol-dependent adults [22]. Through either process, reduced coupling of prefrontal cortical regions from the ventral striatum has been hypothesized to diminish and enhance the capacity of the prefrontal cortex to initiate behaviors in response to natural and alcohol-related reward stimuli, respectively, which in turn drives the cycle of addiction [11].

Developmentally, it is critical to examine alterations in PFC response to reward in alcohol dependence early in adulthood. Not only is this period early in the course of dependence, which provides greater opportunity to examine the development of addiction and less severity of the toxic effects of alcohol exposure [23,24], but early adulthood is a window in which dopamine is exerting a decreasing influence on PFC function [25]. Low VS reponse to monetary reward has been reported in children of alcohol-dependent parents, indicating that this characteristic may be a risk factor for the development of alcohol-related problems [26]. In the PFC, it is especially important to investigate this issue during early adulthood because dopamine influence on PFC function changes across adult development, resulting in changes in function of reward circuitry as well as altered associations between dopamine synthesis and PFC function [25]. Specifically, with adult development, dopamine synthesis decreases in cortex but increases in dorsal striatum, and the shift toward greater dopamine synthesis in the dorsal caudate is associated with lower performance on executive function tasks [27]. These findings suggest that assessing dopamine-related functioning in PFC—for example, during reward processing—is more challenging in older adults, who have experienced declines in PFC dopamine functioning. Thus, to understand dopamine-mediated alterations in PFC control of reward responding, it is optimal to investigate PFC function at a developmental period proximal to development of the dopamine system. Alcohol-dependent young adults in their 20 s provide a valuable group for addressing this research question. Although much of their PFC maturation is completed, their PFC dopamine signaling has not yet declined, they are likely to be early in the clinical course of alcohol dependence, and they are relatively young for people in the alcohol-dependent population.

We examined neural response to monetary reward in 24 young adults with alcohol dependence and 24 healthy young adults. Using a reliable fMRI task involving guessing numbers and winning money, we predicted that alcohol dependence would be related to hypofrontality, defined as low response in OFC, mPFC, and DLPFC. We also predicted that alcohol dependence would be associated with altered frontostriatal functional connectivity, defined as greater negative correlation in task-related functional connectivity between those PFC regions and the nucleus accumbens. Because we focused on monetary reward, we predicted that alcohol dependence would be associated with low VS response. Finally, to address the possible mechanisms leading to group differences, we examined brain-behavior associations involving drinking characteristics such as frequency and quantity of drinking, number of years drinking, and family history of alcohol dependence. Examining associations of these characteristics with neural response and functional connectivity within the alcohol dependent group provided the opportunity to obtain a more detailed understanding of the process by which frontostriatal function could develop from patterns of drinking behavior or genetic vulnerability (in the case of family history).

Materials and Methods

Ethics Statement

Procedures were approved by the University of Pittsburgh Institutional Review Board. All participants provided written informed consent to study procedures.

Participants

Forty-eight young adults (24 with alcohol dependence, 24 healthy controls) underwent fMRI in a Siemens 3 T Trio scanner during a block-design monetary reward task. The groups were matched for age, sex, race, and smoking habits. Sample characteristics are presented in Table 1. As expected, the alcohol dependent group did not differ from the healthy control group in any demographic characteristics. Participants were recruited in the greater Pittsburgh area from a larger PET study and from community advertisements. The original total sample included 59 individuals. Of these, 9 were unable to complete the functional tasks in the fMRI scanner either due to scheduling limitations or

Table 1. Sample Characteristics.

	Alcohol Dependent Group	Healthy Control Group	Group Differences
N	24	24	
Age	27.2±4.9	27.2±3.7	$F(1,46) = .00$, *ns*
Sex	37.5% Female	41.7% Female	$\chi^2 = .09$, *ns*
Race	79.2% Caucasian	79.2% Caucasian	$\chi^2 = .00$, *ns*
Education: Some College	58.3%	83.3%	$\chi^2 = 4.04$, *ns*
Daily Smokers (*n*)	12	12	$\chi^2 = .00$, *ns*
Task Reaction Time (ms)	805.0±161.7	843.4±213.8	$F(1,46) = .49$, *ns*
Frequency of drinking (days/week)	5.83±1.59	N/A	
Severity of Alcohol Dependence	20.21±5.53	N/A	
Drinks/Use	11.61±5.53	N/A	
Years Drinking	10.46±5.69	N/A	
Family History of Alcohol Dependence	79.2%	N/A	
Days since Last Use	48.33±60.54	N/A	

Note: All participants in the alcohol dependent group met DSM-IV criteria for alcohol dependence but had undergone monitored abstinence prior to participating. Severity of alcohol dependence was measured with the Alcohol Dependence Scale [62]. All daily smokers met criteria for nicotine dependence. Family history reflects alcoholism in any first- or second-degree relatives. Groups did not differ significantly for any demographic characteristics. N/A: other than confirming the absence of alcohol use disorders, we did not assess drinking behavior and drinking history in the healthy control group.

scanner malfunction, 2 individuals were excluded for low-response rates in the scanner (less than 50% of total responses), and 1 was excluded for inadequate coverage of prefrontal regions. Exclusion criteria for this study included the following: pregnancy, serious medical or neurological illness, systolic blood pressure > 140 mmHG, diastolic blood pressure <90 mmHG, any current major axis I psychiatric diagnosis (except alcohol and nicotine use disorder), metal implants or paramagnetic objects, employment as a radiation worker or exposure to radiation that exceeds annual dose of radiation, medical history of chronic obstructive pulmonary disease or other chronic respiratory disorders, and renal or liver problems.

Lifetime psychiatric diagnoses in all participants were assessed using the Structured Clinical Interview for DSM-IV [28]. Participants in the alcohol group had current DSM-IV-defined Alcohol Dependence and had undergone a 2-week monitored abstinence. Outpatient monitored abstinence from alcohol and other recreational drugs were confirmed with ethyl glucuronide/ethylsulfate (ETG/ETS) and urine drug screens performed three times/week for two consecutive weeks before assessment. During this monitoring period, participants were paid $75 for each negative ETG/ETS urine to promote abstinence from alcohol. All alcohol dependent subjects were monitored for alcohol withdrawal during the first week of abstinence using the Clinical Institute Withdrawal Assessment of Alcohol Scale (CIWA-Ar). Individuals who scored greater than 19 on the CIWA-Ar during the initial intake evaluation ($n = 0$ for the current study) and/or with a prior history of alcohol withdrawal seizures or delirium tremens were excluded from the research protocol. Participants in the comparison group were free of lifetime psychiatric disorders. All participants were in good medical health and underwent a physical exam and bloodwork prior to entering the study.

Response of Neural Reward Circuitry

Paradigm. The fMRI paradigm was a slow event-related card-guessing game [29] that allows examination of response to monetary reward and reliably engages the striatum (see Figure 1). Participants received win, loss, or a neutral control feedback for each trial. Participants were told that their performance would determine a post-scan monetary reward, with $1 for each win and 50 cents deducted for each loss with no money being gained or deducted for the control blocks. The 45 trials were divided into three different block types: win, loss, and control. These blocks were presented in fixed, pseudorandom order with predetermined outcomes that were identical across participants. During each win and loss trial, participants guessed via button press whether the value of a hidden number was high or low (3 s); learned the value of the hidden number (.5 s); and received outcome feedback (.5 s). Feedback consisted of a green upward-facing arrow for a win outcome and a red downward-facing arrow for a loss outcome. A crosshair was then presented for 3 s (intertrial interval), for a total trial length of 7 s. The motor control aspect of this task operated in the same fashion as the win/loss trials. Participants were asked to press a button when presented with an "X" (3 s), which was followed by an asterisk (.5 s), and were presented with a yellow circle for the neutral outcome (.5 s). The contrast of interest derived from the task for all analyses was *win* > *loss*. The control condition was not included in analyses.

Participants were unaware of fixed outcome probabilities, and their engagement and motivation were maintained by verbal encouragement between runs. Participants practiced the task before the scan and did not exhibit a change in reaction time across task runs during the scan. The alcohol group and comparison group did not differ in mean reaction time during the task.

fMRI acquisition, processing, and analysis

Each participant was scanned using a Siemens Trio 3 T scanner. BOLD functional images were acquired with a gradient echo planar imaging (EPI) sequence and covered 34 axial slices (3 mm thick) beginning at the cerebral vertex and encompassing the entire cerebrum and the majority of the cerebellum (TR/TE = 2000/29 ms, FOV = 200×200, matrix = 64×64). All scanning parameters were selected to optimize the quality of the

BOLD signal while maintaining a sufficient number of slices to acquire whole-brain data. Before the collection of fMRI data for each participant, we acquired a reference EPI scan that we visually inspected for artifacts (e.g., ghosting) and for good signal across the entire volume of acquisition. The fMRI data from all included participants were cleared of such problems.

Whole-brain image analysis was conducted using SPM8 (http://www.fil.ion.ucl.ac.uk/spm). For each scan, images for each participant were realigned to correct for head motion. Data sets were then selected for quality based on our standard small-motion correction (<2 mm) and for signal coverage in the striatal region of interest >80%. Realigned images were co-registered to structural images that had been segmented to select grey matter, then spatially normalized into standard stereotactic space (Montreal Neurological Institute template) using a 12-parameter affine model. Normalized images were smoothed with a 6 mm full-width at half-maximum Gaussian filter. Voxel-wise signal intensities were ratio normalized to the whole-brain global mean.

Preprocessed data sets were then analyzed using first-level random effects models that account for scan-to-scan variability and second-level random effects models that account for participant-to-participant variability to determine task-specific regional responses. For each participant and scan, condition effects (i.e., main effects of task) at each voxel were calculated using a t-statistic, producing a statistical image for the contrast of interest (i.e., win > loss).

Data Analyses

We examined neural response to win vs. loss in the following five *a priori* neural regions of interest (ROIs): (1) ventral and dorsal striatum; (2) mPFC, including medial BA9, medial BA10, and BA32 (24); (3) medial OFC, defined as BAs 11 and 12; (4) lateral OFC, defined as BA47; and (5) DLPFC. We distinguished medial from lateral OFC because of claims that these two subregions differ in function, with medial OFC specializing in value-related choice and lateral OFC specializing in reward learning, inhibitory control, and regulation of reward responding [30,31]. In addition, DLPFC was included because of emerging findings indicating its disruption in addiction, especially during decision-making [32]. ROIs were defined anatomically using the WFU PickAtlas Tool (v3.0.4), either by creating a sphere around a set of central coordinates (for VS, 10 mm radius around [0, 10, −10], [33]; for mPFC, 20 mm radius around [0, 42, 18], [34]) or by selecting a region (i.e., BA47 for lateral OFC; BAs 11 and 12 for medial OFC; BAs 9 and 46 for DLPFC). The mPFC ROI was designed to focus on dorsal mPFC, so that it would not overlap with the medial OFC ROI.

We tested group differences in neural response using second-level random-effects factorial models in SPM. We examined functional connectivity using interaction (PPI) analyses in SPM8, with the bilateral nucleus accumbens, defined by the PickAtlas anatomical region, as the seed region. The psychological variable for PPI was win > loss, which serves to isolate response to reward from response to feedback generally. Because the contrast for PPI involved blocks for which BOLD response would not overlap, our task timing was appropriate for PPI analyses. Sex, race, and daily smoking quantity were included as covariates in analyses for group differences. We investigated brain-behavior analyses focusing on drinking behavior by conducting regressions in SPM within the alcohol dependent group. These regression analyses included age as a covariate. There were no evident sex differences in drinking behaviors, and accordingly we did not include sex as a covariate in these regression analyses. All analyses initially used a voxel-wise threshold of $p<.05$ and a minimum extent of 10 contiguous voxels.

We then used simulations in AlphaSim based on the five-ROI mask to compute minimum cluster sizes in order to adjust for Type I error in all analyses. The minimum extent size of continuous voxels required for a corrected $p<.05$ cutoff using the entire mask was 247 voxels.

Results

Behavior

Participants responded to a high proportion of trials (97.7%±10.0%). As expected, the alcohol dependent and control groups did not differ in reaction time or proportion of trials with responses during the task (Table 1).

Group Differences in Neural Response to Monetary Reward

The alcohol dependent group showed less response in the lateral OFC, mPFC, DLPFC, and VS (anteroventral caudate region, extending into dorsal caudate) than the comparison group to win vs. loss (Table 2; Figure 2). The alcohol dependent group did not exhibit greater response than the comparison group in any of the ROIs. The groups did not differ in medial OFC response. There were no sex differences in neural response. Whole-brain results for group differences confirmed that these ROIs were critical regions in which the groups differed (Table S1).

Group Differences in Frontostriatal Functional Connectivity

Given the role of prefrontal regions in modulating responding in the VS and the pattern of group differences we observed in response of PFC regions, we focused on functional connectivity between the bilateral nucleus accumbens and the lateral OFC, mPFC, and DLPFC during the experience of winning money compared with losing money. The alcohol dependent group displayed stronger negative functional connectivity than the comparison group—that is, a stronger negative correlation in task-related function— between the nucleus accumbens and all 3 prefrontal ROIs tested (see Table 1; Figure 3). That is, the alcohol dependent group showed stronger associations than the comparison group between nucleus accumbens and prefrontal regions during the context of receiving reward vs. losing. Whole-brain analyses confirmed that these PFC regions exhibited negative functional connectivity with the bilateral accumbens. The groups did not differ for positive functional connectivity. There were no sex differences in functional connectivity.

Associations between Drinking Characteristics and Brain Function in Alcohol-Dependent Adults

To investigate the mechanisms of association between alcohol dependence and altered neural response among problem drinkers, we conducted regression analyses with drinking characteristics as regressors. All analyses were conducted within the alcohol dependent group, and they focused on the ROI clusters that emerged from group-difference analyses above. This way, we could examine brain-behavior associations that were relevant to group differences. Age was included as a covariate in these analyses, as it was related to several drinking characteristics (e.g., older participants had spent a greater number of years drinking; $r=.82$ for years drinking, .45 for drinks per use, .45 for frequency of use, .46 for severity, all $ps<.03$). A positive family history of alcohol dependence was associated with low response in anterodorsal cingulate subregion of the mPFC (Table 3; Figure 4).

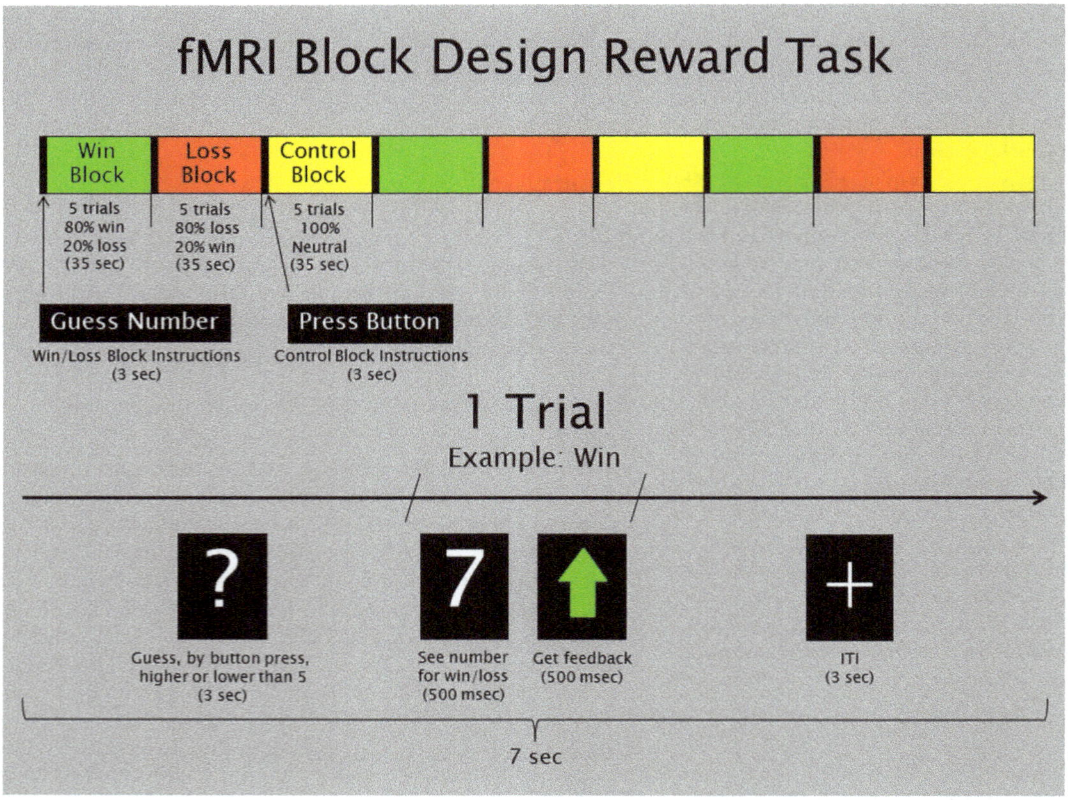

Figure 1. The block-design monetary reward task employed in the current study. Participants were instructed to guess whether a number was low or high and to respond to win outcomes.

Associations between Drinking Characteristics and VS-PFC Functional Connectivity in Alcohol-Dependent Adults

As with our analyses of drinking characteristics and neural response to reward above, we conducted regression analyses with drinking characteristics and functional connectivity between the bilateral nucleus accumbens and the regions that distinguished alcohol and control groups' functional connectivity during the experience of winning money compared with losing money. Frequency of drinking (days/week) was associated with greater functional connectivity between the bilateral nucleus accumbens and a cluster including portions of the perigenual anterior cingulate and rostral mPFC (Table 3; Figure 5). That is, alcohol dependent adults who drank alcohol more often exhibited a stronger association between nucleus accumbens and mPFC in the context of receiving a reward vs. losing.

Discussion

Focusing on the hypothesis that alcohol dependence is accompanied by hypofrontality, we found that young adults with alcohol dependence, compared with healthy young adults, exhibited less response in the lateral OFC, mPFC, and DLPFC in response to monetary reward. In addition, alcohol dependence was associated with a greater negative functional connectivity (i.e., negative correlation in task-related response) between those prefrontal regions and the bilateral nucleus accumbens. Furthermore, suggesting blunted response to non-alcohol reward, young adults with alcohol dependence exhibited less response to monetary reward in the ventral striatum. Relevant to the pathophysiology of alcohol dependence, young adults with alcohol dependence exhibited associations between drinking characteristics and both mPFC response and mPFC-accumbens functional connectivity. Family history of alcohol dependence was related to less mPFC response, and drinking frequency was related to greater negative functional connectivity between the nucleus accumbens and the mPFC. Together, these findings suggest that function in frontostriatal reward circuitry is altered in alcohol dependence, with less response in key PFC regions, disrupted coordination between frontal regions and VS in response to non-alcohol rewards, and associations between drinking characteristics and these frontostriatal alterations. These findings could indicate that alcohol dependence develops through weakened prefrontal regulation of striatal responding, which corresponds to difficulty with behavioral regulation. Because we focused on frontostriatal functional connectivity during winning relative to losing money, our results suggest that altered coordination of VS with mPFC occurs in response to reward rather than to feedback in general. Alternatively, altered coordination between these two reward regions could be weak during rewarding experiences but preserved or strong during loss or punishment experiences. The mechanisms of such weakened prefrontal regulation could include both heritable factors and pattern of exposure to alcohol.

Our findings are consistent with the putative disruptions to components of reward circuitry in addiction. The mPFC was central to our findings, with altered function in response to reward, altered coordination with the nucleus accumbens, and functional associations with pathophysiologic characteristics of alcohol dependence. This region has several key functions in the processing of reward, including both responding directly to reward

Table 2. Differences in Function of Reward Circuitry between Adults with Alcohol Dependence and Healthy Control Adults.

Regions	BA	Cluster Size	*t*-score at peak voxel	Talairach coordinates of peak voxel		
				x	y	z
Alcohol < Control, Neural Response						
Right Lateral OFC	47	780	5.69	32	12	1
mPFC, Right DLPFC	32,8	5782	5.49	2	27	32
Right Lateral OFC	10,11	537	4.89	33	53	1
Left Lateral OFC	13	454	4.86	−36	12	−1
Ventral Striatum, Dorsal Striatum		255	3.88	−10	2	8
Left Lateral OFC	10,11	328	3.99	−23	50	−6
Alcohol > Control, Negative Functional Connectivity with Bilateral Nucleus Accumbens						
Lateral OFC	45,46,47	296	5.12	−53	36	0
DLPFC only	10,9	749	3.99	42	42	16
mPFC	8,10	712	3.45	−16	46	16

Note: Results are from region-of-interest analyses focusing on the OFC, mPFC, DLPFC, and ventral striatum. Analyses were thresholded at $p_{corrected}<0.05$ using AlphaSim. $df = 135$. The contrast generated from the reward task was win > loss. Cluster size is in voxels. There were no regions for which (1) alcohol dependent adults exhibited greater response than healthy adults or (2) less negative functional connectivity with the accumbens than healthy adults. There were null findings for positive functional connectivity. OFC: orbitofrontal cortex. mPFC: medial prefrontal cortex. DLPFC: dorsolateral prefrontal cortex.

as a target of midbrain dopamine neurons and serving as a regulatory region for striatal response to reward [8]. The dorsal mPFC is also thought to work in coordination with the DLPFC to regulate affective response [35]. Thus, our findings of less mPFC response to monetary reward in adults with alcohol dependence—and in those alcohol-dependent adults with a family history of the disorder—suggest that low responding in this region could reflect ineffective modulation of basic reward responding in a way that facilitates addictive behavior. This change in modulation could be a stable vulnerability in those with high familial loading for alcohol-related problems. Our findings of altered mPFC functional connectivity with the nucleus accumbens in alcohol dependent adults, as well as altered functional connectivity in more frequent drinkers in the alcohol-dependent group, occurred during the comparison of receiving money and losing money. Thus, striatal-mPFC coordination could be particularly sensitive to rewarding outcomes rather than outcomes generally. These findings have meaning for the function of reward circuitry associated with alcohol dependence specifically and with addiction in general.

The lateral OFC mediates the influence of rewarding experiences on executive function [36] and appears to play a role in higher-level response to reward. Additionally, baseline function in the lateral OFC is associated with positive emotionality, an affective trait related to reward sensitivity and inversely associated with addiction [37]. Although models of OFC function have postulated that lateral OFC is specialized for processing loss rather than reward, a more recent conceptual stance is that lateral OFC also contributes to reward association learning by assigning credit to rewards and re-evaluating rewards [38]. Less response in this area could thus be interpreted as difficulty with updating the value of rewards, which could lead to reduced flexibility and greater compulsivity in responding.

The DLPFC, while not studied as intensively as other prefrontal regions in relation to reward or in populations with alcohol dependence, has emerged as an important region in addiction. Altered DLPFC function in addiction is thought to reflect disrupted decision-making away from flexible responding and in favor of compulsive behavior [6,39]. In addition, DLPFC is postulated to play a critical role in the self-regulation of reward consumption, for example by modulating the processing of reward value in the service of goals [40,41,42]. Alcohol-dependent adults exhibit reduced DLPFC response to cognitive control [43], and those with greater DLPFC response report greater craving [43] and are more likely to seek treatment [44]. Previous studies of alcohol use disorder have indicated that greater negative functional connectivity between the ventral striatum and DLPFC during operant conditioning is associated with slower learning from reward prediction errors and greater craving [45]. While our task involves other aspects of reward processing rather than learning, our findings could suggest a similar alteration of prefrontal influence over reward processing. That is, instead of reduced prefrontal influence on the efficiency of reward learning, as in that previous study, we could have observed reduced prefrontal influence on another process, the initial response to reward. This process is likely to influence a variety of other reward-related functions, including learning.

In addition, altered PFC response to rewarding events has been reported in both adults with substance dependence and adolescents at risk for alcohol use problems. Bjork et al. [46] reported that substance dependent adults exhibited less response to obtaining risky rewards in a posterior dorsal region of mPFC whose function is associated with conflict monitoring and reward-driven behavior. While the mPFC region distinguishing alcohol dependent and comparison groups in the current study is located in a more anterior area of PFC than the region reported in that previous study, our findings suggest a similar pattern of low PFC engagement during reward processing. In our case, and consistent with the nature of our fMRI task, the mPFC subregion with lower function in alcohol dependence is associated with the expression and regulation of response to pleasant stimuli [47].

Our finding of low dorsal and ventral striatal response to monetary reward in adults with alcohol dependence is consistent with other findings in alcohol dependence, even those focusing on the anticipation of reward rather than rewarding outcomes [20,21]. In the context of the extant literature on response to drug vs. non-drug reward in alcohol dependence, the current findings for VS response provide partial support for the hypothesis that addiction shifts reward function away from natural or non-

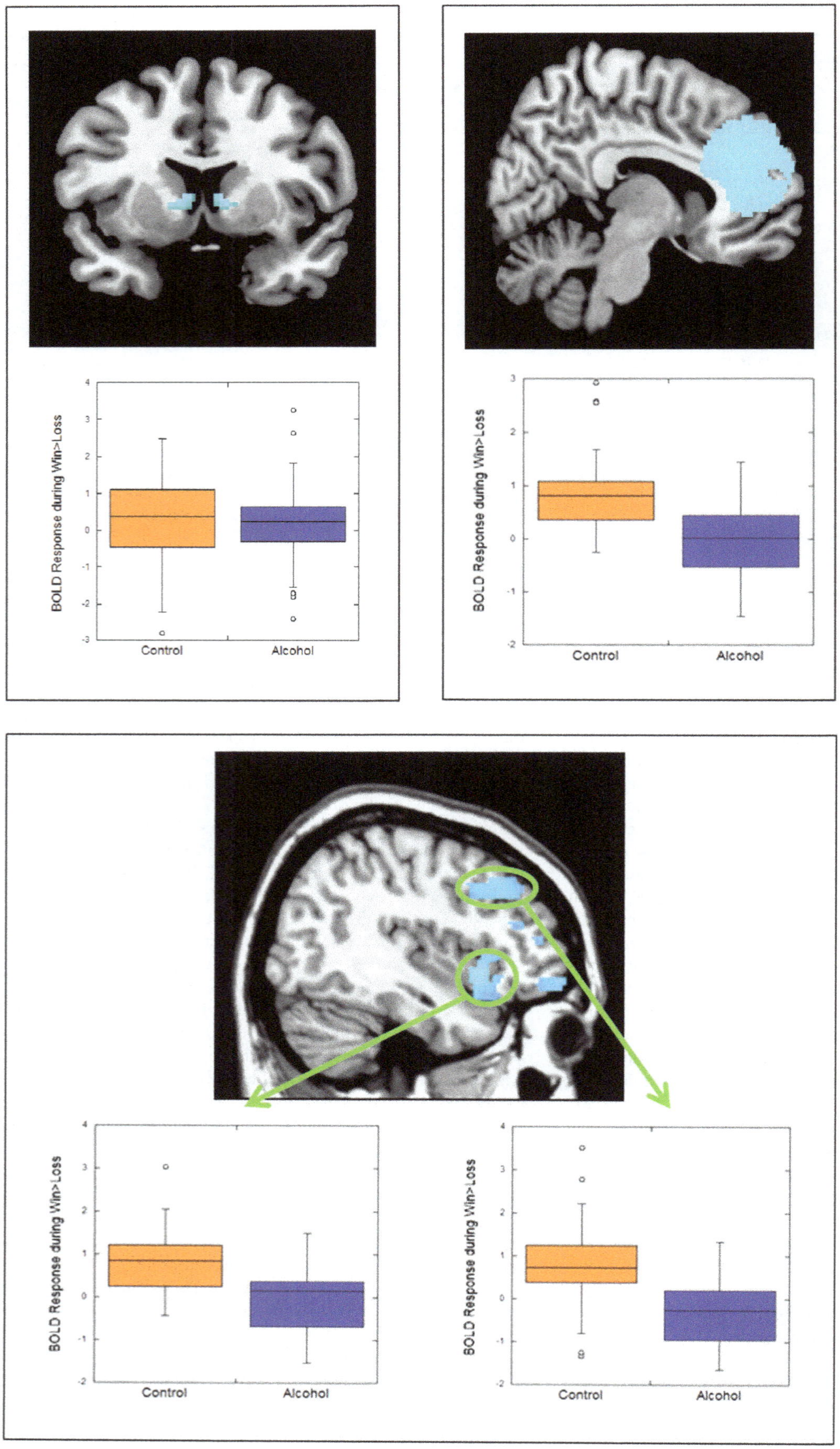
BOLD Response during Win>Loss
Control
Alcohol
BOLD Response during Win>Loss
Control
Alcohol
BOLD Response during Win>Loss
Control
Alcohol
BOLD Response during Win>Loss
Control
Alcohol

Figure 2. Alcohol dependent adults exhibited less response to monetary win vs. loss than healthy adults in three prefrontal regions—the medial prefrontal cortex (top right panel), the lateral orbitofrontal cortex (bottom panel, left boxplot), and the dorsolateral prefrontal cortex (bottom panel, right boxplot)—as well as the ventral striatum (top left). Boxplots illustrate findings by depicting mean BOLD response across the entire indicated functional cluster for each region, by group.

drug rewards—in this case, money—and toward drug rewards [48]. Notably, the accompanying hypothesis that alcohol dependence is associated with altered frontostriatal functional connectivity during reward processing is not inconsistent with low VS response in alcohol dependence. Low response within the VS does not guarantee or preclude altered coordination with frontal regions during the experience of a task. To address this issue in greater depth, research designs that include both drug and non-drug rewards in a single fMRI paradigm will therefore be valuable in future studies. While our findings contribute to what is known about neural response to non-drug rewards in addiction, a more powerful examination of differences in response to drug rewards and non-drug rewards would be provided by fMRI paradigms that incorporate both types of reward.

Notably, we did not find that alcohol dependent adults differed from healthy adults in the response or functional connectivity of the medial OFC. Given the putative role of medial OFC in representing reward value [49], it is possible that our paradigm, with its fixed reward values, did not elicit meaningful differences related to alcohol dependence. The presence of findings for lateral but not medial OFC supports the value of considering these subregions of OFC separately. In addition, our findings for mPFC underscore the importance of considering the medial OFC (or ventral mPFC) distinct from the mPFC, as the two regions differ functionally and have distinct patterns of connectivity with the striatum [8]. Alternatively, alcohol dependence might be more strongly associated with altered function in prefrontal regions with a role in regulating or promoting flexibility in behavior.

Our analyses with drinking characteristics allowed us to elucidate some of the potential mechanisms of group differences between alcohol-dependent and healthy adults. Although we were limited somewhat by not having collected similar data from healthy participants, we were able to investigate the altered frontostriatal function within the alcohol dependent group in greater depth. Our study design did not focus on relapse or on the association of abstinence symptoms with frontostriatal function, but detailed examination of these issues will be worthwhile for future studies. In addition, the individual differences associated with the likelihood and timing of relapse could be a fruitful topic for investigations of the pathophysiology and course of alcohol dependence.

The current sample was somewhat unusual for a study of alcohol dependence because participants were young and high functioning, had no Axis I disorders, and were not seeking treatment. These characteristics allowed us to focus on the function in frontal regions that are components of dopamine systems with minimal confounding by ageing or long-term alcohol exposure. In addition, these sample characteristics allow us to

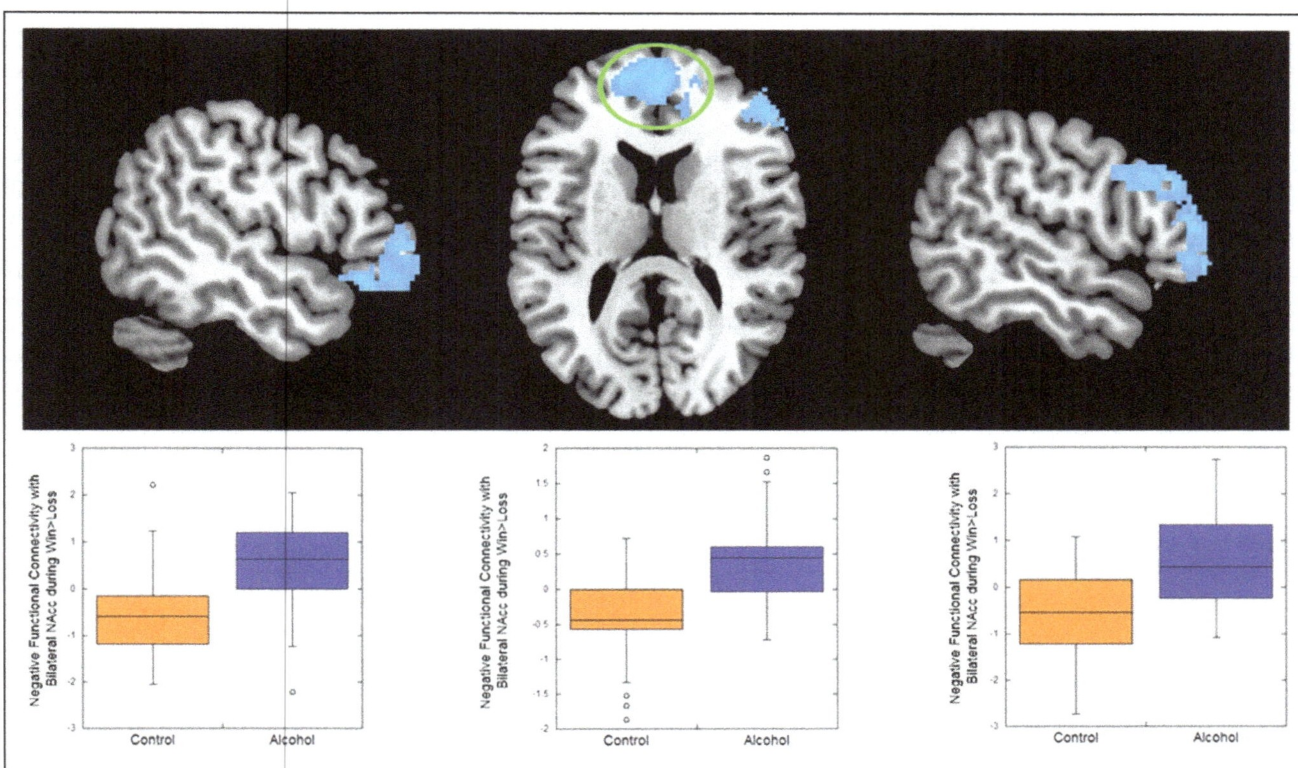

Figure 3. Alcohol dependent adults exhibited stronger negative functional connectivity than healthy adults between the bilateral nucleus accumbens and the lateral orbitofrontal cortex (left), medial prefrontal cortex (center), and the dorsolateral prefrontal cortex (right) during the receipt of monetary reward. Boxplots illustrate findings by depicting mean functional connectivity across the entire indicated functional cluster for each region, by group.

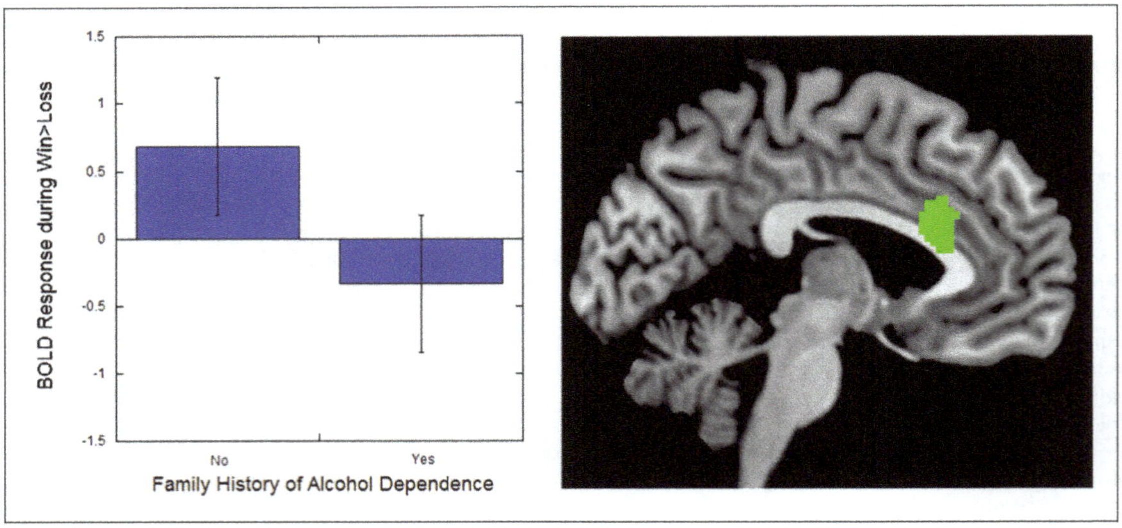

Figure 4. Alcohol dependent adults with a family history of alcohol use disorders exhibited less medial prefrontal response to monetary win vs. loss. The boxplot illustrates findings by depicting mean BOLD response across the entire indicated functional cluster, by family history group.

interpret our findings in light of the literature on frontostriatal function in young people at risk for alcohol dependence. We acknowledge that in many ways, the current study is more an examination of the pathophysiology of alcohol dependence than an examination of its development. Ideally, the field needs prospective studies that include the developmental window allowing assessment of the initiation of alcohol use and development of alcohol dependence. Relevant to this need, findings from the large, multisite IMAGEN consortium have contributed importantly to our understanding of the role of reward circuitry in young people at risk for addiction or early in the process of substance use (e.g., [50,51,52]). This study has reported that adolescents who are smokers [50], had prenatal exposure to nicotine [51], or had "potentially problematic" substance use [52] exhibit low VS responsiveness to reward. Similarly, although we were not able to examine brain function before and after onset of alcohol use or dependence, we note that our sample has unique features that allow us to investigate frontostriatal function early in the course of alcohol use problems.

Recent developmental findings have begun to elucidate the role of reward circuitry in the process of addiction. For instance, adolescents at high familial risk for alcohol use problems exhibit low DLPFC response during risky decision-making [53] and less VS response to reward [26], suggesting that altered prefrontal responding to reward could be an endophenotype present in those who are vulnerable to alcohol use problems before they have used alcohol. However, recent findings of the IMAGEN study indicate that the total contribution of response to reward in a set of reward-related neural regions (including PFC and VS) contributes only modestly to the initiation of alcohol use in early adolescence [54]. The authors of this study interpreted their findings as indicating that the function of reward circuitry contributes more importantly to the processes underlying the development of alcohol dependence than to those underlying the initiation of alcohol use. In distinction to our findings on altered frontostriatal connectivity, young adults at risk for alcohol dependence have been reported to exhibit altered functional connectivity between the accumbens and non-PFC regions such as the precuneus and supplementary sensorimotor area [55]. Together, these findings suggest that response in reward-related neural regions could differ for those with a family history of alcohol dependence but the absence of current problems. In contrast, rather than being a trait-like characteristic or precursor, altered functional connectivity between PFC and accumbens might instead emerge with the process of addiction.

Table 3. Association of Alcohol Dependent Adults' Drinking Characteristics with Function in Reward Circuitry.

Regions	BA	Cluster Size	*t*-score at peak voxel	Talairach coordinates of peak voxel		
				x	y	z
Family History, Negative Correlation						
mPFC	24,32	406	3.48	−1	16	29
Frequency of Use, Negative Functional Connectivity with Bilateral Nucleus Accumbens						
mPFC	10	257	2.99	−1	46	19

Note: Analyses were thresholded at $p_{corrected}<0.05$ using AlphaSim and were constrained using findings for group differences in which the alcohol dependent group exhibited less response than the healthy control group. The contrast generated from the reward task was win > loss. Age was included as a covariate in model of frequency of use. Cluster size is in voxels. mPFC: medial prefrontal cortex.

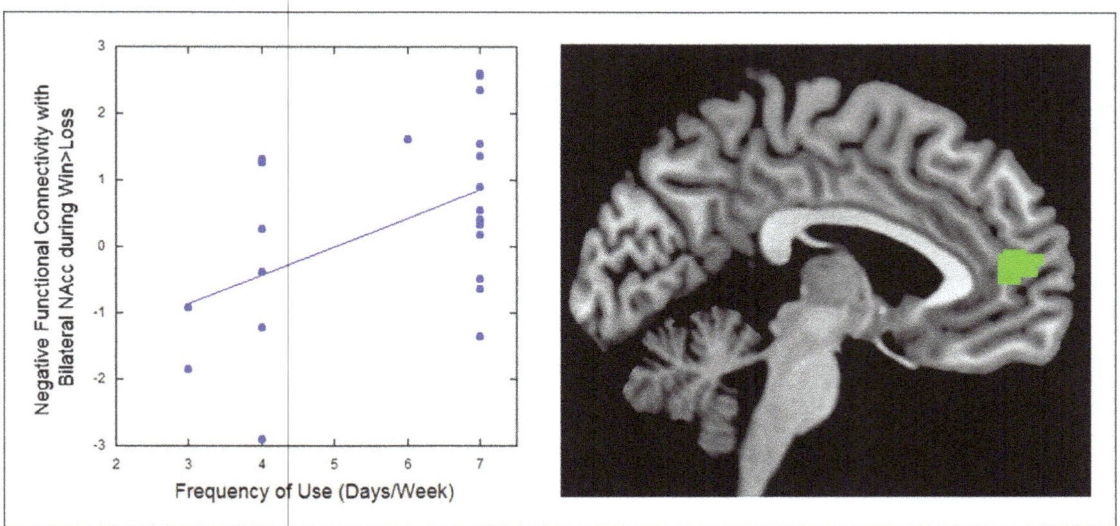

Figure 5. Alcohol dependent adults with more frequent alcohol use exhibited stronger negative connectivity between the bilateral nucleus accumbens and the medial prefrontal cortex and medial orbitofrontal cortex during the receipt of monetary reward. The scatterplot illustrates findings by depicting mean functional connectivity across the entire indicated mPFC functional cluster (y axis) in relation to frequency score (x axis).

Current and past findings cannot definitively settle the meaning of our findings of altered PFC function and frontostriatal connectivity, but they provide a context for understanding these findings. Without a prospective, longitudinal design, it is impossible to separate the role of frontostriatal function as a potential influence on the development of alcohol dependence from its function as a consequence or correlate of alcohol dependence. Indeed, our sample of alcohol-dependent adults, while relatively early in development and relatively young among alcohol-dependent adults, had spent an average of 10 years drinking. This exposure to alcohol is likely to have influenced function in frontostriatal circuitry, especially given its developmental timing. Notably, exposure to alcohol can have particularly pernicious effects on brain development [56,57], and our sample may be valuable for studying the consequences of early-onset alcohol-use problems. Furthermore, given the changes of function in reward circuitry during adolescent development [34,58,59], studies must also account for developmental processes as well as alcohol exposure and addiction as longitudinal influences on reward circuitry. More specifically, prospective studies should examine changes in VS response (i.e., possible decreases in sensitivity to non-drug reward stimuli over time), PFC response (i.e., stably low or decreasing level of response to reward), and frontostriatal connectivity (i.e., negative correlation between VS response and PFC response during reward processing).

Several other factors related to our sample composition constrain our interpretations. We were not able to examine sex differences, as our sampling strategy was designed to minimize differences by matching the alcohol dependent and healthy control groups for this and other demographic characteristics. We did not measure cognitive ability (e.g., IQ) or match groups on it, but this characteristic could have contributed to function in the circuits of interest in the current study. In addition, we did not collect detailed information about family history of alcohol dependence beyond its presence or absence of a first- or second-degree relative. As a result, we were not able to investigate the effects of family history density (e.g., as applied in work by Stoltenberg et al. [60] and Zucker et al. [61]) or of alcohol dependence in particular family members (e.g., mothers) on neural response or functional connectivity. Finally, we did not collect data on alcohol use from participants in our healthy control group, and this would have allowed us to draw stronger conclusions about the mechanisms of group differences in frontostriatal function.

In sum, our findings provide evidence for hypofrontality and altered frontostriatal connectivity in young adults with alcohol dependence. Low responding in these regions, which have roles in self-regulation and higher cognitive function, likely contributes to the compulsive pursuit of alcohol, the poor behavioral flexibility, and the loss of control that accompany this disorder. In addition, altered functional connectivity between prefrontal regions and the VS indicates that coordination within reward circuitry is disrupted in alcohol dependence. Placed in the context of the literature on risk for alcohol dependence, these findings raise the hypothesis that weakening of frontal modulation of VS occurs early in the development of alcohol dependence.

Acknowledgments

We thank Ahmad Hariri for contributions to the development and design of this project. Disclaimer: The content is solely the responsibility of the authors and does not necessarily represent the official views of NIAAA or the National Institutes of Health.

Author Contributions

Conceived and designed the experiments: EEF RN. Performed the experiments: EEF EER RN. Analyzed the data: EEF EER SM. Contributed reagents/materials/analysis tools: EEF. Wrote the paper: EEF EER SM RN.

References

1. Everitt BJ, Robbins TW (2005) Neural systems of reinforcement for drug addiction: from actions to habits to compulsion. Nat Neurosci 8: 1481–1489.
2. Robinson TE, Berridge KC (2008) The incentive sensitization theory of addiction: some current issues. Philos Trans R Soc Lond B Biol Sci 363: 3137–3146.
3. Koob GF, Volkow ND (2010) Neurocircuitry of addiction. Neuropsychopharmacology 35: 217–238.
4. Koob GF (2013) Theoretical frameworks and mechanistic aspects of alcohol addiction: alcohol addiction as a reward deficit disorder. Curr Top Behav Neurosci 13: 3–30.
5. Everitt BJ, Robbins TW (2013) From the ventral to the dorsal striatum: Devolving views of their roles in drug addiction. Neurosci Biobehav Rev. 37: 1946–1954.
6. Goldstein RZ, Volkow ND (2011) Dysfunction of the prefrontal cortex in addiction: neuroimaging findings and clinical implications. Nat Rev Neurosci 12: 652–669.
7. Lodge DJ (2011) The medial prefrontal and orbitofrontal cortices differentially regulate dopamine system function. Neuropsychopharmacology 36: 1227–1236.
8. Haber SN, Knutson B (2010) The reward circuit: linking primate anatomy and human imaging. Neuropsychopharmacology 35: 4–26.
9. Elliott R, Dolan RJ, Frith CD (2000) Dissociable functions in the medial and lateral orbitofrontal cortex: evidence from human neuroimaging studies. Cereb Cortex 10: 308–317.
10. Elliott R, Agnew Z, Deakin JF (2010) Hedonic and informational functions of the human orbitofrontal cortex. Cereb Cortex 20: 198–204.
11. Kalivas PW, Volkow ND (2005) The neural basis of addiction: a pathology of motivation and choice. Am J Psychiatry 162: 1403–1413.
12. Volkow ND, Wang GJ, Telang F, Fowler JS, Logan J, et al. (2007) Profound decreases in dopamine release in striatum in detoxified alcoholics: possible orbitofrontal involvement. J Neurosci 27: 12700–12706.
13. Beck A, Wustenberg T, Genauck A, Wrase J, Schlagenhauf F, et al. (2012) Effect of brain structure, brain function, and brain connectivity on relapse in alcohol-dependent patients. Arch Gen Psychiatry 69: 842–852.
14. Bari A, Robbins TW (2013) Inhibition and impulsivity: Behavioral and neural basis of response control. Prog Neurobiol. 108:44–79.
15. Volkow ND, Fowler JS, Wang GJ, Baler R, Telang F (2009) Imaging dopamine's role in drug abuse and addiction. Neuropharmacology 56 Suppl 1: 3–8.
16. Braus DF, Wrase J, Grusser S, Hermann D, Ruf M, et al. (2001) Alcohol-associated stimuli activate the ventral striatum in abstinent alcoholics. J Neural Transm 108: 887–894.
17. George MS, Anton RF, Bloomer C, Teneback C, Drobes DJ, et al. (2001) Activation of prefrontal cortex and anterior thalamus in alcoholic subjects on exposure to alcohol-specific cues. Arch Gen Psychiatry 58: 345–352.
18. Heinz A, Siessmeier T, Wrase J, Hermann D, Klein S, et al. (2004) Correlation between dopamine D(2) receptors in the ventral striatum and central processing of alcohol cues and craving. Am J Psychiatry 161: 1783–1789.
19. Wrase J, Grusser SM, Klein S, Diener C, Hermann D, et al. (2002) Development of alcohol-associated cues and cue-induced brain activation in alcoholics. Eur Psychiatry 17: 287–291.
20. Beck A, Schlagenhauf F, Wustenberg T, Hein J, Kienast T, et al. (2009) Ventral striatal activation during reward anticipation correlates with impulsivity in alcoholics. Biol Psychiatry 66: 734–742.
21. Wrase J, Schlagenhauf F, Kienast T, Wüstenberg T, Bermpohl F, et al. (2007) Dysfunction of reward processing correlates with alcohol craving in detoxified alcoholics. Neuroimage 35: 787–794.
22. Grüsser SM, Wrase J, Klein S, Hermann D, Smolka MN, et al. (2004) Cue-induced activation of the striatum and medial prefrontal cortex is associated with subsequent relapse in abstinent alcoholics. Psychopharmacology 175: 296–302.
23. Alfonso-Loeches S, Guerri C (2011) Molecular and behavioral aspects of the actions of alcohol on the adult and developing brain. Crit Rev Clin Lab Sci 48: 19–47.
24. Hingson RW, Heeren T, Winter MR (2006) Age at drinking onset and alcohol dependence: age at onset, duration, and severity. Arch Pediatr Adolesc Med 160: 739–746.
25. Dreher JC, Meyer-Lindenberg A, Kohn P, Berman KF (2008) Age-related changes in midbrain dopaminergic regulation of the human reward system. Proc Natl Acad Sci U S A 105: 15106–15111.
26. Yau WY, Zubieta JK, Weiland BJ, Samudra PG, Zucker RA, et al. (2012) Nucleus accumbens response to incentive stimuli anticipation in children of alcoholics: relationships with precursive behavioral risk and lifetime alcohol use. J Neurosci 32: 2544–2551.
27. Braskie MN, Wilcox CE, Landau SM, O'Neil JP, Baker SL, et al. (2008) Relationship of striatal dopamine synthesis capacity to age and cognition. J Neurosci 28: 14320–14328.
28. First MB, Spitzer RL, Gibbon M, Williams JBW (2002) Structured Clinical Interview for DSM-IV-TR Axis I Disorders, Research Version, Non-patient Edition. (SCID-I/NP). New York: Biometrics Research, New York State Psychiatric Institute.
29. Forbes EE, Brown SM, Kimak M, Ferrell RE, Manuck SB, et al. (2009) Genetic variation in components of dopamine neurotransmission impacts ventral striatal reactivity associated with impulsivity. Mol Psychiatry 14: 60–70.
30. Levy DJ, Glimcher PW (2012) The root of all value: a neural common currency for choice. Curr Opin Neurobiol 22: 1027–1038.
31. Rudebeck PH, Murray EA (2011) Balkanizing the primate orbitofrontal cortex: distinct subregions for comparing and contrasting values. Ann N Y Acad Sci 1239: 1–13.
32. Crunelle CL, Veltman DJ, Booij J, Emmerik-van Oortmerssen K, van den Brink W (2012) Substrates of neuropsychological functioning in stimulant dependence: a review of functional neuroimaging research. Brain Behav 2: 499–523.
33. Forbes EE, Hariri AR, Martin SL, Silk JS, Moyles DL, et al. (2009) Altered striatal activation predicting real-world positive affect in adolescent major depressive disorder. Am J Psychiatry 166: 64–73.
34. Forbes EE, Ryan ND, Phillips ML, Manuck SB, Worthman CM, et al. (2010) Healthy adolescents' neural response to reward: associations with puberty, positive affect, and depressive symptoms. J Am Acad Child Adolesc Psychiatry 49: 162–172 e161–165.
35. Phillips ML, Ladouceur CD, Drevets WC (2008) A neural model of voluntary and automatic emotion regulation: implications for understanding the pathophysiology and neurodevelopment of bipolar disorder. Mol Psychiatry 13: 829, 833–857.
36. Wallis JD (2007) Orbitofrontal cortex and its contribution to decision-making. Annu Rev Neurosci 30: 31–56.
37. Volkow ND, Tomasi D, Wang GJ, Fowler JS, Telang F, et al. (2011) Positive emotionality is associated with baseline metabolism in orbitofrontal cortex and in regions of the default network. Mol Psychiatry 16: 818–825.
38. Rushworth MF, Noonan MP, Boorman ED, Walton ME, Behrens TE (2011) Frontal cortex and reward-guided learning and decision-making. Neuron 70: 1054–1069.
39. Fecteau S, Fregni F, Boggio PS, Camprodon JA, Pascual-Leone A (2010) Neuromodulation of decision-making in the addictive brain. Subst Use Misuse 45: 1766–1786.
40. Hare TA, Camerer CF, Rangel A (2009) Self-control in decision-making involves modulation of the vmPFC valuation system. Science 324: 646–648.
41. Dixon ML, Christoff K (2012) The decision to engage cognitive control is driven by expected reward-value: neural and behavioral evidence. PLoS One 7: e51637.
42. Vago DR, Silbersweig DA (2012) Self-awareness, self-regulation, and self-transcendence (S-ART): a framework for understanding the neurobiological mechanisms of mindfulness. Front Hum Neurosci 6: 296.
43. Li CS, Luo X, Yan P, Bergquist K, Sinha R (2009) Altered impulse control in alcohol dependence: neural measures of stop signal performance. Alcohol Clin Exp Res 33: 740–750.
44. Claus ED, Ewing SW, Filbey FM, Sabbineni A, Hutchison KE (2011) Identifying neurobiological phenotypes associated with alcohol use disorder severity. Neuropsychopharmacology 36: 2086–2096.
45. Park SQ, Kahnt T, Beck A, Cohen MX, Dolan RJ, et al. (2010) Prefrontal cortex fails to learn from reward prediction errors in alcohol dependence. J Neurosci 30: 7749–7753.
46. Bjork JM, Knutson B, Hommer DW (2008) Incentive-elicited striatal activation in adolescent children of alcoholics. Addiction 103: 1308–1319.
47. Etkin A, Egner T, Kalisch R (2011) Emotional processing in anterior cingulate and medial prefrontal cortex. Trends Cogn Sci 15: 85–93.
48. Murphy A, Taylor E, Elliott R (2012) The detrimental effects of emotional process dysregulation on decision-making in substance dependence. Front Integr Neurosci 6: 101.
49. Liu X, Hairston J, Schrier M, Fan J (2011) Common and distinct networks underlying reward valence and processing stages: a meta-analysis of functional neuroimaging studies. Neurosci Biobehav Rev 35: 1219–1236.
50. Peters J, Bromberg U, Schneider S, Brassen S, Menz M, et al. (2011) Lower ventral striatal activation during reward anticipation in adolescent smokers. Am J Psychiatry 168: 540–549.
51. Müller KU, Mennigen E, Ripke S, Banaschewski T, Barker GJ, et al. (2013) Altered reward processing in adolescents with prenatal exposure to maternal cigarette smoking. JAMA Psychiatry 70: 847–856.
52. Schneider S, Peters J, Bromberg U, Brassen S, Miedl SF, et al. (2012) Risk taking and the adolescent reward system: a potential common link to substance abuse. Am J Psychiatry 169: 39–46.
53. Cservenka A, Nagel BJ (2012) Risky decision-making: an FMRI study of youth at high risk for alcoholism. Alcohol Clin Exp Res 36: 604–615.
54. Nees F, Tzschoppe J, Patrick CJ, Vollstadt-Klein S, Steiner S, et al. (2012) Determinants of early alcohol use in healthy adolescents: the differential contribution of neuroimaging and psychological factors. Neuropsychopharmacology 37: 986–995.
55. Weiland BJ, Welsh RC, Yau WY, Zucker RA, Zubieta JK, et al. (2013) Accumbens functional connectivity during reward mediates sensation-seeking and alcohol use in high-risk youth. Drug Alcohol Depend 128: 130–139.
56. Selemon LD (2013) A role for synaptic plasticity in the adolescent development of executive function. Transl Psychiatry 3: e238.

57. Spear LP (2013) Adolescents and alcohol: Acute sensitivities, enhanced intake, and later consequences. Neurotoxicol Teratol. 41C: 51–59.
58. Bjork JM, Knutson B, Fong GW, Caggiano DM, Bennett SM, et al. (2004) Incentive-elicited brain activation in adolescents: Similarities and differences from young adults. J Neurosci 24: 1793–1802.
59. Galvan A, Hare TA, Parra CE, Penn J, Voss H, et al. (2006) Earlier development of the accumbens relative to orbitofrontal cortex might underlie risk-taking behavior in adolescents. J Neurosci 26: 6885–6892.
60. Stoltenberg SF, Mudd SA, Blow FC, Hill EM (1998) Evaluating measures of family history of alcoholism: density versus dichotomy. Addiction 93: 1511–1520.
61. Zucker RA, Ellis DA, Fitzgerald HE (1994) Developmental evidence for at least two alcoholisms. I. Biopsychosocial variation among pathways into symptomatic difficulty. Ann N Y Acad Sci 708:134–146.
62. Skinner HA, Horn JL (1984) Alcohol Dependence Scale: Users' Guide. Toronto, Canada: Addiction Research Foundation.

On the Relationship between the Indirectly Measured Attitude Towards Beer and Beer Consumption: The Role of Attitude Accessibility

Mathilde Descheemaeker[1]*, Adriaan Spruyt[2], Dirk Hermans[1]

1 Faculty of Psychology and Educational Sciences, KU Leuven, Leuven, Belgium, **2** Faculty of Psychology and Educational Sciences, Ghent University, Ghent, Belgium

Abstract

Although some studies have demonstrated that the indirectly measured attitude towards alcohol is related to alcohol use, this relationship has not always been confirmed. In the current study, we attempted to shed light on this issue by investigating whether the predictive validity of an indirect attitude measure is dependent upon attitude accessibility. In a sample of 88 students, the picture-picture naming task, an adaptation of the affective priming paradigm, was used to measure the automatically activated attitude towards beer. Attitude accessibility was measured using a speeded evaluative categorization task. Behavioral measures were the amount of beer poured and drunk during a bogus taste test and the choice between a bottle of beer or water at the end of the experiment. In line with our hypothesis, the indirectly measured attitude towards beer predicted behavior during the taste test only when it was highly accessible. In contrast, this attitude was related to choice behavior irrespective of attitude accessibility. This study confirms that indirect attitude measures can be valuable predictors of alcohol-related behavior, but that it is sometimes necessary to take attitude accessibility into account.

Editor: Ingmar H. A. Franken, Erasmus University Rotterdam, Netherlands

Funding: Mathilde Descheemaeker is a research assistant of the Flemish Research Foundation; Adriaan Spruyt is a Postdoctoral Fellow of the Flemish Research Foundation (FWO - Vlaanderen; www.fwo.be). The funders had no role in study design, data collection and analysis, decision to publish, or preparation of the manuscript.

Competing Interests: The authors have declared that no competing interests exist.

* E-mail: mathilde.descheemaeker@ppw.kuleuven.be

Introduction

Alcohol use can lead to a host of negative outcomes, which is most clearly seen in phenomena such as addiction and binge drinking. It is therefore important to study the psychological factors that are related to alcohol use. This knowledge will increase our understanding of the processes at play in alcohol abuse and addiction and will eventually lead to the development of prevention and treatment strategies.

One factor that has been related to alcohol use is the attitude one holds towards alcohol. Traditionally, attitudes are measured directly by means of self-report rating scales. However, the predictive validity of these direct attitude measures can be limited by a lack of introspective capacity [1] and measurement artifacts such as impression management and demand characteristics [2,3]. This is not the case for more recently developed indirect attitude measures, which do not rely on self-report. Instead, an individual's automatically activated attitude towards certain (classes of) stimuli is inferred from the speed or accuracy with which the individual responds to these (classes of) stimuli during certain tasks. Well-known indirect attitude measures are the Implicit Association Test (IAT) [4], the Affective Priming Task (APT) [5], and the affect misattribution procedure [6]. As an example, consider the APT, which is used in the present study. This task requires participants to respond as quickly as possible to positive and negative target stimuli (e.g., to categorize these targets as positive or negative). Each target is preceded by a prime stimulus for which the attitudinal meaning is under investigation. There is reliable evidence showing that the evaluative connotation of the prime is automatically activated and that this leads to an affective priming effect: Performance is faster and more accurate when the prime and the target are affectively congruent than when these stimuli are affectively incongruent ([7,8], see [9] for a meta-analysis). Accordingly, the APT can be used as a measure of participants' automatically activated attitudes towards the prime stimuli (e.g., [10]).

While these indirect attitude measures all aim to measure automatic attitude activation, it is clear that effects on these measures are driven by different underlying processes [11–13]. For example, some studies suggest that the APT captures the automatically activated attitude towards the specific exemplars used, while the IAT is more sensitive to the attitude towards categories of stimuli ([14,15], but see [16,17]).

Recent meta-analyses have demonstrated that indirect attitude measures are predictive of behavior over and above the predictive value of direct attitude measures [18,19]. Also, Greenwald et al. [19] showed that the degree of social sensitivity of a research topic limits the predictive validity of a direct attitude measure to a much greater extent than it does that of an indirect attitude measure. As alcohol use can be a socially sensitive topic and automatic processes have been shown to play an important role in problematic drinking [20,21], indirect attitude measures are increasingly used in this research domain. There is now substantial evidence showing that alcohol use is related to the indirectly measured attitude towards alcohol (mostly measured with the IAT), even after controlling for the variance explained by the self-reported attitude [19,22–24]. Thush and Wiers [25], for example, observed that an IAT measure of the attitude towards alcohol was predictive of the frequency of binge drinking one year later in a sample of adolescents. Moreover, this effect was found over and above the variance explained by a direct measure of alcohol outcome expectancies. Similarly, Payne, Govorun, and Arbuckle ([26], Study 1) showed that the attitude towards beer relative to water as measured by the affect misattribution procedure predicted the choice students made between beer and water.

It may be noted, however, that most studies conducted so far have relied on self-report measures of alcohol use as a dependent variable. Clearly, this type of measure is subject to the same biases and limitations as direct attitude measures [27]. Moreover, the relationship between indirect attitude measures and (often self-reported) alcohol use has not always been confirmed [23,24]. For example, in a recent set of three studies, an IAT measure of the attitude towards alcohol failed to predict alcohol consumption observed in a semi-naturalistic setting, although it was related to self-reported binge drinking and weekly consumption in two of these studies [28].

The mixed evidence concerning the contribution of indirect attitude measures to the prediction of alcohol use has initiated research into the moderators of this relationship. For example, several studies have provided evidence that indirect attitude measures are more predictive of alcohol-related behavior when the capacity for self-control is low [29–31]. Surprisingly little attention has been paid, however, to the extensive literature in the domain of social cognition concerning the determinants of attitude-behavior consistency. In this tradition, attitude characteristics such as attitude stability, ambivalence, and accessibility have repeatedly been shown to moderate the relationship between directly measured attitudes and behavior (see [32–34] for meta-analyses). Nevertheless, this literature is seldom drawn upon in the field of experimental psychopathology in general and when using indirectly measured attitudes as a predictor of alcohol use in particular.

Therefore, the aim of the present study was to examine whether attitude accessibility acts as a moderator of the relationship between the indirectly measured attitude towards alcohol and alcohol use. Attitude accessibility is a component of attitude strength and refers to the ease with which an attitude can be retrieved from memory [35]. Fazio and colleagues (e.g., [5]) proposed an attitude-nonattitude continuum ranging from attitudes that have to be constructed on the spot (because there is no a priori evaluation available) to highly accessible attitudes. Crucially, while there is ample evidence showing that the consistency between self-reported attitudes and behavior is higher when these attitudes are more accessible ([36], see [32–34] for meta-analyses on this topic), it remains largely unexplored whether this is also the case when attitudes are measured indirectly. The only study to our knowledge that relates to this research question showed that a self-activation manipulation (which is assumed to increase the accessibility of self-related knowledge) increased the predictive validity of the IAT for several behaviors, including self-reported alcohol consumption [37].

Current Study

Because alcohol is a heterogeneous category and the attitudes towards subcategories can differ, we decided to focus on beer in the current study. Not only did we investigate the relationship between the indirectly measured attitude towards beer and self-reported beer consumption, we also attempted to predict behavior that was registered during the experiment. More specifically, we registered (a) the amount of beer relative to water participants poured and (b) drank during a bogus taste test and (c) whether participants chose to take home a bottle of beer or water at the end of the experiment. Behaviors during the taste test were relative (beer in comparison to water) to control for factors that can influence beer consumption but are not related to the attitude towards beer (e.g., thirst).

Attitude accessibility is typically measured as the response latency of evaluation: The faster an attitude object can be evaluated, the more accessible the attitude towards this object [36]. In line with previous studies (e.g., [38–40]), we controlled for inter-individual differences in the speed of evaluation that are unrelated to differences in attitude accessibility. This was done by operationalizing the accessibility of the attitude towards beer as the difference in response latency between the evaluative categorization of beer stimuli (positive versus negative) and the non-evaluative categorization of beer stimuli (beer versus water, hereafter referred to as semantic categorization).

As an indirect measure of the attitude towards beer relative to water, we opted for the picture-picture naming task (PPNT) [41]. In this version of the APT, primes and targets are pictures and participants are asked to name the targets as quickly as possible. This task has been shown to predict behavior over and above direct attitude measures in previous research [41–43]. We hypothesized that the predictive validity of the PPNT would be most pronounced in participants whose attitude towards beer was highly accessible.

Method

Ethics Statement

This study was approved by the ethical committee of the KU Leuven and all participants gave written informed consent.

Participants

Eighty-eight first-year psychology students participated in partial fulfillment of a course requirement (70 women; age: $M = 18.6$, $SD = 0.8$). To avoid self-selection bias, students were not informed that they would be asked to taste beer before they signed up. All participants were native Dutch speakers and had normal or corrected-to-normal vision. Because a small amount of alcohol was to be consumed during the experiment, we used the following exclusion criteria: pregnancy, past or current alcohol abuse, use of medication that should not be combined with alcohol, and a medical condition that contraindicates alcohol consumption.

Apparatus and Stimuli

Computer tasks were run on an AMD Athlon XP computer with a 16-inch CRT monitor (85 Hz, resolution 1024×768). Affect 4.0 software [44] controlled stimulus presentation and registered responses. Additionally, we used a response box with two keys during the categorization tasks and an external voice key during the PPNT.

All visual stimuli used during the experiment had a dimension of 512 by 384 pixels and were presented against the black background of the computer monitor. As PPNT targets, we selected four positive pictures (bride, Christmas tree, puppy, sun) and four negative pictures (fire, gun, trash, worms) on the basis of a preliminary study during which 51 students rated the affective connotation of 215 real life color pictures [45]. Each target picture could be named with a single Dutch word. Participants in the current experiment rated the positive targets as significantly more positive than the negative targets on a scale ranging from −10 (*very negative*) to 10 (*very positive*), $M_{positive} = 7.66$ ($SD = 0.65$), $M_{negative} = -7.84$ ($SD = 0.63$), $t(6) = 34.12$, $p < .001$. Primes were eight pictures of beer (seven of which clearly depicted a brand) and eight pictures of still water (seven of which clearly depicted a brand). These beverages were presented on a white background in order to reduce the influence of stimulus characteristics unrelated to the type of beverage. For the practice trials, we used four neutral pictures (cup, glasses, hammer, spoon) as primes. During the attitude accessibility measure (evaluative and semantic categorization tasks), participants were presented with the same eight beer and eight water pictures used during the PPNT. Additionally, during the evaluative categorization task, we used eight clearly positive pictures and eight clearly negative pictures as filler stimuli. We used different stimuli during the practice trials (two positive and two negative pictures for the evaluative categorization task and two beer and two water pictures for the semantic categorization task). Positive, negative, and neutral pictures were also selected on the basis of the previously mentioned study by Spruyt et al. [45].

Procedure

Participants were tested individually in a sound-attenuated room and the lights were dimmed during the computer tasks. The experiment was introduced as an investigation of the evaluation of different brands of beer and still water. The experiment proceeded as follows: Participants first completed the attitude accessibility measure, followed by a filler task, the PPNT, a direct attitude measure, the bogus taste test, a questionnaire concerning beer and alcohol consumption, and the choice of a beverage. To reduce the influence of the time of day on beer consumption during the taste test, the experiment always took place in the afternoon or evening.

To measure *attitude accessibility*, we asked participants to complete two speeded categorization tasks. The first was an evaluative categorization task, during which participants were instructed to categorize stimuli as positive or negative as quickly as possible using the response box. After this, participants completed a semantic categorization task, during which stimuli had to be categorized as beer or water. As described above, these stimuli were eight beer and eight water pictures. During the evaluative categorization task, eight positive and eight negative pictures were added as filler stimuli. Both tasks were made up of two blocks and each stimulus was presented once per block in a semi-random order (no more than two consecutive beer or water stimuli and no more than three consecutive filler stimuli). This resulted in 64 evaluative categorization trials and 32 semantic categorization trials. These trials started with a 500 ms presentation of a fixation cross and a 500 ms interval, followed by the presentation of the stimulus until participants responded. The inter-trial interval varied between 500 and 1500 ms with an average of 1000 ms. The assignment of the left and the right key of the response box to the responses positive/negative and beer/water was counterbalanced across participants. Before the experimental trials, participants received eight practice trials for each task (the practice stimuli described above were all presented twice). The experimenter was not present during the experimental trials.

Because participants expressed their attitude towards beer and water repeatedly during the evaluative categorization task and attitude rehearsal has been shown to strengthen attitude accessibility [36], one might argue that this task was not only a measure, but also an (unintended) manipulation of attitude accessibility. To reduce this influence, we administered a *filler task* (a simple experiment on causal learning of the type reviewed by De Houwer and Beckers [46]) before continuing the experiment. This task lasted approximately 15 minutes.

We used the *PPNT* as an indirect attitude measure. This task started with three series of practice trials. First, participants viewed all the targets (four positive and four negative pictures) one by one, together with their correct name. They were instructed to read the name of each target out loud, to remember it, and to press the space bar when they were ready for the next target. During the second series of practice trials, the targets were presented a second time, but without their corresponding names. Participants were asked to name each target as quickly as possible. During these and all subsequent trials, a trial ended when the voice key was triggered or 2000 ms had elapsed. The experimenter used the keyboard to code whether the voice key had been triggered accurately and whether the participant's response was correct. The third series of practice trials was identical to the actual priming trials, but four neutral pictures were used as primes and each target was presented twice. During the actual priming phase, all primes (eight beer and eight water pictures) and targets were combined, resulting in 128 trials. Participants were instructed to continue naming the targets as quickly as possible, without taking the primes into account. Each trial started with a 500 ms presentation of a fixation cross and a 500 ms interval, after which the prime was presented for 200 ms. Immediately after the prime, the target was presented, resulting in a stimulus onset asynchrony of 200 ms. The inter-trial interval varied between 500 and 1500 ms with an average of 1000 ms. The actual priming trials were divided into four blocks (32 trials per block) in such a way that each block contained the same amount of the different trial types. Within these blocks, trials were presented in a random order. Blocks were separated by instructions reminding participants to name the targets as quickly as possible.

As a final computer task, participants filled out several rating scales. They were asked to evaluate the target and the prime pictures on a scale ranging from −10 (*very negative*) to 10 (*very positive*). On the same scale, they indicated their evaluation of beer, alcohol, and water in general. They also reported how much they liked drinking beer, alcohol, and water on a scale ranging from 0 (*not at all*) to 10 (*very much*). With the exception of the evaluation of the targets, these rating scales were used to *measure attitudes directly*.

Next, during the *bogus taste test*, participants were asked to fill out a form concerning their ratings of three unidentified brands of beer and three unidentified brands of still water on different taste-related characteristics. The order of beer and water on the form was counterbalanced across participants. We used beer low in alcohol content (alcohol by volume < 1%), but participants were not informed of this. At the end of the experiment, participants were asked to estimate the alcohol content of the tasted beers on a scale ranging from 0 (*no alcohol*) to 6 (*very high alcohol content*). Only one participant gave a score of 0, six participants gave a score of 1, and the average rating was 2.87 ($SD = 1.03$). We presented participants with three pitchers of beer and three pitchers of water, each filled with 125 (±2) grams of liquid, and a plastic cup for each beverage. Unbeknown to participants, behavioral measures were the amount of beer drunk and poured subtracted by the amount of water drunk and poured respectively. We told participants that we would throw away what was left in the pitchers and that they could drink more than was necessary to fill out the taste test form. The experimenter was not present during this task and participants could take as much time as they wanted.

At the end of the experiment, participants filled out a *questionnaire about beer and alcohol consumption*. This questionnaire consisted of eight items relating to the frequency, amount, and negative consequences of the consumption of beer and alcohol (assessed separately) in daily life.

As a final behavioral measure, participants were presented with the *choice between a bottle of beer* (with a standard alcohol content) *and a bottle of water* to take home. They were told this was a small token of appreciation for their participation. Participants made this choice when leaving the lab and the experimenter was in an adjacent room at this time.

Results

Data Reduction

Four participants were excluded from the analyses: one participant because of an unusually large amount of errors (50%) during the semantic categorization task, one participant because of an experimenter error during the administration of the taste test, and two participants because we were not able to accurately register a response on more than 25% of the PPNT trials (due to technical errors in the activation of the voice key, naming errors, or the absence of a response within the 2000 ms response window). This resulted in a sample of 84 students (68 women) between 18 and 23 years old ($M = 18.6$, $SD = 0.8$). All data can be obtained by contacting the corresponding author.

With regard to the categorization tasks, two trials with a response latency of 1 ms and two trials during which a participant interrupted the task to ask a question were not included in the analyses. In addition, semantic categorization trials on which an incorrect response was given (categorizing beer as water or vice versa; 1.7%) were excluded. Finally, to reduce the impact of outlying values, we discarded response latencies that deviated more than 2.5 standard deviations from a participant's mean latency for each trial type (e.g., evaluative categorization trials with beer stimuli; 2.6%; see [47]). The accessibility of the attitude towards beer was calculated by subtracting the mean reaction time of semantic categorization of beer stimuli from the mean reaction time of evaluative categorization of beer stimuli (this means that a higher score corresponds with a less accessible attitude). The mean accessibility score was 408 ms with a standard deviation of 300 ms. We performed a tertile split to create a high, a moderate, and a low accessibility group.

We also excluded certain PPNT trials when calculating an affective priming score. If a participant rated a positive target as negative or vice versa, all trials with this target were excluded for this participant (this occurred six times). Trials on which a target was incorrectly named (1.7%), the voice key was not appropriately activated (5.0%), or no response had been given when 2000 ms had elapsed (0.1%) were also excluded. As for the categorization tasks, we discarded response latencies that deviated more than 2.5 standard deviations from a participant's mean latency for each trial type (e.g., trials with a beer prime followed by a positive target; 1.8%; see also [41]). Based on mean reaction times (RT) per trial type, the affective priming score was calculated as follows: (mean RT beer/negative – mean RT beer/positive) – (mean RT water/negative – mean RT water/positive). In this way, higher priming scores reflect a more positive automatically activated attitude towards beer relative to water. The mean priming score was −0.70 ms with a standard deviation of 25.63 ms. The internal consistency of this measure was determined by calculating the priming score for each beer prime relative to water (e.g., Stella: [mean RT Stella/negative – mean RT Stella/positive] – [mean RT water/negative – mean RT water/positive]) and subsequently computing Cronbach's α of a scale consisting of these priming scores. Internal consistency was acceptable for a performance-based measure (Cronbach's α of .63).

A composite score reflecting the directly measured attitude towards beer was calculated by averaging the evaluation of beer, the liking rating of beer (after transformation to a scale ranging from −10 to 10), and the mean evaluation of the beer primes. The directly measured attitude towards water was calculated in the same way. In line with the affective priming score, we used a relative measure that was calculated by subtracting the attitude towards water from the attitude towards beer. The mean of this direct measure of the attitude towards beer relative to water was −4.29 and the standard deviation was 6.02.

Due to the high correlation between the amount of beer relative to water poured ($M = -51.83$ g, $SD = 56.61$ g) and drunk ($M = -54.27$ g, $SD = 52.74$ g) during the taste test, $r(82) = .92$, $p < .001$, we created a composite measure by summing the standardized scores. To obtain a measure of self-reported beer consumption, we calculated the sum score of the standardized beer-related items of the questionnaire about beer and alcohol consumption. This measure demonstrated high internal consistency (Cronbach's α of .92).

Behavioral Prediction

To investigate whether the affective priming score explained unique variance in behavior, we conducted hierarchical regression analyses in which we controlled for the effects of gender and the directly measured attitude, which are known predictors of alcohol use. In this regard, it is relevant to mention that the directly and indirectly measured attitude towards beer relative to water were not correlated, $r(82) = -.00$, $p = .966$. We examined the moderating role of the accessibility of the attitude towards beer by testing whether the interaction effect between the accessibility and the priming score was significant. To that end, predictors were centered at their means in order to avoid multicollinearity. All significance tests were two-tailed.

Behavior during the taste test. Linear regression analysis (see Table 1) indicated that the affective priming score did not predict behavior during the taste test in the group as a whole. Since the interaction effect between the accessibility score and the priming score only just missed the conventional level of significance, we examined the predictive validity of the PPNT in each of the three accessibility groups (see Table 2). In line with our hypothesis, the priming score was a significant predictor of behavior during the taste test in the high accessibility group, but not in the moderate or low accessibility group. The standardized DFBeta statistic revealed one influential case (absolute value larger than 1) in the low accessibility group, but the effect of the priming score remained nonsignificant after excluding this participant.

Choice behavior. Fifty-eight participants chose to take home a bottle of water, 21 participants opted for a bottle of beer, and five participants did not make a choice. Logistic regression analysis (see Table 3) showed that the affective priming score was significantly related to participants' choice. There was no evidence that the accessibility of the attitude towards beer moderated this relationship, as the interaction effect between the accessibility and the priming score was not significant (and results were similar in the three accessibility groups).

Self-reported beer consumption. The affective priming score was not related to beer consumption in daily life as measured by the previously described questionnaire (see Table 4). There was also no evidence for a moderating role of attitude accessibility, as the interaction effect between the accessibility and the priming score was not significant (and results were similar in the three accessibility groups). Conclusions remained the same when we did not control for gender and the direct attitude measure and thus used only the affective priming score as a predictor.

Table 1. Hierarchical multiple linear regression analyses for the prediction of behavior during the taste test.

Predictor	ΔR^2	*P*	β	*t*	*p*
Step 1	.10	.017			
Gender[a]			0.02	0.20	.845
Direct attitude measure: beer relative to water[b]			0.32	2.79	.006
Step 2	.01	.381			
PPNT: beer relative to water			0.09	0.88	.381
Step 3	.00	.715			
Accessibility of the attitude towards beer[c]			−0.04	−0.37	.715
Step 4	.04	.060			
PPNT x Accessibility			−0.26	−1.91	.060

Note. Behavior during the taste test was the sum of the standardized amount of beer relative to water poured and the standardized amount of beer relative to water drunk. Predictors were centered at their means. PPNT = picture-picture naming task.
[a]Coded as 0 = male and 1 = female.
[b]Calculated by averaging the evaluation rating, liking rating (after transformation to a scale ranging from −10 to 10), and mean evaluation rating of the primes for beer and water separately and subsequently subtracting the composite score for water from the composite score for beer.
[c]Calculated by subtracting the mean reaction time of categorization of beer stimuli as beer from the mean reaction time of evaluative categorization of beer stimuli.

Direct attitude measure. Although the predictive validity of the direct attitude measure was not the focus of the present research, it is worth pointing out that, in contrast to what we would have expected, the direct attitude measure was predictive of behavior during the taste test only in the low accessibility group (see Table 2). In line with this finding, the interaction effect between attitude accessibility and the direct attitude measure was significant, $\beta = 0.29$, $t(79) = 2.43$, $p = .017$. To ensure that differences found between the three accessibility groups in the relationship of the PPNT with behavior during the taste test were not due to differences in the amount of variance already explained by the direct attitude measure, we repeated these analyses without controlling for the direct measure. Results were virtually identical:

Table 2. Hierarchical multiple linear regression analyses for the prediction of behavior during the taste test in the three accessibility groups.

Predictor	ΔR^2	*P*	β	*t*	*p*
High accessibility group (*n* = 28)					
Step 1	.04	.621			
Gender[a]			−0.15	−0.72	.476
Direct attitude measure: beer relative to water[b]			0.08	0.38	.705
Step 2	.25	.008			
PPNT: beer relative to water			0.50	2.89	.008
Moderate accessibility group (*n* = 28)					
Step 1	.09	.291			
Gender[a]			0.04	0.19	.855
Direct attitude measure: beer relative to water[b]			0.32	1.58	.128
Step 2	.00	.742			
PPNT: beer relative to water			−0.07	−0.33	.742
Low accessibility group (*n* = 28)					
Step 1	.20	.065			
Gender[a]			0.19	0.96	.346
Direct attitude measure: beer relative to water[b]			0.48	2.47	.021
Step 2	.02	.413			
PPNT: beer relative to water			−0.15	−0.83	.413

Note. Behavior during the taste test was the sum of the standardized amount of beer relative to water poured and the standardized amount of beer relative to water drunk. Groups were created by means of a tertile split. PPNT = picture-picture naming task.
[a]Coded as 0 = male and 1 = female.
[b]Calculated by averaging the evaluation rating, liking rating (after transformation to a scale ranging from −10 to 10), and mean evaluation rating of the primes for beer and water separately and subsequently subtracting the composite score for water from the composite score for beer.

Table 3. Hierarchical multiple logistic regression analyses for the prediction of choice behavior.

Predictor	ΔR^{2a}	χ^2	*p*	*OR*[b]	*Wald*	*p*
Step 1	.26	15.82	<.001			
Gender[c]				0.74	0.19	.664
Direct attitude measure: beer relative to water[d]				3.43	8.27	.004
Step 2	.10	6.65	.010			
PPNT: beer relative to water				2.21	5.76	.016
Step 3	.00	0.10	.755			
Accessibility of the attitude towards beer[e]				0.90	0.09	.759
Step 4	.01	0.45	.502			
PPNT x Accessibility				1.35	0.46	.497

Note. Choice behavior was coded as 0 = water and 1 = beer. Continuous predictors were standardized in order to facilitate the interpretation of the odds ratio. PPNT = picture-picture naming task.
[a]Nagelkerke R^2.
[b]The odds ratio of, for example, the PPNT score can be interpreted as follows: When the PPNT score increases by one standard deviation, the odds of choosing beer increase by a factor of 2.21 (given that gender and the directly measured attitude are held at a fixed value).
[c]Coded as 0 = male and 1 = female.
[d]Calculated by averaging the evaluation rating, liking rating (after transformation to a scale ranging from −10 to 10), and mean evaluation rating of the primes for beer and water separately and subsequently subtracting the composite score for water from the composite score for beer.
[e]Calculated by subtracting the mean reaction time of categorization of beer stimuli as beer from the mean reaction time of evaluative categorization of beer stimuli.

The affective priming score was predictive only in the high accessibility group.

Because of these unexpected results, we also tested this interaction effect for the other dependent variables. The relationship between choice behavior and the direct attitude measure was moderated by attitude accessibility in the expected direction, $OR = 0.27$, $Wald = 6.09$, $p = .014$. The standardized DFBeta statistic for the interaction effect revealed one influential case (absolute value larger than 1), but the interaction effect remained significant after excluding this participant. There was no evidence for a moderating role of attitude accessibility when predicting self-reported beer consumption, $|t| < 1$.

Discussion

Although some studies have shown the indirectly measured attitude towards alcohol to be related to alcohol use (e.g., [25,26]), other studies failed to provide corroborating evidence for this relationship (e.g., [28]; see [23] for a review). Drawing upon the social cognition literature concerning the moderators of the consistency between self-reported attitudes and behavior, we attempted to clarify these inconsistent results by investigating whether the predictive validity of an indirect attitude measure is dependent upon attitude accessibility. Results obtained when predicting the amount of beer poured and drunk during a bogus taste test confirmed our hypothesis: The attitude towards beer as measured by the PPNT was predictive in participants whose attitude towards beer was highly accessible, but not in participants who exhibited moderate or low levels of attitude accessibility. To

Table 4. Hierarchical multiple linear regression analyses for the prediction of self-reported beer consumption.

Predictor	ΔR^2	*p*	β	*t*	*p*
Step 1	.48	<.001			
Gender[a]			−0.04	−0.48	.632
Direct attitude measure: beer relative to water[b]			0.68	7.86	<.001
Step 2	.00	.770			
PPNT: beer relative to water			−0.02	−0.29	.770
Step 3	.02	.071			
Accessibility of the attitude towards beer[c]			−0.15	−1.83	.071
Step 4	.00	.564			
PPNT x Accessibility			0.06	0.58	.564

Note. Self-reported beer consumption was measured with a questionnaire that assessed amount, frequency, and negative consequences of beer consumption. Predictors were centered at their means. PPNT = picture-picture naming task.
[a]Coded as 0 = male and 1 = female.
[b]Calculated by averaging the evaluation rating, liking rating (after transformation to a scale ranging from −10 to 10), and mean evaluation rating of the primes for beer and water separately and subsequently subtracting the composite score for water from the composite score for beer.
[c]Calculated by subtracting the mean reaction time of categorization of beer stimuli as beer from the mean reaction time of evaluative categorization of beer stimuli.

our knowledge, this study is the first to demonstrate that attitude accessibility moderates attitude-behavior consistency when attitudes are measured indirectly. This finding offers a possible explanation as to why previous studies failed to find a relationship between indirectly measured attitudes and observed alcohol consumption, as these studies did not take attitude accessibility into account [28].

We did not find evidence, however, for a similar moderation effect when predicting the choice between a bottle of beer and a bottle of water at the end of the experiment. That is, the indirectly measured attitude towards beer was related to choice behavior irrespective of attitude accessibility. To account for this set of observations, one might argue that attitude accessibility will have less impact on attitude-behavior consistency when there is sufficient motivation and opportunity to engage in deliberative processing [36]. Unlike pouring and drinking behavior, choice behavior requires an explicit consultation of one's attitudes towards the different choice alternatives. As a result, a reduced impact of attitude accessibility can be expected. Alternatively, it could be argued that the absence of a moderation effect when looking at the behavioral choice data simply reflects a type II error. The observation that attitude accessibility did moderate the relationship between choice behavior and the *direct* attitude measure is consistent with this viewpoint. Irrespectively, it would be interesting to investigate whether the degree to which attitude accessibility impacts the relationship between an indirect attitude measure and behavior is itself moderated by the extent to which the criterion behavior requires deliberative processing.

An important advantage of the current study is that we did not rely solely on self-reported alcohol consumption, as was the case in the majority of previous studies on the relationship between indirect attitude measures and alcohol use, but also included measures of alcohol-related behavior registered during the experiment. The present study suggests that this is an important issue. Whereas the PPNT was able to predict behavior registered during the experiment, PPNT scores were unrelated to self-reported beer consumption. This data pattern is in line with the findings of Spruyt et al. [41], who used the PPNT as an indirect measure of the attitudes towards fruit and candy bars. In their study, the PPNT was found to be predictive of the choice between an apple or a Snickers candy bar at the end of the experiment, but was not related to self-reported consumption of these products. Interestingly, Spruyt et al. [41] also administered a candy/fruit IAT and found the exact opposite data pattern with this measure: The IAT was clearly related to self-reported consumption, but not to the actual choice behavior monitored during the experiment. Previous studies that did find evidence for a relationship between the indirectly measured attitude towards alcohol and self-reported drinking and/or drinking problems also used the IAT or the Extrinsic Affective Simon Test as an indirect attitude measure [23]. Taken together, it can be hypothesized that finding a relationship between an indirect attitude measure and self-reported alcohol consumption is dependent on the specific measure used. Evidence that different indirect attitude measures rely on different underlying processes (e.g., [11,12]) is clearly consistent with this reasoning. It would thus be interesting to examine whether different indirect attitude measures are predictive of different outcome measures.

Although not the focus of the current study, it may be noted that the accessibility of the attitude towards beer also moderated the relationship of the direct attitude measure with behavior during the taste test and choice behavior. To our surprise, however, the directly measured attitude towards beer was predictive of behavior during the taste test only in individuals who exhibited a low level of accessibility. This finding contrasts with previous studies showing a stronger relationship between direct attitude measures and behavior when attitudes are more accessible [32–34]. Moreover, when predicting choice behavior, we found a moderating effect in the expected direction. Therefore, it is probably wise not to put too much weight on this isolated finding.

A limitation of the current study is that we used a specific sample of largely female, first-year university students. Even though the processes under study are assumed to be universal, we cannot be sure that our findings generalize to the broader population. In particular, more research is needed to verify whether our findings generalize to a clinical population suffering from alcohol abuse or addiction.

In summary, we demonstrated that attitude accessibility can moderate the predictive validity of an indirect attitude measure. In addition, our findings suggest that the degree to which this moderating effect occurs might itself be dependent upon the precise nature of the behavior being examined. Although further research is needed to substantiate the latter claim, the results of the current study clearly indicate that future research concerning indirectly measured attitudes towards alcohol as a predictor of alcohol use should focus not only on the evaluative quality of these attitudes, but also on their accessibility.

Author Contributions

Conceived and designed the experiments: MD AS DH. Performed the experiments: MD. Analyzed the data: MD. Wrote the paper: MD AS DH.

References

1. Nisbett RE, Wilson TD (1977) Telling more than we can know: Verbal reports on mental processes. Psychol Rev 84: 231–259.
2. Schwarz N (1999) Self-reports: How the questions shape the answers. Am Psychol 54: 93–105.
3. Weber SJ, Cook TD (1972) Subject effects in laboratory research: An examination of subject roles, demand characteristics, and valid inference. Psychol Bull 77: 273–295.
4. Greenwald AG, McGhee DE, Schwartz JLK (1998) Measuring individual differences in implicit cognition: The Implicit Association Test. J Pers Soc Psychol 74: 1464–1480.
5. Fazio RH, Sanbonmatsu DM, Powell MC, Kardes FR (1986) On the automatic activation of attitudes. J Pers Soc Psychol 50: 229–238.
6. Payne BK, Cheng CM, Govorun O, Stewart BD (2005) An inkblot for attitudes: Affect misattribution as implicit measurement. J Pers Soc Psychol 89: 277–293.
7. Fazio RH (2001) On the automatic activation of associated evaluations: An overview. Cognition Emotion 15: 115–141.
8. Hermans D, De Houwer J, Eelen P (2001) A time course analysis of the affective priming effect. Cognition Emotion 15: 143–165.
9. Herring DR, White KR, Jabeen LN, Hinojos M, Terrazas G, et al. (2013) On the automatic activation of attitudes: A quarter century of evaluative priming research. Psychol Bull 139: 1062–1089.
10. Fazio RH, Jackson JR, Dunton BC, Williams CJ (1995) Variability in automatic activation as an unobtrusive measure of racial attitudes: A bona fide pipeline? J Pers Soc Psychol 69: 1013–1027.
11. Deutsch R, Gawronski B (2009) When the method makes a difference: Antagonistic effects on "automatic evaluations" as a function of task characteristics of the measure. J Exp Soc Psychol 45: 101–114.
12. Fazio RH, Olson MA (2003) Implicit measures in social cognition research: Their meaning and use. Annu Rev Psychol 54: 297–327.
13. Spruyt A, Hermans D, De Houwer J, Vandromme H, Eelen P (2007) On the nature of the affective priming effect: Effects of stimulus onset asynchrony and congruency proportion in naming and evaluative categorization. Mem Cognition 35: 95–106.
14. De Houwer J (2001) A structural and process analysis of the Implicit Association Test. J Exp Soc Psychol 37: 443–451.
15. Olson MA, Fazio RH (2003) Relations between implicit measures of prejudice: What are we measuring? Psychol Sci 14: 636–639.

16. Govan CL, Williams KD (2004) Changing the affective valence of the stimulus items influences the IAT by re-defining the category labels. J Exp Soc Psychol 40: 357–365.
17. Mitchell JP, Nosek BA, Banaji MR (2003) Contextual variations in implicit evaluation. J Exp Psychol Gen 132: 455–469.
18. Cameron CD, Brown-Iannuzzi JL, Payne BK (2012) Sequential priming measures of implicit social cognition: A meta-analysis of associations with behavior and explicit attitudes. Pers Soc Psychol Rev 16: 330–350.
19. Greenwald AG, Poehlman TA, Uhlmann EL, Banaji MR (2009) Understanding and using the Implicit Association Test: III. Meta-analysis of predictive validity. J Pers Soc Psychol 97: 17–41.
20. Field M, Wiers RW (2012) Automatic and controlled processes in the pathway from drug abuse to addiction. In: Verster JC, Brady K, Galanter M, Conrod P, editors. Drug Abuse and Addiction in Medical Illness. New York, NY: Springer New York. pp. 35–45.
21. Noël X, Bechara A, Brevers D, Verbanck P, Campanella S (2010) Alcoholism and the loss of willpower: A neurocognitive perspective. J Psychophysiol 24: 240–248.
22. Reich RR, Below MC, Goldman MS (2010) Explicit and implicit measures of expectancy and related alcohol cognitions: A meta-analytic comparison. Psychol Addict Behav 24: 13–25.
23. Roefs A, Huijding J, Smulders FTY, Macleod CM, de Jong PJ, et al. (2011) Implicit measures of association in psychopathology research. Psychol Bull 137: 149–193.
24. Rooke SE, Hine DW, Thorsteinsson EB (2008) Implicit cognition and substance use: A meta-analysis. Addict Behav 33: 1314–1328.
25. Thush C, Wiers RW (2007) Explicit and implicit alcohol-related cognitions and the prediction of future drinking in adolescents. Addict Behav 32: 1367–1383.
26. Payne BK, Govorun O, Arbuckle N (2008) Automatic attitudes and alcohol: Does implicit liking predict drinking? Cognition Emotion 22: 238–271.
27. Davis CG, Thake J, Vilhena N (2010) Social desirability biases in self-reported alcohol consumption and harms. Addict Behav 35: 302–311.
28. Larsen H, Engels RCME, Wiers RW, Granic I, Spijkerman R (2012) Implicit and explicit alcohol cognitions and observed alcohol consumption: Three studies in (semi)naturalistic drinking settings. Addiction 107: 1420–1428.
29. Burton CM, Pedersen SL, McCarthy DM (2012) Impulsivity moderates the relationship between implicit associations about alcohol and alcohol use. Psychol Addict Behav 26: 766–772.
30. Friese M, Bargas-Avila J, Hofmann W, Wiers RW (2010) Here's looking at you, bud: Alcohol-related memory structures predict eye movements for social drinkers with low executive control. Soc Psychol Person Sci 1: 143–151.
31. Friese M, Hofmann W, Wänke M (2008) When impulses take over: Moderated predictive validity of explicit and implicit attitude measures in predicting food choice and consumption behaviour. Brit J Soc Psychol 47: 397–419.
32. Cooke R, Sheeran P (2004) Moderation of cognition-intention and cognition-behaviour relations: A meta-analysis of properties of variables from the theory of planned behaviour. Brit J Soc Psychol 43: 159–186.
33. Glasman LR, Albarracín D (2006) Forming attitudes that predict future behavior: A meta-analysis of the attitude-behavior relation. Psychol Bull 132: 778–822.
34. Kraus SJ (1995) Attitudes and the prediction of behavior: A meta-analysis of the empirical literature. Pers Soc Psychol B 21: 58–75.
35. Krosnick JA, Petty RE (1995) Attitude strength: An overview. In: Petty RE, Krosnick JA, editors. Attitude strength: Antecedents and consequences. Hillsdale, NJ: Erlbaum. pp. 1–24.
36. Fazio RH (1995) Attitudes as object-evaluation associations: Determinants, consequences, and correlates of attitude accessibility. In: Petty RE, Krosnick JA, editors. Attitude strength: Antecedents and consequences. Hillsdale, NJ: Erlbaum. pp. 247–282.
37. Perugini M, O'Gorman R, Prestwich A (2007) An ontological test of the IAT. Exp Psychol 54: 134–147.
38. Cooke R, Sheeran P (2004) Accessibility and temporal stability as moderators of cognition-behaviour relations in the theory of planned behaviour. Irish J Psychol 25: 44–64.
39. Doll J, Ajzen I (1992) Accessibility and stability of predictors in the theory of planned behavior. J Pers Soc Psychol 63: 754–765.
40. Kokkinaki F, Lunt P (1997) The relationship between involvement, attitude accessibility and attitude-behaviour consistency. Brit J Soc Psychol 36: 497–509.
41. Spruyt A, Hermans D, De Houwer J, Vandekerckhove J, Eelen P (2007) On the predictive validity of indirect attitude measures: Prediction of consumer choice behavior on the basis of affective priming in the picture–picture naming task. J Exp Soc Psychol 43: 599–610.
42. Vandromme H, Hermans D, Spruyt A (2011) Indirectly measured self-esteem predicts gaze avoidance. Self Identity 10: 32–43.
43. Verhulst F, Hermans D, Baeyens F, Spruyt A, Eelen P (2006) Determinants and predictive validity of direct and indirect measures of recently acquired food attitudes. Appetite 46: 137–143.
44. Spruyt A, Clarysse J, Vansteenwegen D, Baeyens F, Hermans D (2010) Affect 4.0: A free software package for implementing psychological and psychophysiological experiments. Exp Psychol 57: 36–45.
45. Spruyt A, Hermans D, De Houwer J, Eelen P (2002) On the nature of the affective priming effect: Affective priming of naming responses. Soc Cognition 20: 227–256.
46. De Houwer J, Beckers T (2002) A review of recent developments in research and theories on human contingency learning. Q J Exp Psychol 55B: 289–310.
47. Ratcliff R (1993) Methods for dealing with reaction time outliers. Psychol Bull 114: 510–532.

Permissions

All chapters in this book were first published in PLOS ONE, by The Public Library of Science; hereby published with permission under the Creative Commons Attribution License or equivalent. Every chapter published in this book has been scrutinized by our experts. Their significance has been extensively debated. The topics covered herein carry significant findings which will fuel the growth of the discipline. They may even be implemented as practical applications or may be referred to as a beginning point for another development.

The contributors of this book come from diverse backgrounds, making this book a truly international effort. This book will bring forth new frontiers with its revolutionizing research information and detailed analysis of the nascent developments around the world.

We would like to thank all the contributing authors for lending their expertise to make the book truly unique. They have played a crucial role in the development of this book. Without their invaluable contributions this book wouldn't have been possible. They have made vital efforts to compile up to date information on the varied aspects of this subject to make this book a valuable addition to the collection of many professionals and students.

This book was conceptualized with the vision of imparting up-to-date information and advanced data in this field. To ensure the same, a matchless editorial board was set up. Every individual on the board went through rigorous rounds of assessment to prove their worth. After which they invested a large part of their time researching and compiling the most relevant data for our readers.

The editorial board has been involved in producing this book since its inception. They have spent rigorous hours researching and exploring the diverse topics which have resulted in the successful publishing of this book. They have passed on their knowledge of decades through this book. To expedite this challenging task, the publisher supported the team at every step. A small team of assistant editors was also appointed to further simplify the editing procedure and attain best results for the readers.

Apart from the editorial board, the designing team has also invested a significant amount of their time in understanding the subject and creating the most relevant covers. They scrutinized every image to scout for the most suitable representation of the subject and create an appropriate cover for the book.

The publishing team has been an ardent support to the editorial, designing and production team. Their endless efforts to recruit the best for this project, has resulted in the accomplishment of this book. They are a veteran in the field of academics and their pool of knowledge is as vast as their experience in printing. Their expertise and guidance has proved useful at every step. Their uncompromising quality standards have made this book an exceptional effort. Their encouragement from time to time has been an inspiration for everyone.

The publisher and the editorial board hope that this book will prove to be a valuable piece of knowledge for researchers, students, practitioners and scholars across the globe.

List of Contributors

Tapio Paljärvi and Pia Mäkelä
Alcohol and Drugs Unit, National Institute for Health and Welfare, Helsinki, Finland,

Pekka Martikainen and Taina Leinonen
Population Research Unit, University of Helsinki, Helsinki, Finland

Tiina Pensola
Health and Work Ability, Finnish Institute of Occupational Health, Helsinki, Finland

Aartjan T. F. Beekman and Dick J. Veltman
Department of Psychiatry, Neuroscience Campus Amsterdam, VU University Medical Center, Amsterdam, the Netherlands

Zsuzsika Sjoerds
Department of Psychiatry, Neuroscience Campus Amsterdam, VU University Medical Center, Amsterdam, the Netherlands, Department of Psychiatry, Academic Medical Center, University of Amsterdam, Amsterdam, the Netherlands

Brenda W. J. H. Penninx
Department of Psychiatry, Neuroscience Campus Amsterdam, VU University Medical Center, Amsterdam, the Netherlands
Department of Psychiatry, Leiden University Medical Center, Leiden, the Netherlands, Department of Psychiatry, University Medical Center of Groningen, Groningen, the Netherlands

Wim van den Brink
Department of Psychiatry, Academic
Medical Center, University of Amsterdam, Amsterdam, the Netherlands

Marilyn D. Skinner
Centre de Traitement des Addictions, Hôpital Emile Roux, Assistance Publique-Hôpitaux de Paris, Institut National de la Santé et de la Recherche Médicale U669, Limeil-Brévannes, France

Pierre Lahmek
Centre de Traitement des Addictions, Hôpital Emile Roux, Assistance Publique-Hôpitaux de Paris, Limeil-Brévannes, France

Héloïse Pham
Centre Médical Marmottan Paris, France

Henri-Jean Aubin
Centre d'Enseignement, de Recherche et de Traitement des Addictions, Hôpital Paul Brousse, Assistance Publique-Hôpitaux de Paris, Université Paris-Sud, Institut National de la Santé et de la Recherche Me´dicale U669, Villejuif, France

Jari Lahti, Marius Lahti, Anu-Katriina Pesonen, Kati Heinonen and Katri Räikkönen
Institute of Behavioural Sciences, University of Helsinki, Helsinki, Finland

Eero Kajantie, Tom Forsén and Kristian Wahlbeck
National Public Health Institute, Helsinki, Finland

Johan G. Eriksson
National Public Health Institute, Helsinki, Finland
Department of General Practice and Primary Health Care, University of Helsinki

Clive Osmond and David J. P. Barker
Medical Research Council Lifecourse Epidemiology Unit, University of Southampton, United Kingdom

Christopher J. Hyatt, Shashwath A. Meda and Rachel Jiantonio-Kelly
Olin Neuropsychiatry Research Center, Institute of Living at Hartford Hospital, Hartford, Connecticut, United States of America

Haley L. Yarosh and Michal Assaf
Olin Neuropsychiatry Research Center, Institute of Living at Hartford Hospital, Hartford, Connecticut, United States of America
Department of Psychiatry, Yale University School of Medicine, New Haven, Connecticut, United States of America

Godfrey D. Pearlson
Olin Neuropsychiatry Research Center, Institute of Living at Hartford Hospital, Hartford, Connecticut, United States of America
Department of Psychiatry, Yale University School of Medicine, New Haven, Connecticut, United States of America
Department of Neurobiology, Yale University School of Medicine, New Haven, Connecticut, United States of America

Marc N. Potenza
Department of Psychiatry, Yale University School of Medicine, New Haven, Connecticut, United States of America
Department of Neurobiology, Yale University School of Medicine, New Haven, Connecticut, United States of America
Child Study Center, Yale University School of Medicine, New Haven, Connecticut, United States of America

Cecilie Skule, Hilde Dallavara Lending and Torkil Berge
Community Mental Health Center Vinderen, Diakonhjemmet Hospital, Oslo, Norway

Pål Ulleberg, Tim Brennen and Nils Inge Landrø
Department of Psychology, University of Oslo, Oslo, Norway

Jens Egeland
Department of Psychology, University of Oslo, Oslo, Norway
Vestfold Mental Health Care Trust, Tønsberg, Norway

Minsun Kang and Jae-Hyun Kim
Department of Public Health, Graduate School, Yonsei University, Seoul, Korea, Institute of Health Services Research, Yonsei University, Seoul, Korea

Woo-Hyun Cho
Institute of Health Services Research, Yonsei University, Seoul, Korea
Eulji University, Daejeon, Korea

Eun-Cheol Park
Institute of Health Services Research, Yonsei University, Seoul, Korea
Department of Preventive Medicine, Yonsei University College of Medicine, Seoul, Korea

Eberhard O. Voit
Department of Biomedical Engineering, Georgia Institute of Technology and Emory University Medical School, Atlanta, Georgia, United States of America, Integrative BioSystems Institute, Georgia Institute of Technology, Atlanta, Georgia, United States of America

Zhen Qi
Department of Biomedical Engineering, Georgia Institute of Technology and Emory University Medical School, Atlanta, Georgia, United States of America
Integrative BioSystems Institute, Georgia Institute of Technology, Atlanta, Georgia, United States of America
Center for Neurodegenerative Disease, Emory University School of Medicine, Atlanta, Georgia, United States of America

Felix Tretter
Isar-Amper-Klinikum gemeinnützige GmbH, Klinikum München-Ost, Haar, Landkreis München, Germany

Stephen M. Topper, Sara C. Aguilar, Viktoria Y. Topper, Erin Elbel and Jonathan T. Pierce-Shimomura
Waggoner Center for Alcohol and Addiction Research, Cell & Molecular Biology, Department of Neuroscience, the University of Texas at Austin, Austin, Texas, United States of America

Faten A. Taki and Baohong Zhang
Department of Biology, East Carolina University, Greenville, North Carolina, United States of America

Abdel A. Abdel-Rahman
Department of Pharmacology, East Carolina University, Greenville, North Carolina, United States of America

Shashi Bala, Miguel Marcos, Arijeet Gattu, Donna Catalano and Gyongyi Szabo
Department of Medicine, University of Massachusetts Medical School, Worcester, Massachusetts, United States of America

Frank Qian and Olufunmilayo I. Olopade
Center for Clinical Cancer Genetics and Global Health, Department of Medicine, University of Chicago, Chicago, Illinois, United States of America

Temidayo Ogundiran and Adeyinka Ademola
Department of Surgery, College of Medicine, University of Ibadan, Ibadan, Nigeria

Ningqi Hou and Dezheng Huo
Department of Health Studies, University of Chicago, Chicago, Illinois, United States of America

Paul Ndom
Medical Oncology Service, Yaoundé General Hospital, Yaoundé, Cameroon

Antony Gakwaya and Johashaphat Jombwe
Mulago Hospital, Makerere University, Kampala, Uganda

Imran Morhason-Bello and Oladosu Ojengbede
Center for Population and Reproductive Health, University College Hospital, Ibadan, Nigeria

Clement Adebamowo
Department of Epidemiology and Public Health, University of Maryland, Baltimore, Maryland, United States of America

Erica Rosanna Siu, Luis Paulo Saito, Andressa Kutschenko, Maria Carmen Viana, Yuan-Pang Wang and Laura Helena Andrade
Section of Psychiatric Epidemiology - LIM 23, Institute of Psychiatry, School of Medicine, University of São Paulo, São Paulo, São Paulo, Brazil

Camila Magalhães Silveira
Section of Psychiatric Epidemiology - LIM 23, Institute of Psychiatry, School of Medicine, University of São Paulo, São Paulo, São Paulo, Brazil
Program of the Interdisciplinary Group of Studies on Alcohol and Drugs (GREA), Department and Institute of Psychiatry, School of Medicine, University of São Paulo, São Paulo, São Paulo, Brazil

Arthur Guerra de Andrade
Program of the Interdisciplinary Group of Studies on Alcohol and Drugs (GREA), Department and Institute of Psychiatry, School of Medicine, University of São Paulo, São Paulo, São Paulo, Brazil

James C. Anthony
Department of Epidemiology and Statistics, Michigan State University, East Lansing, Michigan, United States of America

Silvia S. Martins
Department of Epidemiology, Mailman School Of Public Health, Columbia University, New York, New York, United States of America

Mihajlo Jakovljevic
Department of Pharmacology and Toxicology; the Faculty of Medical Sciences, University of Kragujevac, Kragujevac, Serbia

Mirjana Jovanovic
Department of Psychiatry; the Faculty of Medical Sciences, University of Kragujevac, Kragujevac, Serbia

Nemanja Rancic
Centre for Clinical Pharmacology; Medical Faculty Military Medical Academy, University of Defense, Belgrade, Serbia

Benjamin Vyssoki
Department of Psychiatry and Psychotherapy; Medical University of Vienna, Vienna, Austria

Natasa Djordjevic
Department of Pharmacology and Toxicology; the Faculty of Medical Sciences, University of Kragujevac, Kragujevac, Serbia

Ryan P. Vetreno and Fulton T. Crews
Bowles Center for Alcohol Studies, School of Medicine, University of North Carolina at Chapel Hill, Chapel Hill, North Carolina, 27599, United States of America

Margaret Broadwater, Wen Liu and Linda P. Spear
Center for Developmental and Behavioral Neuroscience, Department of Psychology, Binghamton University, Binghamton, New York, 13902, United States of America

Sonia Doallo, Fernando Cadaveira, Montserrat Corral, Nayara Mota, Eduardo López-Caneda and Socorro Rodríguez Holguín
Department of Clinical Psychology and Psychobiology, University of Santiago de Compostela, Santiago de Compostela, Spain

Sara Palm and Ingrid Nylander
Neuropharmacology, Addiction & Behaviour, Department of Pharmaceutical Biosciences, Uppsala University, Uppsala, Sweden

Heleen Riper and Pim Cuijpers
Department of Clinical Psychology and EMGO Institute, VU University Amsterdam, Amsterdam, Netherlands
Division Health Trainings online, EU innovation Incubator, Leuphana University, Lüneburg, Germany

Hana Hadiwijaya
Department of Clinical Psychology and EMGO Institute, VU University Amsterdam, Amsterdam, Netherlands
TS Social and Behavioral Sciences, Department of Developmental Psychology, Tilburg University, Tilburg, the Netherlands

David Ebert
Division Health Trainings online, EU innovation Incubator, Leuphana University, Lüneburg, Germany
Division for Clinical Psychology and Psychotherapy, Department for Psychology, Philipp's University Marburg, Marburg, Germany

Matthijs Blankers
Arkin Mental Health Care, Amsterdam, the Netherlands
Trimbos Institute, Netherlands Institute of Mental Health and Addiction, Utrecht, the Netherlands
Amsterdam Institute for Addiction Research, Department of Psychiatry, Academic Medical Centre, University of Amsterdam, the Netherlands

John Cunningham
Centre for Mental Health Research, the Australian National University, Canberra, Australia
Centre for Addiction and Mental Health, Toronto, Canada

Stella Clarke
NHS Fife, Edinburgh, Scotland, United Kingdom

Reinout Wiers
Addiction, Development and Psychopathology (ADAPT) lab, Department of Psychology, University of Amsterdam, Amsterdam, the Netherlands

Nuzhath Tajuddin, Kwan-Hoon Moon, Edward J. Neafsey and Michael A. Collins
Department of Molecular Pharmacology & Therapeutics, Loyola University Chicago, Stritch School of Medicine, Maywood, Illinois, United States of America

S. Alex Marshall and Kimberly Nixon
Department of Pharmaceutical Sciences, University of Kentucky, Lexington, Kentucky, United States of America

Hee-Yong Kim
Laboratory of Molecular Signaling, NIAAA, National Institutes of Health, Bethesda, Maryland, United States of America

Colin Drummond, Paolo Deluca, Judy Myles, Robert Patton and Katherine Perryman
Addictions Department, Institute of Psychiatry, King's College London, London, United Kingdom

Tom Phillips
Addictions Department, Institute of Psychiatry, King's College London, London, United Kingdom
Humber NHS Foundation Trust, Willerby, United Kingdom

Simon Coulton
Centre for Health Service Studies, University of Kent, Canterbury, United Kingdom

Martin Bland, Christine Godfrey, Veronica Dale and Steve Parrott
Department of Health Sciences, University of York, York, United Kingdom

Paul Cassidy
Teams Family Practice, Gateshead, United Kingdom

Mike Crawford
Department of Psychological Medicine, Imperial College, London, United Kingdom

Ruth McGovern, Dorothy Newbury-Birch and Eileen Kaner
Institute of Health and Society, Newcastle University, Newcastle, United Kingdom

Eilish Gilvarry
Institute of Health and Society, Newcastle University, Newcastle, United Kingdom
Northern Regional Drug and Alcohol Services, Newcastle, United Kingdom

Nick Heather
Faculty of Health and Life Sciences, Northumbria University, Newcastle, United Kingdom

Adenekan Oyefeso
Division of Population Health Sciences and Education, St George's, University of London, London, United Kingdom
Jeesal Cawston Park Hospital, Norfolk, United Kingdom

Jonathan Shepherd
Violence Research Group, Cardiff University, Cardiff, United Kingdom

Robin Touquet
Emergency Department, Kingston Hospital, Kingston upon Thames, London, United Kingdom

Francisco Bruno Teixeira, Luana Nazaréda Silva Santana and Rafael Rodrigues Lima
Laboratory of Functional and Structural Biology, Institute of Biological Sciences, Federal University of Pará, Belém-Pará, Brazil

Fernando Romualdo Bezerra, Sabrina De Carvalho and Cristiane Socorro Ferraz Maia
Laboratory Pharmacology of Inflammation and Behavior, Institute of Health Sciences, Federal University of Pará, Belém-Pará, Brazil

Enéas Andrade Fontes-Júnior
Laboratory Pharmacology of Inflammation and Behavior, Institute of Health Sciences, Federal University of Pará, Belém-Pará, Brazil
Laboratory of Molecular Pharmacology, Institute of Biological
Sciences, Federal University of Pará, Belém-Pará, Brazil

Maria Elena Crespo-Lòpez
Laboratory of Molecular Pharmacology, Institute of Biological
Sciences, Federal University of Pará, Belém-Pará, Brazil

Rui Daniel Prediger
Department of Pharmacology, Center of Biological Sciences, Federal University of Santa Catarina, Florianópolis, Santa Catarina, Brazil

Eric E. Rodriguez and Samuel Musselman
Department of Psychiatry, University of Pittsburgh School of Medicine, Pittsburgh, Pennsylvania, United States of America

Erika E. Forbes
Department of Psychiatry, University of Pittsburgh School of Medicine, Pittsburgh, Pennsylvania, United States of America
Department of Psychology, University of Pittsburgh, Pittsburgh, Pennsylvania, United States of America
Department of Pediatrics, University of Pittsburgh School of Medicine, Pittsburgh, Pennsylvania, United States of America

Rajesh Narendran
Department of Psychiatry, University of Pittsburgh School of Medicine, Pittsburgh, Pennsylvania, United States of America
Department of Radiology, University of Pittsburgh School of Medicine, Pittsburgh, Pennsylvania, United States of America

Mathilde Descheemaeker and Dirk Hermans
Faculty of Psychology and Educational Sciences, KU Leuven, Leuven, Belgium, Adriaan Spruyt
Faculty of Psychology and Educational Sciences, Ghent University, Ghent, Belgium

Index

R

S

T

V

CPSIA information can be obtained
at www.ICGtesting.com
Printed in the USA
BVHW010549050122
625443BV00003B/35

9 781639 270880

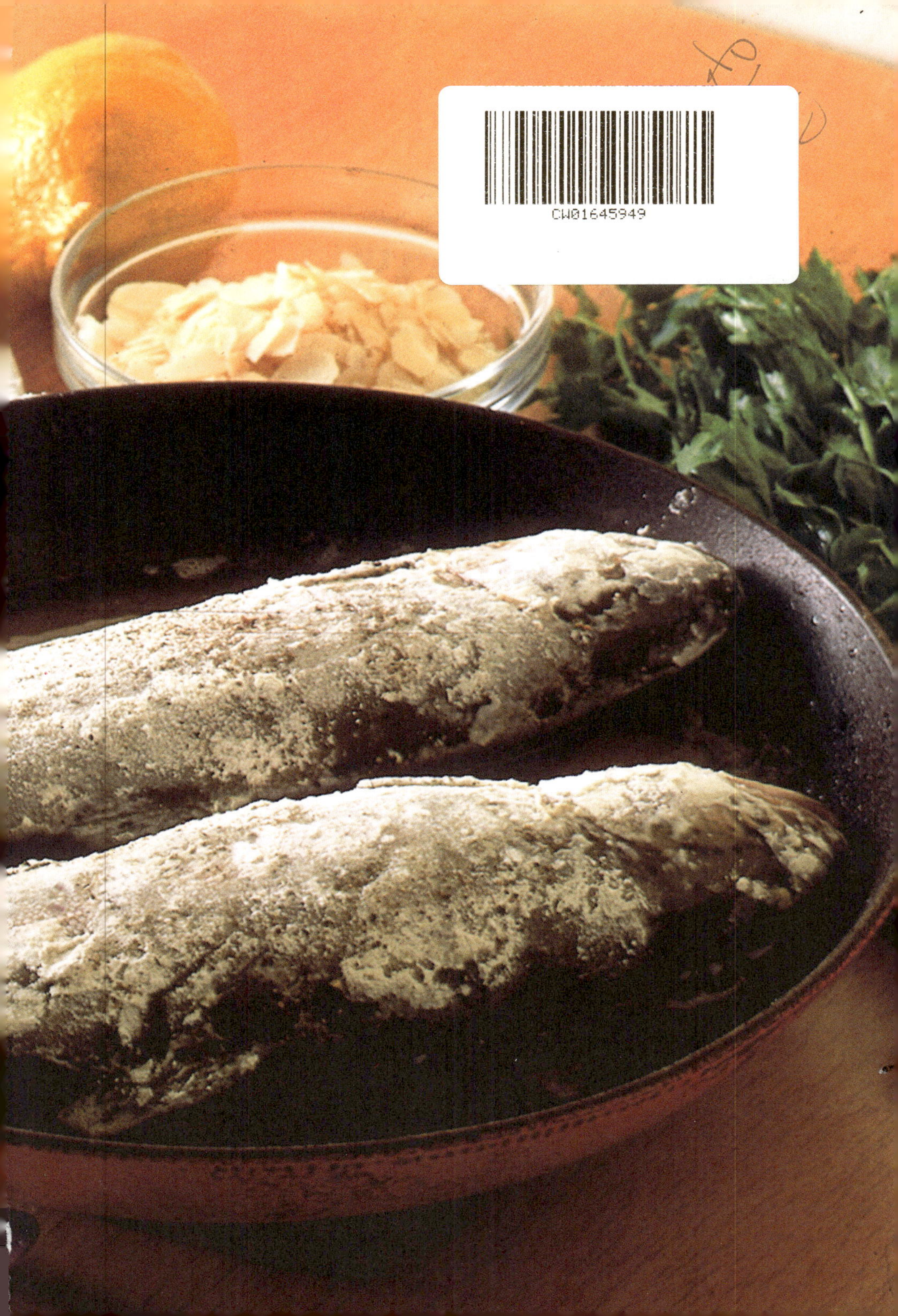

Step by Step

Fish

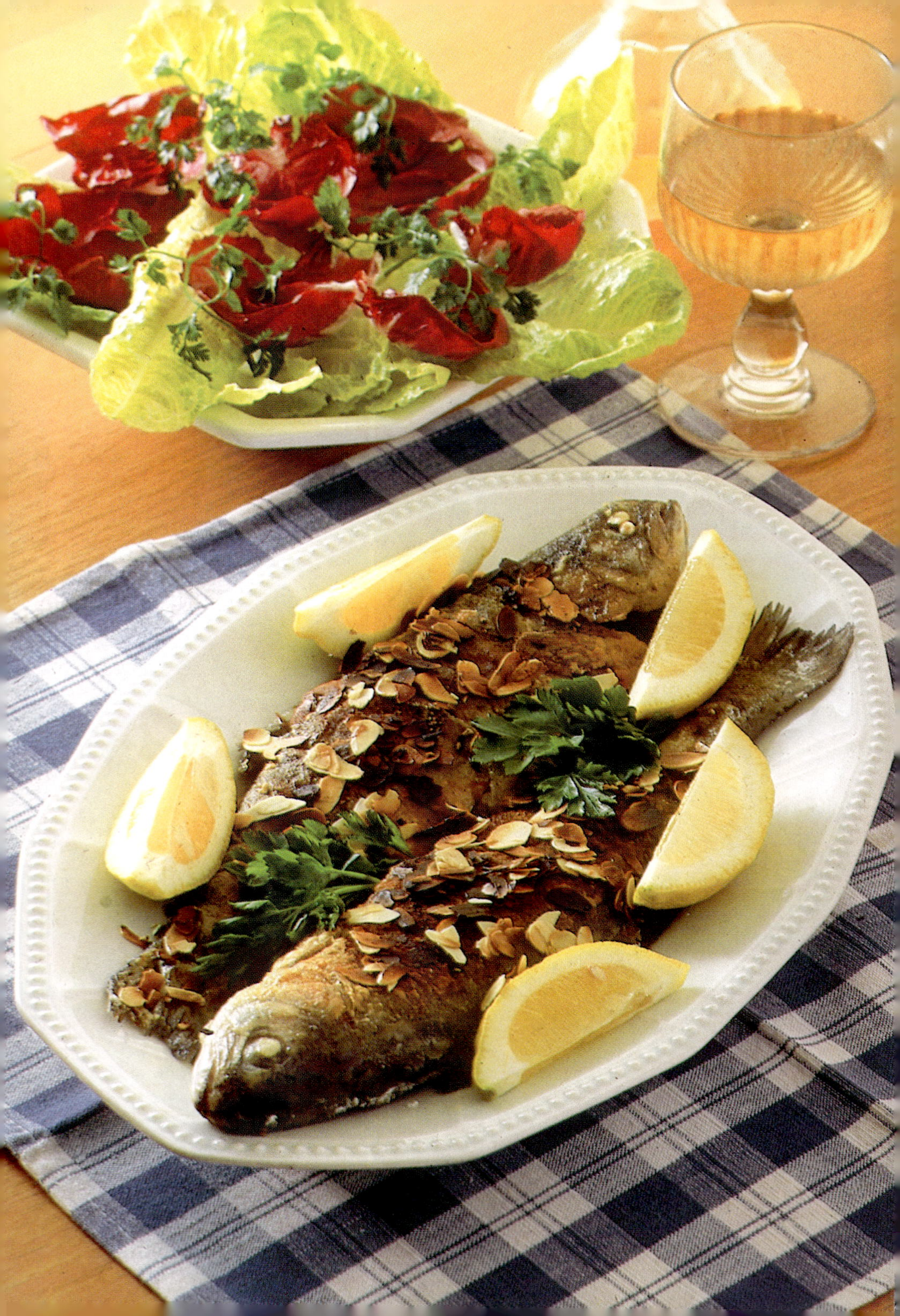

Step by Step

Fish

Janet Marsh Lillie

Bloomsbury Books
London

Page two: Trout with Almonds (p. 11). The secret of success for this succulent dish is to maintain an even heat and to keep the butter bubbling. The endpapers show the preparation for this classic dish.

This edition published in 1994 by
Bloomsbury Books
an imprint of
The Godfrey Cave Group
42 Bloomsbury Street, London. WC1B 3QJ
under license from
Harlaxton Publishing Limited

Harlaxton Publishing Limited
2 Avenue Road, Grantham, Lincolnshire, NG31 6TA
United Kingdom
A Member of the Weldon International Group of Companies

First Published in 1994

Publisher: Robin Burgess
Project Coordinator: Barbara Beckett
Designer: Rachel Rush
Editor: Alison Leach
Illustrator: Maggie Renvoize
Jacket photographer: Rodney Weidland
Inside photography: Jack Sarafian
Food stylist: Janet Marsh Lillie
Produced by Barbara Beckett Publishing
Colour Separation: G.A. Graphics, Stamford, UK
Printer: Imago, Singapore

British Library Cataloguing-in-Publication data.
A catalogue record for this book is available from the British Library

Title: Step by Step, FISH
ISBN: 1 85471 323 X

Step by Step

Contents

Step by Step

Cook's Notes

Measurements

All spoon and cup measurements are level. Standard spoon and cup measures are used in all the recipes. I recommend using a graduated nest of measuring cups: 1 cup, ½ cup, ⅓ cup and ¼ cup. The graduated nest of spoons comprises one tablespoon, 1 teaspoon, ½ teaspoon and ¼ teaspoon. For liquids, use a standard litre or imperial pint measuring jug which also shows cup measurements. As the metric/imperial/US equivalents given are not exact, follow only one system of measurement within each recipe.

Ovens should be preheated to the specified temperature. When cooking on the hob (stove plate), use medium heat where high, low or simmer are not specified.

Ingredients

Fresh fruit and vegetables should be used in the recipes unless otherwise stated. **Herb** quantities are for fresh herbs; if fresh are unobtainable, use half the quantity of dried herbs.Use freshly ground black **pepper** whenever pepper is listed; use **salt** and pepper to individual taste. Use plain (all-purpose) **flour** unless otherwise stated. Fresh **ginger** should be used throughout, unless ground ginger is called for. Use fresh **chillies**; if substituting dried chillies, halve the quantity. Cold-pressed virgin olive **oil** is recommended, but any type may be used. Use unsalted **butter**. Preferably use fermented wine **vinegar**; however, cider vinegar and malt vinegar may be substituted if preferred. White granulated **sugar** is used unless otherwise stated.

Cantonese Steamed Fish (p. 28). To bring out the delicate flavour of this elegant main course, retain the moisture by cooking the fish whole.

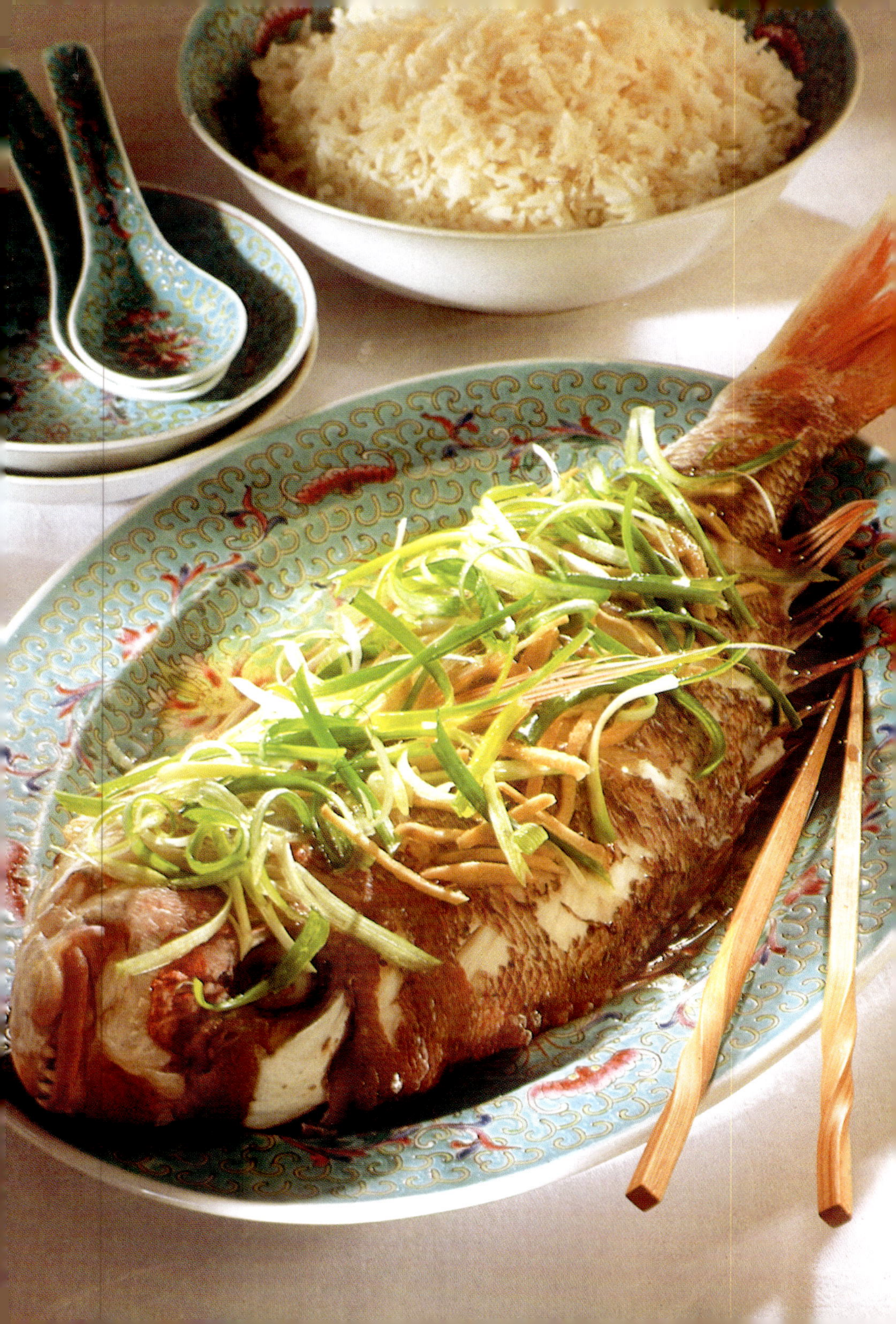

Step by Step

Introduction

When you learn to cook fish, a fantastic diversity of meals is added to your repertoire. The fish may be simply crumbed and pan- or shallow-fried in sizzling butter, dipped in a light batter and deep-fried until crispy and golden, marinated in garlic, ginger and lemon juice and steamed, poached in white wine and stock—even baked whole—every taste can be satisfied.

Nutritionally speaking, fish is an excellent source of protein and is low in calories (kilojoules) and cholesterol. It's easily digested and cooks quickly.

The instructions in this book are all clearly set out. There are step-by-step guides to the different cooking methods, such as poaching, braising and grilling (broiling). Sauces, tips and methods are cross-referenced within the book and there is also a glossary of cooking terms on page 47 so you can look up any term that is unfamiliar.

Be sure to read the information on measurements and ingredients on page 6 and also be aware of an important rule of cooking, which is always to read a recipe through before you start! Check you have all the ingredients called for, the equipment you need and enough time to complete the steps.

Fish cooking relies on a balance between dry goods you will no doubt already have in your cupboard and those familiar fresh produce items you often buy. Staples include flour, in plain (all-purpose), self-raising (self-rising) and cornflour (cornstarch) forms, eggs, caster (superfine) sugar, rice, potatoes, unsalted butter, nuts, seeds, and oil (including olive, peanut and hazelnut). A good stock of lemons is also essential, as is bread for making fresh crumbs.

Some of the more unusual products used in my recipes include tarragon vinegar, poppadums, couscous and curry paste. Aromatic and flavour-enhancing dry spices you'll need include cumin, cardamom, turmeric, oregano, chilli powder and bay leaves.

Handy equipment to have when cooking fish includes a good quality set of sharp knives

Gutting a Fish

Place the tip of the knife into the tiny hole below the tail and cut up towards the gills.

1

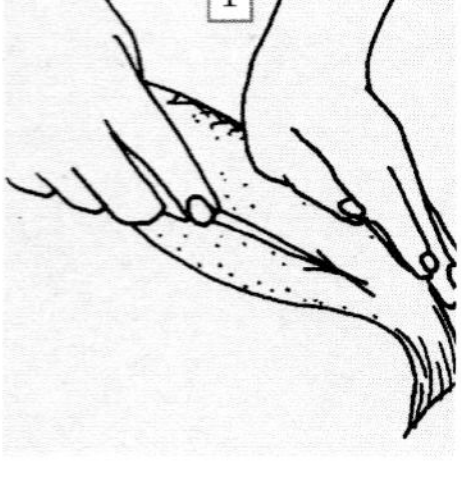

Cut the gills from the backbone with the point of a sharp knife.

2

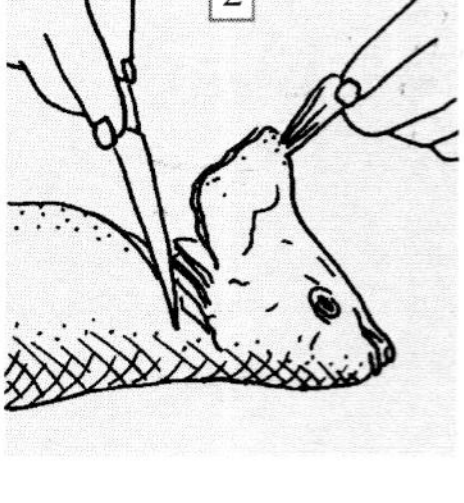

Take out the innards.

3

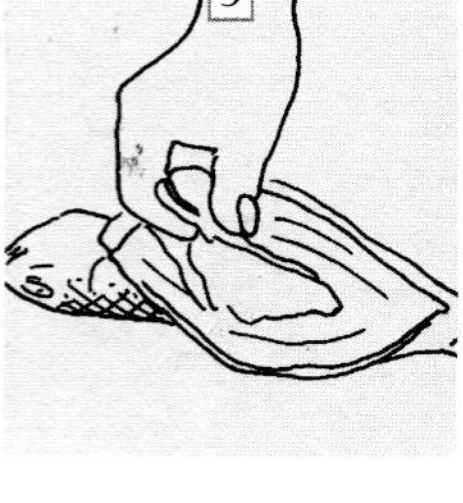

Scrape any further innards out and rinse under cold water.

4

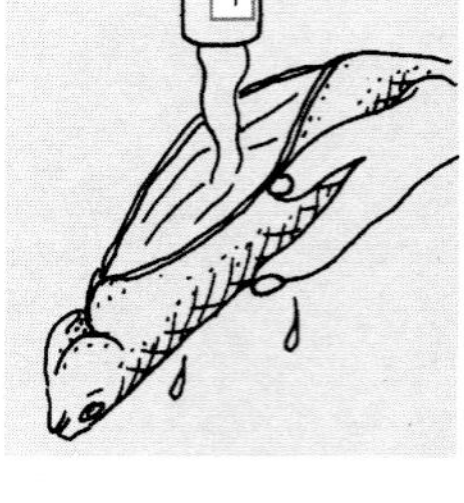

Filleting Fish

Check fish for freshness. It should have bright eyes and firm flesh.	*Make a cut behind the head and cut down to the backbone.*	*Turn the knife and cut carefully towards the tail.*	*Keep the knife close to the backbone.*

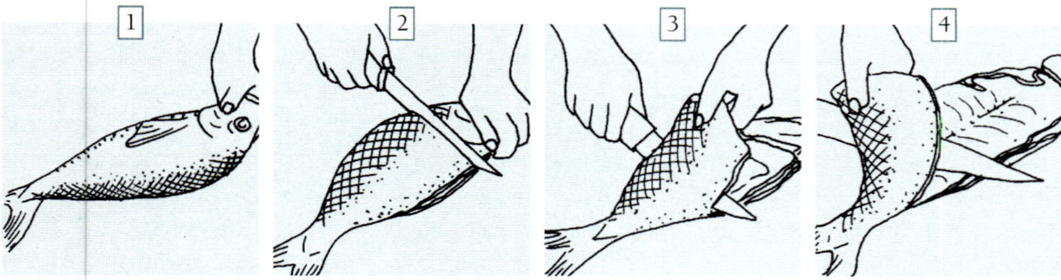

(for chopping, paring and filleting), a couple of frying pans (skillets) and saucepans with lids, a metal or bamboo steamer—even a cake rack can be used for steaming—and a wok is also a desirable utensil. Most other equipment mentioned in this book can be found in the average kitchen.

When a recipe refers to a **fatty** or **oily** fish, varieties fitting this description include tuna, salmon, and mackerel. **Lean** or **firm white** fish varieties include snapper, whiting, bream, trout, sole, flounder, cod, halibut, haddock and varieties of dory.

Enjoy cooking fish. It's so easy—and so tasty!

Preparation of Fish in Beer Batter (p. 18). A delicious contrast in textures results from this combination of crisp light coating with firm fish fillets.

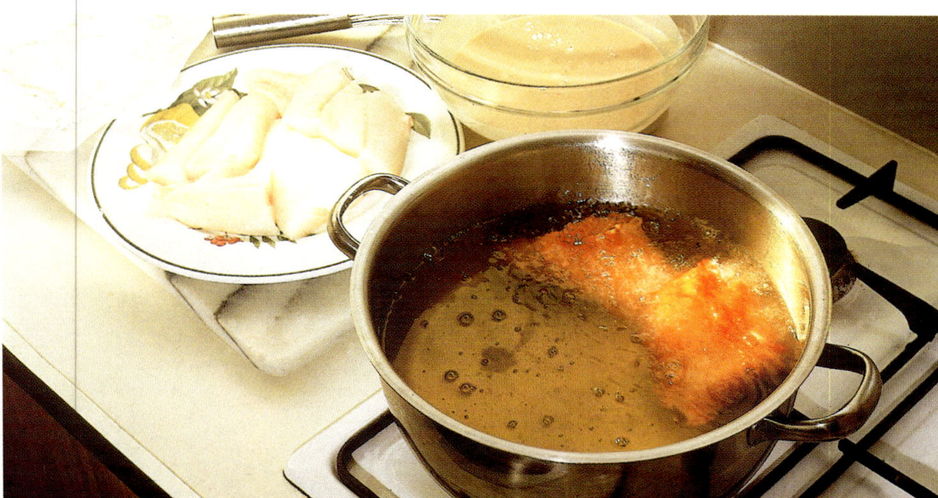

Step by Step

Frying

Frying involves quick cooking in a small amount of fat, usually half butter and half oil, in a frying pan (skillet). The fish is usually added when the butter has melted and starts to foam. You should maintain a moderate temperature and only turn the fish once, very carefully. Cook only until fish is lightly browned and to the point when the flesh is beginning to flake from the bone. As a rule, the presentation side is always fried first. Remember also to dry the fish well before cooking to minimize spitting. It is usual to coat the fish with seasoned flour or a marinade before placing it in the hot pan. In the case of wok cooking or **stir-frying** (as in the Stir-Fried Fish Goujons with Cucumber recipe), the full amount of fat used is oil. Peanut oil is usually chosen because it can be heated to a very high temperature before it starts to smoke, at which point foods burns very quickly. **Shallow-frying** is a variation where just enough oil or a mixture of oil and butter is used to cover coated fish or simple fish cakes.

The fish selected for **deep-frying** should have a low fat content. Choose firm white fillets and dry them completely before coating and cooking. The pan should not be more than ½ to ¾ full of oil. Foods for deep-frying are usually coated in some sort of batter or textured coating. The purpose of this is to provide a golden crust, seal the fish and minimize absorption on immersion in the hot oil. When cooked, the fish should rise to the surface of the oil. Remove and drain immediately on paper towels and keep warm.

Preparation of Crunchy Coconut Fish (p. 16). An important step is to place the coated fish on a plate, cover and chill for 1 hour to set the coating before placing in the pan.

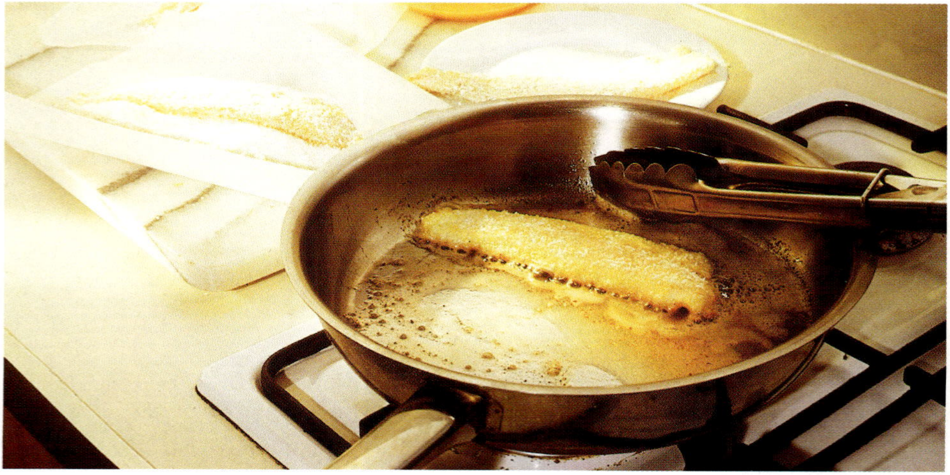

Trout with Almonds

Trout requires an even heat and bubbling butter if it is to cook perfectly. This versatile pan-fried dish can be served with a sprinkling of pepper and a wedge of lemon. This butter sauce with almond flakes is, however, both classic and popular.

4 x 250–300 g/9–11 oz trout, cleaned, head and tail left intact
2–3 tablespoons plain (all-purpose) flour for coating
125 g/4 oz/½ cup butter
Juice of 2 lemons
30 g/1 oz/2 tablespoons butter, extra
30 g/1 oz/¼

Pat the fish dry with paper towels. Put the flour into a polythene bag and season with salt and pepper. Add the trout to the bag and shake carefully.

Melt the 125 g/4 oz/½ cup butter in a frying pan (skillet), add half the lemon juice. When the butter starts to foam, add the flour-coated fish, cover the pan, reduce the heat to low and cook for 5 minutes on each side, or until the flesh is opaque and the skin is a rich, crisp brown.

Transfer each fish to a warmed serving dish and keep hot. Wipe the pan clean and melt the extra butter. Add the remaining lemon juice, almonds, salt and pepper and parsley, bring to the boil and pour over the fish. Serve immediately.

Serves 4

Storing Fish. *For general storage, scale and remove gills and guts if not already done, wash in cold water and dry well, wrap in clingfilm (plastic wrap) or foil and store in the refrigerator for up to 3 days. Freezing fish is not recommended because it loses some of its flavour on thawing. Never re-freeze fish.*

Frying Fish

Wash and dry the fish or fillets. *Melt the butter and oil in the pan.* *Add the fish when butter is foaming.* *Turn the fish once only.*

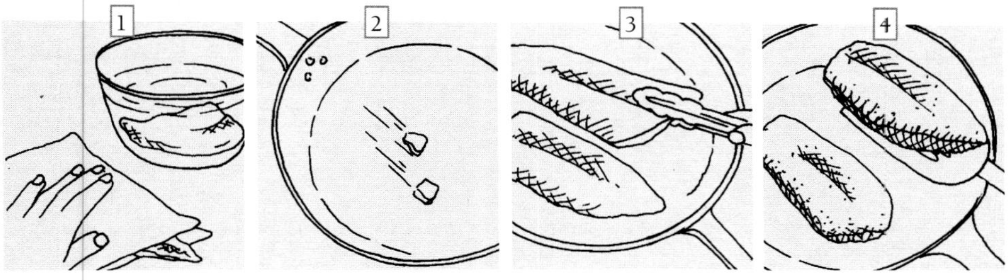

Stir-Fried Fish Goujons with Cucumber

Cod, halibut or red snapper can be used here..

675 g/1½ lb firm white thick-cut fish fillets, cut into 5 x 2.5 cm/2 x 1 inch pieces
2 teaspoons salt
4 tablespoons soy sauce
3 tablespoons dry sherry
2 teaspoons cornflour (cornstarch)
3 tablespoons peanut oil
1 red pepper (capsicum, bell pepper), cut into diamonds or julienne strips
225 g/8 oz cucumber, peeled, sliced in half to remove seeds, cut to the size of the fish pieces
12 mangetout (snow peas), trimmed, cut in half
2 garlic cloves, crushed
2.5 cm/1 inch piece root ginger, cut into julienne strips
250 ml/8 fl oz/1 cup chicken stock
2 teaspoons cornflour (cornstarch), mixed to a paste with 1 tablespoon water
Cooked rice or fried noodles, to serve

Place the fish in a bowl containing a mixture of the salt, 2 tablespoons of the soy sauce, 1 tablespoon of the sherry and the cornflour. Leave to marinate for about 1 hour.

Heat a wok or large frying pan (skillet) and add 2 tablespoons of the peanut oil. Remove the fish pieces from the marinade (reserve) and add the fish pieces to the wok or pan. Stir-fry carefully for about 2 minutes until lightly browned. Remove to paper towels to drain.

Reheat the wok or pan and add the remaining oil. When the oil is hot, add the pepper, cucumber, mangetout, garlic and ginger and stir-fry for 2 minutes. Add the remaining soy sauce and sherry and the chicken stock and cook for a further 3 minutes. Stir in the reserved marinade, return the fish pieces and cook gently until the fish is heated through. Serve with rice or noodles.

Serves 4

Chilli Fish Cakes

Any fish cake is popular–these rely on the fish being blended to a paste with seasonings, making it light and springy in texture. If red curry paste is not available, use a teaspoon of ground coriander.

450 g/1 lb firm white fish fillets, roughly chopped
2 teaspoons red curry paste
1 tablespoon light soy sauce
2–3 tablespoons cornflour (cornstarch)
1 egg, beaten
½–1 teaspoon finely chopped red chilli
2 tablespoons chopped spring onions (scallions)
60 g/2 oz/½ cup finely sliced French (green) beans
Oil for shallow-frying
Lime or lemon wedges, to serve

Stir-Fried Fish Goujons with Cucumber. A handy hint for this exotic fish dish is to work quickly over a high heat.

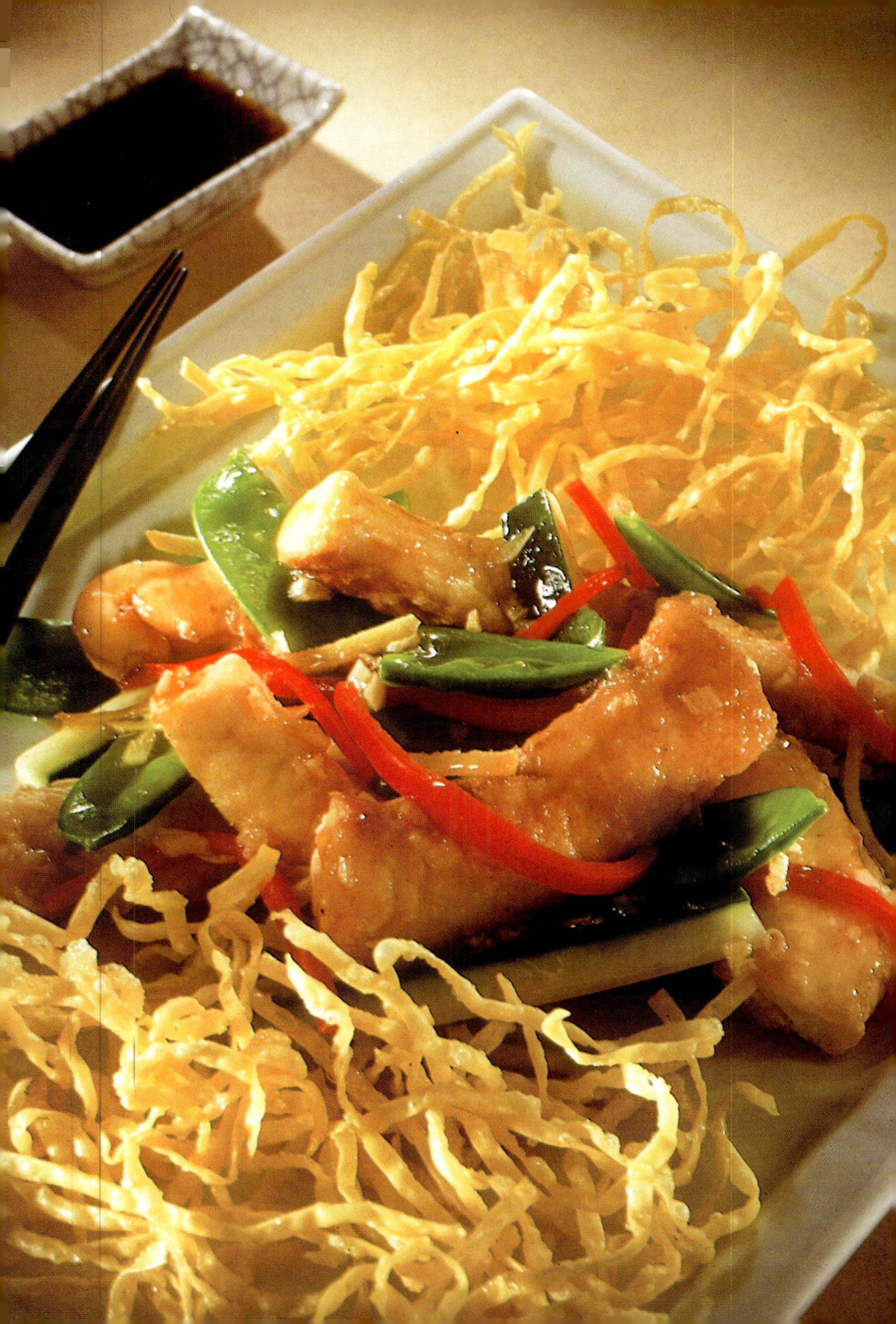

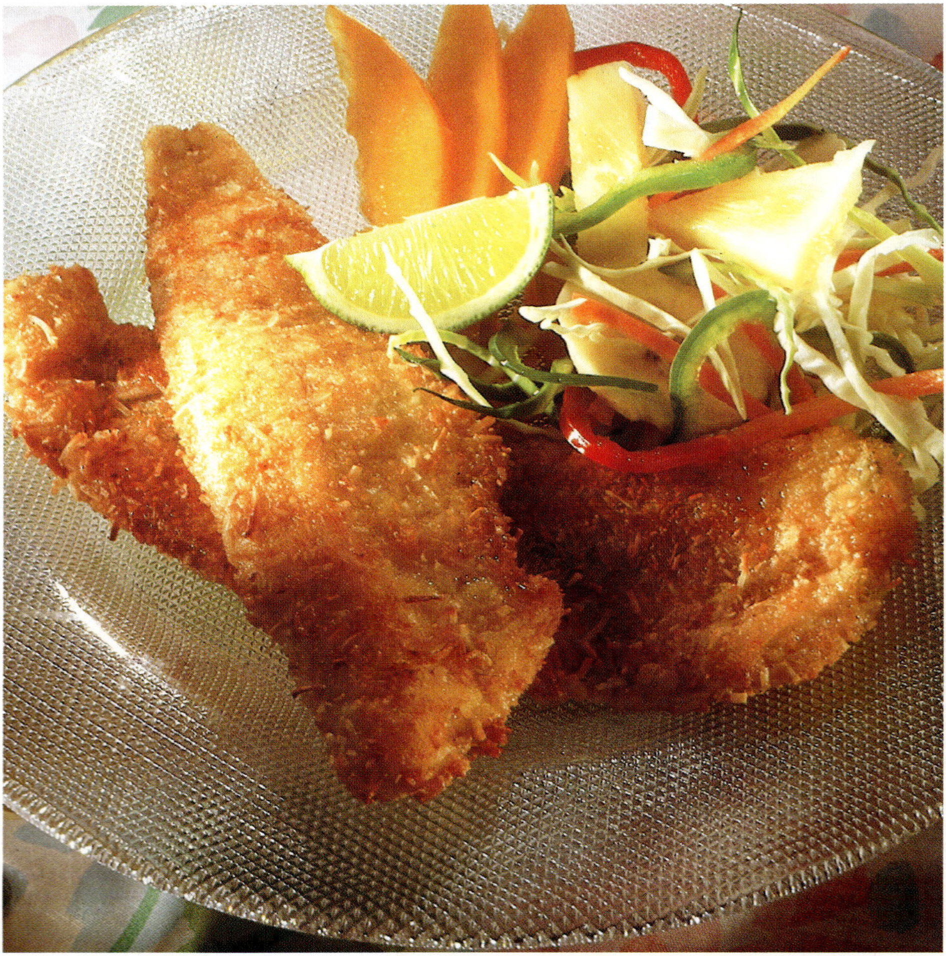

Crunchy Coconut Fish—a tropical delight that requires an egg and breadcrumb coating to ensure easy cooking.

Place the fish in a food processor. Process lightly until smooth. Add the curry paste, soy sauce, cornflour and egg. Process again until well combined. With a spatula, scrape the fish mixture into a bowl and stir in the red chilli, spring onions and beans. With oiled hands, take 3 tablespoons of the mixture at a time and shape into flat, round cakes.

Heat 2.5 cm/1 inch oil in a large frying pan (skillet). Place the cakes into the hot oil 3 at a time, and fry, shaking the pan gently to prevent sticking, until golden brown underneath. Turn the cakes over carefully, using an egg slice, and fry the other side until golden. Remove and drain on paper towels. Serve immediately with lemon or lime wedges or leave to cool.

Makes 6

Vinaigrette Dressing

3 tablespoons olive oil
2 tablespoons vinegar
1 teaspoon Dijon mustard
Salt and pepper

Combine all the ingredients in a small bowl, and whisk together to combine. Alternatively, place the ingredients in a screw-topped jar and shake vigorously to combine.
Makes about 90 ml/3 fl oz/⅓ cup

Crunchy Coconut Fish

8 x 60 g/2 oz firm white fish fillets such as Whiting
Plain (all-purpose) flour for coating
90 g/3 oz/1¾ cups desiccated (shredded) coconut
60 g/2 oz/¼

Roll the fish fillets in the flour, then dip each in the egg. Put the coconut in a polythene bag, add the fillets and shake to coat. Place on a plate, cover and chill for at least 1 hour. This sets the coating and makes the fish easier to cook.

Melt the butter and heat the oil in a large frying pan (skillet). When foaming subsides, add fish fillets and fry until the crust is golden, turning once.
Serves 4

Parmesan Coating. In place of the coconut, a mixture of equal quantities of dried breadcrumbs and grated Parmesan cheese makes an interesting variation.

Fish Grenobloise

Tiny tangy lemon wedges and capers create a quick brown-butter sauce for this interesting pan-fried fish.

175 g/6 oz/¾ cup butter
6 x 200 g/7 oz firm white fish fillets
4 tablespoons plain (all-purpose) flour for coating
60 g/2 oz/ ¼
2 lemons, peeled, pith removed and flesh chopped finely
1 tablespoon chopped parsley

Melt the butter in a frying pan (skillet) over a moderate heat. Pat the fish dry with paper towels, place in a polythene bag with the flour and toss gently to coat. Shake the excess flour from the fish and place in the pan with the butter. Cook, turning once only with an egg slice, until the fish is golden brown and flakes easily. Remove the fish from the pan and keep warm. Add the capers and lemon to the pan and stir to heat through. Place the fish on a serving plate, and sprinkle with the parsley. Season the sauce with salt and pepper and pour over the fish. Serve immediately.
Serves 6

Spicy Blackened Fish

Cajun-creole in style, these fish fillets are coated with a herb and spice marinade, then carefully fried. They are delicious served with an avocado, melon and lettuce salad.

30 g/1 oz/½ cup chopped fresh coriander (cilantro)
4 garlic cloves, crushed
1 tablespoon paprika
¼ teaspoon cayenne pepper
125 ml/4 fl oz/½ cup olive oil
2 tablespoons lemon juice
½ teaspoon black pepper
6 x 200 g/7 oz firm white fish fillets
Oil for shallow-frying
Lime or lemon wedges

Mix the coriander, garlic, paprika, cayenne pepper, olive oil, lemon juice and pepper together in a bowl. Place the fish fillets in a dish and brush liberally with the marinade. Cover and chill overnight. Heat about 2.5 cm/1 inch oil in a frying pan (skillet), and then add the fish in batches. Cook for 2-3 minutes on each side, turning once only, until crisp and lightly browned. Remove and drain on paper towels. Serve immediately with lime or lemon wedges.
Serves 4

Crunchy Almond Fish

Thick fillets of fish are easy to cut into strips (called goujons) for this summer-style recipe. Serve the accompanying salad well chilled so the hot crunchy fish will provide a delicious contrast with the cool green leaves.

150–200 g/5–7 oz firm white fish fillets
3 tablespoons cornflour (cornstarch)
Salt and pepper
3 egg whites, lightly beaten
200 g/7 oz/2 cups unblanched almonds, chopped
Oil for shallow-frying
200 g/7 oz mixed small lettuce leaves
125 g/4 oz mangetout (snow peas) or French (green) beans, blanched (p. 31)
1 red pepper (capsicum, bell pepper), cut into julienne strips
Oil and vinegar dressing (vinaigrette) (p. 14)
Easy Tartare Sauce, to serve (p. 17)

Cut the fish fillets into 24 strips. Place in a polythene bag, add the cornflour, season with salt and pepper. Shake to coat the fish thoroughly, then remove from the bag. Dip in the egg white, then in the almonds, pressing them on firmly.

Heat about 2.5 cm/1 inch oil in a large frying pan (skillet). Fry the fish strips in batches until golden. Drain on paper towels. Keep hot.

Toss the lettuce, vegetables and dressing together in a bowl. Arrange the goujons on top and serve with tartare or soured cream sauce.
Serves 4–6

Fresh Breadcrumbs. *Cut the crusts from a few slices of day-old bread. Place the bread in a food processor or blender and 'pulse' (turn machine on and off every second or two), to obtain roughly chopped crumbs.*

Easy Tartare Sauce

250 ml/8 floz/1 cup soured cream
1 tablespoon snipped chives
1 tablespoon chopped dill
2 finely chopped gherkins
1 teaspoon capers

Combine all the ingredients in a bowl; chill and serve.
Makes about 250 ml/8 fl oz/1 cup

Potato Chips (French Fries)

500 g/18 oz potatoes
Oil for frying

Peel and remove the 'eyes' or holes from the potatoes. Cover with water while you are preparing them to avoid browning. For straight-edged chips, trim the potatoes to straighten the sides. Cut them evenly in to the desired thickness: for French fries, 1 x 1 x 6 cm/½ x ½ x 2½ inches; for matchsticks/shoestrings, 6 mm x 6 mm x 5 cm (¼ x ¼ x 2 inches). Alternatively, slice into thick 'wedges' or paper-thin wafers. Wash the chips under running water to allow some of the starch to escape. Dry well to prevent spitting when frying.

Heat about 7.5 cm/3 inches oil in a large saucepan or wok until it is hot. (The oil is too hot if it starts smoking and rippling on the surface.) Lower the chips into the oil in batches and cook for 5–7 minutes or until golden brown and floating to the top of the oil. Remove with a slotted spoon. Drain on paper towels.
Serves 4–6

Deep-Frying Fish

Coat the fish fillets in flour, yoghurt and then breadcrumbs.

Heat the oil in a large saucepan no more than ⅔ full.

Cook fish until golden and lift out with a slotted spatula.

Drain off fat on paper towels.

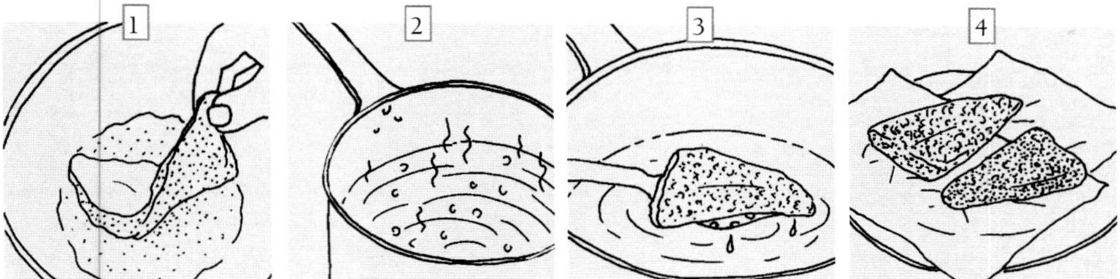

Toasting Nuts and Sesame Seeds. *Spread the nuts or seeds on a baking sheet. Bake in a preheated oven at 180°C/350°F/gas 4 for 4 minutes, remove from the oven, shake the tray or turn the nuts over with a fork. Bake a further 3–4 minutes or until golden. Remove the nuts from the hot tray immediately, or they will continue to cook. Avoid using black baking sheets. Alternatively, dry-fry the nuts by placing them in a frying pan (skillet) over a low to moderate heat for 2–4 minutes, shaking the pan to turn the nuts so that they colour evenly. Pine nuts cook very quickly, so be careful!*

Honey Sesame Fish

Plain yoghurt replaces beaten egg for the coating here. When deep-frying, the amount of oil required will depend on the size of the saucepan or deep-fryer. It is important, however, that the food be completely immersed in the hot oil for the fish to cook quickly and evenly.

2 tablespoons sesame seeds, toasted (above)
90 g/3 oz/1½ cups day-old fresh breadcrumbs (p. 17)
675 g/1½ lb firm white fish fillets, cut into 4 cm/ 1½ inch portions
Plain (all-purpose) flour, seasoned with salt and pepper
400 ml/14 fl oz/1¾ cups plain yoghurt
Vegetable oil for frying
1 tablespoon clear honey

Combine the sesame seeds with the breadcrumbs in a bowl. Coat the fish portions in the seasoned flour, dip in the yoghurt and press the sesame-breadcrumb mixture firmly on to the fish portions.

Heat the oil in a large saucepan. When a cube of bread dropped into it turns golden in about 30 seconds or the oil reaches 130°C/350°F on a thermometer, add the fish, and cook for 4–5 minutes or until the fish is crisp and golden. Lift out with a slotted spoon and drain on paper towels. Combine the remaining yoghurt with the honey. Serve with the fish.

Serves 4

Fish in Beer Batter

A batter prepared with beer makes a very light, crisp coating for any firm white fish fillets such as whiting, grouper or sea bass. A wedge of lemon, a sprinkling of vinegar or tartare sauce and crisp chips are all you need for a scrumptious meal. The fish tastes even better if it is served wrapped in newspaper or butcher's paper.

200 g/7 oz/1¾ cups self-raising (self-rising) flour
½ teaspoon paprika
Salt and pepper
250 ml/8 fl oz/1 cup beer
125 ml/4 fl oz/½ cup water
Vegetable oil for frying
3 tablespoons plain (all-purpose) flour
6 x 200 g/7 oz firm white fish fillets, each cut in half
Potato chips, to serve (p. 17)
Lemon wedges or vinegar, to serve

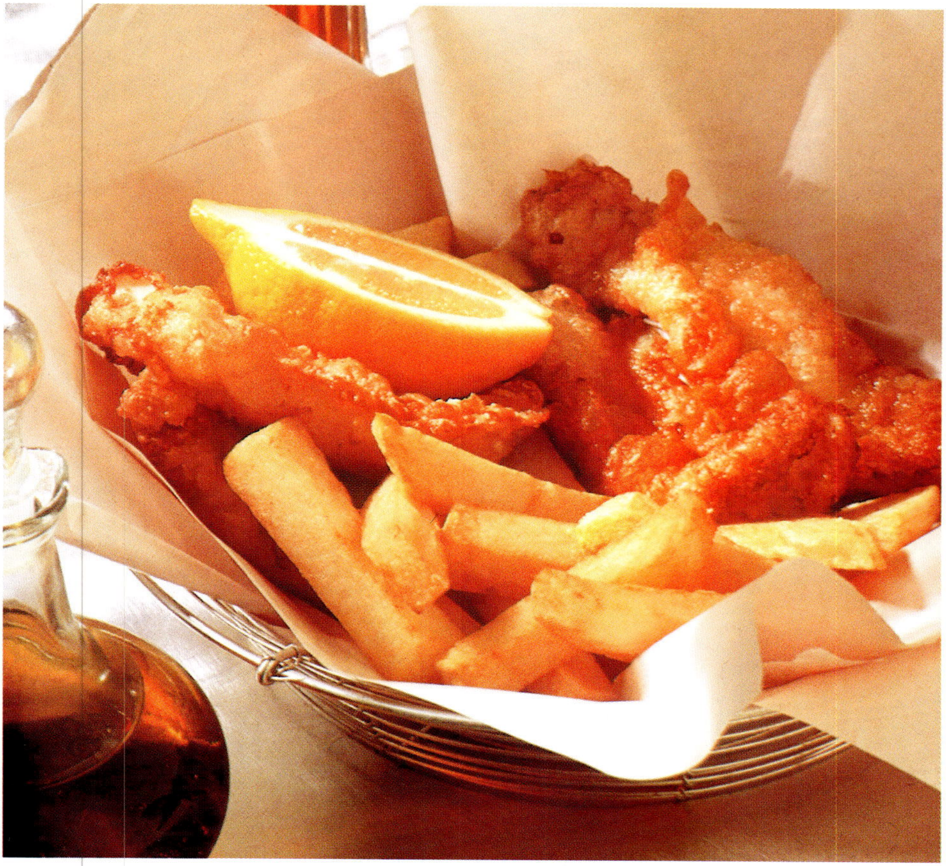

Fish in Beer Batter. The additional tart taste of lemon, vinegar or tartare sauce highlights this delicious meal.

Sift the flour, paprika, salt and pepper into a large bowl and make a well in the centre. Pour in the beer and water and whisk together to make a smooth batter. Allow to stand 1 hour if time permits, so that the batter thickens slightly.

Heat enough oil in a deep-fryer, saucepan or wok to cover the fish portions. When a cube of bread turns golden in about 30 seconds, or the oil reaches 180°C/350°F on a thermometer, it is ready.

Dry the fish portions with paper towels to minimize spitting while frying. Coat four to six fish fillets lightly in the plain flour and dip in the beer batter. Drain the excess on to the rim of the bowl before carefully lowering into the hot oil. Cook for 5–6 minutes or until golden brown. Lift from the oil on to paper towels and leave to drain in a warm oven. Repeat this procedure until all the fillets are cooked. Serve immediately with potato chips (p. 17) and lemon wedges or vinegar.
Serves 4

Step by Step

Grilling (Broiling)

Grilling (broiling) or barbecuing cooks fish very quickly because of the high direct heat involved. These cooking methods are suitable for all types of fish, but particularly for those with a high oil content, such as tuna and salmon. If using whole fish, remember to slash the skin slightly to allow the heat to penetrate. Allow 4 minutes for each 200 g/7 oz and turn only once during that period. For fillets, steaks and cutlets allow 10–12 minutes, again turning only once. The grill pan (broiler) is often greased or lined with foil to prevent sticking. Frequent basting of the fish is essential. Remember that the fish will continue to cook for a few minutes after removal from the heat.

Salmon Steaks with Lemon Parsley Butter

Lemon parsley butter is the simplest sauce you can make to serve with any grilled (broiled) fish–butter mixed with chopped capers, cracked black pepper, snipped chives or dill are alternative flavourings.

4 x 200 g/7 oz salmon steaks
Salt and pepper
60 g/2 oz/¼ cup butter, melted
125 g/4 oz/½ cup extra butter, softened
2 tablespoons finely chopped parsley
2 tablespoons lemon juice
Salt and pepper
Small boiled potatoes, to serve

Season both sides of the salmon steaks with salt and pepper. Place the steaks on a greased grill pan (broiler). Brush the salmon with melted butter and grill (broil) for 3–5 minutes on each side or until cooked (p. 23). Beat the extra butter and parsley together in a bowl until creamy and smooth. Beat in the lemon juice and season with salt and pepper. Serve the salmon steaks and potatoes with the lemon parsley butter.

Serves 4

Bacon Fish Brochettes

Skewer cooking is very popular and easy to prepare in advance. When using wooden skewers, make sure they are soaked in water for 30 minutes or longer before use to prevent them burning when the brochettes are cooked. For this recipe you will need eight 15 cm/6 inch skewers.

Grilling (Broiling) Fish

Make shallow slashes in the skin to allow heat to penetrate. *Brush the fish with melted butter, salt and pepper.* *Put on a greased grill pan (broiler).* *Turn once.*

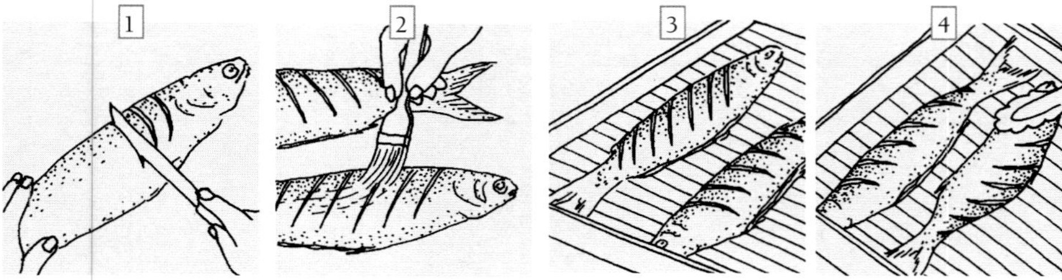

4 x 125 g/4 oz thick firm white fish fillets, each cut into 6 pieces
8 rashers (slices) bacon, rinds removed, each cut into 3 strips
Hollandaise sauce (p. 21)
Oil for basting

Wrap each piece of fish around a strip of bacon and thread three on to each wooden skewer. Place on a grill pan (broiler). Brush the brochettes with a little oil, cook under a preheated grill (broiler), turning once or twice, for 5–10 minutes or until the fish is white in colour and bacon is cooked and slightly crisp. Serve with Hollandaise sauce.
Serves 4

Hollandaise Sauce

4 tablespoons vinegar
5 teaspoons water
12 peppercorns
3 egg yolks
300 g/11 oz/1⅓ cups butter
Juice of 1 lemon
Salt and pepper

Place the vinegar, water and peppercorns in a pan and boil to reduce to a third of its original volume. Allow to cool. Add the yolks and whisk over a gentle heat until creamy. Melt the butter and allow the sediment to settle. Remove the yolk mixture from the heat and whisk in the butter gradually. Add the lemon juice and season with salt and pepper.
Makes about 475 ml/¾ pint/2 cups

Preparation of Fresh Herbs. *Fresh herbs have a tendency to bruise and darken in colour when cut. To avoid this, tear roughly instead.*

Garlic Tuna with Chilli Tomatoes

This robust tomato, pepper and chilli combination, which is Spanish in style, is an ideal sauce for firm oily fish like tuna.

125 ml/4 fl oz/½ cup olive oil
2 onions, sliced
2 small green chillies, seeds removed, finely sliced
3 red peppers (capsicums, bell peppers), cut into julienne strips
1 kg/2¼ lb tomatoes, peeled (p. 45), cut into dice
Salt and pepper
3 tablespoons red wine vinegar
4 x 150 g/5 oz tuna steaks
1–2 tablespoons olive oil
Pepper

SAUCE
2 tablespoons olive oil
2 large garlic cloves, finely chopped

Heat the 125 ml/4 fl oz/½ cup olive oil in a saucepan. Add the onions and cook over a gentle heat for about 5 minutes, or until the onions soften. Add the chillies and red peppers and cook for a further 10 minutes. Add the tomatoes, and cook for another 10 minutes. Season with salt and pepper and leave to stand.

To make the sauce, heat the 2 tablespoons of olive oil in a separate pan and add the garlic. Fry gently for about 3 minutes until golden. Add the red wine vinegar to 'deglaze' the pan, scraping the bottom of the pan to lift any garlic pieces that may have stuck.

Meanwhile, brush each tuna steak with some of the extra olive oil and season with pepper. Place the steaks under a preheated grill (broiler) and cook for 3–5 minutes on each side, or until still a little pink in the centre. Spoon the chilli tomatoes into the centre of each plate, top with the grilled tuna steaks and the combined garlic cloves and olive oil sauce .

Serves 4

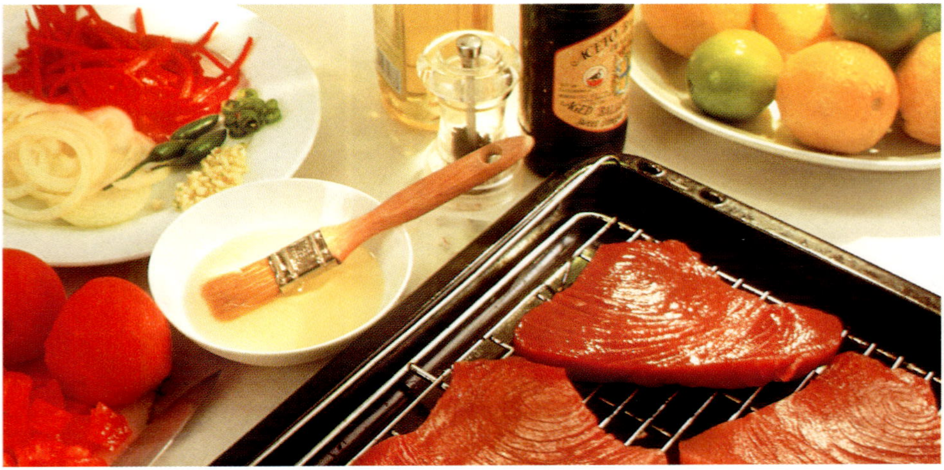

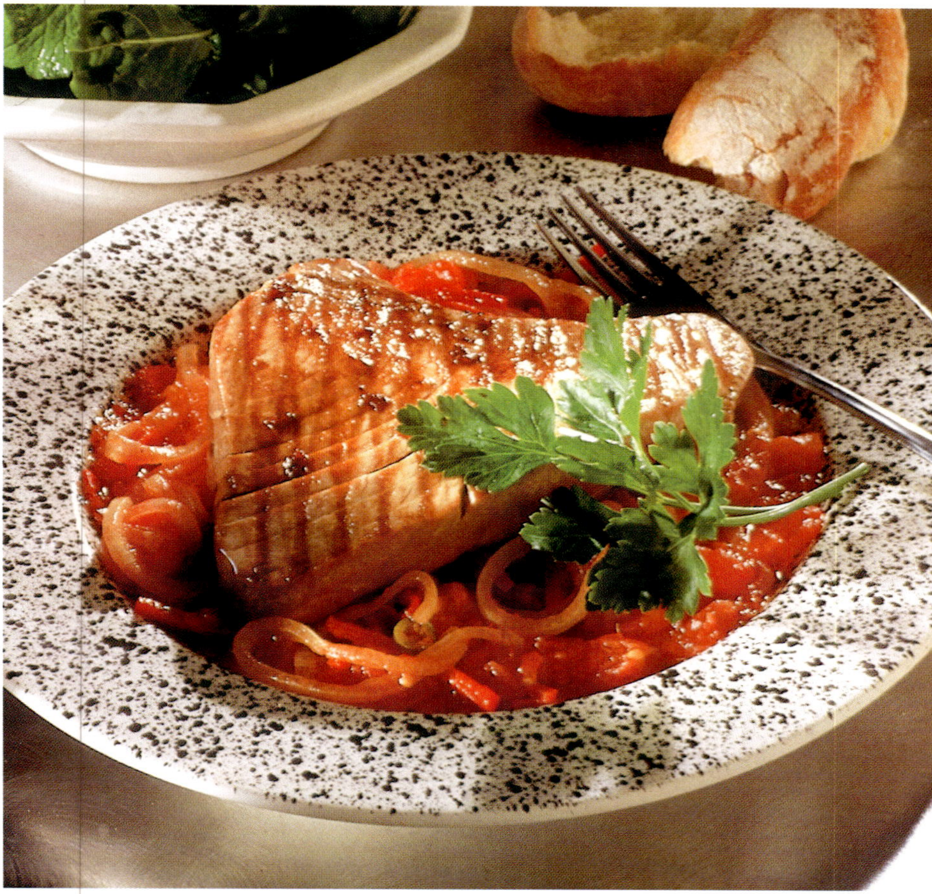

Garlic Tuna with Chilli Tomatoes. The hot and saucy combination of tomato, pepper and chilli sets off the tuna steaks perfectly.To prepare (left) Garlic Tuna with Chilli Tomatoes, place the tuna steaks under a preheated grill (broiler) and cook until a little pink in the centre.
Overleaf: Cantonese Steamed Fish (left)(p. 28), Garlic Tuna with Chilli Tomatoes (right) (left) and Basque Fish Pie (p. 43)—an international trio, offering a variety of exciting and distinctive flavours.

When Is It Cooked? *Fish is cooked when the flesh is opaque (white/cloudy) in colour, the juices run clear and the flesh flakes easily when a fork or tip of a knife is inserted into the thickest section or near the bone. Whole fish, on the other hand, will feel firm to touch and it will continue to cook for a few minutes after being removed from the heat.*

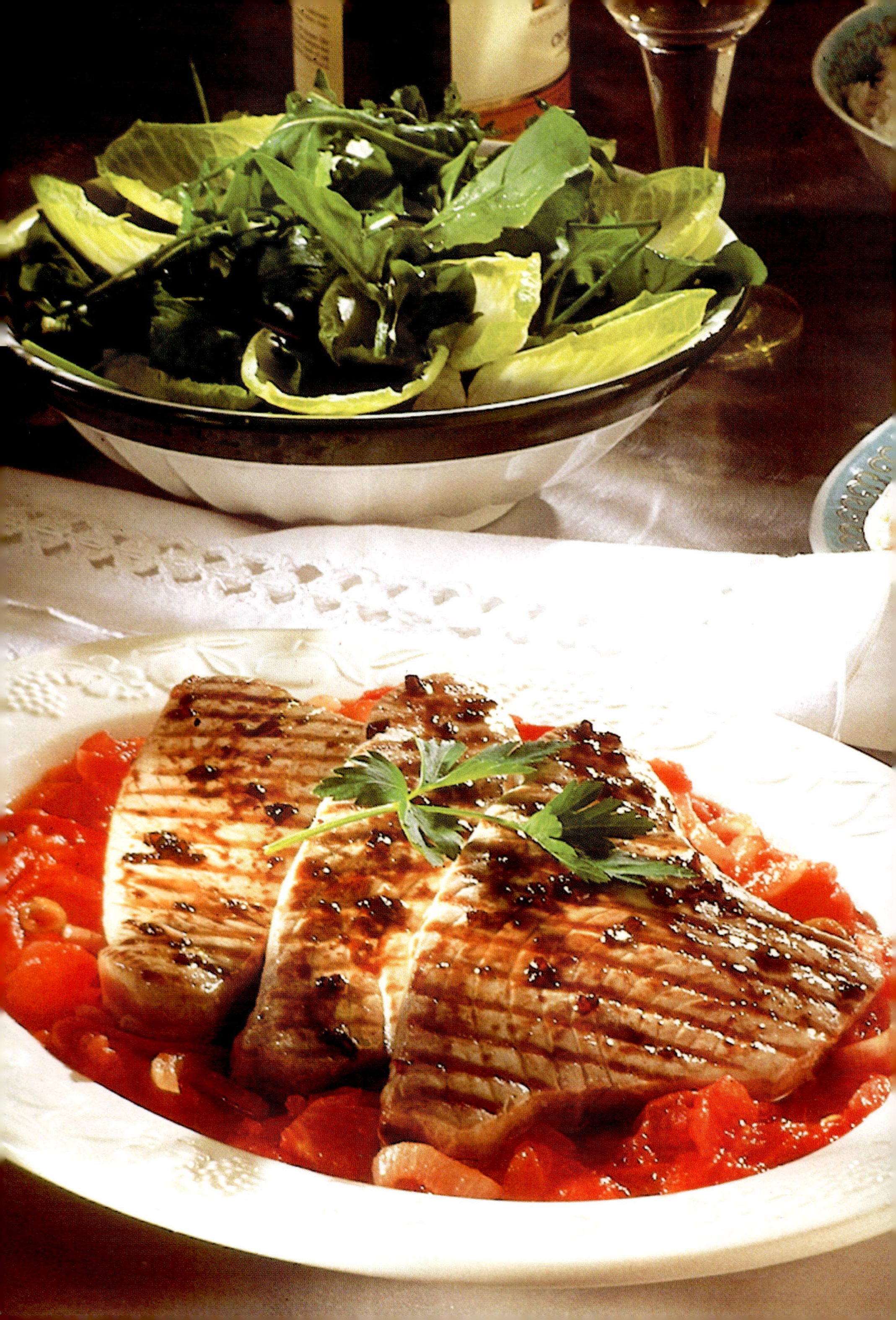

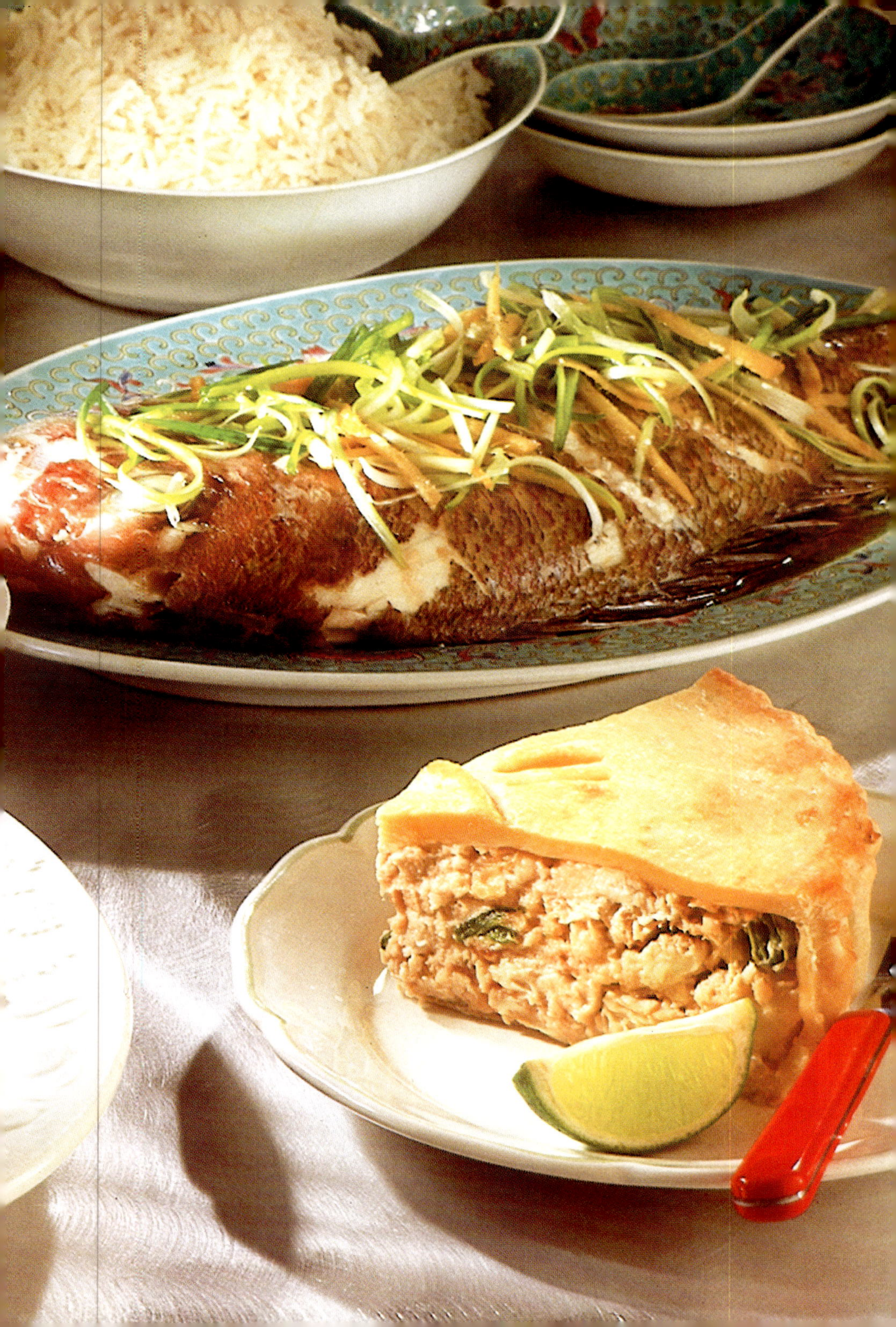

Banana Fish in a Parcel

2 garlic cloves, crushed
1 teaspoon caster (superfine) sugar
2 small red or green chillies, seeds removed and finely chopped
125 ml/4 fl oz/½ cup soy sauce
3 tablespoons lemon juice
4 x 150 g/5 oz whole firm white fish, cleaned and scaled
2 bananas, peeled, skins reserved
2 lemons, thinly sliced

Combine the garlic, sugar, chillies, soy sauce and lemon juice in a bowl. Add the fish and marinate for 30 minutes. Drain and place each fish on a square of foil. Reserve the marinade.

Mash the bananas in a bowl. Place some mashed banana and 1 tablespoon of the marinade over each fish and cover with lemon slices and some banana skin. Wrap completely in the foil. Cook under a preheated hot grill (broiler) for 10 minutes on each side. Place the marinade in a pan and simmer for 3 minutes, adding more sugar and water if necessary. Open the fish parcels, remove the banana skins, pour on some hot marinade and serve.

Serves 4

Whiting with Scallops and Caviar

Plain yoghurt is an excellent marinade base for these skewered, rolled, scallop-stuffed fish fillets which, once grilled (broiled), are served with a caviar yoghurt sauce made from the marinade.

500 g/18 oz whiting or other firm white fish fillets, cut into 12 pieces
12 scallops
200 ml/7 fl oz/¾ cup plain yoghurt
1 tablespoon chopped parsley
1 tablespoon snipped chives
2 spring onions (scallions), finely chopped
1 tablespoon lemon juice
Salt and pepper
30 g/1 oz/2 tablespoons butter
30 g/1 oz red lumpfish caviar
Watercress or dill, to serve

Place a scallop at the end of each whiting fillet and roll up with the scallop coral showing at the side. Secure with a wooden cocktail stick (toothpick). Place in a shallow dish.

Combine the yoghurt, parsley, chives, spring onions and lemon juice. Season lightly with salt and pepper. Spoon over the whiting rolls and marinate for 1–2 hours.

Remove the whiting rolls from the marinade, shake off the excess. Place the rolls in a shallow heatproof dish. Top each with a little piece of butter. Cook under a preheated grill (broiler) for 8–10 minutes, or until the fillets are cooked (p. 23). Remove the cocktail sticks carefully.

Stir half the caviar into the remaining marinade to make a sauce. Spoon a little caviar sauce on to plates and place three whiting rolls on top. Garnish with the remaining caviar and watercress or dill.

Serves 4

Step by Step

Steaming

This method is appropriate for most cuts of fish, particularly those that are firm and white, unlike their oily-natured relatives. The fish is placed in either a bamboo or metal perforated steamer, or for a more modern makeshift approach, a cake rack placed over a wok half-filled with water. As with poaching, the water is kept at simmering point. The fish is always covered, and may be seasoned with a selection of spices. This method is relied upon extensively in Oriental countries.

For whole fish, allow 8–12 minutes for each 200 g/7 oz from the time the water starts simmering. For fillets, steak and cutlets, allow 8–12 minutes.

Steaming Fish

Make shallow slashes on both sides of the fish.

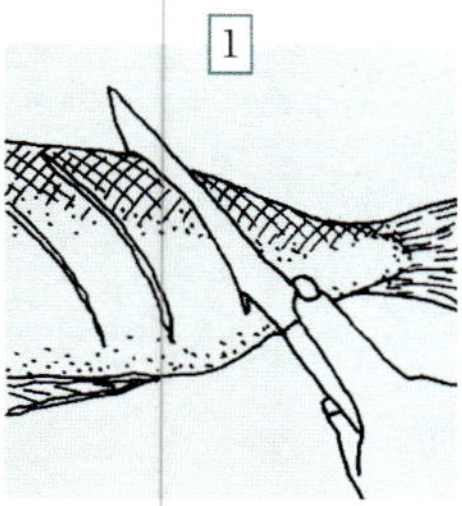

Put on a heatproof plate and garnish.

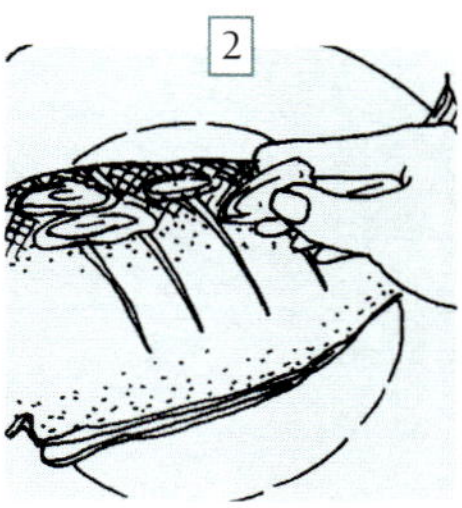

Put in the steamer and cook, covered, for 20 minutes.

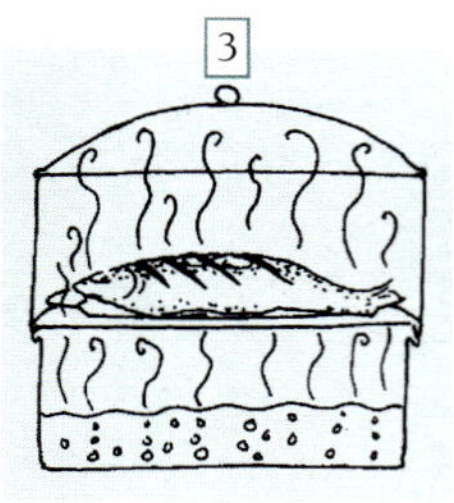

Pour sauce over the fish. Garnish.

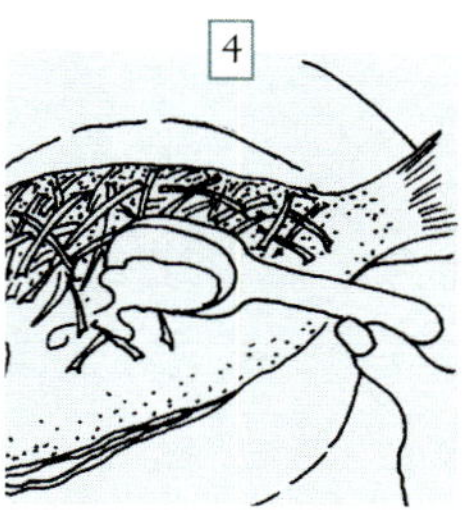

Preparation of Cantonese Steamed Fish (p. 28) Place a rack in a wok, fish kettle or other deep pan.

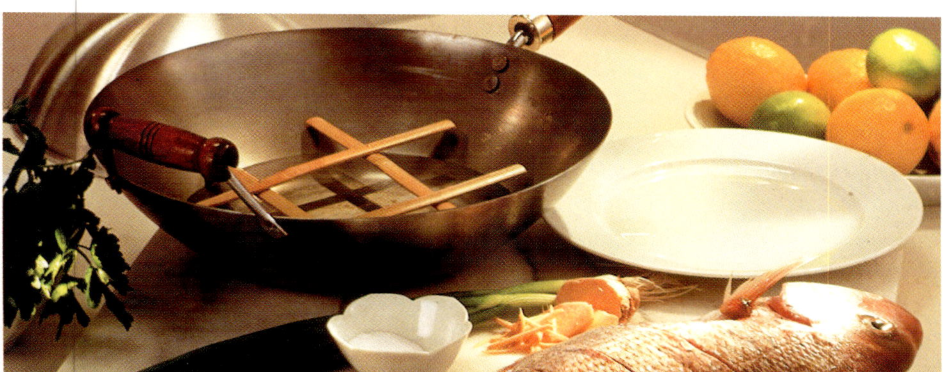

Cantonese Steamed Fish

2 x 1 kg/2¼ lb whole firm white fish
1 teaspoon salt
5 cm/2 inch piece root ginger, peeled, cut into thin slices
2 tablespoons soy sauce
8 spring onions (scallions), finely sliced
4 tablespoons peanut oil
Cooked rice, to serve

Make three or four shallow slashes on each side of the fish. Rub the fish on both sides with the salt and leave to stand for 20 minutes. Place fish on a heatproof platter. Scatter the sliced ginger over the top.

Place a wire or bamboo rack into a wok, fish kettle or other deep pan. Fill with about 5 cm/2 inches of hot water. Bring the water to a simmer. Place the platter holding the fish on to the rack. Cover the wok, fish kettle or pan tightly and steam gently over a medium heat for 20 minutes.

Remove the platter and cooked fish and pour off all the liquid from the platter. Pour the soy sauce over the fish and scatter the spring onions over and around. Heat the oil in a pan until it just smokes, pour this over the fish and serve at once with rice.

Serves 4

Salmon with Roasted Hazelnuts

Salmon fillets are superb when steamed. They will only take a short time to cook. Don't allow the fish to become overcooked–a slightly pink centre is perfect. Serve with hazelnut vinaigrette and steamed potatoes amd steamed potatoes.

150 g/5 oz/1¼ cups hazelnuts

HAZELNUT DRESSING
125 ml/4 fl oz/½ cup hazelnut oil
Juice of ¼ lemon
Salt and pepper

2 x 500 g/18 oz whole salmon fillets, cut through on an angle into 2 portions
2 courgettes (baby marrows, zucchini), cut into fine julienne strips
½ bunch chives, snipped
Small steamed potatoes, to serve

Roast the hazelnuts in a preheated oven at 200°C/400°F/Gas 8 for 10–15 minutes or until the skins are toasted. Cool and rub off the skins. Chop the hazelnuts finely.

To make the dressing, whisk the hazelnut oil, lemon juice, salt and pepper together in a bowl.

Using a bamboo or metal steamer or a cake rack in a wok or deep pan, arrange salmon fillets, skinned side down, and top with the courgettes. Add about 5 cm/2 inch water. Steam for about 5 minutes or until the fish is sealed on the outside but still a little pink in the centre. Remove, using an egg slice.

Place each fillet on a warmed serving plate. Spoon over 2 tablespoons of the hazelnut dressing and scatter over the chopped hazelnuts and snipped chives. Serve immediately.

Serves 4

Step by Step

Poaching

This method of cooking is particularly suitable for whole fish or smaller cuts. The fish and the flavouring ingredients are placed in a pan and covered with water which is then brought to the boil. The pan is either removed from the heat or held at simmering point for a short period. A court bouillon is commonly used for poaching fish. It consists of water, wine or vinegar, roughly chopped vegetables, such as onion, carrot and celery, herbs and peppercorns. This poaching liquid can subsequently be reserved as the basis for an accompanying sauce.

Lemon Ginger Turbans

½ red pepper (capsicum, bell pepper), cut into julienne strips
1 carrot, cut into julienne strips
2 celery sticks, cut into julienne strips
8 x 60 g/2 oz firm white fish fillets, skins removed
250 ml/8 fl oz/1 cup water
3 tablespoons dry white wine
1 thyme sprig
1 bay leaf
5 peppercorns
2 tablespoons clear honey
3 tablespoons lemon juice
2 tablespoons sherry
1 garlic clove, crushed
12 mm/½ inch piece fresh root ginger, grated
Steamed rice, to serve

Preparation of Fish in Caper Butter Sauce (p. 31). The subtly piquant sauce complements these delicious fish steaks perfectly.

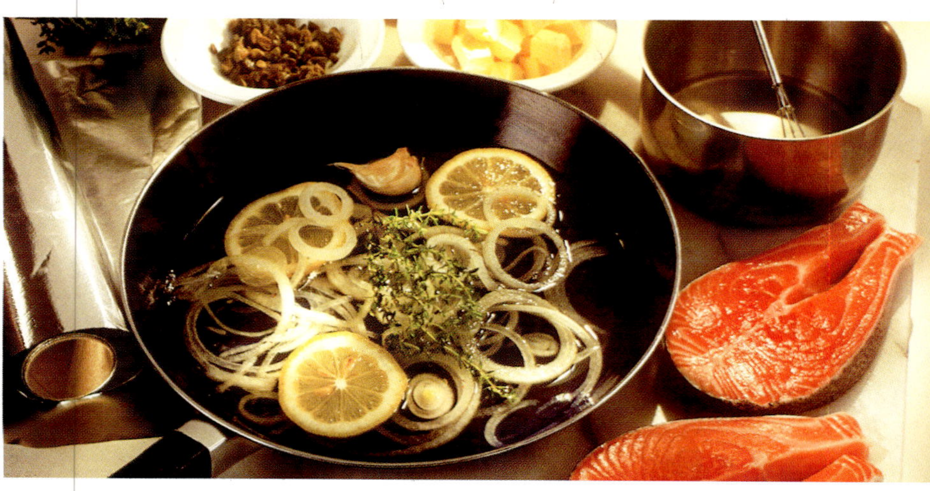

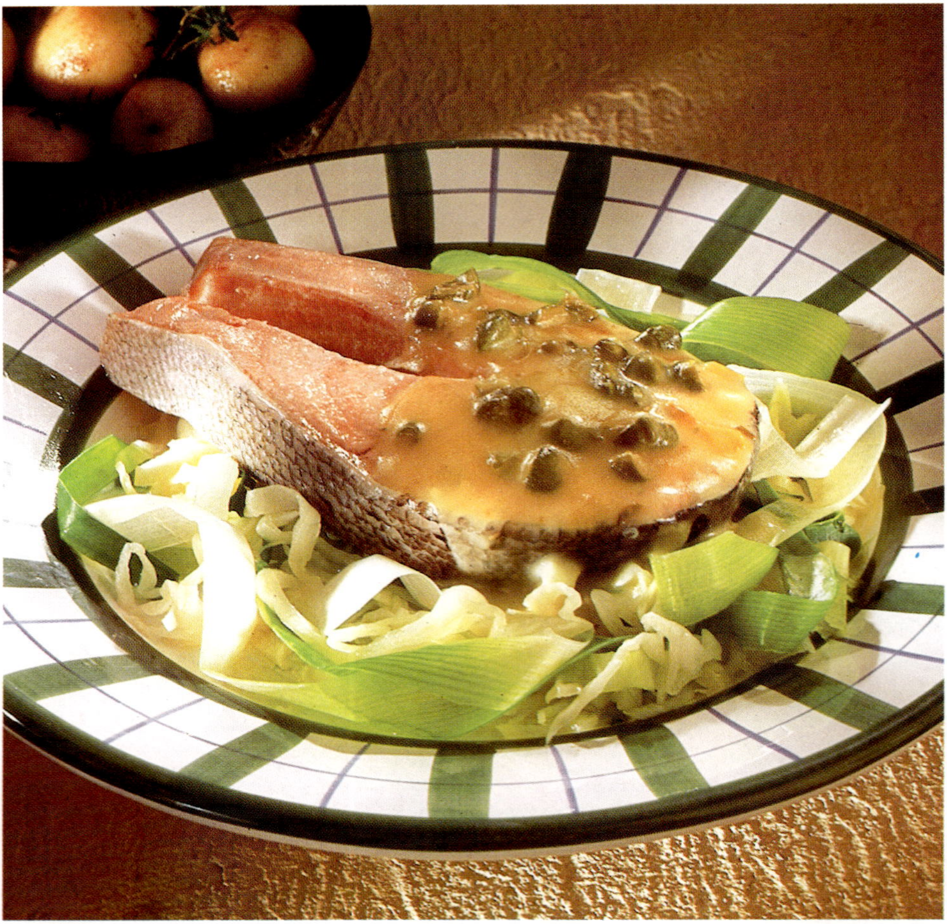

Fish in Caper Butter Sauce.

Combine the julienne vegetables and place some on the tail end of each fillet. Roll up and secure with wooden cocktail sticks (toothpicks).

Put the water, wine, thyme, bay leaf and peppercorns in a large frying pan (skillet). Place the fish rolls in the liquid and poach for about 3 minutes, or until they are white in colour throughout. Drain the fish on paper towels and transfer to a warmed serving dish.

Place the honey, lemon juice, sherry, garlic and ginger in a small saucepan and stir continuously until the sauce thickens slightly. Remove the wooden cocktail sticks from the fish and serve with the sauce. Accompany with steamed rice.

Serves 4

Blanching Vegetables. *Bring a large saucepan of water to the boil. Cut vegetables into the desired shape (florets, if broccoli or cauliflower, or if celery, carrot or courgette, into sticks of about 9 mm x 9 mm x 7.5 cm ($\frac{3}{8}$ x $\frac{3}{8}$ x 3 inches). Put the vegetables into a strainer or colander that will fit into your saucepan. Plunge the vegetables into boiling water for about 20 seconds, drain and plunge immediately into iced water to arrest further cooking so the vegetables will retain their crispness. Drain and use as required. This process is used to soften vegetables slightly and bring out their colour.*

Fish in Caper Butter Sauce

2 brown onions, finely sliced
4 sprigs thyme
1 unpeeled garlic clove, crushed
1 teaspoon salt
$\frac{1}{4}$ teaspoon pepper
1 lemon, cut into slices
4 x 200 g/7 oz thick, firm, white fish steaks
1 litre/1$\frac{3}{4}$ pints/4$\frac{1}{4}$ cups water
125 ml/4 fl oz/$\frac{1}{2}$ cup tarragon or wine vinegar
125 g/4 oz/$\frac{1}{2}$ cup butter, cut into small pieces
2 tablespoons capers, finely chopped
1 wedge cabbage, central core removed, finely sliced, blanched (above), to serve
1 leek, cut into ribbons, blanched (above), to serve

Combine the onions, thyme, garlic, salt, pepper and lemon slices in a pan. Add the fish and cover with water. Cover and bring to simmering point, remove from the heat. Reserve 250 ml/8 fl oz/1 cup of the liquid and leave the fish to stand in the remaining liquid for about 10 minutes.

Place the reserved liquid in a saucepan, cook over a high heat for about 5 minutes until reduced by half. Add the tarragon or wine vinegar and boil for about 1 minute. Reduce the heat to low and whisk in the butter gradually, ensuring each piece is mixed in before adding more. Add the capers and season with salt and pepper.

Remove the fish from the pan. Place the blanched cabbage and leek on warm serving plates, top with the fish, and pour over the sauce.

Serves 4

Poaching Fish

Put the wine, herbs and pepper into a pan.

Place the fish in the pan and cover with water.

Cover the pan and bring to the boil. Remove from heat.

Leave fish to stand in the liquid for10 minutes to finish cooking.

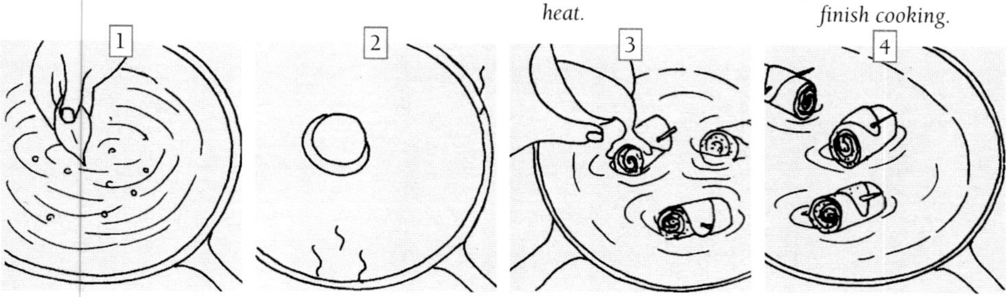

Step by Step

Baking

This method of cooking is suitable for all cuts of fish—both whole and portions. Because fish flesh is so delicate and lean, it is recommended that oil or melted butter be brushed over regularly during the cooking process to protect the fish from drying out. Rapid cooking by this method helps to keep particularly lean fish moist. Some of the following recipes have either liquid or a topping poured over them for added protection. Always preheat your oven to a moderate temperature (180°C/350°F/gas 4, as a guide) for best results. For whole fish, allow 10 minutes for each 200 g/7 oz. For fillets or steaks, 20–30 minutes.

The foil baking method is an excellent way of retaining flavour and moisture. The physical barrier reduces greatly the evaporation of juices and in effect serves as a steaming implement. The fish is placed on a section of foil large enough to enclose the fish. It is seasoned and topped with vegetables or herbs, nuts and fruit, or even seafood, as you will see in the following recipes. The foil is gathered around the fish and its accompaniments, sealed tightly into an 'envelope' and baked in the oven for a designated time, which is usually only up to 10 minutes.

Tomato-Lemon Fish

Select firm fish fillets or cutlets for this dish. Serve with steamed potatoes or rice and a salad.

1 lemon, cut into 8 thin slices
4 x 200 g/7 oz firm white fish fillets or cutlets
2 tomatoes, each cut into 4 slices
2 courgettes (baby marrows, zucchini), thinly sliced
Pepper
A few sprigs Italian (flat leafed) parsley or basil leaves

Cut four matching squares of foil and place two lemon slices in the centre of each. Place a fish fillet or cutlet on top, add two slices of tomato and some slices of courgette, season with pepper and top with parsley or basil leaves. Fold over the foil to seal the fish into tight parcels. Place on a hot barbecue/grill (broiler) for 4–10 minutes depending on their thickness, or bake in a preheated oven at 180°C/350°F/gas 4 for 6–10 minutes.
Serves 4

Tomato-Lemon Fish. You would be forgiven for thinking this dish had Mediterranean origins—perhaps it's the Italian parsley!

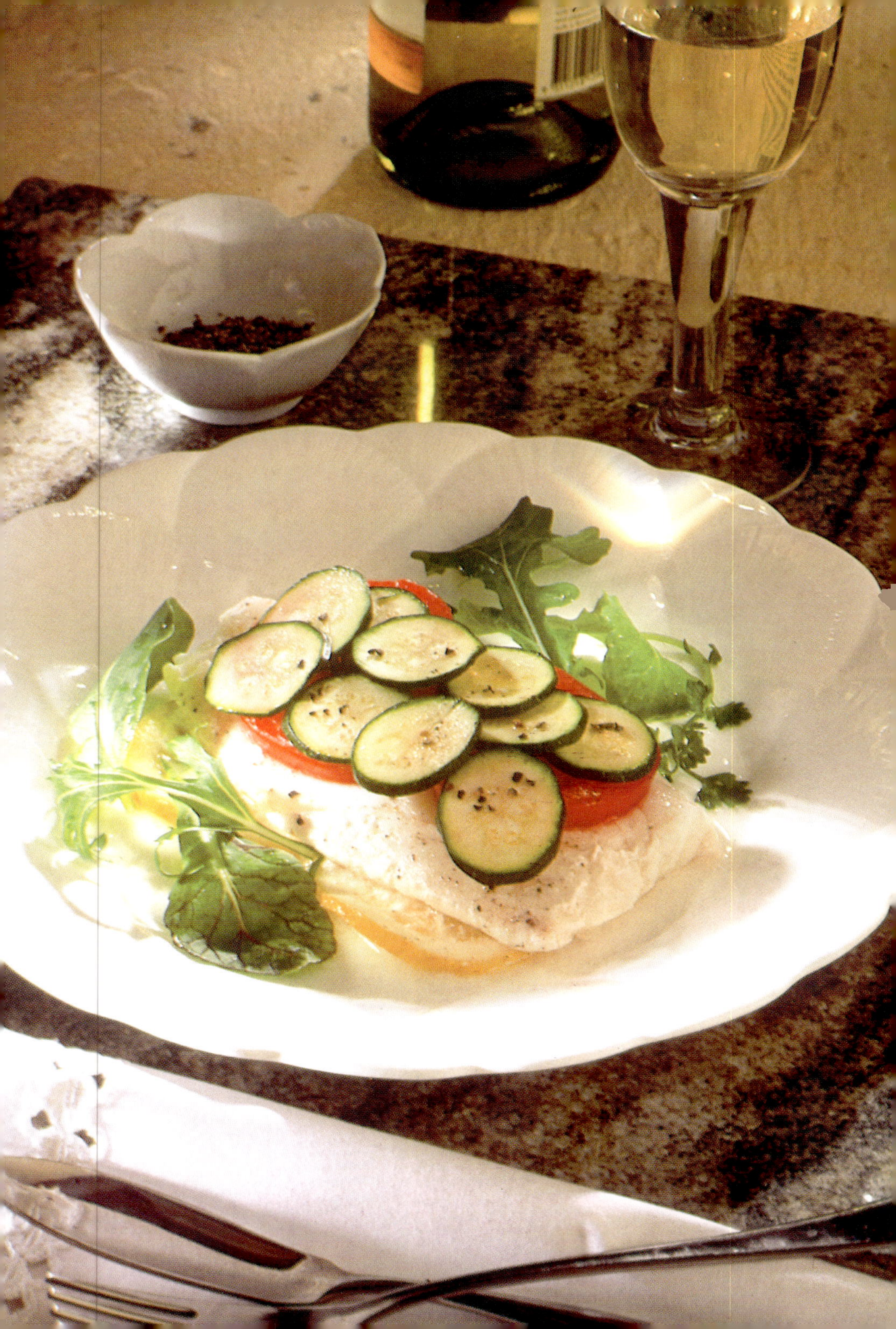

Variations. Ingredients are listed in the order in which they are placed on the foil:

Sliced tomatoes, breadcrumbs, a little curry powder, sultanas, fish, pepper, a little dry white wine.

Olive oil and a little lemon juice or sherry brushed on to both sides of fish.

Very thinly sliced mushrooms, thin strips of celery and carrot, fish, lemon juice or white wine.

Very thinly sliced leeks, fish, more leeks and a little dry white wine.

Foil Baking or En Papillote

Cut a foil square large enough to contain each fish.

Place seasoning vegetables in centre of foil.

Place fish fillet on top with herbs and lemon slices.

Fold the foil over to seal the fish in secure parcels.

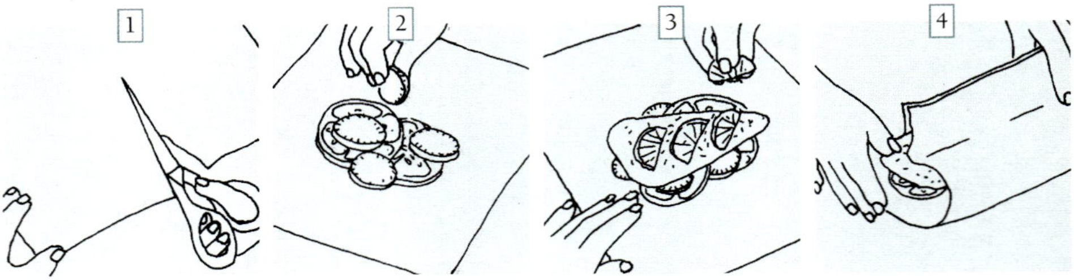

Preparation of Tomato-Lemon Fish (p. 32). Foil is used in this dish to protect the fish during cooking and to retain the moisture and delicious flavour.

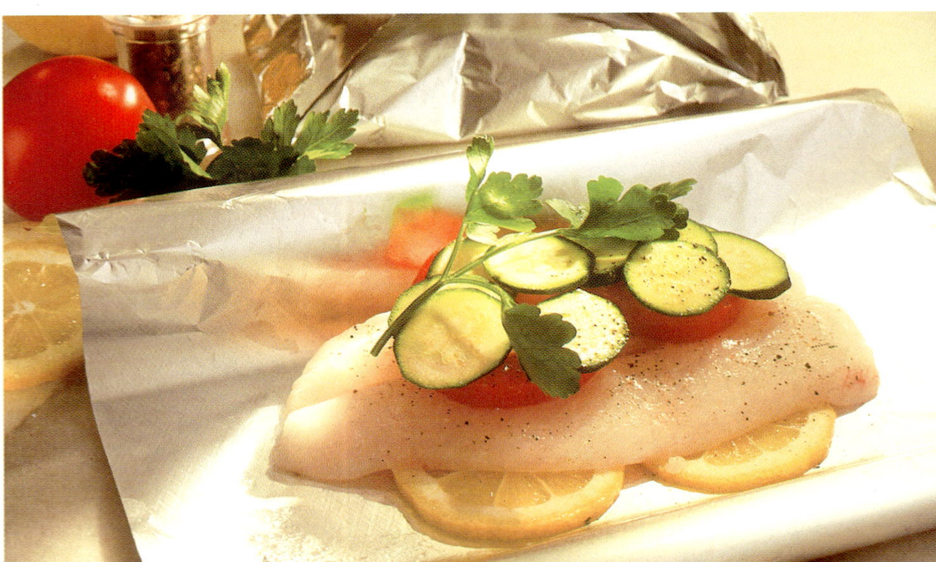

Cleaning Leeks. *Cut off and discard any dark green leaves. They're too tough and can be bitter. If using as a whole vegetable, cut down the middle of the leek to about 2.5 cm/1 inch of the root end. Wash thoroughly under cold water, spreading the layers gently, making sure all the grit is washed out. Slice or chop as required.*

Seafood Snapper in Foil

If prawns (shrimp) and scallops are not available, substitute thin strips of blanched celery, carrot and leek.

2 leeks, cut into thin slices and blanched (above)
4 x 200 g/7 oz snapper fillets
12 scallops
8 large green prawns (shrimp), peeled and cleaned
2.5 cm/1 inch piece root ginger, cut into julienne strips
1 teaspoon lemon peel
4 teaspoons lemon juice
60 g/2 oz/¼ cup butter, melted
Salt and pepper

Cut foil into four 30 cm/12 inch diameter circles. Place blanched leeks in the centre of each foil circle and lay a fish fillet on top. Arrange the scallops and prawns on top and sprinkle with the ginger and lemon peel. Spoon over the lemon juice and butter. Season with salt and pepper.

Gather up the edges of foil and fold over to seal the parcels. Place on a baking sheet and bake in a preheated oven at 200°C/400°F/gas 6 for 10–12 minutes, or until cooked (p. 23).

Place each fish parcel on an individual plate. Fold back the edges of the foil and serve at once or slide the contents of the parcel on to the plate.

Serves 4

Date and Almond Baked Fish

This unusual stuffing mixture adds a Middle Eastern flavour to whole fish. Wrapped in foil, this dish can be prepared in advance.

250 g/9 oz/1¾ cups roughly chopped dates
125 g/4 oz/1 cup ground blanched almonds
3 tablespoons butter, melted
½ teaspoon ground cinnamon
1 tablespoon chopped coriander (cilantro)
2.5 cm/1 inch piece root ginger, finely chopped
5 tablespoons lemon juice
Pepper
6 x 350–425 g/12–15 oz whole firm white fish, cleaned and scaled (p. 36)
Oil for brushing
Cooked rice or couscous, to serve

Combine the dates, almonds, butter, cinnamon, coriander, ginger and lemon juice in a bowl, season with pepper. Mix well.

Pat the fish dry with paper towels. Cut six sheets of foil large enough to wrap each fish completely. Brush with oil. Divide the date mixture between the sheets of foil, place the fish on top and sprinkle over any remaining mixture.

Wrap the foil tightly around the fish and bake in a preheated oven at 180°C/350°/gas 4 for 20 minutes, or until cooked (p. 23). Cut open the foil, serve with cooked rice or couscous.

Serves 6

Scaling Fish. *To scale, hold the fish by the tail and scrape with a knife from the tail to the head. Repeat with the other side of the backbone over a large sheet of paper. Remove any fins with a sharp pair of scissors, being careful as they may be quite spiky.*

Baking a Whole Fish

Place fish in a baking dish and pour over wine and melted butter.

Sprinkle on spring onions (scallions) and carrot. Cover with foil. Bake for 15 minutes.

Remove from oven. Pour pan juices into a saucepan to make sauce.

Place fish on a warm plate and serve the sauce separately.

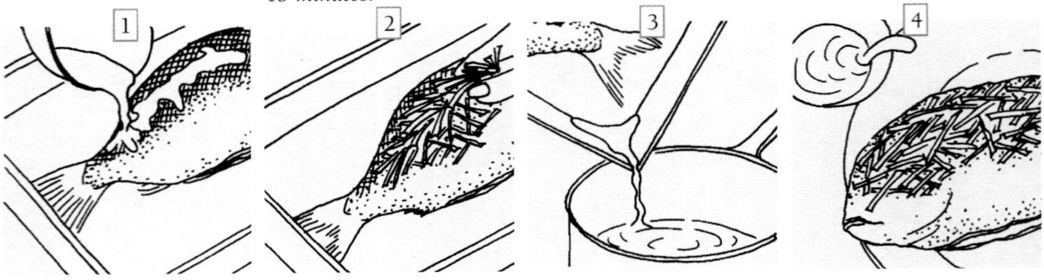

Snapper Calabrese

Olives and capers in this tomato sauce add a robust Italian flavour to any baked firm, white whole fish.

4 x 350–450 g/17 oz–1 lb whole snapper, scaled (above)
Salt and pepper
1 lemon, thinly sliced
90 g/3 oz/6 tablespoons butter
3 tablespoons capers, drained
10 black olives or stuffed olives, sliced
1 tablespoon oregano leaves
400 g/14 oz canned peeled tomatoes or fresh tomatoes, peeled (p. 45)
6 tablespoons tomato paste
3 tablespoons lemon juice
3 tablespoons water

Lemon Twist Garnish. *Slice a lemon thinly with a sharp knife. Make a small cut into one side of the slice and twist outwards.*

Pat the fish dry with paper towels, season the cavities with salt and pepper and tuck two lemon slices into each fish.

Melt 60 g/2 oz/¼ cup of the butter in a large roasting pan. Roll each snapper in the butter to coat both sides. Bake in a preheated oven at 180°C/350°F/gas 4 for 20 minutes or until cooked (p. 23). Lift the fish on to a heated platter and keep warm.

Melt the remaining butter in a saucepan, add the remaining ingredients and stir until combined, breaking up the tomatoes with the edge of a spoon. Simmer for 5 minutes and spoon the sauce over the snapper.

Serves 4

Tarragon Fish Gratin

If fresh tarragon is not available, use half the quantity of dried or substitute dill, another excellent herb used frequently when cooking fish.

4 x 200 g/7 oz firm white fish fillets
Salt and pepper
150 ml/1/4 pint/2/3 cup white wine
1 sprig of tarragon
30 g/1 oz/2 tablespoons butter
30 g/1 oz/2 tablespoons plain (all-purpose) flour
200 ml/7 fl oz/3/4 cup single (light) cream
1 tablespoon chopped tarragon
4 tablespoons fresh breadcrumbs (p. 17)
60 g/2 oz/¼ cup butter, melted
Creamed potatoes, to serve
Steamed vegetables, to serve

Place the fish fillets in a greased baking dish. Season with salt and pepper. Pour over the wine and add the sprig of tarragon. Cover with foil and bake in a preheated oven at 180°C/350°F/gas 4 for about 10 minutes.

Melt the butter in a saucepan, add the flour to make a roux (p. 48). Cook for about 2 minutes, stirring continuously, then set aside to cool. Heat the cream, simmer for 3 minutes until it thickens slightly. Whisk or stir the hot cream into the roux until the sauce combines. Set aside.

Remove the fish from the oven. Pour the pan juices into another saucepan and boil to reduce by half. Add slowly to the cream sauce over a moderate heat, whisking or stirring continuously until sauce boils. Add the chopped tarragon.

Pour the sauce over the fish, sprinkle with the breadcrumbs and melted butter and grill (broil) or return to the oven until golden brown.

Serve with creamed potatoes and a colourful combination of steamed seasonal vegetables.

Serves 4

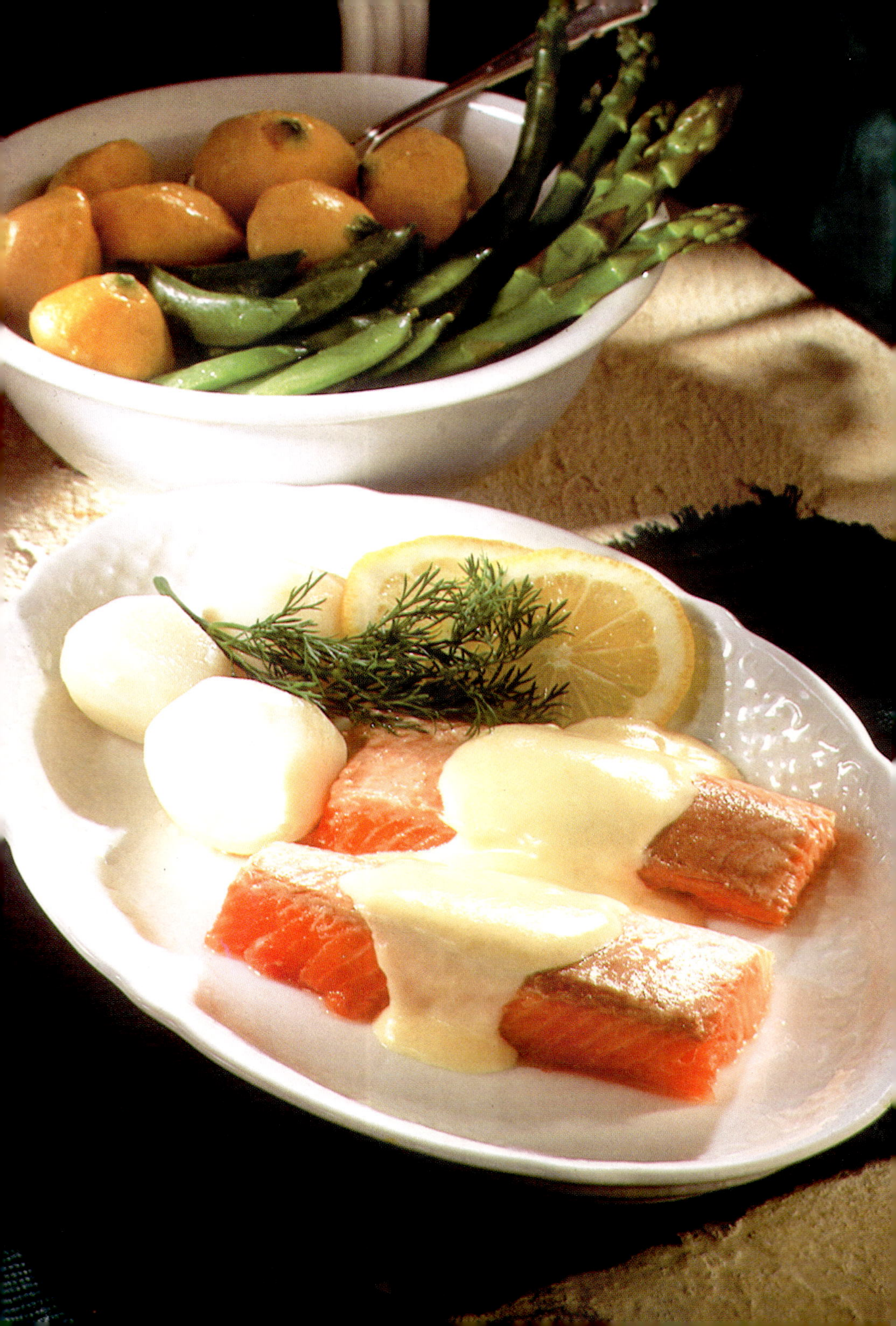

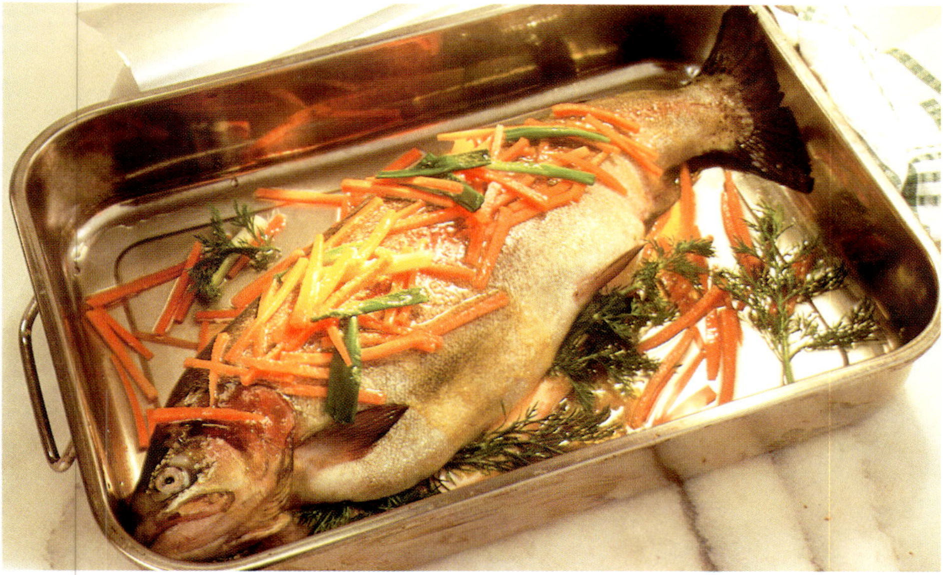

Above: Preparation of Baked Trout with Lemon Cream Sauce. Add the cooking juices to cream and lemon juice for this wonderful sauce. Left: This is a simply delicious dish which can be adapted to larger or smaller fish varieties.

Baked Trout with Lemon Cream Sauce

This simple dish can be adapted to the size of the fish you're able to get. Alter the quantities and adjust the baking time if necessary.

1 x 800 g/13⁄4 lb (or 2 x 375 g/12 oz) whole salmon trout
250 ml/8 fl oz/1 cup white wine
125 g/4 oz/1/2 cup butter, melted
Salt and pepper
3 spring onions (scallions), cut into 7.5 cm/3 inch lengths, blanched (p. 31)
2 carrots, cut into julienne strips, blanched (p. 31)
3 tablespoons single (light) cream
1–2 tablespoons lemon juice

Place the fish in a large baking dish, pour over the white wine and melted butter. Season with salt and pepper.

Place the spring onions and carrot on top of the fish, cover with foil and bake in a preheated oven at 230°C/450°F/gas 8 for 15–20 minutes or until cooked (p. 23). Remove from the oven and keep warm while you make the sauce.

Pour the cooking juices from the fish into a saucepan and boil to reduce slightly. Add the cream and lemon juice and reduce until it has thickened. Serve with the trout.

Serves 4

Pine Nut-Crumb Baked Mackerel

A Sicilian-style crumb crust incorporating pine nuts and raisins and the citrus flavour of orange. It's perfect with any oily type of fish.

4 x 250 g/9 oz mackerel, cleaned
Salt and pepper
5 tablespoons fresh breadcrumbs (p. 17)
2 oranges
125 g/4 oz/1 cup raisins, soaked in water for about 10 minutes
125 g/4 oz/1/2 cup pine nuts
6 tablespoons virgin olive oil

Season the mackerel with salt and pepper. Arrange in a greased casserole dish.

Mix the breadcrumbs with the grated peel of 1 orange, the raisins and pine nuts. Squeeze the juice from the orange and pour 3 tablespoons over the mackerel. Pour over the olive oil and cover with the breadcrumb mixture. Bake in a preheated oven at 200°C/400°F/gas 8 for 20–25 minutes. Remove from the oven. Cut the remaining orange into thin slices to garnish the mackerel and serve.

Serves 6

Baked Fish in Filo

This is a simple oven-baked surprise. Filo pastry layers are wrapped around whiting or other similar fillets. The pastry not only protects but provides moisture and flavour to the fish.

8 sheets filo pastry
90 g/3 oz/6 tablespoons butter, melted
4 x 150–200 g/5–7 oz firm white long fish fillets, cut in half horizontally
2 tablespoons lemon juice
30 g/1 oz/2 tablespoons butter, extra
8 spring onions (scallions), finely chopped
125 g/4 oz mushrooms, finely chopped
Lemon twists (p. 37) and parsley, to garnish

Brush two sheets of filo pastry lightly with the melted butter. Place one on top of the other. Place two fish fillets in the centre of the pastry square and sprinkle with lemon juice. Repeat for the remaining fillets.

Melt the extra butter in a frying pan (skillet) and fry the spring onions and mushrooms over a moderate heat for 5 minutes. Spoon over the fish fillets and fold the pastry into an envelope enclosing the fish fillets. Place on a greased baking sheet and brush with melted butter. Bake in the upper half of a preheated oven at 200°C/400°F/gas 6 for 15 minutes or until pastry is golden brown. Garnish with lemon and the parsley and serve with seasonal vegetables or tossed salad.

Serves 4

Basque Fish Pie (p. 43). This delectable Spanish-style pie can be devoured hot or cold at a picnic or on the patio.

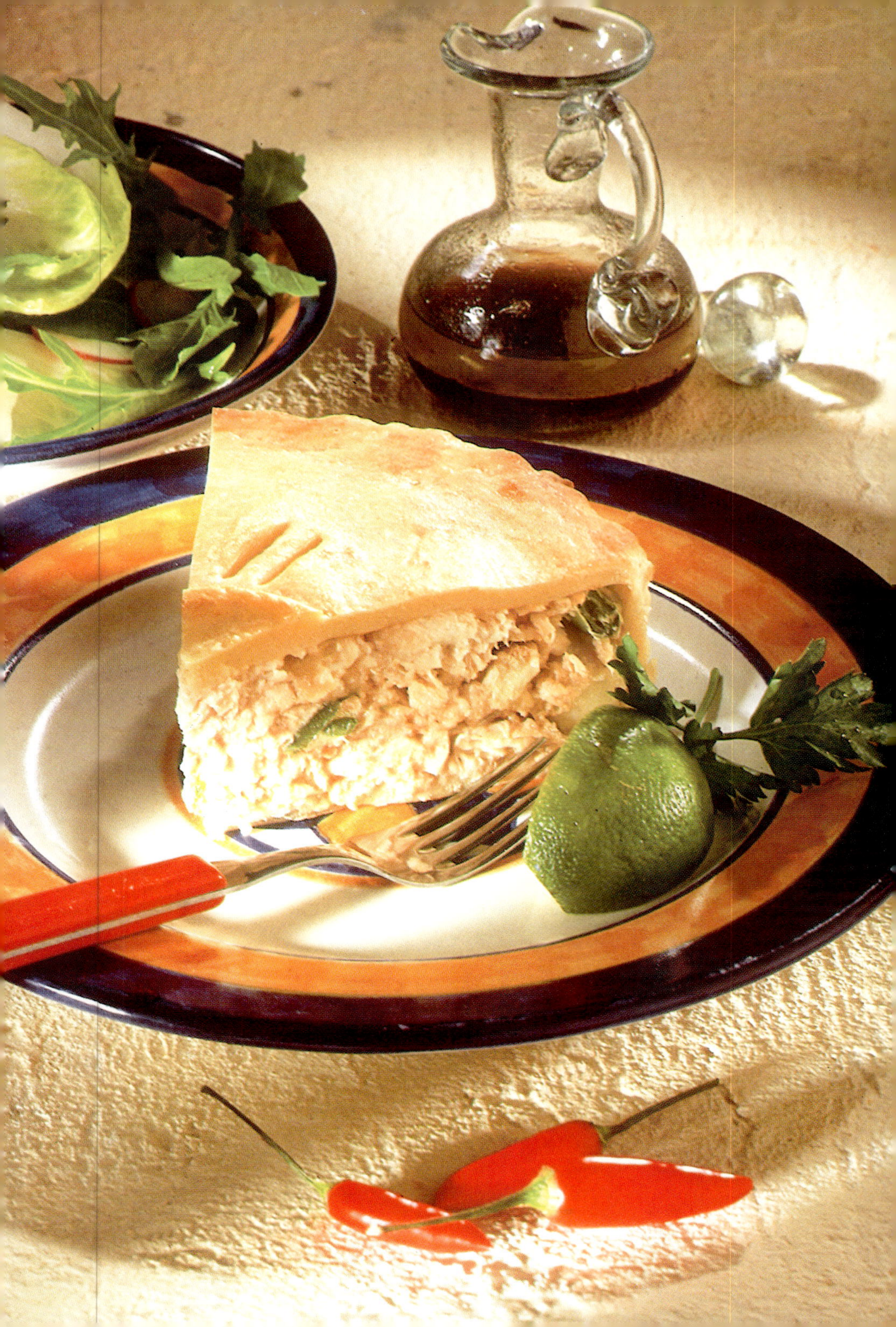

How To Bake Pastry Blind. *Line a pan as directed in the recipe. Place a piece of lightly greased foil on top of the pastry (shiny side down). Top the covered pastry case with rice or pasta as a weight. Bake in a preheated oven at 200°C/400°F/gas 6 for about 10 minutes. Remove foil and rice or pasta, reduce the temperature to 180°C/350°F/gas 4, prick the base lightly with a fork and continue baking for another 15 minutes or until the pastry is lightly browned and crisp. Use as required. This is done to firm the base up before adding a pie filling, which may be heavy and interfere with the cooking of the pastry.*

Preparation of Basque Fish Pie. When the fish is added to the pan, cover, reduce the heat and cook until the fish is opaque.

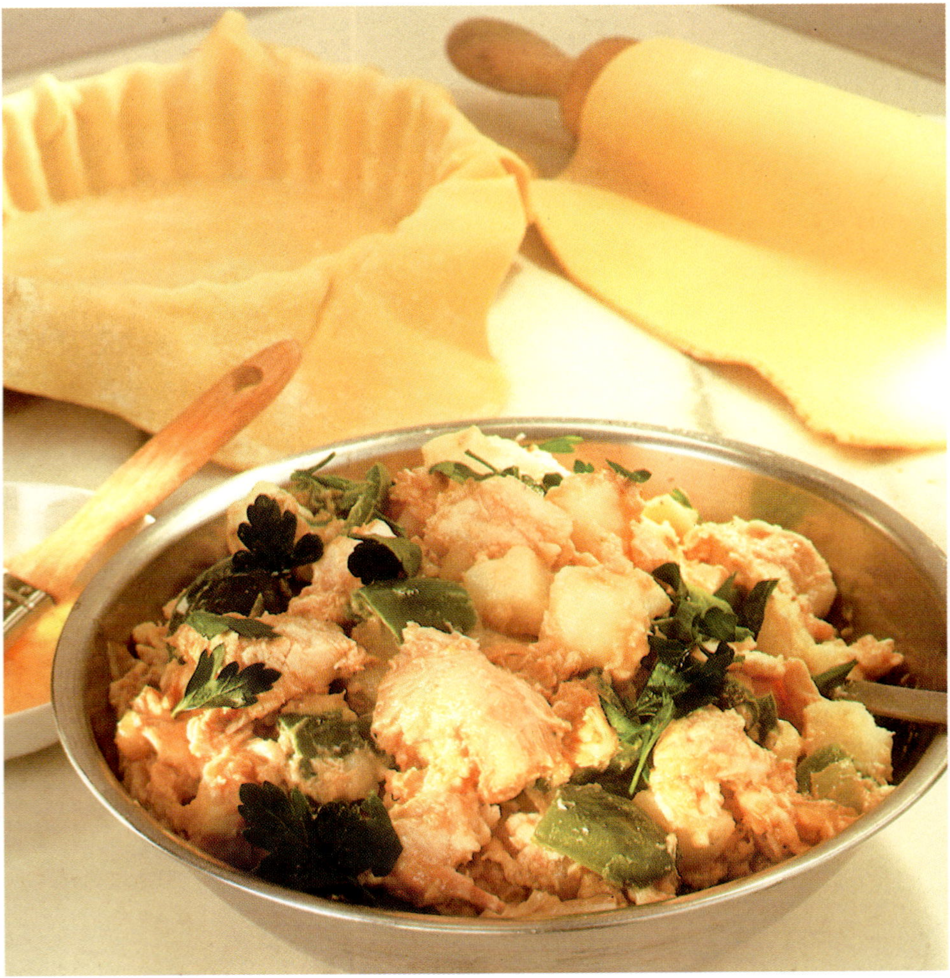

Basque Fish Pie

A pie baked in a fluted flan tin (pie pan) produces a fish, pepper and potato combination.

500 g/18 oz shortcrust pastry (basic pie dough)
2 tablespoons olive oil
1 large brown onion, thinly sliced
575 g/11/4 lb green pepper (capsicum, bell pepper), cut into julienne strips
2 garlic cloves, crushed
1 kg/21/4 lb tuna or firm white fish fillets, cut into large dice
1 kg/21/4 lb potatoes, cut into dice
1 litre/13/4 pints/41/4 cups water
3 tablespoons tomato paste
1/2 teaspoon paprika
Salt and pepper
2 tablespoons roughly chopped parsley
1 egg yolk
2 tablespoons milk
Lemon wedges, to serve

Roll out two-thirds of the pastry and line a deep 25 cm/10 inch flan tin (pie pan) with a removable base. Trim the edges and bake blind (left) in a preheated oven at 220°C/425°F/gas 7 for 10 minutes. Remove from oven. Reduce the oven temperature to 190°C/375°F/gas 5.

Heat the oil in a large saucepan, add the onion, peppers and garlic. Fry for 4–5 minutes or until the vegetables soften. Add the fish, cover, reduce the heat to low and cook for 5–6 minutes or until opaque.

Meanwhile, place the diced potato in a large saucepan and cover with the water. Bring to the boil and simmer for 15 minutes. Drain the potato and add to the fish mixture. Add the paprika, salt, pepper, parsley and tomato paste, with a little water if the mixture seems dry. Spoon into the baked pie shell.

Roll the remaining pastry and any trimmings out into a circle. Place on top of the pie, and trim the edges. Brush with the combined egg yolk and milk. Place in the oven and bake for 20–25 minutes or until the pastry is golden. Leave to stand for 5 minutes and then cut into wedges. Serve with lemon wedges and salad.

Serves 6

Making a Fish Pie

Line a fluted flan tin (pie pan) with half the pastry.

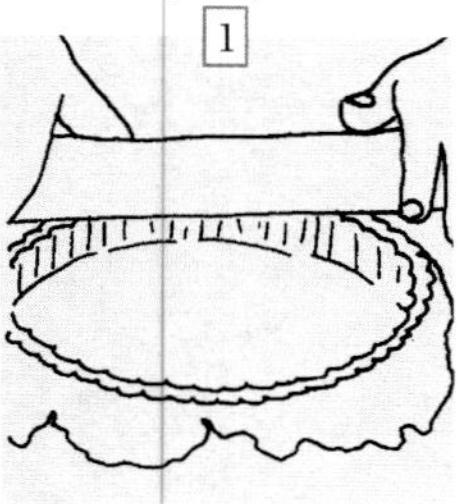

Cook vegetables in a pan, then cook fish fillets until just opaque.

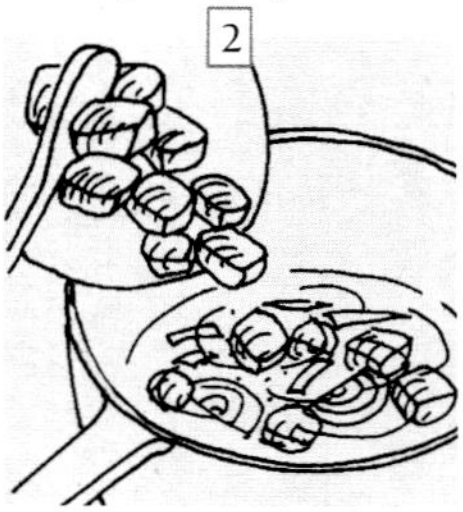

Put potatoes, tomato paste, seasonings, fish and vegetables in pie.

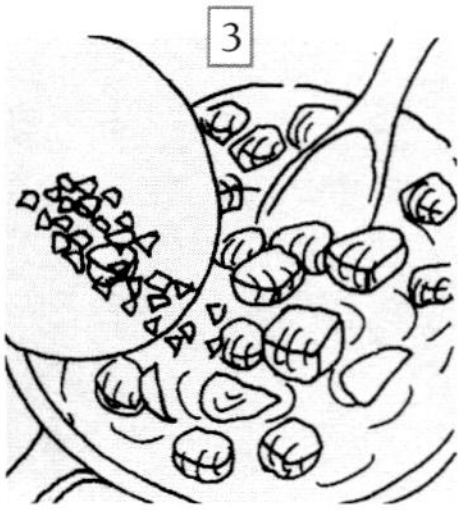

Cover with pastry, trim and brush with eggwash.

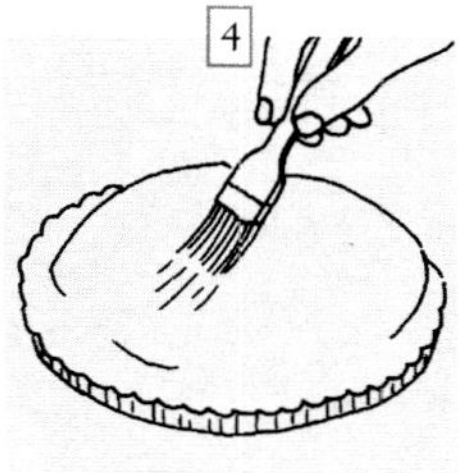

Step by Step

Braising

When braising fish, the time involved must be minimal or overcooking will result in fish that is crumbly and dry. Spices or flavourings are pan-fried first, liquid is usually added and the fish is tossed in towards the end of the cooking time. The liquid used is maintained at a simmer. Liquid that boils rapidly over a period will break up and overcook the fish. The method of layering the potatoes in the following Boullinada recipe gives more than interest to the dish—it acts as a protective barrier too.

Boullinada

This is a Spanish version of a Bouillabaisse and is a hearty fish stew you can prepare easily.

1 teaspoon butter
4 garlic cloves, crushed
200 g/7 oz red pepper (capsicum, bell pepper), cut into julienne strips
2 onions, coarsely chopped
1-2 red chillies, seeds removed, sliced
1 cup chopped parsley
Salt and pepper
1 kg/21/4 lb potatoes, thinly sliced
800 g/13/4 lb firm white fish fillets
1 litre/13/4 pints/41/4 cups water
2 tablespoons olive oil
Garlic bread, to serve (p. 44)

Melt the butter in a large saucepan, add the garlic, red peppers, onions, chillies and parsley. Season with salt and pepper. Cook for about 5 minutes, stirring continuously until the onions soften.

Layer half the potato slices on top of the parsley mixture, followed by half the fish, more potatoes, the remaining fish and potatoes. Pour in the water, cover and bring to the boil, over a high heat. Add the oil and cook rapidly for 15 minutes to reduce the liquid and thicken the sauce. Serve with garlic bread.

Serves 4

Garlic Bread. *Cut a small loaf of French or Italian bread into fairly thick slices, cutting all the way through. Spread the cut surfaces with garlic butter (see recipe above). Re-assemble the loaf and wrap it in foil. Bake in a preheated oven at 190°C/375°F/gas 5 for 20 minutes, open foil and bake a further 5 minutes, or until crunchy. Serve immediately.*

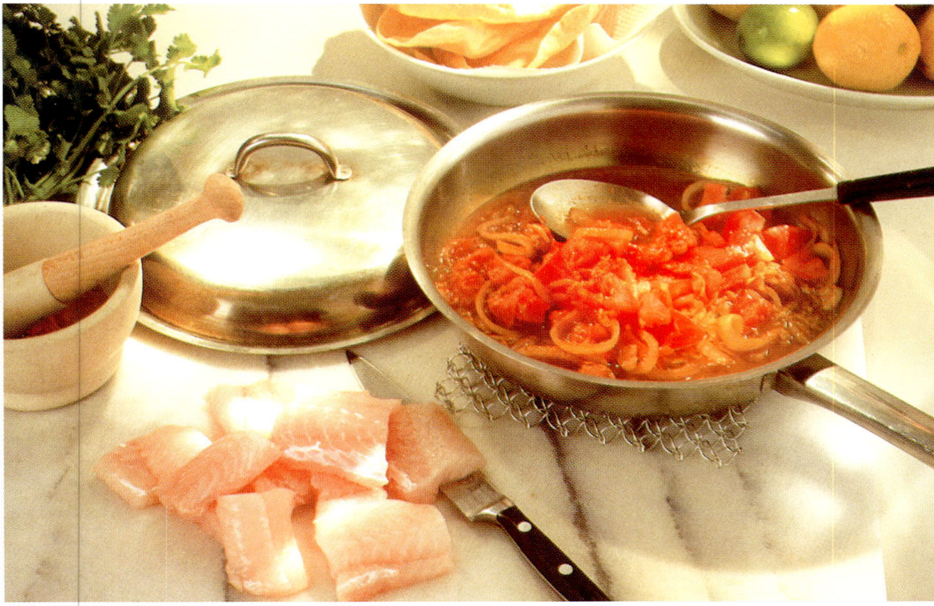

Preparation of Spicy Fish Curry. Here's an important hint—always cook ground spices to release their aromatic flavour.

Spicy Fish Curry

You can add some coconut cream or plain yoghurt as a variation and serve with crisp poppadums and fruit chutney.

675 g/1½ lb firm white fish fillets
2 tablespoons oil
2 onions, sliced
12 mm/½ inch piece fresh root ginger, grated
2 garlic cloves, crushed
1 teaspoon turmeric
½ teaspoon chilli powder
A pinch each of ground coriander, cloves, cumin, cardamom, paprika and cinnamon
3 tomatoes, peeled (below), chopped
Grated peel of 1 lemon
125 ml/4 fl oz/½ cup water
Cooked rice, to serve

Peeling Tomatoes. *Use ripe tomatoes only! Cut out the core, using a small knife. Plunge into boiling water for 1–2 minutes. The skin will start to lift (assisted if you prick the skin with a fork beforehand). Refresh under cold water, peel off the skin. Use as needed.*

Peeled and Seeded Tomatoes (Concasse). *Cut each peeled tomato in half. Squeeze gently, or scoop out the seeds with a teaspoon. Flatten each half gently and cut into small cubes.*

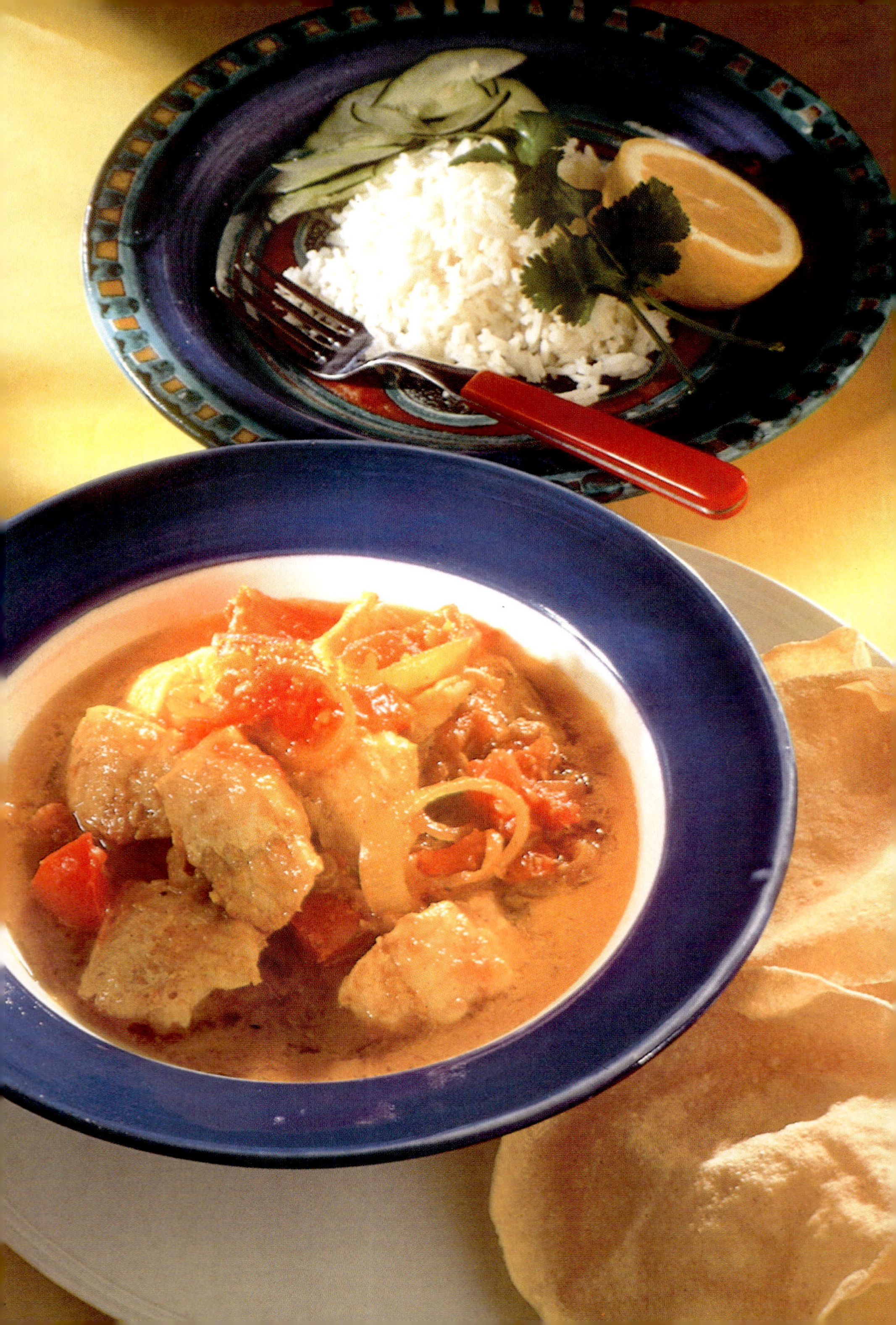

Spicy Fish Curry (p. 43). Served with rice and tasty curry accompaniments, this Asian dish will leave your taste buds tingling.

Wash the fish fillets and dry with paper towels. Cut into largish serving pieces.

Heat the oil in a heavy-based pan (skillet), add the onions and fry over a low heat for 4–5 minutes or until soft. Add the ginger, garlic and all the spices. Cook for 2 minutes, stirring continuously. Add the tomatoes, lemon peel and water, cover and simmer for 15 minutes.

Add the fish pieces, cover and simmer for a further 10 minutes or until fish is cooked (p. 23). Serve with rice and suggested curry accompaniments.

Step by Step

Glossary

Batter A mixture of flour and liquid beaten together until it is smooth and at pouring consistency, used to coat food. The addition of egg whites makes it lighter.

Blanch To place vegetables to boiling water for a few seconds and then refresh them under cold water to stop any further cooking. This process brings out their colour and softens them slightly.

Capers Pickled buds of a Mediterranean shrub.

Cardamom Commonly used to flavour rice dishes. The pods are the dried fruits of a plant found in India, related to the ginger family. Available in either seed or ground form.

Cayenne pepper The ground dried pods of a red chilli pepper.

Coriander (cilantro) A very aromatic herb used extensively in curries. It is a member of the parsley family.

Couscous A cereal often used in North Africa. It is processed from semolina into tiny grain-like particles.

Cumin A spice used in Mexican, Indian and Latin American cooking. This ground, dried seed of a plant belonging to the carrot family is highly aromatic.

Curry paste A blend of different spices such as cumin, coriander, ginger, chilli, garlic and turmeric in an oil, such as rapeseed. It comes in different strengths.

Deglaze To add stock or wine to a pan after excess fat has been poured off and to incorporate pan residues into the liquid—usually to make a sauce.

Dice To cut into small even cubes.

Dill A herb from the parsley family. The leaves are used fresh or dried.

Dijon mustard A hot mustard, containing wine, which makes it suitable for use in sauces and dressings.

Filo A pastry with many thin layers of incorporated fat. It is very fragile and dries out quickly, so requires care when handling.

Flake To separate or break into small pieces with a fork.

Ginger Commonly used in Asian cuisine, it is the highly aromatic root stem of a south-east Asian plant.

Goujon. A thin strip of fish or meat.

Julienne strips Even-sized sticks of vegetables or fruit. The thickness depends on the dish and use.

Marinate To let food stand in a marinade to season and tenderize. The marinade usually contains an acid for this purpose as well as other flavourings which penetrate the food immersed in it.

Poppadums Thin wafers, commonly consumed with curries, made from lentil flour, spices and salt. Some contain raising agents and spices.

Paupiette A thin strip of fish or meat rolled around a filling or stuffing.

Pine nuts Small, oval, cream-coloured kernels.

Reduce To boil liquid for the purpose of evaporating some of its water, thus concentrating flavours and consistency.

Reduction The liquid from the process of reducing.

Roux Melted butter and flour which is cooked over a fairly low heat, to which milk, wine or stock is added. This forms the basis of many sauces and soups.

Soured cream A thick, commercially cultured cream.

Soy sauce Used extensively in Asian cooking, made from fermented soya beans.

Tarragon A very aromatic herb, with a slightly tart flavour. Often used to flavour marinades and vinegars. Its flavour complements fish.

Turmeric A bright yellow powder produced from the dried root stem of a plant related to the ginger family. Commonly used in curries.

Vinaigrette A salad dressing based on a combination of oil, vinegar and seasonings.

Whisk To beat at high speed, with a fork or wire whisk, using a circular motion to combine ingredients.

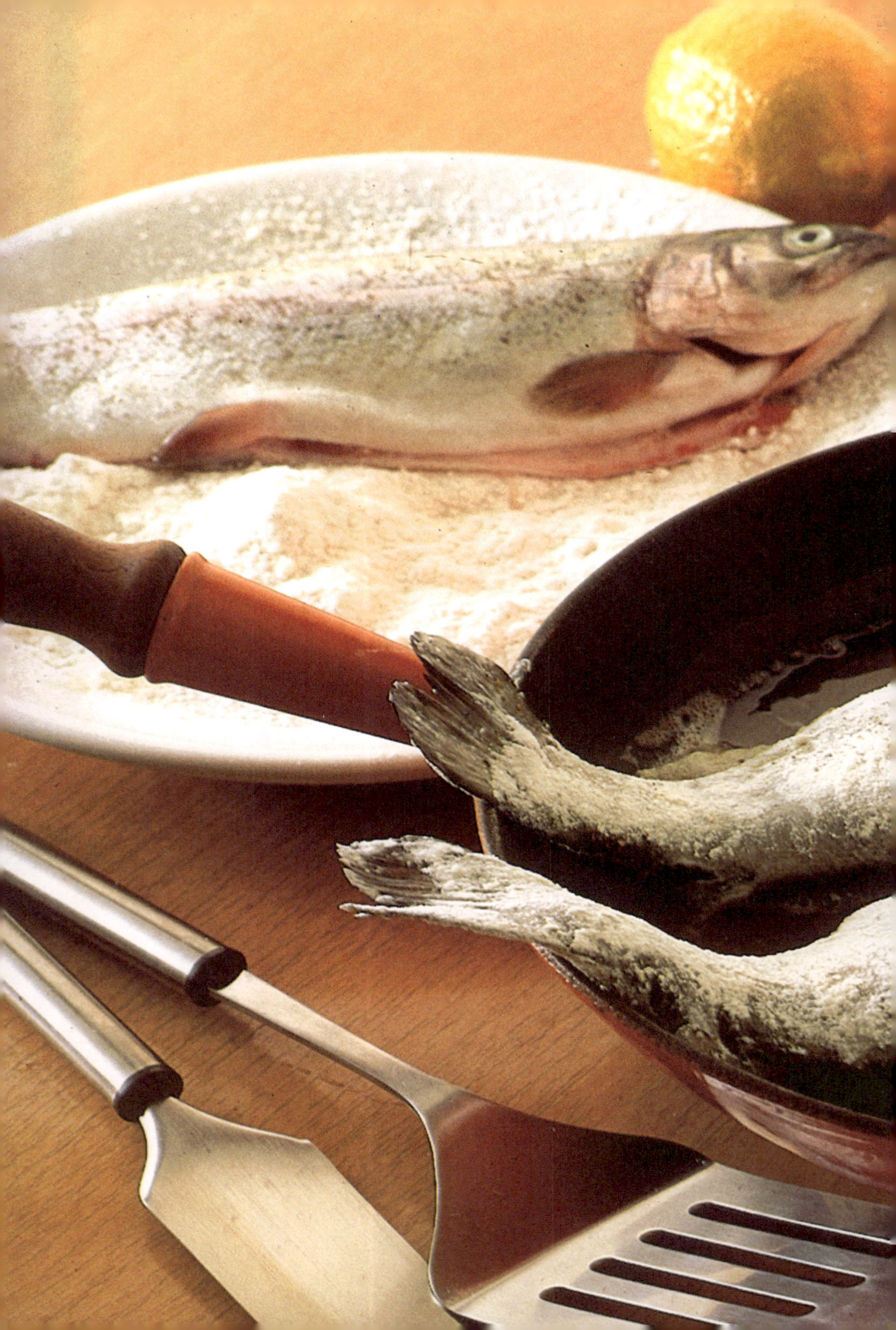